Colorectal Cancer: From Pathophysiology to Novel Therapeutic Approaches

Colorectal Cancer: From Pathophysiology to Novel Therapeutic Approaches

Editor

Valeria Barresi

MDPI • Basel • Beijing • Wuhan • Barcelona • Belgrade • Manchester • Tokyo • Cluj • Tianjin

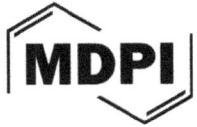

Editor
Valeria Barresi
University of Verona
Italy

Editorial Office
MDPI
St. Alban-Anlage 66
4052 Basel, Switzerland

This is a reprint of articles from the Special Issue published online in the open access journal *Biomedicines* (ISSN 2227-9059) (available at: https://www.mdpi.com/journal/biomedicines/special_issues/colorectal_cancer_pathophysiol_ther).

For citation purposes, cite each article independently as indicated on the article page online and as indicated below:

LastName, A.A.; LastName, B.B.; LastName, C.C. Article Title. *Journal Name* **Year**, *Volume Number*, Page Range.

ISBN 978-3-0365-2922-6 (Hbk)
ISBN 978-3-0365-2923-3 (PDF)

Cover image courtesy of Valeria Barresi

© 2022 by the authors. Articles in this book are Open Access and distributed under the Creative Commons Attribution (CC BY) license, which allows users to download, copy and build upon published articles, as long as the author and publisher are properly credited, which ensures maximum dissemination and a wider impact of our publications.
The book as a whole is distributed by MDPI under the terms and conditions of the Creative Commons license CC BY-NC-ND.

Contents

About the Editor vii

Valeria Barresi
Colorectal Cancer: From Pathophysiology to Novel Therapeutic Approaches
Reprinted from: *Biomedicines* 2021, 9, 1858, doi:10.3390/biomedicines9121858 1

Marco Vacante, Roberto Ciuni, Francesco Basile and Antonio Biondi
Gut Microbiota and Colorectal Cancer Development: A Closer Look to the Adenoma-Carcinoma Sequence
Reprinted from: *Biomedicines* 2020, 8, 489, doi:10.3390/biomedicines8110489 5

Jan Philipp Dobert, Anne-Sophie Cabron, Philipp Arnold, Egor Pavlenko, Stefan Rose-John and Friederike Zunke
Functional Characterization of Colon-Cancer-Associated Variants in *ADAM17* Affecting the Catalytic Domain
Reprinted from: *Biomedicines* 2020, 8, 463, doi:10.3390/biomedicines8110463 27

Marco Vacante, Roberto Ciuni, Francesco Basile and Antonio Biondi
The Liquid Biopsy in the Management of Colorectal Cancer: An Overview
Reprinted from: *Biomedicines* 2020, 8, 308, doi:10.3390/biomedicines8090308 43

Alessandro Parisi, Giampiero Porzio, Fanny Pulcini, Katia Cannita, Corrado Ficorella, Vincenzo Mattei and Simona Delle Monache
What Is Known about Theragnostic Strategies in Colorectal Cancer
Reprinted from: *Biomedicines* 2021, 9, 140, doi:biomedicines9020140 65

Giulia Turri, Valeria Barresi, Alessandro Valdegamberi, Gabriele Gecchele, Cristian Conti, Serena Ammendola, Alfredo Guglielmi, Aldo Scarpa and Corrado Pedrazzani
Clinical Significance of Preoperative Inflammatory Markers in Prediction of Prognosis in Node-Negative Colon Cancer: Correlation between Neutrophil-to-Lymphocyte Ratio and Poorly Differentiated Clusters
Reprinted from: *Biomedicines* 2021, 9, 94, doi:biomedicines9010094 95

Kyusang Hwang, Jin Hwan Yoon, Ji Hyun Lee and Sukmook Lee
Recent Advances in Monoclonal Antibody Therapy for Colorectal Cancers
Reprinted from: *Biomedicines* 2021, 9, 39, doi:biomedicines9010039 107

Ugo Testa, Germana Castelli and Elvira Pelosi
Genetic Alterations of Metastatic Colorectal Cancer
Reprinted from: *Biomedicines* 2020, 8, 414, doi:10.3390/biomedicines8100414 131

Kristian Urh, Margareta Žlajpah, Nina Zidar and Emanuela Boštjančič
Identification and Validation of New Cancer Stem Cell-Related Genes and Their Regulatory microRNAs in Colorectal Cancerogenesis
Reprinted from: *Biomedicines* 2021, 9, 179, doi:10.3390/biomedicines9020179 161

Flaviana Marzano, Mariano Francesco Caratozzolo, Graziano Pesole, Elisabetta Sbisà and Apollonia Tullo
TRIM Proteins in Colorectal Cancer: TRIM8 as a Promising Therapeutic Target in Chemo Resistance
Reprinted from: *Biomedicines* 2021, 9, 241, doi:10.3390/biomedicines9030241 181

Jachym Rosendorf, Marketa Klicova, Lenka Cervenkova, Jana Horakova, Andrea Klapstova, Petr Hosek, Richard Palek, Jan Sevcik, Robert Polak, Vladislav Treska, Jiri Chvojka and Vaclav Liska
Reinforcement of Colonic Anastomosis with Improved Ultrafine Nanofibrous Patch: Experiment on Pig
Reprinted from: *Biomedicines* **2021**, *9*, 102, doi:10.3390/biomedicines9020102 203

Raffaella Liccardo, Antonio Nolano, Matilde Lambiase, Carlo Della Ragione, Marina De Rosa, Paola Izzo and Francesca Duraturo
MSH2 Overexpression Due to an Unclassified Variant in 3'-Untranslated Region in a Patient with Colon Cancer
Reprinted from: *Biomedicines* **2020**, *8*, 167, doi:10.3390/biomedicines8060167 221

Helle Samdal, Lene C Olsen, Knut S Grøn, Elin S Røyset, Therese S Høiem, Ingunn Nervik, Pål Sætrom, Arne Wibe, Svanhild A Schønberg and Caroline H H Pettersen
Establishment of a Patient-Derived Xenograft Model of Colorectal Cancer in CIEA NOG Mice and Exploring Smartfish Liquid Diet as a Source of Omega-3 Fatty Acids
Reprinted from: *Biomedicines* **2021**, *9*, 282, doi:10.3390/biomedicines9030282 231

Carolina Peixoto, Marta B. Lopes, Marta Martins, Luís Costa and Susana Vinga
TCox: Correlation-Based Regularization Applied to Colorectal Cancer Survival Data
Reprinted from: *Biomedicines* **2020**, *8*, 488, doi:10.3390/biomedicines8110488 259

About the Editor

Valeria Barresi is Associate Professor of Pathology at the University of Verona, Italy. She has authored more than 200 papers in international peer-reviewed journals with impact factors. Her research interests mainly involve colorectal cancer and brain tumors. Her research in colorectal cancer has been focused on the identification of factors able to predict the risk of progression in early-stage tumors. In particular, she has been studying the significance of tumor budding and poorly differentiated clusters in the process of the metastatization of colorectal carcinoma, also participating in the International Consensus on Tumor Budding in colorectal cancer.

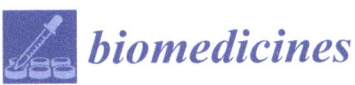

Editorial

Colorectal Cancer: From Pathophysiology to Novel Therapeutic Approaches

Valeria Barresi

Dipartimento di Diagnostica e Sanità Pubblica, Sezione di Anatomia Patologica, Università di Verona, 37134 Verona, Italy; valeria.barresi@univr.it; Tel.: +39-04-5812-4809

Citation: Barresi, V. Colorectal Cancer: From Pathophysiology to Novel Therapeutic Approaches. *Biomedicines* **2021**, *9*, 1858. https://doi.org/10.3390/biomedicines9121858

Received: 1 December 2021
Accepted: 3 December 2021
Published: 8 December 2021

Publisher's Note: MDPI stays neutral with regard to jurisdictional claims in published maps and institutional affiliations.

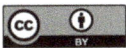

Copyright: © 2021 by the author. Licensee MDPI, Basel, Switzerland. This article is an open access article distributed under the terms and conditions of the Creative Commons Attribution (CC BY) license (https://creativecommons.org/licenses/by/4.0/).

According to the Global Cancer Statistics 2020, colorectal cancer (CRC) represents the third most frequent malignancy worldwide, and is the second in terms of mortality [1].

Its higher prevalence in geographic areas with a high human development index is connected with dietary habits such as a high consumption of red meat and alcohol, and with a sedentary lifestyle [1]. Since the early 2000s, screening programs and the consequent early identification and removal of pre-cancerous lesions, together with the shift to a healthier lifestyle, have reduced the frequency of CRC cases in high-incidence areas [2,3]. In addition, the development of targeted therapies has given novel therapeutic opportunities for patients affected by this malignancy [4].

Ongoing scientific research, by increasing the knowledge of the pathogenetic mechanisms and identifying novel prognostic and predictive biomarkers, might lead to a further progressive reduction in the incidence and mortality of CRC.

A relevant concept, which emerged in recent years, is the key role of inflammation in in the tumorigenesis, progression, and metastasization of CRC [5]. The induction of an inflammatory status of the colorectal mucosa is the way in which environmental or dietary habits may trigger colorectal carcinogenesis [5,6]. Indeed, a high consumption of alcohol or red meat may alter the composition of the gut microbiota—so-called dysbiosis—with a decrease in commensal bacterial species (i.e., butyrate-producing bacteria) and the growth of detrimental bacterial strains (i.e., pro-inflammatory opportunistic pathogens) [7]. Aside from a role in the initiation of CRC, dysbiosis seems also to be involved in the resistance to some chemotherapeutic agents, due to its ability to modulate the immune response, and is associated with shorter cancer-specific survival [6,8]. Therefore, probiotics, prebiotics, or antibiotics capable of restoring the normal equilibrium of gut microbiota (eubiosis) could open new scenarios for the prevention or treatment of CRC [6,8].

Notably, assessment of the gut microbiota could represent a non-invasive diagnostic tool for the early identification of CRC [6]. Indeed, some microbial species, including *Escherichia coli, Streptococcus gallolyticus, Bacteroides fragilis, Fusobacterium nucleatum*, and *Enterococcus faecalis*, among others, were found in the stools of patients with colorectal adenoma or carcinoma, but not in heathy subjects [9].

The likely role of inflammation in the progression of CRC is also suggested by the prognostic significance of the blood count of neutrophils in patients with this neoplasia [10]. Of note, a high neutrophil-to-lymphocyte ratio (H-NLR) was found to be significantly associated with shorter overall survival in patients with non-metastatic CRC at diagnosis (pathological TNM Stages I and II) [10]. The mechanism by which a high H-NLR could influence disease progression is still to be clarified; however, its association with histopathological features connected with tumor de-differentiation (e.g., poorly differentiated clusters) [10] suggests that an inflammatory status may induce the activation of pathways connected to the epithelial mesenchymal transition in CRC.

The notion that a percentage of CRCs are inflammation-induced has prompted the investigation of the tumorigenic role of some pro-inflammatory proteins, such as the membrane-bound metalloproteinase ADAM17, which induces the release of TNF-α and regulates IL-6 signaling [11].

In spite of the development of novel therapeutic strategies for CRC, there are still several open questions. A dilemma is whether and which patients with non-metastatic CRC could benefit from adjuvant post-surgical therapies. Indeed, the treatment decision regarding patients with CRC is currently based on the pTNM stage, which is regarded as the main prognostic factor. However, a percentage of non-metastatic CRCs unexpectedly progress [12]; therefore, additional prognostic markers are urgently needed to identify high-risk patients who could benefit from adjuvant treatments. In this regard, several histopathological factors, including lympho-vascular invasion, poor tumor differentiation according to the World Health Organization (WHO) grading system, perineural invasion, tumor budding, and poorly differentiated clusters (PDC) are considered high-risk factors for the progression of non-metastatic CRC [13]. A recent consensus on best practice established that pTNM Stage II CRC should be considered at a high risk of progression, even if tumor budding is the only histopathological risk factor present [14].

If confirmed in other studies, H-NLR may also represent a prognostic biomarker of a higher risk of progression in patients with non-metastatic CRC and may therefore be used for the identification of subjects who may benefit from adjuvant treatments [10].

Liquid biopsy might also be a promising tool for the identification of CRC patients at a high risk of progression [8,15]. This represents the isolation of cancer-derived components, such as circulating tumor cells (CTC), circulating tumor DNA (ctDNA), microRNAs (miRNAs), long non-coding RNAs (lncRNAs), and proteins, from the peripheral blood or other body fluids [8,15]. Although its use in routine practice is still limited by the lack of validation, the demonstration of cancer-derived components in the blood of patients with non-metastatic CRC may be relevant to identifying patients at a high risk of progression.

In the last two decades, the discovery of molecular therapeutic targets in CRC allowed the development of several targeted therapies based on the use of monoclonal antibodies [4]. Although these are more effective and display lower toxicity compared with traditional chemotherapy [16], they have not produced a substantial increase in the 5-year survival rate of patients with metastatic (Stage IV) CRC, which is still less than 10% [17]. The failure of targeted therapies may be due to several reasons. First, in most cases, the presence of the target, or of eventual resistance-related mutations, is assessed in the primary tumor and not in the metastases, which actually represent the neoplastic diseases to be treated. Therefore, targeted therapy's inefficacy may be due to a dissimilarity in the genetic abnormalities between the primary CRC and the matched metastases, as reported in several studies [18]. The discordance between the primary tumor and the metastases may be due to a subclonal evolution during metastasization, or to the genetic heterogeneity of the primary tumor [18]. A study analyzing matched samples showed that the genetic alterations in lymph node metastases reflect those found in the invasive front rather than in the main tumor mass of primary CRC, suggesting that the assessment of molecular targets should be preferentially carried out in this part of the primary tumor [19]. However, discordant alterations may also be present among the different metastases [18].

Another mechanism of drug resistance may also be related to the therapy-induced selection of cancer stem cells, which represent tumor cells that are able to self-renew and to generate tumor cells harboring different genetic alterations [20]. Therefore, understanding their molecular features may be useful for developing therapeutic strategies that are able to target cancer stem cells and to overcome drug resistance.

In conclusion, although the knowledge of the mechanisms underlying the pathogenesis, progression, and metastasization of CRC has greatly expanded in recent decades, many aspects still remain to be clarified. This Special Issue represents a collection of original and review articles focused on recent advances in CRC, providing new insights for future research in this field.

Funding: No funding was required for this manuscript.

Conflicts of Interest: The author declares no conflict of interest.

References

1. Sung, H.; Ferlay, J.; Siegel, R.L.; Laversanne, M.; Soerjomataram, I.; Jemal, A.; Bray, F. Global cancer statistics 2020: GLOBOCAN estimates of incidence and mortality worldwide for 36 cancers in 185 countries. *CA Cancer J. Clin.* **2021**, *71*, 209–249. [CrossRef] [PubMed]
2. Arnold, M.; Abnet, C.C.; Neale, R.E.; Vignat, J.; Giovannucci, E.L.; McGlynn, K.A.; Bray, F. Global burden of 5 major types of gastrointestinal cancer. *Gastroenterology* **2020**, *159*, 335–349. [CrossRef] [PubMed]
3. Schreuders, E.H.; Ruco, A.; Rabeneck, L.; Schoen, R.E.; Sung, J.J.; Young, G.P.; Kuipers, E.J. Colorectal cancer screening: A global overview of existing programmes. *Gut* **2015**, *64*, 1637–1649. [CrossRef] [PubMed]
4. Hwang, K.; Yoon, J.H.; Lee, J.H.; Lee, S. Recent advances in monoclonal antibody therapy for colorectal cancers. *Biomedicines* **2021**, *9*, 39. [CrossRef] [PubMed]
5. Schmitt, M.; Greten, F.R. The inflammatory pathogenesis of colorectal cancer. *Nat. Rev. Immunol.* **2021**, *21*, 653–667. [CrossRef] [PubMed]
6. Vacante, M.; Ciuni, R.; Basile, F.; Biondi, A. Gut microbiota and colorectal cancer development: A closer look to the adenoma-carcinoma sequence. *Biomedicines* **2020**, *8*, 489. [CrossRef] [PubMed]
7. Sanchez-Alcoholado, L.; Ramos-Molina, B.; Otero, A.; Laborda-Illanes, A.; Ordonez, R.; Medina, J.A.; Gomez-Mill, J.; Queipo-Ortu, M.I. The role of the gut microbiome in colorectal cancer development and therapy response. *Cancers* **2020**, *12*, 1406. [CrossRef] [PubMed]
8. Parisi, A.; Porzio, G.; Pulcini, F.; Cannita, K.; Ficorella, C.; Mattei, V.; Delle Monache, S. What is known about theragnostic strategies in colorectal cancer. *Biomedicines* **2021**, *9*, 140. [CrossRef] [PubMed]
9. Mangifesta, M.; Mancabelli, L.; Milani, C.; Gaiani, F.; de'Angelis, N.; de'Angelis, G.L.; van Sinderen, D.; Ventura, M.; Turroni, F. Mucosal microbiota of intestinal polyps reveals putative biomarkers of colorectal cancer. *Sci. Rep.* **2018**, *8*, 13974. [CrossRef] [PubMed]
10. Turri, G.; Barresi, V.; Valdegamberi, A.; Gecchele, G.; Conti, C.; Ammendola, S.; Guglielmi, A.; Scarpa, A.; Pedrazzani, C. Clinical significance of preoperative inflammatory markers in prediction of prognosis in node-negative colon cancer: Correlation between neutrophil-to-lymphocyte ratio and poorly differentiated clusters. *Biomedicines* **2021**, *9*, 94. [CrossRef] [PubMed]
11. Dobert, J.P.; Cabron, A.S.; Arnold, P.; Pavlenko, E.; Rose-John, S.; Zunke, F. Functional characterization of colon-cancer-associated variants in adam17 affecting the catalytic domain. *Biomedicines* **2020**, *8*, 463. [CrossRef] [PubMed]
12. Siegel, R.L.; Miller, K.D.; Jemal, A. Cancer statistics, 2018. *CA Cancer J. Clin.* **2018**, *68*, 7–30. [CrossRef] [PubMed]
13. Barresi, V.; Reggiani Bonetti, L.; Ieni, A.; Branca, G.; Tuccari, G. Histologic prognostic markers in stage IIA colorectal cancer: A comparative study. *Scand. J. Gastroenterol.* **2016**, *51*, 314–320. [CrossRef] [PubMed]
14. Haddad, T.S.; Lugli, A.; Aherne, S.; Barresi, V.; Terris, B.; Bokhorst, J.M. Improving tumor budding reporting in colorectal cancer: A Delphi consensus study. *Virchows Arch.* **2021**, *479*, 459–469. [CrossRef] [PubMed]
15. Vacante, M.; Ciuni, R.; Basile, F.; Biondi, A. The Liquid biopsy in the management of colorectal cancer: An overview. *Biomedicines* **2020**, *8*, 308. [CrossRef] [PubMed]
16. Rosa, B.; de Jesus, J.P.; de Mello, E.L.; Cesar, D.; Correia, M.M. Effectiveness and safety of monoclonal antibodies for metastatic colorectal cancer treatment: Systematic review and meta-analysis. *Ecancermedicalscience* **2015**, *9*, 582. [CrossRef] [PubMed]
17. Miller, K.D.; Nogueira, L.; Mariotto, A.B.; Rowland, J.H.; Yabroff, K.R.; Alfano, C.M.; Jemal, A.; Kramer, J.L.; Siegel, R.L. Cancer treatment and survivorship statistics, 2019. *CA Cancer J. Clin.* **2019**, *69*, 363–385. [CrossRef] [PubMed]
18. Testa, U.; Castelli, G.; Pelosi, E. Genetic alterations of metastatic colorectal cancer. *Biomedicines* **2020**, *8*, 414. [CrossRef] [PubMed]
19. Reggiani Bonetti, L.; Barresi, V.; Bettelli, S.; Caprera, C.; Manfredini, S.; Maiorana, A. Analysis of KRAS, NRAS, PIK3CA, and BRAF mutational profile in poorly differentiated clusters of KRAS-mutated colon cancer. *Hum. Pathol.* **2017**, *62*, 91–98. [CrossRef] [PubMed]
20. Urh, K.; Zlajpah, M.; Zidar, N.; Bostjancic, E. Identification and validation of new cancer stem cell-related genes and their regulatory microRNAs in colorectal cancerogenesis. *Biomedicines* **2021**, *9*, 179. [CrossRef] [PubMed]

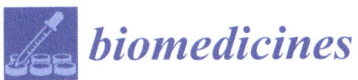

Review

Gut Microbiota and Colorectal Cancer Development: A Closer Look to the Adenoma-Carcinoma Sequence

Marco Vacante *, Roberto Ciuni, Francesco Basile and Antonio Biondi

Department of General Surgery and Medical-Surgical Specialties, University of Catania, Via S. Sofia 78, 95123 Catania, Italy; ciuni.r@gmail.com (R.C.); fbasile@unict.it (F.B.); abiondi@unict.it (A.B.)
* Correspondence: marcovacante@yahoo.it

Received: 26 October 2020; Accepted: 8 November 2020; Published: 10 November 2020

Abstract: There is wide evidence that CRC could be prevented by regular physical activity, keeping a healthy body weight, and following a healthy and balanced diet. Many sporadic CRCs develop via the traditional adenoma-carcinoma pathway, starting as premalignant lesions represented by conventional, tubular or tubulovillous adenomas. The gut bacteria play a crucial role in regulating the host metabolism and also contribute to preserve intestinal barrier function and an effective immune response against pathogen colonization. The microbiota composition is different among people, and is conditioned by many environmental factors, such as diet, chemical exposure, and the use of antibiotic or other medication. The gut microbiota could be directly involved in the development of colorectal adenomas and the subsequent progression to CRC. Specific gut bacteria, such as *Fusobacterium nucleatum*, *Escherichia coli*, and enterotoxigenic *Bacteroides fragilis*, could be involved in colorectal carcinogenesis. Potential mechanisms of CRC progression may include DNA damage, promotion of chronic inflammation, and release of bioactive carcinogenic metabolites. The aim of this review was to summarize the current knowledge on the role of the gut microbiota in the development of CRC, and discuss major mechanisms of microbiota-related progression of the adenoma-carcinoma sequence.

Keywords: colorectal cancer; gut microbiota; colorectal adenoma; polyps; bacteria

1. Introduction

Colorectal cancer (CRC) is a leading cause of cancer mortality worldwide with approximately 900,000 deaths every year, and the increasing age-standardized incidence rate of CRC in most countries represents an important public health challenge [1]. Indeed, the global incidence of CRC was 1.8 million (95% UI 1.8–1.9) in 2017, with an age-standardized incidence rate of 23.2 per 100,000 person-years that raised by 9.5% (4.5–13.5) between 1990 and 2017 [2]. There is wide evidence that CRC risk is highly modifiable through diet and lifestyle [3]. Several studies suggested that a significant number of CRC cases could be prevented by regular physical activity, keeping a healthy body weight, and following a healthy and balanced diet [4–6].

Around 60–90% of sporadic CRCs arise via the traditional adenoma-carcinoma pathway, starting as premalignant lesions represented by conventional, tubular, or tubulovillous adenomas [7]. Cancers that derive from this pathway are frequently associated with male sex, and located in the distal colon. These tumors are characterized by chromosomal instability (CIN), inactivating mutations or losses in the adenomatous polyposis coli (APC) tumor suppressor gene, and in some cases mutations in the *KRAS* oncogene, *SMAD4*, *PIK3CA*, and *TP53* genes [8,9].

The term "gut microbiota" indicates the collection of microorganisms (bacteria, archaea and eukarya) colonizing the human gastrointestinal tract. Overall, the number of these microorganisms has been calculated to exceed 10^{14}, with a ratio of human:bacterial cells closer to 1:1 [10,11]. The gut bacteria play a crucial role in regulating host metabolism (i.e., absorption of indigestible carbohydrates and fat-soluble vitamins, and stimulation of innate and cell-mediated immunity) and also contribute to preserve intestinal barrier function and an effective immune response against pathogen colonization [12–14]. The microbiota composition is different among people, and is conditioned by many environmental factors, such as diet, chemical exposure, and the use of antibiotic or other medication [15].

Several studies suggested that the gut microbiota could be directly involved in the development of colorectal adenomas and the subsequent progression to CRC [16]. Patients with CRC could present changes in microbial composition and ecology, and functional studies in animal models underlined the importance of certain bacteria, such as *Fusobacterium nucleatum*, *Escherichia coli*, and *Bacteroides fragilis*, in colorectal carcinogenesis [17,18]. Possible mechanisms of CRC progression may include DNA damage, promotion of chronic inflammation, and release of bioactive carcinogenic metabolites [19–21].

The aim of this review was to summarize the current knowledge on the role of the gut microbiota in the development of CRC, including major mechanisms of microbiota-related progression of the adenoma-carcinoma sequence.

2. Risk Factors for the Development of Adenomas and CRC

Genetic alterations play a key role in the progression of adenomas to CRC; for instance, mutations may occur in oncogenes (i.e., *KRAS*), tumor suppressor genes such as *APC*, *p53*, and *CTNNB1*, as well as in pathways associated with CpG island methylation (CIMP), mismatch repair (MMR), and chromosomal and microsatellite instability (CIN and MSI) [22–24]. Ageing and family history have been also correlated with higher risk of adenomas and CRC [25–27].

It has been suggested that genetic predisposition and somatic mutations in combination with environmental factors could be responsible for CRC, in the way of a complex disease [28–30]. Lifestyle and dietary habits represent the most common environmental factors associated with colorectal adenomas and CRC [31–33]. Even if it is difficult to analyze the single dietary risk factors in epidemiological studies, preclinical animal models have shown the key role of nutrition in tumor development [34,35]. Nutrition may affect the incidence, natural progression and therapeutic response of cancer, modulating the release of endocrine factors, modifying inflammatory and immunological pathways, or by changing the gut microbiota composition [36–38].

An increased risk of adenomas and CRC has been observed in subjects consuming diets high in red meat or processed meat, food with a high glycemic index, salt and alcohol, and low daily water and fiber intake [39,40]. On the contrary, the consumption of white meat, vegetables and fish oils with a high omega-3 polyunsaturated fatty acids (PUFA) to omega-6 PUFA ratio could lower the risk of CRC [41–43]. A diet rich in fiber, vitamin B6, C, D, E, folic acid, magnesium and selenium, has also been suggested to decrease the risk of CRC [44]. Other risk factors that may contribute to the development of CRC are obesity, smoking, male sex, non-hispanic black ethnicity, and lack of physical activity [45–47].

There is growing evidence that diet may select for the microbiota composition, thus regulating many beneficial or harmful effects of gut bacteria [15,48]. For instance, dietary fiber are able to stimulate the colonic microbial production of anti-proliferative and counter carcinogenic substances, especially butyrate [49]. The adoption of a healthy lifestyle, and a diet rich in fiber, vegetables and fruit, could decrease the risk of CRC. Moreover, a recent study showed that higher fiber intake after the diagnosis of non-metastatic CRC (non-mCRC) was associated with decreased CRC-specific and overall mortality. Indeed, an increased fiber intake after CRC diagnosis could give supplementary advantages to patients with CRC due to the interaction with gut microbiota [50,51].

3. Dysbiosis, Inflammation and Toxic Bacterial Metabolites

The adenomas are the most frequent premalignant precursor lesions of almost all the sporadic CRCs [52]. Up to 40% of individuals aged 60 years or older may present adenomatous polyps, with a transformation rate into CRC of approximately 0.25% per year [53,54]. Inactivating mutations of the *APC* gene are considered as the initial step of the adenoma-carcinoma sequence. A loss of *APC* gene activity results in the accumulation of β-catenin, that leads to abnormal cell proliferation, and formation of adenomatous polyposis [55]. There is evidence that an interaction between gut microbiota and genetic could contribute to the genetic pattern of the adenoma-carcinoma sequence; indeed, bacterial drivers could be responsible for the initiation of precancerous lesions and the subsequent accumulation of gene mutations [56–58].

Chronic inflammation has also been suggested to play a crucial role in many aspects of CRC initiation, promotion, and progression [59,60]. A meta-analysis confirmed the association between circulating levels of C-reactive protein (CRP), a non-specific marker of systemic inflammation, and risk of colorectal adenoma [61]. Also, higher levels of pro-inflammatory cytokines, such as tumor necrosis factor-alpha (TNF-α) and interleukin-6 (IL-6), have been observed within adenoma tissues as an expression of an inflammatory state. TNF-α and IL-6 are also involved in cell growth, differentiation, and apoptosis [62,63].

At the phyla level, the colonic microbiota of healthy individuals usually shows a predominance of Gram-positive Firmicutes and Gram-negative Bacteroidetes, with a less presence of Verrucomicrobia and Actinobacteria. The Firmicutes phylum is represented by more than 200 different genera including *Clostridium, Lactobacillus, Enterococcus, Bacillus,* and *Ruminicoccus*. The Actinobacteria phylum mainly consists of the *Bifidobacterium* genus [64,65]. Variation in the composition of gut microbiota between phenotypically similar and healthy subjects may be influenced by age, gender, genetics, diet and diseases [66].

Some studied reported abnormalities in the normal bacterial community composition, known as dysbiosis, in CRC patients [67]. Dysbiosis of the gut microbiota is characterized by the reduction in commensal bacterial species (i.e., butyrate-producing bacteria) and the growth of detrimental bacterial strains (i.e., pro-inflammatory opportunistic pathogens) [68].

Changes in the balance of commensal bacteria may lead to a raise in mucosal permeability, bacterial translocation, and activation of factors of the innate and adaptive immune system to stimulate chronic inflammation [69]. Over-expression of proinflammatory cytokines, such as IL-12, IL-23, IFNγ and TNF-α by dendritic cells, macrophages, and natural killer (NK) cells, may further promote the activation of T and B cells and different inflammatory mediators. The activation of signaling pathways by transcription factors such as NF-κB and signal transducer and activator of transcription 3 (STAT3) in colonic epithelial cells, the production of reactive oxygen species (ROS) and the related oxidative stress, DNA damage, and abnormal cell proliferation, may favor the development of colorectal adenomas and cancer [70–72] (Figure 1).

During chronic inflammation, there is a general imbalance in the gut due to release of toxic compounds and procarcinogens. Actually, an abnormal generation of bacterial metabolites directly involved in tumor metabolism, such as polyamines and short-chain fatty acids (i.e., butyrate, propionate and acetate), has been observed in patients with adenomas and CRC [15,73]. Under homeostasis, the gut microbiota is metabolized to generate many beneficial compounds for the host, whereas under an unbalanced state, the bacterial growth and health of the host may be negatively influenced [74].

The microbiota initiates and supports the hypoxic environment of the gut that is fundamental for nutrient absorption, epithelial barrier function, and immune response. The response to hypoxia is regulated by hypoxia-inducible factors (HIFs), which modulate the expression of genes, including the ones involved in metabolism, that promote adaptation to hypoxia. Chronic HIF activation may aggravate disease conditions, leading to intestinal damage, inflammation, and CRC [75–77].

Overall, the fermentation of carbohydrates produces short-chain fatty acids, especially butyrate, which can be utilized by the host and shows antineoplastic properties, while proteolytic fermentation generates ammonia, sulphides, phenols, and cresols, which may exert a pro-inflammatory effect, increase tissue permeability and in turn contribute to the development of adenomas and CRC [78,79]. Great amounts of specific strains of bacteria may lead to the generation of other substances with anti- and/or pro-carcinogenic effects, such as enterotoxins, B vitamins, urolithins, cyclomodulins, lignans, and equol [16,80].

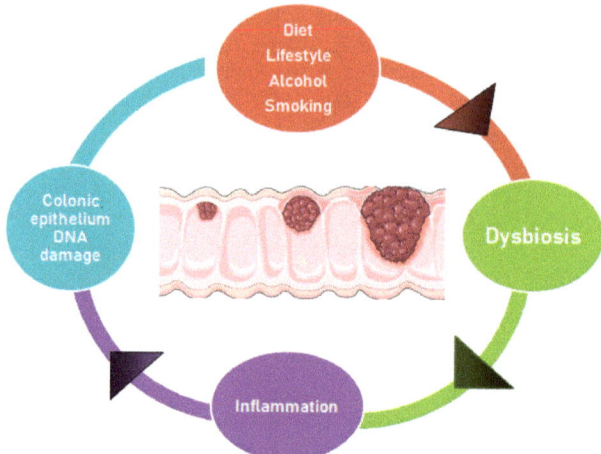

Figure 1. Dysbiosis and other factors contributing to the adenoma-carcinoma progression. The adenoma-carcinoma progression may occur because of the genomic instability caused by alterations in the gut microbiota. These changes may be supported by diet and lifestyle, which promote dysbiosis, inflammatory state and epithelial DNA damage, thus contributing to CRC development. The carcinogenesis leads to gut niche changes, which may favor the proliferation of opportunistic pathogens.

Changes of the microbiota profile in adenomas could enhance the production of primary and secondary bile acids, as well as sucrose, lipid, starch, and phenylpropanoid metabolism, thus supporting an intestinal environment that favors the growth of bile-resistant and sulfidogenic microorganisms including *Desulfovibrio* and *Bilophilia* [81,82].

It is well recognized that hydrogen sulfide (H_2S) generated by bacteria in the gut is related to adenoma development and eventually CRC [83]. Many anaerobic bacterial strains such as *Salmonella enterica, Clostridia, Escherichia coli,* and *Enterobacter aerogenes* are able to convert cysteine to H_2S, ammonia and pyruvate by cysteine desulfhydrase; moreover some gut bacteria (i.e., *Escherichia coli, Salmonella, Enterobacter, Staphylococcus, Bacillus, Klebsiella, Corynebacterium,* and *Rhodococcus*) may generate H_2S by sulfite reduction [84]. H_2S modulates inflammation, ischemia and/or perfusion injury and motility, and exerts a toxic activity on the colonic epithelium [85]. Phenolic substances such as amines, N-nitroso compounds (NOCs) found in processed meat, may also exert toxic activities favoring carcinogenesis [86,87].

Colibactin is a genotoxin produced by certain strains of bacteria, such as B2 phylogroup *E. coli* strains that colonize the human gut [88]. The synthesis of colibactin by the polyketide synthetase (*pks*) genomic island, especially in members of the family *Enterobacteriaceae*, may lead to chromosomal instability and DNA damage in eukaryotic cells, apoptosis of immune cells, and in turn the development of CRC [89].

4. Specific Bacteria Associated with Colorectal Adenoma and Cancer Development

Numerous studies have identified tumour-specific bacteria present in colorectal mucosal and/or faecal samples, and not detectable in healthy controls or tumour tissue versus the bordering healthy mucosa [90] (Table 1). A metagenome-wide association study (MGWAS) on stools from advanced adenoma and CRC patients and from healthy individuals, detected microbial genes, strains and functions enriched in each group. High consumption of red meat relative to fruits and vegetables seems to be associated with development of specific bacteria that could contribute to a more hostile intestinal milieu [91]. In general, microbial species associated with CRC development are represented by specific strains of *Escherichia coli*, *Streptococcus gallolyticus*, *Bacteroides fragilis*, *Fusobacterium nucleatum*, and *Enterococcus faecalis* among others [16].

Hale et al. observed significant abundances of multiple taxa in subjects with adenomas, such as *Bilophila*, *Desulfovibrio*, pro-inflammatory bacteria in the genus *Mogibacterium*, and *Bacteroidetes* spp. On the other hand, *Veillonella*, Firmicutes (class Clostridia), and Actinobacteria (family *Bifidobacteriales*) were more represented in patients without adenomas [81].

A study by Peters et al. analyzed for the first time the link between the gut microbiota and specific colorectal polyp types in 540 subjects, and showed that conventional adenomas (CA) cases had lower species diversity in faeces compared to controls ($p = 0.03$), especially with regard to advanced CA cases ($p = 0.004$). Only subjects with distal or advanced CA showed significant differences in general microbiota composition compared to controls ($p = 0.02$ and $p = 0.002$). Faeces of CA cases were characterized by the reduction in *Clostridia* from families *Ruminococcaceae*, *Clostridiaceae*, and *Lachnospiraceae*, and the increase in the classes Gammaproteobacteria and Bacilli, order Enterobacteriales, and genera *Streptococcus* and *Actinomyces*. There were not significant differences between sessile serrated adenoma (SSA) and hyperplastic polyps (HP) cases in diversity or composition compared to controls [92].

Feng et al. detected a great amount of *Bacteroides* and *Parabacteroides*, together with *Bilophila wadsworthia*, *Lachnospiraceae bacterium*, *Alistipes putredinis*, and *Escherichia coli* in CRC compared with both healthy and advanced adenoma. Also, gut commensals such as *Bifidobactium animalis* and *Streptococcus thermophilus*, were diminished in stools from adenoma or CRC patients, thus highlighting a divergence from healthy microbiota. Patients with advanced adenoma or CRC seem to be lacking in lactic acid-producing commensals such as *Bifidobacterium* that could facilitate epithelium regeneration and inhibition of opportunistic pathogens [91].

Table 1. Studies of gut bacteria associated with the development of adenoma and/or CRC

Authors (Year).	Bacteria	Methods	Sample Size	Statistical Significance (p Value, Odds Ratio, and/or Hazard Ratio)	Clinical Evidence
Hale et al. (2017) [81]	*Bilophila, Desulfovibrio, Mogibacterium, Bacteroidetes* spp.	16S rRNA gene sequencing	233 adenomas, 547 controls	AUC of 0.6599, ($p = 0.001$)	Adenoma and CRC development
Kasai et al. (2016) [90]	*Actinomyces, Atopobium, Fusobacterium,* and *Haemophilus* spp.	T-RFLP and NGS	49 controls, 50 adenomas, 9 CRC (3/9 invasive cancer and 6/9 carcinoma in adenoma	*Actinomyces odontolyticus* ($p = 0.007$), *Bacteroides fragile* ($p = 0.004$), *Clostridium nexile* ($p = 0.036$), *Fusobacterium varium* ($p = 0.022$), *Haemophilus parainfluenzae* ($p = 0.020$), *Prevotella stercorea* ($p = 0.022$), *Streptococcus gordonii* ($p = 0.014$), and *Veillonella dispar* ($p = 0.042$)	Association with CRC development
Feng et al. (2015) [91]	*Bacteroides, Prevotella,* and *Parabacteroides* spp. *Alistipes putredinis, Bilophila wadsworthia, Lachnospiraceae bacterium, Fusobacterium, E. coli*	MGWAS on stools	55 controls, 42 advanced adenoma, 41 CRC	$p = 0.005$, $p < 0.001$ (among the groups respectively, Kruskal–Wallis test)	Development of advanced adenoma and CRC
Peters et al. (2016) [92]	Reduction in Clostridia (*Clostridiaceae,* and *Lachnospiraceae*), and enrichment in Bacilli and Gammaproteobacteria, (Enterobacteriales), *Actinomyces* and *Streptococcus*	16S rRNA gene sequencing	540 total: 144 CA, 73 serrated polyps, 323 polyp-free controls	CA $p = 0.03$; advanced CA $p = 0.004$. Distal or advanced CA vs. controls ($p = 0.02$ and $p = 0.002$)	Early stages of carcinogenesis and development of CAs
Li et al. (2016) [93]	*F. nucleatum*	FQ-PCR in CRC and normal tissues, FISH analysis (to confirm 22 cases)	101 CRC	CRC vs. controls: 0.242 (95% C.I. 0.178–0.276) vs. 0.050 (95% C.I. 0.023–0.067), $p < 0.001$	Association with CRC development and metastasis
Fukugaiti et al. (2015) [94]	*F. nucleatum* and *Clostridium difficile*	qRT-PCR	17 total: 7 CRC	*F. nucleatum* ($p < 0.01$); *Clostridium difficile* ($p < 0.04$)	Possible role of in CRC carcinogenesis

Table 1. *Cont.*

Authors (Year).	Bacteria	Methods	Sample Size	Statistical Significance (*p* Value, Odds Ratio, and/or Hazard Ratio)	Clinical Evidence
Yu et al. (2015) [95]	*Fusobacterium, Streptococcus* and *Enterococcus* spp.	Pyrosequencing of the 16S ribosome RNA (rRNA) from fecal samples	52 controls, 47 advanced adenoma, 42 CRC	Increase of the three bacteria groups during the adenoma-carcinoma sequence: $p < 0.05$. Increase of the Fusobacterial phylum: from normal (0.27%) to adenoma (0.61%) to CRC (1.69%) ($p = 0.016$)	*F. nucleatum* colonization in the gut may favor colorectal tumorigenesis
Yu et al. (2016) [96]	*F. nucleatum*	16S rRNA FISH	35 HPs, 33 SSAs, 48 proximal CRCs, and 10 matched metastatic lymph nodes	Higher *Fusobacterium* in proximal HPs and SSAs vs. proximal TAs and distal TAs ($p < 0.05$). Higher *Fusobacterium* in more proximal CRCs vs. distal CRCs ($p < 0.05$), and in matched metastatic lymph nodes vs. nonmetastatic lymph nodes ($p < 0.001$).	Carcinogenesis of proximal colon through the serrated neoplasia pathway. Less important role in the TA-carcinoma sequence.
Mima et al. (2016) [97]	*F. nucleatum*	Assessment of DNA in CRC tissue	1069 CRC in the Nurses' Health Study and the Health Professionals Follow-up Study	HRs for CRC-specific mortality in *F. nucleatum*-low cases and *F. nucleatum*-high cases:1.25 (95% C.I. 0.82 to 1.92) and 1.58 (95% C.I. 1.04 to 2.39), respectively, (p for trend = 0.020). Association with MSI-high OR 5.22 (95% C.I. 2.86 to 9.55)	Evidence of poorer survival, and potential use as prognostic biomarker
Yu et al. (2017) [98]	*Fusobacterium, Anaerosporobacter, Parvimonas, Peptostreptococcus,* and *Prevotella*	Pyrosequence (Roche 454 GS FLX)	Phase I: 16 CRC with recurrence and 15 CRC without recurrence Phase II: 48 CRC without recurrence and 44 CRC with recurrence	Recurrence rate in the high-risk vs. low-risk group (73.4% vs. 30.9%, $p < 0.001$)	High amount of *F. nucleatum* could favor CRC chemoresistance and predict potential CRC recurrence
Little et al. (2019) [99]	*S. bovis*	*S. bovis*-positive blood cultures	86 patients with *S. bovis* bacteriemia	30 patients underwent colonoscopy with 3 (10%) having adenocarcinoma and 11 (37%) having adenomatous polyps. Gastroenterology consultation was significantly associated with having a colonoscopy ($p = 0.001$).	Association between *S. bovis* bacteriemia and CRC risk.

Table 1. *Cont.*

Authors (Year).	Bacteria	Methods	Sample Size	Statistical Significance (*p* Value, Odds Ratio, and/or Hazard Ratio)	Clinical Evidence
Corredoira-Sánchez et al. (2012) [100]	*S. gallolyticus*	*S. gallolyticus* positive blood cultures	109 patients with *S. gallolyticus* bacteriemia and 196 controls	98 patients underwent colonoscopy: 57 had adenomas (39 advanced adenomas) and 12 had invasive carcinomas. Total colorectal neoplasia in patients with *S. gallolyticus* bacteriemia vs. controls: 70% vs. 32%; OR 5.1, 95% C.I. 3.0–8.6). For advanced adenomas: 40% vs. 16%; OR 3.5, 95% C.I. 2.0–6.1. For invasive carcinomas: 12% vs. 5%; OR 2.9, 95% C.I. 1.2–6.9.	*S. gallolyticus* infection could represent a valuable marker for detection of occult CRC
Butt et al. (2016) [101]	*S. gallolyticus*	Antibody responses to recombinant affinity-purified *S. gallolyticus* pilus proteins Gallo1569, 2039, 2178 and 2179 were analysed by multiplex serology	576 CRC and 576 controls	Antibody responses to Gallo2039 (OR 1.58, 95% C.I. 1.09–2.28), Gallo2178 (OR 1.58, 95% C.I. 1.09–2.30) and Gallo2179 (OR 1.45, 95% C.I. 1.00–2.11) were significantly associated with CRC risk. The association was stronger for positivity to two or more pilus proteins of Gallo1569, Gallo2178 and Gallo2179 (OR 1.93, 95% C.I. 1.04-3.56) and for double-positivity to Gallo2178 and Gallo2179 (OR 3.54, 95% C.I. 1.49-8.44)	Association between *S. gallolyticus* infection and CRC risk
Purcell et al. (2017) [102]	ETBF	Quantitative PCR	150 consecutive patients who underwent colonoscopy	Associations with low-grade dysplasia ($p = 0.007$), tubular adenomas ($p = 0.027$), and serrated polyps ($p = 0.007$)	Potential marker of early colorectal carcinogenesis
Xie et al. (2016) [103]	ETBF and *pks + E. coli*	Quantitative real time PCR	36 adenoma, 18 controls	Increase of toxin produced by ETBF in adenoma vs. controls ($p = 0.003$) and in *pks + E. coli* ($p < 0.001$)	Possible relationship with carcinogenesis in adenomas
Zamani et al. (2020) [104]	ETBF	Quantitative real-time PCR	68 precancerous and CRC condition, 52 controls	Positivity of *bft* gene in patients vs. controls $p = 0.00$. OR 22.22 (95% C.I. 5-98.74)	Risk factor and screening marker for developing CRC

Table 1. Cont.

Authors (Year).	Bacteria	Methods	Sample Size	Statistical Significance (p Value, Odds Ratio, and/or Hazard Ratio)	Clinical Evidence
Viljoen, et al. (2015) [105]	*Fusobacterium* spp., *Streptococcus gallolyticus*, *Enterococcus faecalis*, ETBF, Enteropathogenic *E. coli*, and afaC− or pks + *E. coli*	Quantitative PCR	Paired tumor and normal tissue samples from 55 CRC	*Fusobacterium* was significantly higher in CRC vs. controls ($p < 0.001$). ETBF (FDR = 0.04 and 0.002 for controls and CRC, respectively) and *Fusobacterium* spp. (FDR = 0.03 CRC) levels were significantly higher in stage III/IV CRC	Associations with clinicopathological features, mainly for *Fusobacterium* and ETBF
Ambrosi et al. (2019) [106]	*E. coli*	16S rRNA gene sequencing and PCR	Phase I: 20 adenomatous polyps, 20 polyps, 20 adjacent tissue close to polyps (5–7 cm), 10 controls Phase II: total 1500 biopsies, 600 adenomatous polyps, 600 adjacent non-adenomatous tissues, 300 controls	In polyps, prevalence of phylogroup A and B2, strong biofilm and poor protease producers ($p < 0.05$). Phylogroup B2 showed highest isolates with virulence factor score ≥10 ($p = 0.0034$).	Association of specific phenotypes of *E. coli* with adenomatous polyps
Iyadorai et al. (2020) [107]	Pks + *E. coli*	16S rRNA gene sequencing and PCR	Phase I: Primary colon epithelial and CRC (HCT116) cell lines Phase II: 48 CRC (48 tumor and 48 matching non-malignant tissue), 23 controls (23 proximal and 23 distal biopsies)	16.7% of CRC patients were positive for pks + *E. coli* vs. 4.35% of controls ($p = 0.144$). Pks + *E. coli* was observed in 1/26 colonoscopy biopsies from controls vs. 16/96 tissue samples from CRC ($p = 0.01$)	Initiation and development of CRC

Abbreviations: T-RFLP: terminal restriction fragment length polymorphism, NGS: next-generation sequencing, MGWAS: metagenome-wide association study, CA: conventional adenoma, FQ-PCR: fluorescent quantitative polymerase chain reaction, FISH: fluorescence in situ hybridization, C.I.: confidence interval, qRT-PCR: real-time quantitative reverse transcription polymerase chain reaction, HP: proximal hyperplastic polyp, SSA: sessile serrated adenoma, TA: traditional adenoma, HR: hazard ratio, OR: odds ratio, ETBF: enterotoxigenic *Bacteroides fragilis*, afaC: afimbrial adhesin, pks: polyketide synthase, FDR: false discovery rate.

4.1. Fusobacterium nucleatum

F. nucleatum is an oral symbiont, and opportunistic pathogen that has been detected in intestinal cancers [93,94]. *F. nucleatum* may enhance CRC carcinogensis by stimulating the production of interleukin (IL)-17F/21/22/23/31/cluster of differentiation (CD)40L and protein expression of phospho-STAT3 (p-STAT3), p-STAT5, and phospho-extracellular regulated protein kinases (p-ERK)1/2 [95]. A great amount of *Fusobacteria* has been observed in SSA [108,109]; a study by Yu et al. reported that the prevalence of invasive *Fusobacteria* within proximal SSAs (78.8%) and HPs (65.7%) was significantly more elevated than that of proximal and distal traditional adenomas (28.9% and 24.4% respectively; $p < 0.05$) [96]. The presence of *F. nucleatum* has been associated with poor prognosis in CRC patients and development of chemoresistance [97,98]. *F. nucleatum* binds E-cadherin in the clonic epithelium and stimulates colorectal carcinogenesis through the fusobacterial adhesin FadA [110,111]. The interplay between Gal-GalNAc, a host polysaccharide, with fusobacterial lectin (Fap2) may promote the increase of *F. nucleatum* in colorectal adenoma and cancer [112]. A study by Mima et al. showed that multivariable hazard ratios (HRs) for CRC-specific mortalityin *F. nucleatum*-low subjects and *F. nucleatum*-high subjects, compared with *F. nucleatum*-negative subjects, were 1.25 (95% C.I. 0.82 to 1.92) and 1.58 (95% C.I. 1.04 to 2.39), respectively (p for trend = 0.020). The quantity of *F. nucleatum* was correlated with microsatellite instability (MSI)-high (multivariable odd ratio (OR), 5.22; 95% CI 2.86 to 9.55) independent of the presence of CIMP and BRAF mutation. A significant association between CIMP and BRAF mutation with *F. nucleatum* was observed only in univariate analyses ($p < 0.001$) but not in multivariate analysis that adjusted for MSI status [97].

Yang et al. observed that an infection of CRC cells lines (HCT116, HT29, LoVo, and SW480) with *F. nucleatum* increased cell growth, invasiveness, and capability to form xenograft cancers in mice. *F. nucleatum* promoted Toll-like receptor 4 (TLR4) signaling to myeloid differentiation factor 88 (MYD88), activating NFκB signaling pathways and increasing the expression of microRNA-21 (miR21), which reduced the levels of the RAS GTPase p21 protein activator 1 (RASA1). Shorter survival times were observed for tumors with high amounts of *F. nucleatum* DNA and miR21 [113].

It has been also observed that *F. nucleatum* may promote LC3-II protein expression, autophagy pathway, and autophagosome production in CRC cells. *F. nucleatum* may favor the release of the autophagy-related proteins, pULK1, ULK1, and ATG7, contributing to the resistance to oxaliplatin and 5-fluorouracil regimens in CRC cells [98].

A study by Bullman et al. showed the persistance of F. nucleatum also in distal metastatic lesions of CRC patients. Administration of metronidazole in mice bearing a colon cancer xenograft decreased *F. nucleatum* load, tumor cell proliferation, and overall cancer development, thus suggesting that specific antibiotics could potentially be used to treat patients with *Fusobacterium*-associated CRC [114].

4.2. Streptococcus gallolyticus (Formerly S. bovis)

Streptococcus gallolyticus subsp. gallolyticus (SGG), formerly known as *S. bovis* biotype I, represents a common causative agent for bacteremia and endocarditis in older adults. Gut colonization by SGG is strongly correlated with the development of CRC [99,115]. Indeed, both American and European guidelines recommended colonoscopy in patients with SGG bacteremia [116,117].

A case-control study by Corredoira-Sánchez et al. carried out on 109 cases showed that the prevalence of CRC was higher in patients with SGG bacteremia compared to controls (70% vs. 32%; OR, 5.1; 95% CI 3.0–8.6). The study did not show significant differences when comparing nonadvanced adenomas (19% vs. 12%). However, significant differences were observed in advanced adenomas (40% vs. 16%; OR 3.5, 95% C.I. 2.0–6.1) and invasive CRC (12% vs. 5%, OR 2.9, 95% C.I. 1.2–6.9) [100].

A large epidemiological study by Butt et al. showed for the first time a statistically significant association between exposure to SGG antigens and CRC, and pointed out that the risk for CRC was stronger among subjects younger than 65 years [101].

Aymeric et al. observed that CRC-specific conditions may favor SGG colonization of the gut at the expense of commensal enterococci. Indeed, gut colonization by SGG is promoted by a bacteriocin called "gallocin", which is enhanced by bile acids and may exert toxic activity to enterococci. Also, the stimulation of the Wnt pathway, and the reduced expression of the bile acid apical transporter gene *Slc10A2*, may act on the *APC* founding mutation, supporting the gut colonization by SGG [115].

4.3. Enterotoxigenic Bacteroides fragilis (ETBF)

Enterotoxigenic *B. fragilis* (ETBF) may support colorectal carcinogenesis by the production of pro-inflammatory cytokines and the stimulation of Wnt signaling. Expression of *B. fragilis* toxin (BFT), a 20 kDa metalloprotease produced by ETBF, is able to promote persistent colitis in mice, damage E-cadherin junctions, as well as stimulate B-catenin signaling and IL-8 production in colonic epithelial cells [118].

A study by Purcell et al. underlined the key role of ETBF in the development of colorectal low-grade dysplasia, tubular adenomas, and serrated polyps (*p*-values of 0.007, 0.027 and 0.007, respectively) [102]. Similar findings were reported in a study of patients with colonic adenomas that presented higher expression of the *B. fragilis* toxin gene (*bft*) associated with adenoma tissue compared to normal healthy mucosa [103].

Zamani et al. reported an increased positivity of ETBF in patients with precancerous and cancerous lesions compared to healthy controls. Higher ORs of ETBF were significantly associated with serrated lesions and adenoma with low-grade dysplasia. The most common subtype of *bft* gene was the *bft1* gene, followed by the *bft2* gene. An assessment of ETBF could represent a marker of CRC prognosis, especially in the precancerous lesions, and could be used for the screening of these conditions [104].

4.4. Enterococcus faecalis

E. faecalis is a Gram-positive commensal bacterium, that may be responsible for human disease through translocation from intestinal wall, oral cavity, and genito-urinary mucosa, leading to a systemic infection [119]. *E. faecalis* represents one of the most frequent causes of infection in older adults, and some studies underlined its importance for the development of cancer [120]. It has also been reported an association between enterococcal endocarditis and hidden CRC [119,121]. On the other hand, *E. faecalis* showed anti-inflammatory properties and probiotic activity, and is frequently administered in subjects with chronic sinusitis and bronchitis or in infant acute diarrhea [122].

Actually, there is no consensus on the role of *E. faecalis* in CRC: some studies highlighted its protective role or no role in CRC, whereas others reported potential pro-carcinogenic effects [123].

A study by Viljoen et al. carried out on 55 patients, did not highlight any significant clinical association between *E. faecalis* and CRC. However, the same study showed a relevant association bewteen clinicopathological features of CRC and *Fusobacterium* spp. and ETBF [105]. Miyamoto et al. observed that heat-killed *E. faecalis* strain EC-12 could suppress intestinal polyp development in Apc mutant Min mice. Administration of heat-killed EC-12 reduced the levels of c-Myc and cyclin D1 mRNA expression in intestinal polyps, by blocking the transcriptional activity of the T-cell factor/lymphoid enhancer factor [124].

E. faecalis could play a role in inducing CRC by activation of Wnt/β-catenin signaling and induction of pluripotent transcription factors linked to dedifferentiation. Indeed, exposure of murine primary colon epithelial cells to *E. faecalis*-infected macrophages contributed to CRC initiation through gene mutation, chromosomal instability, and endogenous cell transformation, which involved the transcription factors c-Myc, Klf4, Oct4, and Sox2i [125].

Perhaps, these controversial data could be explained taking into account the different geographical origin of the isolated strain, and dysbiosis due to the use of antibiotics or changes in diet [126,127].

4.5. Escherichia coli

Classification of the Gram negative bacterium *E. coli* includes 8 phylogenetic groups (A, B1, B2, C, D, E, F and clade I). Commensal strains are commonly represented by A and B1 groups, being the largest part of the fecal flora of healthy individuals. Extraintestinal pathogenic strains (ExPEC) include mainly B2 and D groups, and may be responsible for many extraintestinal infections, due to the achievement of numerous virulence factors that potentially support the colonization of extraintestinal tissues [128]. However, both commensals and ExPEC are considered as a part of the normal gut microbiota in healthy subjects [129].

There is evidence that *E. coli* could play a role in the development of CRC [106,130]. Indeed, some patients with CRC may show an excessive growth of *E. coli* strains, mainly B2, characterized by high expression of virulence genes, including those encoding toxins and effectors that may induce carcinogenesis, such as colibactin, cytolethal distending toxins, cytotoxic necrotizing factors, and cycle-inhibiting factor [131,132]. In vitro studies showed that colibactin could be involved in DNA alkylation on adenine residues, leading to double-strand breaks [133,134]. Pleguezuelos-Manzano et al. demonstrated that exposure to genotoxic *pks + E. coli*, could be responsible for specific mutational signature in human intestinal organoids; indeed, an identical mutational signature was observed in 5876 human cancer genomes from two independent study cohorts, mostly in CRC [135].

Ambrosi et al. analyzed 272 *E. coli* isolates from colonoscopy biopsies, and showed that *E. coli* strains colonizing adenomatous polyps were characterized by specific phenotypes compared to those from normal mucosa, which included lack of motility, moderate to strong biofilm forming activity, and poor proteolytic capability [106].

In a study by Iyadorai et al. *pks + E. coli* was detected more frequently in CRC patients compared to healthy subjects. In vitro assays carried out on primary colon epithelial (PCE) and CRC (HCT116) cell lines, highlighted that the cytopathic effect of *pks + E. coli* strains could support the initiation and development of CRC [107].

5. Future Perspectives

Modulation of the gut microbiota, aiming to reverse microbial dysbiosis, could represent a new tool for prevention and treatment of CRC. The strategies could include the use of probiotics, prebiotics, postbiotics, antibiotics, and fecal microbiota transplantation (FMT) [136–139].

Overall, the effects of microbiota modulation on CRC prevention could be due to many mechanisms, such as the suppression of inflammatory state, stimulation of apoptosis of early cancer cells, re-establishment of intestinal barrier function and correction of microbiota composition [140,141]. Also, manipulation of the gut microbiota could alleviate chemotherapy-induced side effects, such as mucositis, as confirmed by a decreased incidence of diarrhea and weight loss after the administration of several probiotics strains in animal models [142,143].

There is growing evidence that modifications of microbial abundances in some pathological conditions could affect their co-abundance interactions; indeed, Chen et al. observed specific gut microbial co-abundance networks in patients with inflammatory bowel disease (IBD) and obesity. These findings underlined the importance of microbial dysbiosis in the pathogenesis of some diseases, and suggested that even the development of CRC could share similar mechanisms [144–146].

Promising preclinical studies suggested that modulation of gut microbiota could increase therapeutic efficacy of anticancer drugs. There is evidence that the administration of antibiotics could lead to clinical benefits to CRC patients by gut microbiota depletion and subsequent reduction of chemotherapeutic resistance. Indeed, a study by Geller et al. observed that intratumor bacteria could favor gemcitabine resistance through enzymatic inactivation, and therefore the administration of a gemcitabine-ciprofloxacin combination therapy could enhance the efficacy of chemotherapy [147].

Some studies demonstrated that the gut microbiota is also able to affect chemotherapy and/or immunotherapy efficacy by modulating immune response [148]. Oral administration of some probiotics, such as *Bifidobacterium* spp. and *Akkermansia muciniphila*, or FMT from treatment-responsive patients, stimulated the programmed cell death protein 1 ligand 1 (PD-L1)-based immunotherapy, thus blocking cancer development through the increase of dendritic cell and T cell response [149–151].

There is growing evidence that microbial shift markers could be used succesfully for non-invasive early diagnosis and/or prognostic assessment of CRC and advanced adenomas [81,152]. Mangifesta et al. performed a metataxonomic analysis based on 16S rRNA gene sequencing approach, and showed that some microbial taxa such as *Bacteroides*, *Faecalibacterium*, and *Romboutsia*, seem to be reduced in cancerogenic mucosa and in adenomatous polyps, thus representing potential new biomarkers of early carcinogenesis. Furthermore, the detection of high amounts of *F. nucleatum* in polyps, underlined the key role of this microorganism as a microbial biomarker for early diagnosis of CRC [153].

A study by Hale et al. showed that the composition of the gut microbiota in subjects with adenomas is significantly different from that of healthy subjects, and is similar to the microbiota of subjects with CRC. These changes could be a consequence of the Western diet and could result in metabolic changes leading to intestinal cellular damage and mutagenesis [81,154].

The combined assessment of heterogeneous CRC cohorts detected reproducible microbiota biomarkers and disease-predictive models that could represent useful tools for clinical prognostic tests and future research. A meta-analysis of 969 stool metagenomes carried out using data from five open access datasets and two new cohorts, showed that the gut microbiota in CRC was characterized by more richness than controls ($p < 0.01$), partly due to the growth of some species originating from the oral cavity. The results also highlighted an association between gluconeogenesis, putrefaction and fermentation processes with CRC, while the starch and stachyose degradation were associated with controls. A significant association between microbiota choline metabolism and CRC was also observed ($p = 0.001$) [155]. Another meta-analysis of eight stool metagenomic studies of CRC (n = 768) from different geographical areas, reported a significant enrichment in a group of 29 species in CRC metagenomes (FDR $< 1 \times 10^{-5}$). An elevated production of secondary bile acids from CRC metagenomes, higher expression of mucin and protein catabolism genes and reduction of carbohydrates degradation genes were observed, thus underlying a metabolic relationship between gut microbiota in CRC and a diet rich in meat and fat [156].

A study by Poore et al. carried out on The Cancer Genome Atlas (TCGA) detected specific microbial signatures in blood and tissue of different types of tumors, including CRC, which were predictive for patients with stage Ia-IIc tumor and tumors without any genomic modifications as detected by cell-free tumor DNA assessment. These findings could pave the way to a novel type of microbial-based CRC diagnostics [157].

Currently, there is a great limitation in availability of mouse models to study the interaction between gut microbiota and CRC. Zeb2$^{IEC-Tg/+}$ (intestinal epithelial cell-specific transgenic expression of the epithelial-to-mesenchymal transition regulator Zeb2) mice represented the first and only microbiota-dependent CRC mouse model available so far. Specific characteristics of Zeb2$^{IEC-Tg/+}$ mice included the presence of gut dysbiosis, and the preventive effect on carcinogenesis through the microbiota reduction by broad-spectrum antibiotics or germ-free rederivation [158].

6. Conclusions

In conclusion, detecting key relationships between diet, gut microbiota, and metabolites involved in the adenoma-carcinoma sequence could provide important basis for personalized medicine aimed at preventing and managing CRC. Secondary bile acids, H_2S, and other bacterial metabolites could exert genotoxic activities and should be kept into account when investigating the adenoma and carcinoma development. Nonetheless, further studies are needed to evaluate the effects of diet, lifestyle, or medications on the gut metabolic environment and the microbiota. Finally, the identification of global microbiota signatures specific for CRC represents a promising tool in CRC diagnosis and therapy.

Author Contributions: Conceptualization, M.V. and A.B.; writing—original draft preparation, M.V.; writing—review and editing, M.V., R.C., F.B., and A.B. All authors have read and agreed to the published version of the manuscript.

Funding: This research received no external funding.

Acknowledgments: The images used in the figure and graphical abstract are distributed under Creative Commons License and can be freely available at the following link: https://smart.servier.com/.

Conflicts of Interest: The authors declare no conflict of interest.

References

1. Fitzmaurice, C.; Abate, D.; Abbasi, N.; Abbastabar, H.; Abd-Allah, F.; Abdel-Rahman, O.; Abdelalim, A.; Abdoli, A.; Abdollahpour, I.; Global Burden of Disease Cancer Collaboration; et al. Global, Regional, and National Cancer Incidence, Mortality, Years of Life Lost, Years Lived with Disability, and Disability-Adjusted Life-Years for 29 Cancer Groups, 1990 to 2017: A Systematic Analysis for the Global Burden of Disease Study. *JAMA Oncol.* **2019**, *5*, 1749–1768. [CrossRef] [PubMed]
2. Safiri, S.; Sepanlou, S.G.; Ikuta, K.S.; Bisignano, C.; Salimzadeh, H.; Delavari, A.; Ansari, R.; Roshandel, G.; Merat, S.; Fitzmaurice, C.; et al. The global, regional, and national burden of colorectal cancer and its attributable risk factors in 195 countries and territories, 1990–2017: A systematic analysis for the Global Burden of Disease Study 2017. *Lancet Gastroenterol. Hepatol.* **2019**, *4*, 913–933. [CrossRef]
3. Hou, N.; Huo, D.; Dignam, J.J. Prevention of colorectal cancer and dietary management. *Chin. Clin. Oncol.* **2013**, *2*, 13. [CrossRef] [PubMed]
4. Hughes, L.A.E.; Simons, C.C.J.M.; Brandt, P.A.; van den Engeland, M.; van Weijenberg, M.P. Lifestyle, Diet, and Colorectal Cancer Risk According to (Epi)genetic Instability: Current Evidence and Future Directions of Molecular Pathological Epidemiology. *Curr. Colorectal Cancer Rep.* **2017**, *13*, 455. [CrossRef]
5. Schlesinger, S.; Lieb, W.; Koch, M.; Fedirko, V.; Dahm, C.C.; Pischon, T.; Nöthlings, U.; Boeing, H.; Aleksandrova, K. Body weight gain and risk of colorectal cancer: A systematic review and meta-analysis of observational studies. *Obes Rev.* **2015**, *16*, 607–619. [CrossRef]
6. Shahjehan, F.; Merchea, A.; Cochuyt, J.J.; Li, Z.; Colibaseanu, D.T.; Kasi, P.M. Body Mass Index and Long-Term Outcomes in Patients with Colorectal Cancer. *Front. Oncol.* **2018**, *8*. [CrossRef]
7. Bae, J.M.; Kim, J.H.; Kang, G.H. Molecular Subtypes of Colorectal Cancer and Their Clinicopathologic Features, with an Emphasis on the Serrated Neoplasia Pathway. *Arch. Pathol. Lab. Med.* **2016**, *140*, 406–412. [CrossRef]
8. Vacante, M.; Borzì, A.M.; Basile, F.; Biondi, A. Biomarkers in colorectal cancer: Current clinical utility and future perspectives. *World J. Clin. Cases* **2018**, *6*, 869–881. [CrossRef]
9. Sievers, C.K.; Grady, W.M.; Halberg, R.B.; Pickhardt, P.J. New insights into the earliest stages of colorectal tumorigenesis. *Expert Rev. Gastroenterol. Hepatol.* **2017**, *11*, 723–729. [CrossRef]
10. Sender, R.; Fuchs, S.; Milo, R. Revised Estimates for the Number of Human and Bacteria Cells in the Body. *PLoS Biol.* **2016**, *14*, e1002533. [CrossRef]
11. Thursby, E.; Juge, N. Introduction to the human gut microbiota. *Biochem. J.* **2017**, *474*, 1823–1836. [CrossRef] [PubMed]
12. Pickard, J.M.; Zeng, M.Y.; Caruso, R.; Núñez, G. Gut Microbiota: Role in Pathogen Colonization, Immune Responses and Inflammatory Disease. *Immunol. Rev.* **2017**, *279*, 70–89. [CrossRef] [PubMed]
13. Yoshii, K.; Hosomi, K.; Sawane, K.; Kunisawa, J. Metabolism of Dietary and Microbial Vitamin B Family in the Regulation of Host Immunity. *Front. Nutr.* **2019**, *6*. [CrossRef] [PubMed]
14. Zhang, Z.; Tang, H.; Chen, P.; Xie, H.; Tao, Y. Demystifying the manipulation of host immunity, metabolism, and extraintestinal tumors by the gut microbiome. *Signal Transduct. Target. Ther.* **2019**, *4*, 1–34. [CrossRef] [PubMed]
15. Sánchez-Alcoholado, L.; Ramos-Molina, B.; Otero, A.; Laborda-Illanes, A.; Ordóñez, R.; Medina, J.A.; Gómez-Millán, J.; Queipo-Ortuño, M.I. The Role of the Gut Microbiome in Colorectal Cancer Development and Therapy Response. *Cancers* **2020**, *12*, 1406. [CrossRef] [PubMed]
16. Alhinai, E.A.; Walton, G.E.; Commane, D.M. The Role of the Gut Microbiota in Colorectal Cancer Causation. *Int. J. Mol. Sci.* **2019**, *20*, 5295. [CrossRef]
17. Wong, S.H.; Yu, J. Gut microbiota in colorectal cancer: Mechanisms of action and clinical applications. *Nat. Rev. Gastroenterol. Hepatol.* **2019**, *16*, 690–704. [CrossRef]
18. Sun, T.; Liu, S.; Zhou, Y.; Yao, Z.; Zhang, D.; Cao, S.; Wei, Z.; Tan, B.; Li, Y.; Lian, Z.; et al. Evolutionary biologic changes of gut microbiota in an 'adenoma-carcinoma sequence' mouse colorectal cancer model induced by 1, 2-Dimethylhydrazine. *Oncotarget* **2016**, *8*, 444–457. [CrossRef]
19. Arends, M.J. Pathways of colorectal carcinogenesis. *Appl. Immunohistochem. Mol. Morphol.* **2013**, *21*, 97–102. [CrossRef]

20. Kidane, D.; Chae, W.J.; Czochor, J.; Eckert, K.A.; Glazer, P.M.; Bothwell, A.L.M.; Sweasy, J.B. Interplay between DNA repair and inflammation, and the link to cancer. *Crit. Rev. Biochem. Mol. Biol.* **2014**, *49*, 116–139. [CrossRef]
21. Saus, E.; Iraola-Guzmán, S.; Willis, J.R.; Brunet-Vega, A.; Gabaldón, T. Microbiome and colorectal cancer: Roles in carcinogenesis and clinical potential. *Mol. Aspects Med.* **2019**, *69*, 93–106. [CrossRef] [PubMed]
22. Hu, Y.; Chen, Y.; Guo, H.; Yu, J.; Chen, Y.; Liu, Y.; Lan, L.; Li, J.; Wang, H.; Zhang, H. Molecular Alterations in Circulating Cell-Free DNA in Patients with Colorectal Adenoma or Carcinoma. *Cancer Manag. Res.* **2020**, *12*, 5159–5167. [CrossRef] [PubMed]
23. Al-Sohaily, S.; Biankin, A.; Leong, R.; Kohonen-Corish, M.; Warusavitarne, J. Molecular pathways in colorectal cancer. *J. Gastroenterol. Hepatol.* **2012**, *27*, 1423–1431. [CrossRef] [PubMed]
24. Koveitypour, Z.; Panahi, F.; Vakilian, M.; Peymani, M.; Seyed Forootan, F.; Nasr Esfahani, M.H.; Ghaedi, K. Signaling pathways involved in colorectal cancer progression. *Cell Biosci.* **2019**, *9*. [CrossRef] [PubMed]
25. Valli, A.; Harris, A.L.; Kessler, B.M. Hypoxia metabolism in ageing. *Aging* **2015**, *7*, 465–466. [CrossRef] [PubMed]
26. Henrikson, N.B.; Webber, E.M.; Goddard, K.A.; Scrol, A.; Piper, M.; Williams, M.S.; Zallen, D.T.; Calonge, N.; Ganiats, T.G.; Janssens, A.C.J.W.; et al. Family history and the natural history of colorectal cancer: Systematic review. *Genet. Med.* **2015**, *17*, 702–712. [CrossRef] [PubMed]
27. Rametta, S.; Grosso, G.; Galvano, F.; Mistretta, A.; Marventano, S.; Nolfo, F.; Buscemi, S.; Gangi, S.; Basile, F.; Biondi, A. Social disparities, health risk behaviors, and cancer. *BMC Surg.* **2013**, *13* (Suppl. 2), S17. [CrossRef]
28. Valle, L. Genetic predisposition to colorectal cancer: Where we stand and future perspectives. *World J. Gastroenterol.* **2014**, *20*, 9828–9849. [CrossRef]
29. Schubert, S.A.; Morreau, H.; de Miranda, N.F.C.C.; van Wezel, T. The missing heritability of familial colorectal cancer. *Mutagenesis* **2020**, *35*, 221–231. [CrossRef]
30. Esteban-Jurado, C.; Garre, P.; Vila, M.; Lozano, J.J.; Pristoupilova, A.; Beltrán, S.; Abulí, A.; Muñoz, J.; Balaguer, F.; Ocaña, T.; et al. New genes emerging for colorectal cancer predisposition. *World J. Gastroenterol.* **2014**, *20*, 1961–1971. [CrossRef]
31. Pietrzyk, Ł. Food properties and dietary habits in colorectal cancer prevention and development. *Int. J. Food Prop.* **2017**, *20*, 2323–2343. [CrossRef]
32. Quang, L.N.; Hien, N.Q.; Quang, N.T.; Chung, N.T. Active Lifestyle Patterns Reduce the Risk of Colorectal Cancer in the North of Vietnam: A Hospital-Based Case–Control Study. *Cancer Control* **2019**, *26*. [CrossRef] [PubMed]
33. Nolfo, F.; Rametta, S.; Marventano, S.; Grosso, G.; Mistretta, A.; Drago, F.; Gangi, S.; Basile, F.; Biondi, A. Pharmacological and dietary prevention for colorectal cancer. *BMC Surg.* **2013**, *13*, 1–11. [CrossRef] [PubMed]
34. Deng, T.; Lyon, C.J.; Bergin, S.; Caligiuri, M.A.; Hsueh, W.A. Obesity, Inflammation, and Cancer. *Annu. Rev. Pathol.* **2016**, *11*, 421–449. [CrossRef] [PubMed]
35. Grosso, G.; Buscemi, S.; Galvano, F.; Mistretta, A.; Marventano, S.; La Vela, V.; Drago, F.; Gangi, S.; Basile, F.; Biondi, A. Mediterranean diet and cancer: Epidemiological evidence and mechanism of selected aspects. *BMC Surg.* **2013**, *13* (Suppl. 2), S14. [CrossRef]
36. Zitvogel, L.; Pietrocola, F.; Kroemer, G. Nutrition, inflammation and cancer. *Nat. Immunol.* **2017**, *18*, 843–850. [CrossRef]
37. De Almeida, C.V.; de Camargo, M.R.; Russo, E.; Amedei, A. Role of diet and gut microbiota on colorectal cancer immunomodulation. *World J. Gastroenterol.* **2019**, *25*, 151–162. [CrossRef]
38. Grosso, G.; Biondi, A.; Galvano, F.; Mistretta, A.; Marventano, S.; Buscemi, S.; Drago, F.; Basile, F. Factors associated with colorectal cancer in the context of the mediterranean diet: A case-control study. *Nutr. Cancer* **2014**, *66*, 558–565. [CrossRef]
39. Turner, N.D.; Lloyd, S.K. Association between red meat consumption and colon cancer: A systematic review of experimental results. *Exp. Biol. Med.* **2017**, *242*, 813–839. [CrossRef]
40. Fung, T.T.; Brown, L.S. Dietary Patterns and the Risk of Colorectal Cancer. *Curr. Nutr. Rep.* **2013**, *2*, 48–55. [CrossRef]
41. Kantor, E.D.; Lampe, J.W.; Peters, U.; Vaughan, T.L.; White, E. Long-chain omega-3 polyunsaturated fatty acid intake and risk of colorectal cancer. *Nutr. Cancer* **2014**, *66*, 716–727. [CrossRef] [PubMed]
42. Volpato, M.; Hull, M.A. Omega-3 polyunsaturated fatty acids as adjuvant therapy of colorectal cancer. *Cancer Metastasis Rev.* **2018**, *37*, 545–555. [CrossRef] [PubMed]

43. Borzì, A.M.; Biondi, A.; Basile, F.; Luca, S.; Vicari, E.S.D.; Vacante, M. Olive oil effects on colorectal cancer. *Nutrients* **2019**, *11*, 32. [CrossRef] [PubMed]
44. Pericleous, M.; Mandair, D.; Caplin, M.E. Diet and supplements and their impact on colorectal cancer. *J. Gastrointest. Oncol.* **2013**, *4*, 409–423. [CrossRef] [PubMed]
45. Low, E.E.; Demb, J.; Liu, L.; Earles, A.; Bustamante, R.; Williams, C.D.; Provenzale, D.; Kaltenbach, T.; Gawron, A.J.; Martinez, M.E.; et al. Risk Factors for Early-Onset Colorectal Cancer. *Gastroenterology* **2020**, *159*, 492–501.e7. [CrossRef] [PubMed]
46. Jackson, C.S.; Oman, M.; Patel, A.M.; Vega, K.J. Health disparities in colorectal cancer among racial and ethnic minorities in the United States. *J. Gastrointest. Oncol.* **2016**, *7*, S32–S43. [CrossRef] [PubMed]
47. Demb, J.; Earles, A.; Martínez, M.E.; Bustamante, R.; Bryant, A.K.; Murphy, J.D.; Liu, L.; Gupta, S. Risk factors for colorectal cancer significantly vary by anatomic site. *BMJ Open Gastroenterol.* **2019**, *6*. [CrossRef] [PubMed]
48. Vipperla, K.; O'Keefe, S.J. Diet, microbiota, and dysbiosis: A 'recipe' for colorectal cancer. *Food Funct.* **2016**, *7*, 1731–1740. [CrossRef] [PubMed]
49. Wu, X.; Wu, Y.; He, L.; Wu, L.; Wang, X.; Liu, Z. Effects of the intestinal microbial metabolite butyrate on the development of colorectal cancer. *J. Cancer* **2018**, *9*, 2510–2517. [CrossRef] [PubMed]
50. Yang, J.; Yu, J. The association of diet, gut microbiota and colorectal cancer: What we eat may imply what we get. *Protein Cell* **2018**, *9*, 474–487. [CrossRef] [PubMed]
51. Song, M.; Wu, K.; Meyerhardt, J.A.; Ogino, S.; Wang, M.; Fuchs, C.S.; Giovannucci, E.L.; Chan, A.T. Fiber intake and survival after colorectal cancer diagnosis. *JAMA Oncol.* **2018**, *4*, 71–79. [CrossRef] [PubMed]
52. Müller, M.F.; Ibrahim, A.E.K.; Arends, M.J. Molecular pathological classification of colorectal cancer. *Virchows Arch.* **2016**, *469*, 125–134. [CrossRef] [PubMed]
53. Zhiqiang, F.; Jie, C.; Yuqiang, N.; Chenghua, G.; Hong, W.; Zheng, S.; Wanglin, L.; Yongjian, Z.; Liping, D.; Lizhong, Z.; et al. Analysis of population-based colorectal cancer screening in Guangzhou, 2011–2015. *Cancer Med.* **2019**, *8*, 2496–2502. [CrossRef] [PubMed]
54. Conteduca, V.; Sansonno, D.; Russi, S.; Dammacco, F. Precancerous colorectal lesions (Review). *Int. J. Oncol.* **2013**, *43*, 973–984. [CrossRef]
55. Zhang, L.; Shay, J.W. Multiple Roles of APC and its Therapeutic Implications in Colorectal Cancer. *J. Natl. Cancer Inst.* **2017**, *109*. [CrossRef]
56. Liu, W.; Zhang, R.; Shu, R.; Yu, J.; Li, H.; Long, H.; Jin, S.; Li, S.; Hu, Q.; Yao, F.; et al. Study of the Relationship between Microbiome and Colorectal Cancer Susceptibility Using 16SrRNA Sequencing. *Biomed. Res. Int.* **2020**, *2020*, 7828392. [CrossRef]
57. Gao, R.; Gao, Z.; Huang, L.; Qin, H. Gut microbiota and colorectal cancer. *Eur. J. Clin. Microbiol. Infect. Dis.* **2017**, *36*, 757–769. [CrossRef]
58. Liang, S.; Mao, Y.; Liao, M.; Xu, Y.; Chen, Y.; Huang, X.; Wei, C.; Wu, C.; Wang, Q.; Pan, X.; et al. Gut microbiome associated with APC gene mutation in patients with intestinal adenomatous polyps. *Int. J. Biol. Sci.* **2020**, *16*, 135–146. [CrossRef]
59. Piotrowski, I.; Kulcenty, K.; Suchorska, W. Interplay between inflammation and cancer. *Rep. Pract. Oncol. Radiother.* **2020**, *25*, 422–427. [CrossRef]
60. Lucas, C.; Barnich, N.; Nguyen, H.T.T. Microbiota, Inflammation and Colorectal Cancer. *Int. J. Mol. Sci.* **2017**, *18*, 1310. [CrossRef]
61. Godos, J.; Biondi, A.; Galvano, F.; Basile, F.; Sciacca, S.; Giovannucci, E.L.; Grosso, G. Markers of systemic inflammation and colorectal adenoma risk: Meta-analysis of observational studies. *World J. Gastroenterol.* **2017**, *23*, 1909–1919. [CrossRef] [PubMed]
62. Luo, Y.; Zheng, S.G. Hall of Fame among Pro-inflammatory Cytokines: Interleukin-6 Gene and Its Transcriptional Regulation Mechanisms. *Front. Immunol.* **2016**, *7*, 604. [CrossRef] [PubMed]
63. Comstock, S.S.; Xu, D.; Hortos, K.; Kovan, B.; McCaskey, S.; Pathak, D.R.; Fenton, J.I. Association of serum cytokines with colorectal polyp number and type in adult males. *Eur. J. Cancer Prev.* **2016**, *25*, 173–181. [CrossRef] [PubMed]
64. Rinninella, E.; Raoul, P.; Cintoni, M.; Franceschi, F.; Miggiano, G.A.D.; Gasbarrini, A.; Mele, M.C. What is the Healthy Gut Microbiota Composition? A Changing Ecosystem across Age, Environment, Diet, and Diseases. *Microorganisms* **2019**, *7*, 14. [CrossRef]

65. Magne, F.; Gotteland, M.; Gauthier, L.; Zazueta, A.; Pesoa, S.; Navarrete, P.; Balamurugan, R. The Firmicutes/Bacteroidetes Ratio: A Relevant Marker of Gut Dysbiosis in Obese Patients? *Nutrients* **2020**, *12*, 1474. [CrossRef]
66. Tuddenham, S.; Sears, C.L. The intestinal microbiome and health. *Curr. Opin. Infect. Dis.* **2015**, *28*, 464–470. [CrossRef]
67. Lu, Y.; Chen, J.; Zheng, J.; Hu, G.; Wang, J.; Huang, C.; Lou, L.; Wang, X.; Zeng, Y. Mucosal adherent bacterial dysbiosis in patients with colorectal adenomas. *Sci. Rep.* **2016**, *6*, 26337. [CrossRef]
68. DeGruttola, A.K.; Low, D.; Mizoguchi, A.; Mizoguchi, E. Current understanding of dysbiosis in disease in human and animal models. *Inflamm. Bowel. Dis.* **2016**, *22*, 1137–1150. [CrossRef]
69. Keku, T.O.; Dulal, S.; Deveaux, A.; Jovov, B.; Han, X. The gastrointestinal microbiota and colorectal cancer. *Am. J. Physiol. Gastrointest. Liver Physiol.* **2015**, *308*, G351–G363. [CrossRef]
70. Liu, T.; Zhang, L.; Joo, D.; Sun, S.-C. NF-κB signaling in inflammation. *Signal Transduct. Target Ther.* **2017**, *2*, 17023. [CrossRef]
71. Hnatyszyn, A.; Hryhorowicz, S.; Kaczmarek-Ryś, M.; Lis, E.; Słomski, R.; Scott, R.J.; Pławski, A. Colorectal carcinoma in the course of inflammatory bowel diseases. *Hered. Cancer Clin. Pract.* **2019**, *17*. [CrossRef] [PubMed]
72. Cheng, W.T.; Kantilal, H.K.; Davamani, F. The Mechanism of Bacteroides fragilis Toxin Contributes to Colon Cancer Formation. *Malays. J. Med. Sci.* **2020**, *27*, 9–21. [CrossRef] [PubMed]
73. Ramos-Molina, B.; Queipo-Ortuño, M.I.; Lambertos, A.; Tinahones, F.J.; Peñafiel, R. Dietary and Gut Microbiota Polyamines in Obesity- and Age-Related Diseases. *Front. Nutr.* **2019**, *6*. [CrossRef] [PubMed]
74. Wang, X.; Zhang, A.; Miao, J.; Sun, H.; Yan, G.; Wu, F.; Wang, X. Gut microbiota as important modulator of metabolism in health and disease. *RSC Adv.* **2018**, *8*, 42380–42389. [CrossRef]
75. Singhal, R.; Shah, Y.M. Oxygen battle in the gut: Hypoxia and hypoxia-inducible factors in metabolic and inflammatory responses in the intestine. *J. Biol. Chem.* **2020**, *295*, 10493–10505. [CrossRef]
76. Valli, A.; Morotti, M.; Zois, C.E.; Albers, P.K.; Soga, T.; Feldinger, K.; Fischer, R.; Frejno, M.; McIntyre, A.; Bridges, E.; et al. Adaptation to HIF1α Deletion in Hypoxic Cancer Cells by Upregulation of GLUT14 and Creatine Metabolism. *Mol. Cancer Res.* **2019**, *17*, 1531–1544. [CrossRef]
77. Valli, A.; Rodriguez, M.; Moutsianas, L.; Fischer, R.; Fedele, V.; Huang, H.-L.; Van Stiphout, R.; Jones, D.; Mccarthy, M.; Vinaxia, M.; et al. Hypoxia induces a lipogenic cancer cell phenotype via HIF1α-dependent and -independent pathways. *Oncotarget* **2014**, *6*, 1920–1941. [CrossRef]
78. Diether, N.E.; Willing, B.P. Microbial Fermentation of Dietary Protein: An Important Factor in Diet–Microbe–Host Interaction. *Microorganisms* **2019**, *7*, 19. [CrossRef]
79. Baxter, N.T.; Schmidt, A.W.; Venkataraman, A.; Kim, K.S.; Waldron, C.; Schmidt, T.M. Dynamics of Human Gut Microbiota and Short-Chain Fatty Acids in Response to Dietary Interventions with Three Fermentable Fibers. *mBio* **2019**, *10*. [CrossRef]
80. Gaya, P.; Medina, M.; Sánchez-Jiménez, A.; Landete, J.M. Phytoestrogen Metabolism by Adult Human Gut Microbiota. *Molecules* **2016**, *21*, 1034. [CrossRef]
81. Hale, V.L.; Chen, J.; Johnson, S.; Harrington, S.C.; Yab, T.C.; Smyrk, T.C.; Nelson, H.; Boardman, L.A.; Druliner, B.R.; Levin, T.R.; et al. Shifts in the fecal microbiota associated with adenomatous polyps. *Cancer Epidemiol. Biomark. Prev.* **2017**, *26*, 85–94. [CrossRef] [PubMed]
82. Feng, Y.; Stams, A.J.M.; de Vos, W.M.; Sánchez-Andrea, I. Enrichment of sulfidogenic bacteria from the human intestinal tract. *FEMS Microbiol. Lett.* **2017**, *364*. [CrossRef] [PubMed]
83. Guo, F.-F.; Yu, T.-C.; Hong, J.; Fang, J.-Y. Emerging Roles of Hydrogen Sulfide in Inflammatory and Neoplastic Colonic Diseases. *Front. Physiol.* **2016**, *7*. [CrossRef] [PubMed]
84. Tomasova, L.; Konopelski, P.; Ufnal, M. Gut Bacteria and Hydrogen Sulfide: The New Old Players in Circulatory System Homeostasis. *Molecules* **2016**, *21*, 1558. [CrossRef]
85. Singh, S.B.; Lin, H.C. Hydrogen Sulfide in Physiology and Diseases of the Digestive Tract. *Microorganisms* **2015**, *3*, 866–889. [CrossRef]
86. Herrmann, S.S.; Duedahl-Olesen, L.; Christensen, T.; Olesen, P.T.; Granby, K. Dietary exposure to volatile and non-volatile N-nitrosamines from processed meat products in Denmark. *Food Chem. Toxicol.* **2015**, *80*, 137–143. [CrossRef]
87. Steinberg, P. Red Meat-Derived Nitroso Compounds, Lipid Peroxidation Products and Colorectal Cancer. *Foods* **2019**, *8*, 252. [CrossRef]

88. Wernke, K.M.; Xue, M.; Tirla, A.; Kim, C.S.; Crawford, J.M.; Herzon, S.B. Structure and bioactivity of colibactin. *Bioorg. Med. Chem. Lett.* **2020**, *30*, 127280. [CrossRef]
89. Faïs, T.; Delmas, J.; Barnich, N.; Bonnet, R.; Dalmasso, G. Colibactin: More Than a New Bacterial Toxin. *Toxins* **2018**, *10*, 151. [CrossRef]
90. Kasai, C.; Sugimoto, K.; Moritani, I.; Tanaka, J.; Oya, Y.; Inoue, H.; Tameda, M.; Shiraki, K.; Ito, M.; Takei, Y.; et al. Comparison of human gut microbiota in control subjects and patients with colorectal carcinoma in adenoma: Terminal restriction fragment length polymorphism and next-generation sequencing analyses. *Oncol. Rep.* **2016**, *35*, 325–333. [CrossRef]
91. Feng, Q.; Liang, S.; Jia, H.; Stadlmayr, A.; Tang, L.; Lan, Z.; Zhang, D.; Xia, H.; Xu, X.; Jie, Z.; et al. Gut microbiome development along the colorectal adenoma-carcinoma sequence. *Nat. Commun.* **2015**, *6*, 6528. [CrossRef] [PubMed]
92. Peters, B.A.; Dominianni, C.; Shapiro, J.A.; Church, T.R.; Wu, J.; Miller, G.; Yuen, E.; Freiman, H.; Lustbader, I.; Salik, J.; et al. The gut microbiota in conventional and serrated precursors of colorectal cancer. *Microbiome* **2016**, *4*, 69. [CrossRef] [PubMed]
93. Li, Y.-Y.; Ge, Q.-X.; Cao, J.; Zhou, Y.-J.; Du, Y.-L.; Shen, B.; Wan, Y.-J.Y.; Nie, Y.-Q. Association of Fusobacterium nucleatum infection with colorectal cancer in Chinese patients. *World J. Gastroenterol.* **2016**, *22*, 3227–3233. [CrossRef] [PubMed]
94. Fukugaiti, M.H.; Ignacio, A.; Fernandes, M.R.; Ribeiro Júnior, U.; Nakano, V.; Avila-Campos, M.J. High occurrence of Fusobacterium nucleatum and Clostridium difficile in the intestinal microbiota of colorectal carcinoma patients. *Braz. J. Microbiol.* **2015**, *46*, 1135–1140. [CrossRef]
95. Yu, Y.-N.; Yu, T.-C.; Zhao, H.-J.; Sun, T.-T.; Chen, H.-M.; Chen, H.-Y.; An, H.-F.; Weng, Y.-R.; Yu, J.; Li, M.; et al. Berberine may rescue Fusobacterium nucleatum-induced colorectal tumorigenesis by modulating the tumor microenvironment. *Oncotarget* **2015**, *6*, 32013–32026. [CrossRef]
96. Yu, J.; Chen, Y.; Fu, X.; Zhou, X.; Peng, Y.; Shi, L.; Chen, T.; Wu, Y. Invasive Fusobacterium nucleatum may play a role in the carcinogenesis of proximal colon cancer through the serrated neoplasia pathway. *Int. J. Cancer* **2016**, *139*, 1318–1326. [CrossRef]
97. Mima, K.; Nishihara, R.; Qian, Z.R.; Cao, Y.; Sukawa, Y.; Nowak, J.A.; Yang, J.; Dou, R.; Masugi, Y.; Song, M.; et al. Fusobacterium nucleatum in colorectal carcinoma tissue and patient prognosis. *Gut* **2016**, *65*, 1973–1980. [CrossRef]
98. Yu, T.; Guo, F.; Yu, Y.; Sun, T.; Ma, D.; Han, J.; Qian, Y.; Kryczek, I.; Sun, D.; Nagarsheth, N.; et al. Fusobacterium nucleatum Promotes Chemoresistance to Colorectal Cancer by Modulating Autophagy. *Cell* **2017**, *170*, 548–563.e16. [CrossRef]
99. Little, D.H.W.; Onizuka, K.M.; Khan, K.J. Referral for Colonoscopy in Patients with Streptococcus bovis Bacteremia and the Association with Colorectal Cancer and Adenomatous Polyps: A Quality Assurance Study. *Gastrointest. Disord.* **2019**, *1*, 385–390. [CrossRef]
100. Corredoira-Sánchez, J.; García-Garrote, F.; Rabuñal, R.; López-Roses, L.; García-País, M.J.; Castro, E.; González-Soler, R.; Coira, A.; Pita, J.; López-Álvarez, M.J.; et al. Association between bacteremia due to Streptococcus gallolyticus subsp. gallolyticus (Streptococcus bovis I) and colorectal neoplasia: A case-control study. *Clin. Infect. Dis.* **2012**, *55*, 491–496. [CrossRef]
101. Butt, J.; Romero-Hernández, B.; Pérez-Gómez, B.; Willhauck-Fleckenstein, M.; Holzinger, D.; Martin, V.; Moreno, V.; Linares, C.; Dierssen-Sotos, T.; Barricarte, A.; et al. Association of Streptococcus gallolyticus subspecies gallolyticus with colorectal cancer: Serological evidence. *Int. J. Cancer* **2016**, *138*, 1670–1679. [CrossRef] [PubMed]
102. Purcell, R.V.; Pearson, J.; Aitchison, A.; Dixon, L.; Frizelle, F.A.; Keenan, J.I. Colonization with enterotoxigenic Bacteroides fragilis is associated with early-stage colorectal neoplasia. *PLoS ONE* **2017**, *12*, e0171602. [CrossRef] [PubMed]
103. Xie, L.L.; Wu, N.; Zhu, Y.M.; Qiu, X.Y.; Chen, G.D.; Zhang, L.M.; Liu, Y.L. [Expression of enterotoxigenic Bacteroides fragilis and polyketide synthase gene-expressing Escherichia coli in colorectal adenoma patients]. *Zhonghua Yi Xue Za Zhi* **2016**, *96*, 954–959. [CrossRef] [PubMed]
104. Zamani, S.; Taslimi, R.; Sarabi, A.; Jasemi, S.; Sechi, L.A.; Feizabadi, M.M. Enterotoxigenic Bacteroides fragilis: A Possible Etiological Candidate for Bacterially-Induced Colorectal Precancerous and Cancerous Lesions. *Front. Cell Infect Microbiol.* **2020**, *9*. [CrossRef] [PubMed]

105. Viljoen, K.S.; Dakshinamurthy, A.; Goldberg, P.; Blackburn, J.M. Quantitative profiling of colorectal cancer-associated bacteria reveals associations between fusobacterium spp., enterotoxigenic Bacteroides fragilis (ETBF) and clinicopathological features of colorectal cancer. *PLoS ONE* **2015**, *10*, e0119462. [CrossRef]
106. Ambrosi, C.; Sarshar, M.; Aprea, M.R.; Pompilio, A.; Di Bonaventura, G.; Strati, F.; Pronio, A.; Nicoletti, M.; Zagaglia, C.; Palamara, A.T.; et al. Colonic adenoma-associated Escherichia coli express specific phenotypes. *Microbes Infect.* **2019**, *21*, 305–312. [CrossRef]
107. Iyadorai, T.; Mariappan, V.; Vellasamy, K.M.; Wanyiri, J.W.; Roslani, A.C.; Lee, G.K.; Sears, C.; Vadivelu, J. Prevalence and association of pks+ Escherichia coli with colorectal cancer in patients at the University Malaya Medical Centre, Malaysia. *PLoS ONE* **2020**, *15*, e0228217. [CrossRef]
108. IJspeert, J.E.G.; Vermeulen, L.; Meijer, G.A.; Dekker, E. Serrated neoplasia-role in colorectal carcinogenesis and clinical implications. *Nat. Rev. Gastroenterol. Hepatol.* **2015**, *12*, 401–409. [CrossRef]
109. Güven, D.C.; Dizdar, O. Fusobacterium and colorectal carcinogenesis. *Carcinogenesis* **2018**, *39*, 84. [CrossRef]
110. Rubinstein, M.R.; Wang, X.; Liu, W.; Hao, Y.; Cai, G.; Han, Y.W. Fusobacterium nucleatum promotes colorectal carcinogenesis by modulating E-cadherin/β-catenin signaling via its FadA adhesin. *Cell Host. Microbe* **2013**, *14*, 195–206. [CrossRef]
111. Ma, C.-T.; Luo, H.-S.; Gao, F.; Tang, Q.-C.; Chen, W. Fusobacterium nucleatum promotes the progression of colorectal cancer by interacting with E-cadherin. *Oncol. Lett.* **2018**, *16*, 2606–2612. [CrossRef] [PubMed]
112. Abed, J.; Emgård, J.E.M.; Zamir, G.; Faroja, M.; Almogy, G.; Grenov, A.; Sol, A.; Naor, R.; Pikarsky, E.; Atlan, K.A.; et al. Fap2 Mediates Fusobacterium nucleatum Colorectal Adenocarcinoma Enrichment by Binding to Tumor-Expressed Gal-GalNAc. *Cell Host. Microbe* **2016**, *20*, 215–225. [CrossRef] [PubMed]
113. Yang, Y.; Weng, W.; Peng, J.; Hong, L.; Yang, L.; Toiyama, Y.; Gao, R.; Liu, M.; Yin, M.; Pan, C.; et al. Fusobacterium nucleatum Increases Proliferation of Colorectal Cancer Cells and Tumor Development in Mice by Activating Toll-Like Receptor 4 Signaling to Nuclear Factor-κB, and Up-regulating Expression of MicroRNA-21. *Gastroenterology* **2017**, *152*, 851–866.e24. [CrossRef] [PubMed]
114. Bullman, S.; Pedamallu, C.S.; Sicinska, E.; Clancy, T.E.; Zhang, X.; Cai, D.; Neuberg, D.; Huang, K.; Guevara, F.; Nelson, T.; et al. Analysis of Fusobacterium persistence and antibiotic response in colorectal cancer. *Science* **2017**, *358*, 1443–1448. [CrossRef]
115. Aymeric, L.; Donnadieu, F.; Mulet, C.; du Merle, L.; Nigro, G.; Saffarian, A.; Bérard, M.; Poyart, C.; Robine, S.; Regnault, B.; et al. Colorectal cancer specific conditions promote Streptococcus gallolyticus gut colonization. *Proc. Natl. Acad. Sci. USA* **2018**, *115*, E283–E291. [CrossRef]
116. Baddour, L.M.; Wilson, W.R.; Bayer, A.S.; Fowler, V.G.; Tleyjeh, I.M.; Rybak, M.J.; Barsic, B.; Lockhart, P.B.; Gewitz, M.H.; Levison, M.E.; et al. Infective Endocarditis in Adults: Diagnosis, Antimicrobial Therapy, and Management of Complications: A Scientific Statement for Healthcare Professionals from the American Heart Association. *Circulation* **2015**, *132*, 1435–1486. [CrossRef]
117. Habib, G.; Lancellotti, P.; Antunes, M.J.; Bongiorni, M.G.; Casalta, J.-P.; Del Zotti, F.; Dulgheru, R.; El Khoury, G.; Erba, P.A.; Iung, B.; et al. 2015 ESC Guidelines for the management of infective endocarditis: The Task Force for the Management of Infective Endocarditis of the European Society of Cardiology (ESC). Endorsed by: European Association for Cardio-Thoracic Surgery (EACTS), the European Association of Nuclear Medicine (EANM). *Eur. Heart J.* **2015**, *36*, 3075–3128. [CrossRef]
118. Allen, J.; Hao, S.; Sears, C.L.; Timp, W. Epigenetic Changes Induced by Bacteroides fragilis Toxin. *Infect. Immun.* **2019**, *87*. [CrossRef]
119. Khan, Z.; Siddiqui, N.; Saif, M.W. Enterococcus Faecalis Infective Endocarditis and Colorectal Carcinoma: Case of New Association Gaining Ground. *Gastroenterol. Res.* **2018**, *11*, 238–240. [CrossRef]
120. Goh, H.M.S.; Yong, M.H.A.; Chong, K.K.L.; Kline, K.A. Model systems for the study of Enterococcal colonization and infection. *Virulence* **2017**, *8*, 1525–1562. [CrossRef]
121. Alozie, A.; Köller, K.; Pose, L.; Raftis, M.; Steinhoff, G.; Westphal, B.; Lamprecht, G.; Podbielski, A. Streptococcus bovis infectious endocarditis and occult gastrointestinal neoplasia: Experience with 25 consecutive patients treated surgically. *Gut. Pathog.* **2015**, *7*. [CrossRef] [PubMed]
122. Gong, J.; Bai, T.; Zhang, L.; Qian, W.; Song, J.; Hou, X. Inhibition effect of Bifidobacterium longum, Lactobacillus acidophilus, Streptococcus thermophilus and Enterococcus faecalis and their related products on human colonic smooth muscle in vitro. *PLoS ONE* **2017**, *12*, e0189257. [CrossRef] [PubMed]
123. De Almeida, C.V.; Taddei, A.; Amedei, A. The controversial role of Enterococcus faecalis in colorectal cancer. *Ther. Adv. Gastroenterol.* **2018**, *11*. [CrossRef] [PubMed]

124. Miyamoto, S.; Komiya, M.; Fujii, G.; Hamoya, T.; Nakanishi, R.; Fujimoto, K.; Tamura, S.; Kurokawa, Y.; Takahashi, M.; Ijichi, T.; et al. Preventive Effects of Heat-Killed Enterococcus faecalis Strain EC-12 on Mouse Intestinal Tumor Development. *Int. J. Mol. Sci.* **2017**, *18*, 826. [CrossRef] [PubMed]
125. Wang, X.; Yang, Y.; Huycke, M.M. Commensal-infected macrophages induce dedifferentiation and reprogramming of epithelial cells during colorectal carcinogenesis. *Oncotarget* **2017**, *8*, 102176–102190. [CrossRef] [PubMed]
126. Iebba, V.; Totino, V.; Gagliardi, A.; Santangelo, F.; Cacciotti, F.; Trancassini, M.; Mancini, C.; Cicerone, C.; Corazziari, E.; Pantanella, F.; et al. Eubiosis and dysbiosis: The two sides of the microbiota. *New Microbiol.* **2016**, *39*, 1–12.
127. Flandroy, L.; Poutahidis, T.; Berg, G.; Clarke, G.; Dao, M.-C.; Decaestecker, E.; Furman, E.; Haahtela, T.; Massart, S.; Plovier, H.; et al. The impact of human activities and lifestyles on the interlinked microbiota and health of humans and of ecosystems. *Sci. Total Environ.* **2018**, *627*, 1018–1038. [CrossRef]
128. Vila, J.; Sáez-López, E.; Johnson, J.R.; Römling, U.; Dobrindt, U.; Cantón, R.; Giske, C.G.; Naas, T.; Carattoli, A.; Martínez-Medina, M.; et al. Escherichia coli: An old friend with new tidings. *FEMS Microbiol. Rev.* **2016**, *40*, 437–463. [CrossRef]
129. Poolman, J.T.; Wacker, M. Extraintestinal Pathogenic Escherichia coli, a Common Human Pathogen: Challenges for Vaccine Development and Progress in the Field. *J. Infect. Dis.* **2016**, *213*, 6–13. [CrossRef]
130. Gagnière, J.; Raisch, J.; Veziant, J.; Barnich, N.; Bonnet, R.; Buc, E.; Bringer, M.-A.; Pezet, D.; Bonnet, M. Gut microbiota imbalance and colorectal cancer. *World J. Gastroenterol.* **2016**, *22*, 501–518. [CrossRef]
131. Khan, A.A.; Khan, Z.; Malik, A.; Kalam, M.A.; Cash, P.; Ashraf, M.T.; Alshamsan, A. Colorectal cancer-inflammatory bowel disease nexus and felony of Escherichia coli. *Life Sci.* **2017**, *180*, 60–67. [CrossRef] [PubMed]
132. Bleich, R.M.; Arthur, J.C. Revealing a microbial carcinogen. *Science* **2019**, *363*, 689–690. [CrossRef] [PubMed]
133. Wilson, M.R.; Jiang, Y.; Villalta, P.W.; Stornetta, A.; Boudreau, P.D.; Carrá, A.; Brennan, C.A.; Chun, E.; Ngo, L.; Samson, L.D.; et al. The human gut bacterial genotoxin colibactin alkylates DNA. *Science* **2019**, *363*. [CrossRef] [PubMed]
134. Xue, M.; Kim, C.; Healy, A.; Wernke, K.; Wang, Z.; Frischling, M.; Shine, E.; Wang, W.; Herzon, S.; Crawford, J. Structure elucidation of colibactin and its DNA cross-links. *Science* **2019**, *365*. [CrossRef] [PubMed]
135. Pleguezuelos-Manzano, C.; Puschhof, J.; Rosendahl Huber, A.; van Hoeck, A.; Wood, H.M.; Nomburg, J.; Gurjao, C.; Manders, F.; Dalmasso, G.; Stege, P.B.; et al. Mutational signature in colorectal cancer caused by genotoxic pks + E. coli. *Nature* **2020**, *580*, 269–273. [CrossRef]
136. Fong, W.; Li, Q.; Yu, J. Gut microbiota modulation: A novel strategy for prevention and treatment of colorectal cancer. *Oncogene* **2020**, *39*, 4925–4943. [CrossRef]
137. Ambalam, P.; Raman, M.; Purama, R.K.; Doble, M. Probiotics, prebiotics and colorectal cancer prevention. *Best Pract. Res. Clin. Gastroenterol.* **2016**, *30*, 119–131. [CrossRef]
138. Malaguarnera, G.; Leggio, F.; Vacante, M.; Motta, M.; Giordano, M.; Biondi, A.; Basile, F.; Mastrojeni, S.; Mistretta, A.; MalaGuarnera, M.; et al. Probiotics in the gastrointestinal diseases of the elderly. *J. Nutr. Health Aging* **2012**, *16*, 402–410. [CrossRef]
139. Uccello, M.; Malaguarnera, G.; Basile, F.; Dagata, V.; Malaguarnera, M.; Bertino, G.; Vacante, M.; Drago, F.; Biondi, A. Potential role of probiotics on colorectal cancer prevention. *BMC Surg.* **2012**, *12*, S35. [CrossRef]
140. Gamallat, Y.; Meyiah, A.; Kuugbee, E.D.; Hago, A.M.; Chiwala, G.; Awadasseid, A.; Bamba, D.; Zhang, X.; Shang, X.; Luo, F.; et al. Lactobacillus rhamnosus induced epithelial cell apoptosis, ameliorates inflammation and prevents colon cancer development in an animal model. *Biomed. Pharmacother.* **2016**, *83*, 536–541. [CrossRef]
141. Kuugbee, E.D.; Shang, X.; Gamallat, Y.; Bamba, D.; Awadasseid, A.; Suliman, M.A.; Zang, S.; Ma, Y.; Chiwala, G.; Xin, Y.; et al. Structural Change in Microbiota by a Probiotic Cocktail Enhances the Gut Barrier and Reduces Cancer via TLR2 Signaling in a Rat Model of Colon Cancer. *Dig. Dis. Sci.* **2016**, *61*, 2908–2920. [CrossRef] [PubMed]
142. Yeung, C.-Y.; Chan, W.-T.; Jiang, C.-B.; Cheng, M.-L.; Liu, C.-Y.; Chang, S.-W.; Chiang Chiau, J.-S.; Lee, H.-C. Amelioration of Chemotherapy-Induced Intestinal Mucositis by Orally Administered Probiotics in a Mouse Model. *PLoS ONE* **2015**, *10*, e0138746. [CrossRef] [PubMed]

143. Mi, H.; Dong, Y.; Zhang, B.; Wang, H.; Peter, C.C.K.; Gao, P.; Fu, H.; Gao, Y. Bifidobacterium Infantis Ameliorates Chemotherapy-Induced Intestinal Mucositis Via Regulating T Cell Immunity in Colorectal Cancer Rats. *Cell Physiol. Biochem.* **2017**, *42*, 2330–2341. [CrossRef] [PubMed]
144. Montalban-Arques, A.; Scharl, M. Intestinal microbiota and colorectal carcinoma: Implications for pathogenesis, diagnosis, and therapy. *EBioMedicine* **2019**, *48*, 648–655. [CrossRef] [PubMed]
145. Chen, L.; Collij, V.; Jaeger, M.; van den Munckhof, I.C.L.; Vich Vila, A.; Kurilshikov, A.; Gacesa, R.; Sinha, T.; Oosting, M.; Joosten, L.A.B.; et al. Gut microbial co-abundance networks show specificity in inflammatory bowel disease and obesity. *Nat. Commun.* **2020**, *11*, 4018. [CrossRef]
146. Flemer, B.; Lynch, D.B.; Brown, J.M.R.; Jeffery, I.B.; Ryan, F.J.; Claesson, M.J.; O'Riordain, M.; Shanahan, F.; O'Toole, P.W. Tumour-associated and non-tumour-associated microbiota in colorectal cancer. *Gut* **2017**, *66*, 633–643. [CrossRef]
147. Geller, L.T.; Barzily-Rokni, M.; Danino, T.; Jonas, O.H.; Shental, N.; Nejman, D.; Gavert, N.; Zwang, Y.; Cooper, Z.A.; Shee, K.; et al. Potential role of intratumor bacteria in mediating tumor resistance to the chemotherapeutic drug gemcitabine. *Science* **2017**, *357*, 1156–1160. [CrossRef]
148. Viaud, S.; Saccheri, F.; Mignot, G.; Yamazaki, T.; Daillère, R.; Hannani, D.; Enot, D.P.; Pfirschke, C.; Engblom, C.; Pittet, M.J.; et al. The intestinal microbiota modulates the anticancer immune effects of cyclophosphamide. *Science* **2013**, *342*, 971–976. [CrossRef]
149. Sivan, A.; Corrales, L.; Hubert, N.; Williams, J.B.; Aquino-Michaels, K.; Earley, Z.M.; Benyamin, F.W.; Lei, Y.M.; Jabri, B.; Alegre, M.-L.; et al. Commensal Bifidobacterium promotes antitumor immunity and facilitates anti-PD-L1 efficacy. *Science* **2015**, *350*, 1084–1089. [CrossRef]
150. Gopalakrishnan, V.; Spencer, C.N.; Nezi, L.; Reuben, A.; Andrews, M.C.; Karpinets, T.V.; Prieto, P.A.; Vicente, D.; Hoffman, K.; Wei, S.C.; et al. Gut microbiome modulates response to anti-PD-1 immunotherapy in melanoma patients. *Science* **2018**, *359*, 97–103. [CrossRef]
151. Routy, B.; Le Chatelier, E.; Derosa, L.; Duong, C.P.M.; Alou, M.T.; Daillère, R.; Fluckiger, A.; Messaoudene, M.; Rauber, C.; Roberti, M.P.; et al. Gut microbiome influences efficacy of PD-1-based immunotherapy against epithelial tumors. *Science* **2018**, *359*, 91–97. [CrossRef] [PubMed]
152. Villéger, R.; Lopès, A.; Veziant, J.; Gagnière, J.; Barnich, N.; Billard, E.; Boucher, D.; Bonnet, M. Microbial markers in colorectal cancer detection and/or prognosis. *World J. Gastroenterol.* **2018**, *24*, 2327–2347. [CrossRef] [PubMed]
153. Mangifesta, M.; Mancabelli, L.; Milani, C.; Gaiani, F.; de'Angelis, N.; de'Angelis, G.L.; van Sinderen, D.; Ventura, M.; Turroni, F. Mucosal microbiota of intestinal polyps reveals putative biomarkers of colorectal cancer. *Sci. Rep.* **2018**, *8*. [CrossRef] [PubMed]
154. Conlon, M.A.; Bird, A.R. The Impact of Diet and Lifestyle on Gut Microbiota and Human Health. *Nutrients* **2014**, *7*, 17–44. [CrossRef]
155. Thomas, A.M.; Manghi, P.; Asnicar, F.; Pasolli, E.; Armanini, F.; Zolfo, M.; Beghini, F.; Manara, S.; Karcher, N.; Pozzi, C.; et al. Metagenomic analysis of colorectal cancer datasets identifies cross-cohort microbial diagnostic signatures and a link with choline degradation. *Nat. Med.* **2019**, *25*, 667–678. [CrossRef]
156. Wirbel, J.; Pyl, P.T.; Kartal, E.; Zych, K.; Kashani, A.; Milanese, A.; Fleck, J.S.; Voigt, A.Y.; Palleja, A.; Ponnudurai, R.; et al. Meta-analysis of fecal metagenomes reveals global microbial signatures that are specific for colorectal cancer. *Nat. Med.* **2019**, *25*, 679–689. [CrossRef]
157. Poore, G.D.; Kopylova, E.; Zhu, Q.; Carpenter, C.; Fraraccio, S.; Wandro, S.; Kosciolek, T.; Janssen, S.; Metcalf, J.; Song, S.J.; et al. Microbiome analyses of blood and tissues suggest cancer diagnostic approach. *Nature* **2020**, *579*, 567–574. [CrossRef]
158. Slowicka, K.; Petta, I.; Blancke, G.; Hoste, E.; Dumas, E.; Sze, M.; Vikkula, H.; Radaelli, E.; Haigh, J.J.; Jonckheere, S.; et al. Zeb2 drives invasive and microbiota-dependent colon carcinoma. *Nat. Cancer* **2020**, *1*, 620–634. [CrossRef]

Publisher's Note: MDPI stays neutral with regard to jurisdictional claims in published maps and institutional affiliations.

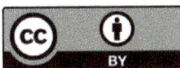

© 2020 by the authors. Licensee MDPI, Basel, Switzerland. This article is an open access article distributed under the terms and conditions of the Creative Commons Attribution (CC BY) license (http://creativecommons.org/licenses/by/4.0/).

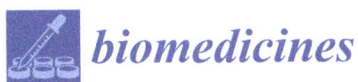

Article

Functional Characterization of Colon-Cancer-Associated Variants in *ADAM17* Affecting the Catalytic Domain

Jan Philipp Dobert [1], Anne-Sophie Cabron [1], Philipp Arnold [2], Egor Pavlenko [1], Stefan Rose-John [1] and Friederike Zunke [1,3,*]

1. Institute of Biochemistry Christian-Albrechts-Universität zu Kiel, 24118 Kiel, Germany; stu118262@mail.uni-kiel.de (J.P.D.); acabron@biochem.uni-kiel.de (A.-S.C.); stu119549@mail.uni-kiel.de (E.P.); rosejohn@biochem.uni-kiel.de (S.R.-J.)
2. Institute of Anatomy, Christian-Albrechts-Universität zu Kiel, 24118 Kiel, Germany; p.arnold@anat.uni-kiel.de
3. Department of Molecular Neurology, University Hospital Erlangen, Friedrich-Alexander-Universität Erlangen-Nürnberg, 91054 Erlangen, Germany
* Correspondence: friederike.zunke@fau.de; Tel.: +49-9131-85-39324; Fax: +49-9131-85-3467

Received: 21 September 2020; Accepted: 29 October 2020; Published: 30 October 2020

Abstract: Although extensively investigated, cancer is still one of the most devastating and lethal diseases in the modern world. Among different types, colorectal cancer (CRC) is most prevalent and mortal, making it an important subject of research. The metalloprotease ADAM17 has been implicated in the development of CRC due to its involvement in signaling pathways related to inflammation and cell proliferation. ADAM17 is capable of releasing membrane-bound proteins from the cell surface in a process called *shedding*. A deficiency of ADAM17 activity has been previously shown to have protective effects against CRC in mice, while an upregulation of ADAM17 activity is suspected to facilitate tumor development. In this study, we characterize ADAM17 variants found in tissue samples of cancer patients in overexpression studies. We here focus on point mutations identified within the catalytic domain of ADAM17 and could show a functional dysregulation of the CRC-associated variants. Since the catalytic domain of ADAM17 is the only region structurally determined by crystallography, we study the effect of each point mutation not only to learn more about the role of ADAM17 in cancer, but also to investigate the structure–function relationships of the metalloprotease.

Keywords: ADAM17; colorectal cancer (CRC); TNFα; IL-6R; AREG; shedding

1. Introduction

Cancer is one of the leading causes of death in modern society. In 2019, over 1.7 million new cases and over 600,000 deaths were reported in the US alone. Colorectal cancer (CRC) cancer is among the more common and also lethal forms of it, being ranked third in terms of incidence for both males and females [1]. The highest non-genetic risk factor for developing CRC is a chronic inflammation of the gut, generally known as inflammatory bowel disease (IBD) [2,3], which includes a subset of diseases resulting in chronic inflammation of the gastrointestinal tract, such as ulcerative colitis or Crohn's disease [4]. Although many susceptibility genes for IBDs are known, most cases can be linked to a variety of different environmental factors, including diet, smoking, stress and many more [5]. A so-called "Western diet" (high fat, low fiber) has been associated with a higher risk of developing IBD and CRC in humans and mice alike [6–8]. In recent years, the membrane-bound metalloprotease ADAM17 (a disintegrin and metalloprotease 17) has been identified as a key player in the development of colon cancer. First discovered as the protease responsible for cleaving proTNFα at the cell surface [9],

ADAM17 has since been found to cleave over 80 substrates and thus being involved in almost all parts of cell homeostasis [10]. This includes inflammation, regeneration, differentiation and immunity. Underlining the important role of ADAM17 in vivo, *ADAM17* knock out mice are not viable and die prenatally [11]. A hypomorphic mouse model expressing very low levels of ADAM17 (~5%) is viable, but highly compromised [12]. Due to its wide range of functions and its almost ubiquitous expression throughout the organism, a pathophysiological role of ADAM17 has long been implicated [13]. ADAM17 is expressed as a zymogen and consists of six major domains: an inhibitory pro-domain that also functions as a chaperone [14], a catalytic domain (CD), a disintegrin domain, a membrane-proximal domain harboring the CANDIS region [15], a transmembrane domain and a small cytosolic tail. During the maturation process, the pro-domain is cleaved by furin in the trans-Golgi network, exposing the catalytic site and enabling protease activity [16]. ADAM17 is then transported to the cell surface where it acts as sheddase [10].

In addition to activation by furin, regulation of ADAM17 can take place by phosphorylation of the cytoplasmic domain [17–20], cellular localization [21], composition of the cell membrane [22] and/or activation/inactivation by protein-disulfide isomerase [23]. Another regulatory mechanism is substrate recognition, which is thought to be facilitated mainly by the membrane-proximal domain. In addition, the transmembrane proteins iRhom1 and iRhom2 have been found to be crucial for ADAM17 substrate selectivity, trafficking and activation [24–27]. Other studies have shown that even after maturation, the cleaved pro-domain can function as a potent inhibitor of ADAM17 [28]. Given its importance in such fundamental cellular pathways, it is no surprise that ADAM17 is highly regulated by so many different mechanisms. Interestingly, no protein structure of full-length ADAM17 has been obtained yet. Single domain structures have been solved only for the catalytic domain [29] as well as the membrane-proximal domain [23]. Among the many signaling pathways ADAM17 is involved in, the most prominent ones are connected to inflammation and regeneration. In inflammation, ADAM17 is responsible for the release of TNFα and its receptors TNFR1 and TNFR2, which are essential for an inflammatory response [30]. High levels of soluble TNFα are associated with an inflammatory state and are a hallmark of IBD [31]. Many other proteins involved in leukocyte activation are also shed by ADAM17, such as L-selectin, VCAM-1, ICAM-1 and more [32–35]. ADAM17 also influences the Interleukin 6 (IL-6) pathway by shedding the Interleukin 6 receptor (IL-6R) from the cell surface [36]. IL-6-mediated pathways are also heavily involved in inflammation, acting in both a pro- and anti-inflammatory manner [37,38]. Almost all inflammatory diseases are associated with an upregulation of IL-6. Signaling can be induced in two different way, typically described as classic and trans-signaling. In classic signaling, IL-6 binds to IL-6R at the cell surface, then a gp130 homodimer is recruited to form the signaling complex [39]. However, if IL-6R has been shed from the cell surface, IL-6 can still bind to the shed ectodomain of IL-6R, forming a soluble ligand–receptor complex. This complex can then bind to a gp130 homodimer on any type of cell (even those not expressing IL-6R) to form the trans-signaling complex [40]. While classic IL-6 signaling is associated with anti-inflammatory properties, trans-signaling has been shown to have a pro-inflammatory effect and play a major role in the development of cancer [41–43].

In regeneration, ADAM17 is capable of regulating cell proliferation by cleaving and releasing EGF-R ligands like Amphiregulin (AREG), TGF-α, Hb-EGF and EREG [44]. The EGF receptor (ErbB1) is a transmembrane tyrosine kinase receptor capable of binding different ligands [45]. Activation of EGF-R can induce a variety of signaling cascades involved in cell survival, proliferation and differentiation [46]. EGF-R overexpression, as well as increased activation of EGF-R pathways, are high risk factors for developing cancer and EGF-R signaling is often highly upregulated in human carcinomas [47–49]. Previous studies have shown that ADAM17 is upregulated in colon tumor tissue [50]. In mice, ADAM17-deficiency has a protective effect on tumor burden in an induced genetic colon cancer model [51]. Thus, ADAM17 activation seems to play a key role in the development of CRC. The specific role of ADAM17 in CRC, however, appears to be multifaceted as all three major ADAM17-regulated pathways (TNFα-, EGF-R- and IL-6-signaling) on different cell types are implicated in tumor progression. A recent study has found that both the activation of EGF-R pathways, as well as IL-6 trans signaling can be observed during tumor development, and both require ADAM17 [51]. Release of sIL-6R by ADAM17 to promote IL-6 trans-signaling can be facilitated by tumor cells and macrophages [52,53], whereas ADAM17 on myeloid cells is speculated to release EGF-R ligands and activate EGF-R signaling in an autocrine manner, as well as on macrophages. This in turn leads to the production of IL-6, further promoting IL-6 trans-signaling [43,54].

In this study, we analyzed naturally occurring mutations within the *ADAM17* gene found in colon cancer tissues, utilizing databases (IntOGen, COSMIC, TCGA and ICGC) [55–60] containing sequence data of patient tumor samples. Interestingly, single nucleotide variations (SNVs) could be found distributed all over the *ADAM17* gene and are hence found within all protein domains of the metalloprotease.

We here selected three ADAM17 missense point mutations from colon cancer tissue (E319G, E406X, M435I) as well as one variant found within pancreatic cancer (P417Q). All these variants are found within the catalytic domain of the translated protein. The E406X mutation is located right at the beginning of the Zn^{2+} binding motif and introduces an early stop codon. The resulting truncated protein thus consists of only the pro-domain and a small part of the catalytic domain. Out of the four selected mutants, only the M435I variant has been subject to research before. This variant was found to be catalytically inactive as the methionine at this position is part of a highly conserved loop structure integral for enzymatic function [61]. Utilizing an ADAM10/17 deficient HEK293 cell line, we characterized these ADAM17 variants based on their expression, cellular localization as well as their ability to cleave substrates implicated in cancer.

2. Experimental Section

2.1. Database Analysis

The ADAM17 variants were found by screening for cancer-associated mutations in the catalytic domain. The databases used are the following: IntOGen (Integrative Onco Genomics, Barcelona Biomedical Genomics Lab, Barcelona, Spain), Cosmic (Catalogue of Somatic Mutations in Cancer; Sanger Institute, Cambridge, UK), The Cancer Genome Atlas Program (TCGA; National Institutes of Health, Bethesda, MD, USA) and the International Cancer Genome Consortium (ICGC). These databases provide somatically acquired mutations found in tumor tissue of cancer patients (the project identification code, Date Month Year).

2.2. cDNA Constructs and Cloning

Expression plasmids of murine (m) ADAM17 wild type (wt), as well as the colon cancer-associated mutants (E319G, E406X, M435I, P417Q), were assembled using mADAM17 cDNA and the pcDNA3.1 (+) vector (#V79020, Thermo Fisher Scientific Inc., Waltham, MA, USA). Mutations were introduced via site-directed mutagenesis PCR. The generated constructs were verified by using Sanger sequencing (Eurofins Genomics, Ebersberg, Germany). Expression plasmids of ADAM17 substrates (murine AREG, IL-6R and proTNFα) were also based on pcDNA3.1 (+) and were used for co-transfection experiments in order to analyze ADAM17 enzymatic activity. For staining of the plasma membrane in immunofluorescence analysis (see Section 2.7), a custom made eGFP construct was used. It comprises the coding sequence of eGFP with an added farnesylation motif for membrane anchoring, cloned into pcDNA3.1 (+).

2.3. Cell Culture

HEK cells deficient for ADAM10 and ADAM17 (A10/A17 dKO) were used for overexpression experiments as recently described [14]. Cells were cultivated in Dulbecco's Modified Eagle's medium (DMEM; #D6429, Sigma-Aldrich, Munich, Germany) supplemented with 10% heat-inactivated fetal calf serum (FCS) (#3306-PI31004, PAA Laboratories, Pasching, Austria) and 1× penicillin/streptomycin (Pen/Strep; #P0781, Sigma-Aldrich, Munich, Germany). Passaging of the cells was required every 3–4 days once they reached a confluency of 80–90%.

2.4. Transfection

Prior to transfection, the cell count of the respective cell line was determined via Cellometer Auto T4 Plus (Nexcelom Bioscience, Lawrence, MA, USA). The HEK A10/17 dKO cells were then plated at a density of 2.2×10^6 per 10 cm plate and 2×10^5 per 6-well and cultivated overnight. The next day, cells were transfected with a mixture of polyethylenimine (PEI, 1 µg/µL) (#24765-1, Polysciences, Warrington, PA, USA) and DNA (1 µg/µL) in a ratio of 3:1 diluted in DMEM. Per plasmid, 1 µg of DNA was used for transfection of a 10 cm dish and 0.5 µg of DNA per well of a 6-well plate. The cells were harvested after 48 h and, where indicated, stimulated with 200 nM phorbol 12-myristate 13-acetate (PMA; #P8139, Sigma-Aldrich, Munich, Germany) for 2 h prior to harvesting.

2.5. Western Blot Analysis

HEK A10/A17 dKO cells were transfected as described above and harvested by mechanically detaching from the culture dish. Afterwards, the cells were washed twice with cold PBS and lysed in lysis buffer (1% Triton X-100, 150 mM NaCl, 50 mM Tris-HCl pH 7.4), 10 mM 1.10-phenanthroline (#841491, Merck, Darmstadt, Germany) and 1× cOmplete protease inhibitor cocktail (#11697498001, Roche, Basel, Switzerland) for 60 min at 4 °C. The protein concentration was determined by BCA assay (#23225, Thermo Fisher Scientific Inc., Waltham, MA, USA). Then, 40 µg of total protein was supplemented with 5× SDS sample buffer (0.3 M Tris-HCl, pH 6.8, 10% SDS, 50% glycerol, 5% β-mercaptoethanol, 5% bromophenol blue) and denatured at 95 °C for 5 min. The samples were then run in an SDS-PAGE and transferred to a PVDF-membrane (#IPFL00010, Merck Millipore, Burlington, MA, USA). The membrane was blocked in TBS containing 6% milk powder and incubated with primary antibodies overnight at 4 °C. Secondary antibodies were applied for 1 h at room temperature.

The following primary antibodies were used: anti-ADAM17 10.1 (binding epitope between aa 290–309; Pineda Antikörper-Service, Berlin, Germany), anti-TNFα (Pineda Antikörper-Service, Berlin, Germany), anti-IL-6R C#1 (Pineda Antikörper-Service, Berlin, Germany), anti-myc (Cell Signaling, Frankfurt am Main, Germany; clone 9B11 #2276), anti-transferrin receptor (#ab84036, abcam, Cambridge, UK) and anti-β-actin (#A5441, Sigma-Aldrich, Darmstadt, Germany). As secondary antibodies, goat anti-rabbit HRP and sheep anti-mouse HRP (#111-035-144, #515-035-062, both Dianova, Hamburg, Germany), as well as IRDye 800CW donkey anti-rabbit and IRDye 680RD Donkey anti-Mouse (#926-32213, #926-68072, both LI-COR Biosciences, Lincoln, Nebraska) were used.

2.6. Biotinylation

First, 2×10^6 HEK A10/A17 dKO cells were transfected as described above. Twenty-four hours after transfection, the cells were cooled to 4 °C, washed twice with ice-cold PBS-CM (PBS with 0.1 mM $CaCl_2$ and 1 mM $MgCl_2$ added) and afterwards incubated with 1 mg/mL Sulfo-NHS-SS-Biotin (#21331, Thermo Fisher Scientific Inc., Waltham, MA, USA) in PBS-CM for 30 min at 4 °C. Simultaneously, control cells were incubated in only PBS-CM. The solutions were removed and ice-cold quenching buffer (PBS plus 50 mM Tris-HCl; pH 8.0 in PBS-CM) was added for 10 min. After three washing steps with PBS-CM the cells were lysed in biotinylation lysis buffer (1% Triton X-100, 0.1% SDS, 150 mM NaCl, 50 mM Tris-HCl pH 7.4 and 1× complete protease cocktail inhibitor) for 30 min at 4 °C. The protein amount was determined by BCA and an aliquot of 20 µg of total protein was taken as a lysate control sample and prepared for SDS-PAGE. An equal amount of total protein from each sample was then diluted to a volume of 250 µL using biotinylation lysis buffer. Then, 75 µL of streptavidin beads (#20359, Thermo Fisher Scientific Inc., Waltham, MA, USA) per sample were washed three times with 100 µL biotinylation lysis buffer and added to the diluted samples. After an incubation of 1 h at 4 °C, the supernatant was removed and the beads were washed several times with 500 µL of biotinylation lysis buffer. Afterwards, all supernatant was removed and 40 µL 1× SDS sample buffer were added to the beads of each sample and heated up to 60 °C for 20 min. All samples were then analyzed via SDS-PAGE and Western blot.

2.7. Immunofluorescence Analysis

HEK A10/A17 dKO cells were seeded in a 6-well plate (2.0×10^5 cells per well) containing glass cover slips and transfected as previously described. The cells were then washed with PBS, fixed with 4% PFA in PBS for 15 min at room temperature and permeabilized with 0.3% Triton X-100 (Sigma-Aldrich, Darmstadt, Germany) in PBS for 30 min. Subsequently, cells were blocked in blocking buffer (2% BSA, 5% heat-inactivated FCS and 0.3% Triton in PBS) for 60 min and then incubated at 4 °C overnight with the primary antibodies. All antibodies were diluted in blocking buffer to their working concentrations (see below). Afterwards, the cells were washed three times with PBS containing 0.3% Triton X-100, then incubated with secondary antibodies for 60 min at room temperature. Finally, cells were washed three more times with 0.3% Triton X-100 in PBS, once with PBS and stained with DAPI as part of the mounting mix consisting of Dabco (Sigma-Aldrich, Darmstadt, Germany) and Mowiol (Merck Millipore, Burlington, MA, USA). Immunofluorescence analyses were performed with a confocal laser scanning microscope (FV1000, Olympus, Tokyo, Japan) equipped with a U Plan S Apo 100× oil immersion objective. Digital images were analyzed using FV10-ASW Viewer version 4.2 (Olympus, Tokyo, Japan). Primary antibodies used: anti-PDI (1:100, abcam, Cambridge, UK; #ab13506), anti-ADAM17 10.1 (1:100, Pineda Antikörper-Service, Berlin, Germany). Secondary antibodies were purchased from Thermo Fisher Scientific (Waltham, MA, USA): goat-anti-mouse Alexa Fluor 594 (#A11032) and goat-anti-rabbit Alexa Fluor 488 (#A11037).

2.8. Enzyme-Linked Immunosorbent Assay (ELISA)

First, 3.5×10^5 cells were transfected as previously described with each ADAM17 variant and the respective substrate (mAREG, mIL-6R or mpro-TNFα). The shed cytokines were determined in the cell-free supernatant by ELISA according to the manufacturer's instructions (mTNFα: #11560637 eBioscience, Frankfurt am Main, Germany; mIL-6R and mAREG: #DY1830 and #DY989, R and D Systems, Minneapolis, MN, USA).

2.9. Live Cell Surface ADAM17 Activity Assay

First, 2×10^6 HEK A10/A17 dKO cells were seeded onto a 10 cm culture dish and transfected the next day. Twenty-four hours after transfection the cells were detached from the culture dish using trypsin and seeded onto a 96-well plate (2×10^5 cells per well). The following day, ADAM17 surface activity was measured by removing the culturing media and supplying the cells with PBS containing 20 µM of a quenched fluorogenic peptide (Abz-LAQAVRSSSR-Dpa; ADAM17 (TACE) substrate IV (Calbiochem, Merck, Darmstadt, Germany; #616407)). The fluorescence (λ_{Ex}: 320 nm; λ_{Em}: 405 nm) was measured every 30 s over a total of 120 min using a Tecan plate reader (Tecan Infinite 200 Pro, TECAN, Männedorf, Switzerland). ADAM17 surface activity was represented by the area under curve (fluorescence over time) and normalized to wt.

2.10. Structural Analysis

The catalytic domain of ADAM17 was visualized based on the crystal structure published by Mazzola et al. (PDB: 3E8R) [29]. Molecular graphics and analyses were performed with UCSF Chimera (version 1.14), developed by the Resource for Biocomputing, Visualization, and Informatics at the University of California, San Francisco, with support from NIH P41-GM103311 [62]. Solvent-excluded molecular surfaces were created with the help of the MSMS package [63].

2.11. Data Analysis and Statistic

All values are expressed as the mean ± SEM. For data analysis Excel (Microsoft, Redmond, WA, USA) and GraphPad Prism version 7 (GraphPad Software, San Diego, CA, USA) were used. Differences among mean values were analyzed by two-tailed, unpaired Student t test or one-way ANOVA, followed by Tukey's multiple comparison test where applicable. In all analyses, the null hypothesis was rejected at $p < 0.05$ with * < 0.05, ** < 0.01, *** < 0.001, **** < 0.0001.

3. Results

3.1. Cloning and Expression of ADAM17 Mutations

We searched the databases IntOGen, COSMIQ, TCGA and ICGC for mutations within the *ADAM17* gene. These databases are listing somatic mutations found in tumor tissue of cancer patients. The search for ADAM17 came up with 175 results of single nucleotide variations (SNVs) within unique cancer tissue samples (Figure S1A). In this study, we focused on missense point mutations identified in colon cancer samples (in total 11 different ADAM17 variants were found; Figure S1B). Interestingly, colon cancer-associated point mutations are distributed over the whole protein, located in following domains: pro-, catalytic-, disintegrin-, membrane proximal and cytoplasmic domain (Figure S1B). Most variants were found within the catalytic and membrane proximal domain (both three different mutations; Figure S1B), underlining the importance of both domains for proper enzymatic function.

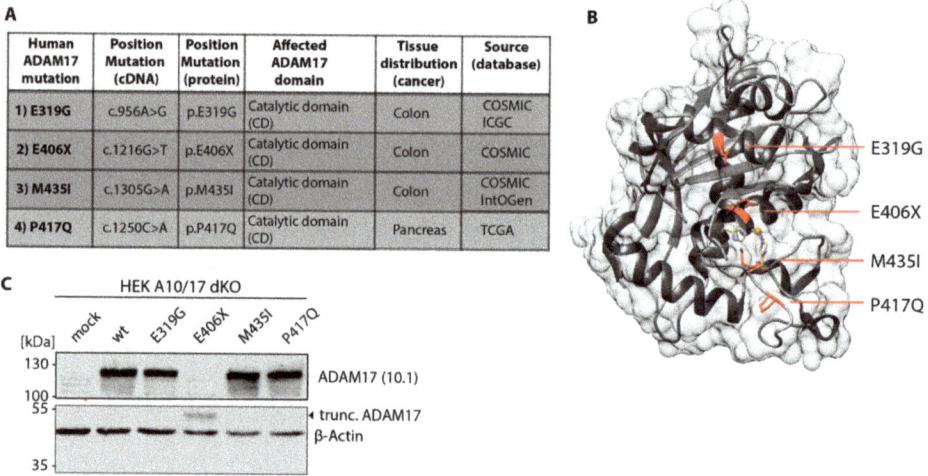

Figure 1. Overview and expression of cancer-associated ADAM17 variants within the catalytic domain. (**A**) Table and description of somatic mutations in human ADAM17 found within tumor tissue of colon and pancreatic cancer patients. Listed is also the position in the cDNA and amino acid sequence as well as the database (COSMIQ, ICGC, IntOGen or TCGA) in which there were found. (**B**) Structural model of catalytic domain (CD) of ADAM17 including mutations highlighted in red (structure derived from PDB: 3E8R). The three histidine residues coordinating the zinc ion in the active center are also highlighted in orange. (**C**) Overexpression of ADAM17 variants in ADAM10/ADAM17 double-deficient HEK cells (HEK A10/A17 dKO). Representative immunoblot showing equal protein levels of ADAM17 wild type (wt) and the ADAM17 variants after overexpression. Only the truncated variant E406X (black arrow, ~50 kDa) exhibits a lower expression level. β-actin was used as a loading control.

We here analyzed four cancer-associated missense mutations located within the catalytic domain of the ADAM17 protein (Figure 1A). First, we focused on the point mutation E319G (c.956A>G; p.E319G) found in tumor tissue of colon cancer patients. The negatively charged glutamic acid at position 319 is replaced by a glycine, which is located in an α-helix offside the active center (Figure 1B). Next, the colon cancer-associated E406X (c.1216G>T; E406X) mutation was studied (Figure 1A). The mutation leads to a premature stop after His405, resulting in a truncated ADAM17 protein lacking the last 422 amino acids, which includes the three histidines that form the active center (Figure 1B). The M435I (c.1305G>A; p.M435I) variant, which was also found in colon cancer samples, was the third mutation analyzed in this study (Figure 1A). Here, the methionine of the Met-turn structure near the active site is replaced by an isoleucine (Figure 1B). Last, the P417Q (c.1250C>T; p.P417Q) variant was examined in this study. Its point mutation is located right next to the histidines (His405, His409 and His415) of the active center and the coordinated zinc ion (Figure 1B). In comparison to the other mutants, this variant was found in pancreatic tumor tissue and was included to this study because of its unique location within the catalytic domain.

All ADAM17 variants were generated by mutagenesis PCR and inserted into a pcDNA3.1 expression plasmid containing the mADAM17 cDNA. Afterwards, ADAM10 and ADAM17 double deficient HEK cells (HEK A10/17 dKO) were reconstituted with the ADAM17 variants and the wild type by transient overexpression. The expression was analyzed via SDS-PAGE and Western blot using an anti-ADAM17 antibody (10.1 antibody) (Figure 1C). The epitope region recognized by this antibody is still intact in the truncated ADAM17 variant E406X, hence this variant can be detected as a smaller protein at ~50 kDa. However, the E406X variant showed decreased protein levels compared to the other analyzed variants and the wild type (Figure 1C). This suggest stable protein expression of the variants E319G, M435I and P417Q, but not E406X. This truncation probably results in an unstable ADAM17 protein, making it prone for degradation processes.

3.2. Proteolytic Activity of Cancer-Associated ADAM17 Variants

Next, we performed functional analyses of the aforementioned ADAM17 variants to study how the inserted point mutations affect the proteolytic activity of the enzyme. To do this, we co-transfected HEK A10/A17 dKO cells with respective ADAM17 variants along with one of the following ADAM17 substrates: pro-TNFα, IL-6 receptor (IL-6R) or amphiregulin (AREG). All of these substrates are shed by ADAM17 and the soluble (s) ectodomain is released into the cell supernatant. We then measured the amount of sTNFα (Figure 2A), sIL-6R (Figure 2B) and sAREG (Figure 2C) in the media utilizing ELISA assays. In addition, we stimulated the cells with the protein kinase C activator PMA (200 nM, 2 h), which is described to increase ADAM17-mediated shedding [36]. For HEK A10/A17 dKO cells transfected with wild type ADAM17, higher levels of sTNFα (Figure 2A), sIL-6R (Figure 2B) and sAREG (Figure 2C) could be measured in comparison to mock transfected cells. Interestingly, PMA treatment only resulted in increased shedding of IL-6R (Figure 2B), and AREG (Figure 2C), but not TNFα (Figure 2A). Equal protein expression of the substrates was verified via SDS-PAGE and Western blot: TNFα (Figure 2D); IL-6R (Figure 2E) and myc-tagged AREG (Figure 2F). All three co-transfected substrates together with the E406X variant showed slightly reduced protein expression (Figure 2D–F). The E406X variant also showed no activity towards any of the analyzed substrates measured by ELISA assay (Figure 2A–C). This was expected since this variant lacks the active center and zinc-binding motif. Interestingly, the variant E319G seemed to be partially active and exhibited shedding activity towards TNFα (Figure 2A) and AREG (Figure 2C). This variant only exhibited partial enzymatic shedding activity towards IL-6R when stimulated with PMA (Figure 2B). The M435I variant presented with significantly decreased enzymatic activity towards IL-6R (Figure 2C) and AREG (Figure 2E) even after PMA stimulation. Only the P417Q variant showed shedding activity towards all here analyzed substrates (TNFα, IL-6R, AREG) at comparable levels as the ADAM17 wild type (Figure 2A–C).

To further study the enzymatic activity of the ADAM17 variants, a live-cell surface activity assay of ADAM17 was performed by utilizing a quenched fluorogenic TNFα peptide. Intriguingly, all three colon cancer-associated mutants (E319G, E406X, M435I) showed diminished enzymatic activity on the cell surface comparable to the mock control, whereas the pancreatic cancer variant P417Q exhibited peptide cleavage even above ADAM17 wild type level (Figure 2G).

Taken together, these results show that the point mutation E319G, E406X and M435I in close proximity to the active center have a negative influence on the shedding activity of ADAM17. In contrast, the variant P417Q seemed to be as active as the wild type.

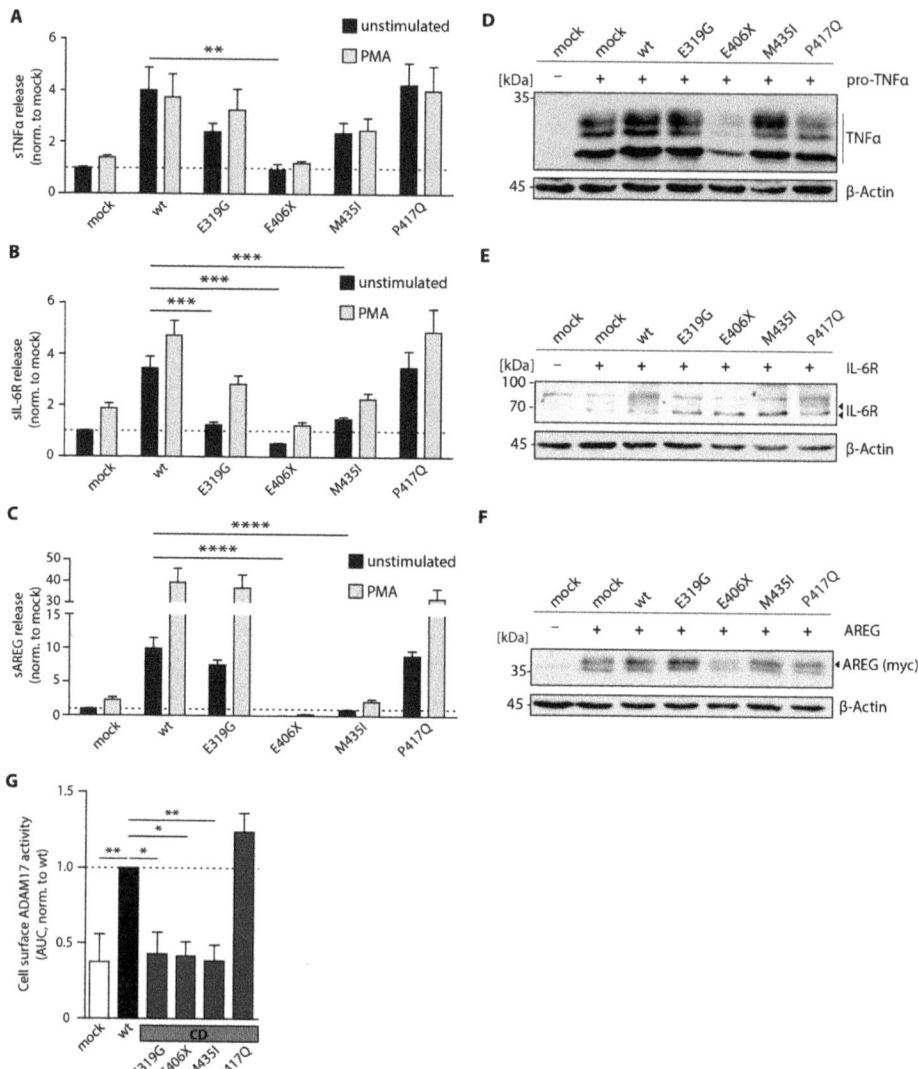

Figure 2. Proteolytic activity of ADAM17 variants. Enzyme-linked Immunosorbent Assay (ELISA) of soluble (s) TNFα (**A**), IL-6R (**B**) and AREG (**C**) measured in cell-free supernatants of HEK A10/17 dKO cells overexpressing ADAM17 wt and ADAM17 variants. Values have been normalized to mock transfected cells. Shown is the summary of three independent experiments statistically analyzed utilizing a one-way ANOVA together with a Tukey's multiple comparison test. *** $p < 0.005$, **** $p < 0.001$. Representative immunoblots show expression of analyzed substrates TNFα (**D**), IL-6R (**E**) und AREG (**F**) in HEK A10/A17 dKO after co-transfection with ADAM17 variants. The here utilized AREG construct exhibits an N-terminal myc-tag, which was used for detection (anti-myc). β-actin was used as a loading control. (**G**) Cell surface activity assay of ADAM17 variants (wt and four mutations within the catalytic domain (CD): E319G, E406X, M435I, P417Q) in living HEK A10/A17 dKO. A quenched fluorogenic TNFα peptide was used and the increase in fluorescence was measured every 30 s for 120 min. Activity was determined as area under curve. Shown are normalized values (to mock) of three independent experiments. The statistical analysis was performed utilizing a one-way-ANOVA together with a Tukey's multiple comparison test. * $p < 0.05$, ** $p < 0.01$, *** $p < 0.001$, **** $p < 0.0001$.

3.3. Cellular Localization of ADAM17 Variants

An impaired trafficking during maturation of the protein within the secretory pathway, for example between endoplasmic reticulum (ER) and cell surface could be an explanation for the decreased ADAM17 shedding activity of the variants E319G, E406X and M435I. Therefore, we performed immunofluorescence (IF) stainings of HEK A10/A17 dKO cells reconstituted with the respective variants (Figure 3A,B). In Figure 3A, ADAM17 (red) was stained using the anti-ADAM17 antibody 10.1. As reference the ER (green) was co-stained using an anti-PDI antibody. The wild type and the variant P417Q co-localized with the ER, but also partly appeared on the cell surface (Figure 3A) and seemed to reach the cell surface to a similar extent. The truncated variant E406X exhibited accumulation within the ER, indicated by a strong co-localization with PDI and the appearance of clumpy ER structures, suggesting impaired trafficking out of the ER. This seems to be also true for the E319G variant (Figure 3A). However, the accumulation of the E319G within ER structures was not as prominent as for the E406X variant. Interestingly, in some cells the M435I showed an excessive amount of ADAM17 outside of the ER (Figure 3A).

For better visualization of ADAM17 on the cell surface, a second immunofluorescence experiment was conducted (Figure 3B), in which HEK A10/A17 dKO cells were co-transfected with a membrane-targeted GFP construct (farnesylated eGFP, green channel) in addition to ADAM17 reconstitution (red). For the wild type, as well as the mutants E319G, M435I and P417Q, ADAM17 signal could be observed at the cell surface (Figure 3B). In comparison, the E406X variant appeared to localize towards the center of the cell with the ADAM17 signal not fully extending to the plasma membrane, further suggesting accumulation in the ER and no cell surface expression.

For quantitative analysis of ADAM17 cell surface transport, a biotinylation and pulldown of cell surface proteins from transfected HEK A10/A17 dKO cells was performed, followed by Western blot analysis (Figure 3C). As a positive control for the pulldown, we stained for the cell surface protein transferrin receptor. A biotin-negative control (- Biotin) was used to show specificity and sensitivity of the analysis (Figure 3C). Moreover, the lysate control confirmed similar input/expression of ADAM17 protein (Figure 3C). Except for the truncated E406X mutant, all here analyzed ADAM17 variants, including the wild type, were detectable at the cell surface. It seems that the E406X is not transported to the cell surface, as already indicated by the IF analysis (Figure 3A,B). This was expected as this variant lacks a transmembrane domain and therefore cannot be anchored to the membrane. To quantify the amount of ADAM17 on the cell surface, the band intensity of each of the biotinylated samples was normalized to the respective lysate control and is expressed relative to the wild type (Figure 3D). The E319G, P417Q and M435I variant showed a similar band intensity to the wild type after normalization, indicating that all three reach the cell surface.

Overall, our data indicate that colon cancer-associated ADAM17 variants (E319G, E406X, M435I) exhibit diminished substrate recognition and/or enzymatic activity towards physiological substrates of the metalloprotease (TNFα, IL-6R, AREG). Although the E319G and M435I variants were found to be localized at cell membrane, they did not show any activity on the cell surface towards a fluorogenic TNFα peptide. This indicates that both point mutations within the catalytic domain do not influence intracellular protein trafficking pathways, but rather affect enzymatic function. Intriguingly, the pancreatic cancer-associated variant P417Q was neither impaired in shedding activity nor in intracellular trafficking, as it was found on the cell membrane and active towards all tested substrates.

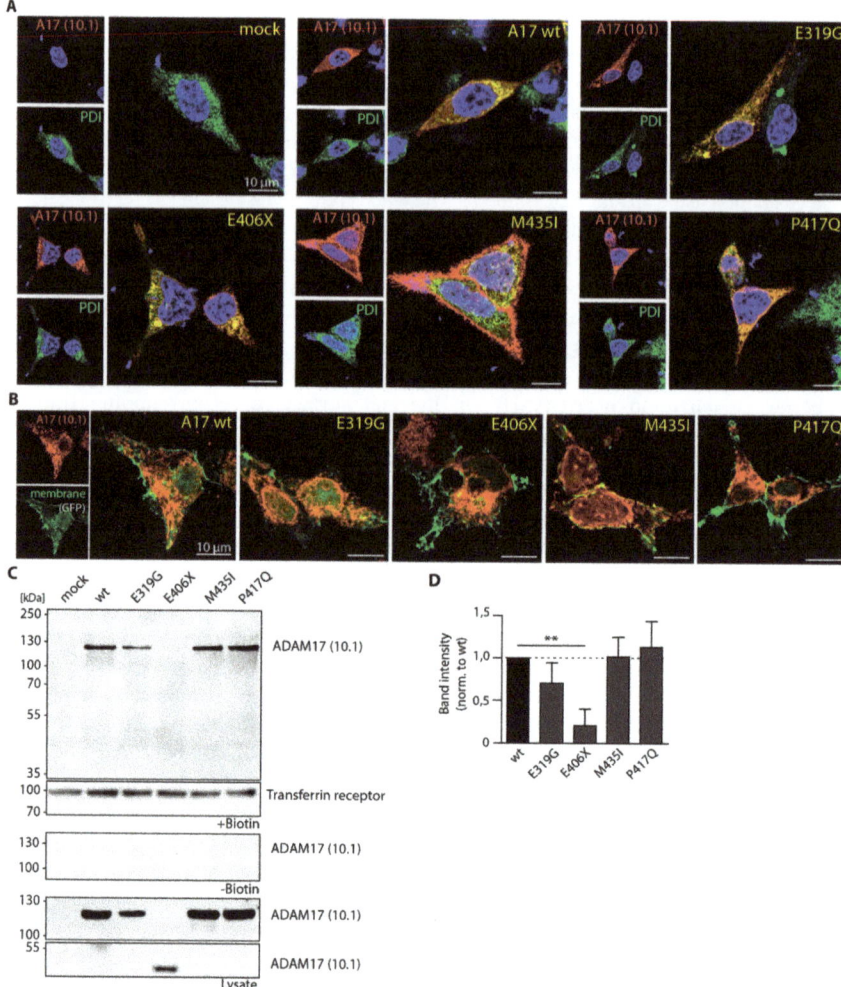

Figure 3. Cellular localization of ADAM17 variants. (**A**) Representative immunofluorescence pictures of HEK A10/A17 dKO cells transfected with the ADAM17 variants (red; antibody: 10.1). As reference, the ER was stained (green) using an anti-PDI antibody. Scale bar: 10 μm. (**B**) Representative immunofluorescence pictures of HEK A10/A17 dKO cells transfected with ADAM17 variants (red; antibody: 10.1), as well as a membrane targeted eGFP construct (green) to visualize ADAM17 on the cell surface. (**C**) Representative immunoblots of biotinylated HEK A10/A17 dKO cells transfected with the ADAM17 variants. The transferrin receptor was used as a control for positive pull-down of cell surface proteins. Also shown are HEK A10/A17 dKO incubated without biotin as a negative control. The lysate control (first and second to last blot) shows the input of the biotinylation assay. (**D**) Quantification of biotinylation. The values shown are derived from three independent experiment and normalized first to expression level in cell lysates and then shown relative to wt. A one-way-ANOVA together with Tukey's multiple comparison test was performed. ** $p < 0.01$.

4. Discussion

Recent in vitro and mouse studies have shown the involvement of ADAM17 in inflammation and cancer pathways [12,43,51–53,64]. The role of ADAM17 in colon cancer is thought to be linked to

ADAM17-mediated shedding of EGF-R activating ligands, as well as IL-6 trans-signaling, which is also promoted by ADAM17 via the shedding of IL-6R [43]. Upregulation of both pathways are hallmarks and high risk factors of colon cancer and their activation is mediated and regulated by ADAM17 [51], underlining its role in pathology.

In this study, we analyzed cancer-associated ADAM17 variants to gain further insight into the role of ADAM17 in disease pathways and the effect of these mutations on the protein. We screened multiple human cancer databases for variants found in tumor tissue of cancer patients [55–60]. Among this dataset, a large percentage (34.9%) of ADAM17 mutations was found in cancer of the gastrointestinal tract. Colon cancer-associated mutations were of especially high incidence, making up 13.1% of the total dataset and 37.7% of the GIT-associated subset. Another large subset of variants was found in lung cancer (10.3%), in which ADAM17 has also been implicated [65]. In this study, we chose four ADAM17 variants located within the catalytic domain for analysis: three were found in colon cancer samples (E319G, E406X, M435I) and one in pancreatic cancer (P417Q), all of them resulting in an amino acid change or the introduction of an early stop codon. We postulated that these mutations would affect ADAM17 activity due to being localized in the catalytic domain of the protein and their proximity to the active site.

Our results show that indeed, overall ADAM17 activity is significantly altered in the E319G, E406X and M435I variants, while the P417Q variant does not differ from the wild type. In case of the E406X and M435I mutation, we observed significantly reduced activity towards all tested substrates (TNFα, IL-6-R, AREG and a fluorogenic peptide). For the M435I variant, the data correspond with the findings of Perez et al. [61], supporting their hypothesis that this variant is impaired in shedding substrates due to the importance of the Met-turn structure for proteolytic activity. Interestingly, we could observe changes in the cellular trafficking of this variant. Although our biotinylation experiments show that the M435I variant still reaches the cell surface, we could observe an intracellular signal of ADAM17 divergent from the wild type. By utilizing immunofluorescence techniques (co-staining with ER marker PDI as well as cell surface GFP construct), the M435I seems to strongly localize around the perimeter of the cell. Since there was no significant difference of ADAM17 protein level on the cell surface after biotinylation in comparison to the wild type, the M435I seems to accumulate in other cell compartments, but outside of ER-structures.

The E406X mutant is a truncated ADAM17 variant, consisting of only the pro-domain and part of the catalytic domain. Due to the truncation, this variant is lacking the zinc binding motif, as well as all downstream domains including the transmembrane domain. To no surprise, this variant showed a complete lack of proteolytic activity towards all tested substrates. The lack of its transmembrane domain led to impaired intracellular transport and absence of cell surface expression. Immunofluorescence data suggest that this variant was mostly ER-localized. In co-expression analyses, where E406X was transfected together with a substrate, we could consistently observe lower expression levels of the co-transfected substrates (TNFα, IL-6-R, AREG). It seems that in the context of overexpression, this variant influences overall protein expression, which could be explained by its accumulation inside the ER and a potential activation of protein degradation pathways, like for example the ERAD pathway [66].

Interestingly, the ADAM17 E319G variant exhibited intriguing results. Although showing significantly impaired activity towards TNFα, IL-6R and the TNFα-derived fluorogenic peptide, this variant was fully capable of shedding AREG. This indicates that the mutation does not directly affect catalytic activity, but rather substrate recognition and specificity, leading to selective inactivity towards certain substrates. Cellular localization of this variant is comparable to the wild type, although we observed a slight, non-significant decrease in surface localization and increase in ER co-localization compared to the wild type. In all conducted experiments, the pancreatic cancer-associated variant P417Q was indistinguishable from the wild type protein. Even though the amino acid change (position 417) is adjacent to the zinc binding motif (405–416), the change from proline to glutamine appears to have no significant effect on the enzymatic function in our experimental context.

Altogether, the colon cancer-associated ADAM17 mutations analyzed in this study either negatively affected shedding ability and/or intracellular trafficking. These findings are contradictory to the current dogma about the relationship between ADAM17 and cancer, in which an activation and upregulation of ADAM17 is thought to promote tumor development via EGF-R activation and IL-6 trans-signaling [41,43,51,52]. For the variants characterized in this study, their specific role in the development of cancer remains unclear. Most notably, no detailed information about the patient, its symptoms or the genetic background was available. Therefore, no statement can be made about whether these mutations are actually driver mutations and actively promote tumor development, or are rather passenger mutations that occurred by chance along other more detrimental mutations. It is, however, notable that almost all cancer-associated ADAM17 mutations analyzed in this study, as well as in our previous study [14], seem to have a negative effect of proteolytic activity in some way. It remains unknown whether this downregulation of ADAM17 activity can positively influence the development and progression of CRC. It is known that in the hypomorphic ADAM17$^{ex/ex}$ mouse model, regeneration of the intestinal epithelium is severely compromised due to reduced EGF-R signaling, leading to significantly higher and more prolonged inflammation in a DSS-induced colitis model [12]. Since chronic inflammation is one of highest risk factors for developing CRC, further studies investigating the role of ADAM17 downregulation in intestinal regeneration and chronic inflammation, utilizing suitable animal models and more physiological experimental approaches, might shed more light on the complex role of ADAM17 in cancer pathology. Moreover, a better understanding of ADAM17 (dys)function within the development and progression of this devastating disease might reveal novel possible approaches for treatment and prevention.

Supplementary Materials: Supplementary materials can be found at http://www.mdpi.com/2227-9059/8/11/463/s1.

Author Contributions: Conceptualization, F.Z.; Experiments, J.P.D., A.-S.C., E.P., F.Z.; Data Analysis, J.P.D., A.-S.C., P.A. and F.Z.; Writing—Original Draft Preparation, J.P.D., A.-S.C. and F.Z.; Writing—Review and Editing, J.P.D., F.Z.; Visualization, J.P.D., P.A., F.Z.; Supervision, F.Z.; Funding Acquisition, S.R.-J., P.A. and F.Z. All authors have read and agreed to the published version of the manuscript.

Funding: This research was funded by the Deutsche Forschungsgemeinschaft (DFG, German Research Foundation), grant number 125440785—SFB 877 (project A1 to S.R.-J., A13 to P.A. and B11 to F.Z.).

Acknowledgments: We thank Melanie Boss and Dwayne Götze for excellent technical assistance. Further, we thank Jörn Rabe for kindly providing the HEK A10/A17 dKO cells. The farnesylated eGFP construct used for membrane staining in immunofluorescence was made and kindly provided to us by Bernd Schröder and Torben Mentrup (both Institute of Physiological Chemistry, TU Dresden). The results shown here are in part based upon data generated by the TCGA Research Network: https://www.cancer.gov/tcga. We thank the "Colon Adenocarcinoma" (COAD-US) project of the ICGC and TCGA and all associated investigators.

Conflicts of Interest: The authors declare no conflict of interest with the contents of this article.

Abbreviations

ADAM17	A Disintegrin and Metalloproteinase 17
AREG	Amphiregulin
CD	catalytic domain
CRC	colorectal cancer
dKO	double knock-out
EGF-R	epidermal growth factor receptor
ELISA	Enzyme-Linked Immunosorbent Assay
ER	endoplasmatic reticulum
HEK	human embryonic kidney cells
IL-6R	interleukin-6 receptor
kDa	kilo Dalton
m	murine
PDI	protein disulfide isomerase
PMA	phorbol 12-myristate 13-acetate
sTNFα	soluble tumor necrosis factor alpha
wt	wild type

References

1. Cancer Facts & Figures 2019. Available online: https://www.cancer.org/research/cancer-facts-statistics/all-cancer-facts-figures/cancer-facts-figures-2019.html (accessed on 23 March 2020).
2. Johnson, C.M.; Wei, C.; Ensor, J.E.; Smolenski, D.J.; Amos, C.I.; Levin, B.; Berry, D.A. Meta-analyses of colorectal cancer risk factors. *Cancer Causes Control* **2013**, *24*, 1207–1222. [CrossRef] [PubMed]
3. Terzic, J.; Grivennikov, S.; Karin, E.; Karin, M. Inflammation and colon cancer. *Gastroenterology* **2010**, *138*, 2101–2114.e2105. [CrossRef] [PubMed]
4. Ponder, A.; Long, M.D. A clinical review of recent findings in the epidemiology of inflammatory bowel disease. *Clin. Epidemiol.* **2013**, *5*, 237–247. [CrossRef] [PubMed]
5. Ye, Y.; Pang, Z.; Chen, W.; Ju, S.; Zhou, C. The epidemiology and risk factors of inflammatory bowel disease. *Int. J. Clin. Exp. Med.* **2015**, *8*, 22529–22542. [PubMed]
6. Amre, D.K.; D'Souza, S.; Morgan, K.; Seidman, G.; Lambrette, P.; Grimard, G.; Israel, D.; Mack, D.; Ghadirian, P.; Deslandres, C.; et al. Imbalances in dietary consumption of fatty acids, vegetables, and fruits are associated with risk for Crohn's disease in children. *Am. J. Gastroenterol.* **2007**, *102*, 2016–2025. [CrossRef] [PubMed]
7. Christ, A.; Lauterbach, M.; Latz, E. Western Diet and the Immune System: An Inflammatory Connection. *Immunity* **2019**, *51*, 794–811. [CrossRef]
8. O'Neill, A.M.; Burrington, C.M.; Gillaspie, E.A.; Lynch, D.T.; Horsman, M.J.; Greene, M.W. High-fat Western diet-induced obesity contributes to increased tumor growth in mouse models of human colon cancer. *Nutr. Res.* **2016**, *36*, 1325–1334. [CrossRef]
9. Black, R.A.; Rauch, C.T.; Kozlosky, C.J.; Peschon, J.J.; Slack, J.L.; Wolfson, M.F.; Castner, B.J.; Stocking, K.L.; Reddy, P.; Srinivasan, S.; et al. A metalloproteinase disintegrin that releases tumour-necrosis factor-alpha from cells. *Nature* **1997**, *385*, 729–733. [CrossRef]
10. Zunke, F.; Rose-John, S. The shedding protease ADAM17: Physiology and pathophysiology. *Biochim. Biophys Acta Mol. Cell Res.* **2017**, *1864*, 2059–2070. [CrossRef]
11. Peschon, J.J.; Slack, J.L.; Reddy, P.; Stocking, K.L.; Sunnarborg, S.W.; Lee, D.C.; Russell, W.E.; Castner, B.J.; Johnson, R.S.; Fitzner, J.N.; et al. An essential role for ectodomain shedding in mammalian development. *Science* **1998**, *282*, 1281–1284. [CrossRef]
12. Chalaris, A.; Adam, N.; Sina, C.; Rosenstiel, P.; Lehmann-Koch, J.; Schirmacher, P.; Hartmann, D.; Cichy, J.; Gavrilova, O.; Schreiber, S.; et al. Critical role of the disintegrin metalloprotease ADAM17 for intestinal inflammation and regeneration in mice. *J. Exp. Med.* **2010**, *207*, 1617–1624. [CrossRef]
13. Gooz, M. ADAM-17: the enzyme that does it all. *Crit. Rev. Biochem. Mol. Biol.* **2010**, *45*, 146–169. [CrossRef]
14. Pavlenko, E.; Cabron, A.-S.; Arnold, P.; Dobert, J.; Rose-John, S.; Zunke, F. Functional Characterization of Colon Cancer-Associated Mutations in ADAM17: Modifications in the Pro-Domain Interfere with Trafficking and Maturation. *Int. J. Mol. Sci.* **2019**, *20*, 2198. [CrossRef] [PubMed]
15. Düsterhöft, S.; Michalek, M.; Kordowski, F.; Oldefest, M.; Sommer, A.; Röseler, J.; Reiss, K.; Grötzinger, J.; Lorenzen, I. Extracellular Juxtamembrane Segment of ADAM17 Interacts with Membranes and Is Essential for Its Shedding Activity. *Biochemistry* **2015**, *54*, 5791–5801. [CrossRef] [PubMed]
16. Peiretti, F.; Canault, M.; Deprez-Beauclair, P.; Berthet, V.; Bonardo, B.; Juhan-Vague, I.; Nalbone, G. Intracellular maturation and transport of tumor necrosis factor alpha converting enzyme. *Exp. Cell Res.* **2003**, *285*, 278–285. [CrossRef]
17. Soond, S.M.; Everson, B.; Riches, D.W.; Murphy, G. ERK-mediated phosphorylation of Thr735 in TNFalpha-converting enzyme and its potential role in TACE protein trafficking. *J. Cell Sci.* **2005**, *118*, 2371–2380. [CrossRef]
18. Schwarz, J.; Schmidt, S.; Will, O.; Koudelka, T.; Kohler, K.; Boss, M.; Rabe, B.; Tholey, A.; Scheller, J.; Schmidt-Arras, D.; et al. Polo-like kinase 2, a novel ADAM17 signaling component, regulates tumor necrosis factor alpha ectodomain shedding. *J. Biol. Chem.* **2014**, *289*, 3080–3093. [CrossRef] [PubMed]
19. Xu, P.; Derynck, R. Direct activation of TACE-mediated ectodomain shedding by p38 MAP kinase regulates EGF receptor-dependent cell proliferation. *Mol. Cell* **2010**, *37*, 551–566. [CrossRef]
20. Diaz-Rodriguez, E.; Montero, J.C.; Esparis-Ogando, A.; Yuste, L.; Pandiella, A. Extracellular signal-regulated kinase phosphorylates tumor necrosis factor alpha-converting enzyme at threonine 735: A potential role in regulated shedding. *Mol. Biol. Cell* **2002**, *13*, 2031–2044. [CrossRef]

21. Lorenzen, I.; Lokau, J.; Korpys, Y.; Oldefest, M.; Flynn, C.M.; Künzel, U.; Garbers, C.; Freeman, M.; Grötzinger, J.; Düsterhöft, S. Control of ADAM17 activity by regulation of its cellular localisation. *Sci. Rep.* **2016**, *6*, 35067. [CrossRef]
22. Tellier, E.; Canault, M.; Rebsomen, L.; Bonardo, B.; Juhan-Vague, I.; Nalbone, G.; Peiretti, F. The shedding activity of ADAM17 is sequestered in lipid rafts. *Exp. Cell Res.* **2006**, *312*, 3969–3980. [CrossRef]
23. Düsterhöft, S.; Jung, S.; Hung, C.W.; Tholey, A.; Sönnichsen, F.D.; Grötzinger, J.; Lorenzen, I. Membrane-proximal domain of a disintegrin and metalloprotease-17 represents the putative molecular switch of its shedding activity operated by protein-disulfide isomerase. *J. Am. Chem. Soc.* **2013**, *135*, 5776–5781. [CrossRef] [PubMed]
24. Adrain, C.; Zettl, M.; Christova, Y.; Taylor, N.; Freeman, M. Tumor Necrosis Factor Signaling Requires iRhom2 to Promote Trafficking and Activation of TACE. *Science* **2012**, *335*, 225. [CrossRef] [PubMed]
25. Düsterhöft, S.; Babendreyer, A.; Giese, A.A.; Flasshove, C.; Ludwig, A. Status update on iRhom and ADAM17: It's still complicated. *Biochim Biophys Acta Mol. Cell Res.* **2019**, *1866*, 1567–1583. [CrossRef]
26. McIlwain, D.R.; Lang, P.A.; Maretzky, T.; Hamada, K.; Ohishi, K.; Maney, S.K.; Berger, T.; Murthy, A.; Duncan, G.; Xu, H.C.; et al. iRhom2 Regulation of TACE Controls TNF-Mediated Protection Against *Listeria* and Responses to LPS. *Science* **2012**, *335*, 229. [CrossRef] [PubMed]
27. Tang, B.; Li, X.; Maretzky, T.; Perez-Aguilar, J.M.; McIlwain, D.; Xie, Y.; Zheng, Y.; Mak, T.W.; Weinstein, H.; Blobel, C.P. Substrate-selective protein ectodomain shedding by ADAM17 and iRhom2 depends on their juxtamembrane and transmembrane domains. *FASEB J.* **2020**, *34*, 4956–4969. [CrossRef]
28. Gonzales, P.E.; Solomon, A.; Miller, A.B.; Leesnitzer, M.A.; Sagi, I.; Milla, M.E. Inhibition of the tumor necrosis factor-alpha-converting enzyme by its pro domain. *J. Biol. Chem.* **2004**, *279*, 31638–31645. [CrossRef]
29. Mazzola, R.D., Jr.; Zhu, Z.; Sinning, L.; McKittrick, B.; Lavey, B.; Spitler, J.; Kozlowski, J.; Neng-Yang, S.; Zhou, G.; Guo, Z.; et al. Discovery of novel hydroxamates as highly potent tumor necrosis factor-alpha converting enzyme inhibitors. Part II: optimization of the S3' pocket. *Bioorg. Med. Chem. Lett.* **2008**, *18*, 5809–5814. [CrossRef]
30. Birkedal-Hansen, H. Role of cytokines and inflammatory mediators in tissue destruction. *J. Periodontal Res.* **1993**, *28*, 500–510. [CrossRef]
31. Papadakis, K.A.; Targan, S.R. Role of Cytokines in the Pathogenesis of Inflammatory Bowel Disease. *Annu. Rev. Med.* **2000**, *51*, 289–298. [CrossRef]
32. Garton, K.J.; Gough, P.J.; Blobel, C.P.; Murphy, G.; Greaves, D.R.; Dempsey, P.J.; Raines, E.W. Tumor Necrosis Factor-α-converting Enzyme (ADAM17) Mediates the Cleavage and Shedding of Fractalkine (CX3CL1). *J. Biol. Chem.* **2001**, *276*, 37993–38001. [PubMed]
33. Garton, K.J.; Gough, P.J.; Philalay, J.; Wille, P.T.; Blobel, C.P.; Whitehead, R.H.; Dempsey, P.J.; Raines, E.W. Stimulated shedding of vascular cell adhesion molecule 1 (VCAM-1) is mediated by tumor necrosis factor-alpha-converting enzyme (ADAM 17). *J. Biol. Chem.* **2003**, *278*, 37459–37464. [CrossRef] [PubMed]
34. Tsakadze, N.L.; Sithu, S.D.; Sen, U.; English, W.R.; Murphy, G.; D'Souza, S.E. Tumor Necrosis Factor-α-converting Enzyme (TACE/ADAM-17) Mediates the Ectodomain Cleavage of Intercellular Adhesion Molecule-1 (ICAM-1). *J. Biol. Chem.* **2006**, *281*, 3157–3164. [CrossRef] [PubMed]
35. Lisi, S.; D'Amore, M.; Sisto, M. ADAM17 at the interface between inflammation and autoimmunity. *Immunol. Lett.* **2014**, *162*, 159–169. [CrossRef] [PubMed]
36. Müllberg, J.; Schooltink, H.; Stoyan, T.; Günther, M.; Graeve, L.; Buse, G.; Mackiewicz, A.; Heinrich, P.C.; Rose-John, S. The soluble interleukin-6 receptor is generated by shedding. *Eur. J. Immunol.* **1993**, *23*, 473–480. [CrossRef]
37. Wolf, J.; Rose-John, S.; Garbers, C. Interleukin-6 and its receptors: A highly regulated and dynamic system. *Cytokine* **2014**, *70*, 11–20. [CrossRef]
38. Scheller, J.; Chalaris, A.; Schmidt-Arras, D.; Rose-John, S. The pro- and anti-inflammatory properties of the cytokine interleukin-6. *Biochim. Biophys. Acta (BBA) Mol. Cell Res.* **2011**, *1813*, 878–888. [CrossRef]
39. Heinrich, P.C.; Behrmann, I.; MÜLler-Newen, G.; Schaper, F.; Graeve, L. Interleukin-6-type cytokine signalling through the gp130/Jak/STAT pathway1. *Biochem. J.* **1998**, *334*, 297–314. [CrossRef]
40. Rose-John, S.; Heinrich, P.C. Soluble receptors for cytokines and growth factors: generation and biological function. *Biochem. J.* **1994**, *300 (Pt. 2)*, 281–290. [CrossRef]
41. Chalaris, A.; Garbers, C.; Rabe, B.; Rose-John, S.; Scheller, J. The soluble Interleukin 6 receptor: Generation and role in inflammation and cancer. *Eur. J. Cell Biol.* **2011**, *90*, 484–494. [CrossRef]

42. Rose-John, S. IL-6 Trans-Signaling via the Soluble IL-6 Receptor: Importance for the Pro-Inflammatory Activities of IL-6. *Int. J. Biol. Sci.* **2012**, *8*, 1237–1247. [CrossRef] [PubMed]
43. Schumacher, N.; Rose-John, S. ADAM17 Activity and IL-6 Trans-Signaling in Inflammation and Cancer. *Cancers* **2019**, *11*, 1736. [CrossRef]
44. Blobel, C.P. ADAMs: key components in EGFR signalling and development. *Nat. Rev. Mol. Cell. Biol.* **2005**, *6*, 32–43. [CrossRef]
45. Sibilia, M.; Kroismayr, R.; Lichtenberger, B.M.; Natarajan, A.; Hecking, M.; Holcmann, M. The epidermal growth factor receptor: from development to tumorigenesis. *Differentiation* **2007**, *75*, 770–787. [CrossRef]
46. Al Moustafa, A.E.; Achkhar, A.; Yasmeen, A. EGF-receptor signaling and epithelial-mesenchymal transition in human carcinomas. *Front. Biosci (Sch. Ed.)* **2012**, *4*, 671–684. [CrossRef] [PubMed]
47. Adriano, A.; Giovanni Luca, G.; Nadia, R.; Danilo, M.; Claudio, F.; Paola, M.; Anna, T.; Carlo, V.; Mauro, B. Suppression of EGF-R signaling reduces the incidence of prostate cancer metastasis in nude mice. *Endocr. -Relat. Cancer Endocr. Relat. Cancer* **2006**, *13*, 197–210. [CrossRef]
48. Malecka-Panas, E.; Kordek, R.; Biernat, W.; Tureaud, J.; Liberski, P.P.; Majumdar, A.P. Differential activation of total and EGF receptor (EGF-R) tyrosine kinase (tyr-k) in the rectal mucosa in patients with adenomatous polyps, ulcerative colitis and colon cancer. *Hepatogastroenterology* **1997**, *44*, 435–440. [CrossRef]
49. Berasain, C.; Castillo, J.; Prieto, J.; Avila, M.A. New molecular targets for hepatocellular carcinoma: the ErbB1 signaling system. *Liver Int.* **2007**, *27*, 174–185. [CrossRef]
50. Blanchot-Jossic, F.; Jarry, A.; Masson, D.; Bach-Ngohou, K.; Paineau, J.; Denis, M.G.; Laboisse, C.L.; Mosnier, J.F. Up-regulated expression of ADAM17 in human colon carcinoma: co-expression with EGFR in neoplastic and endothelial cells. *J. Pathol.* **2005**, *207*, 156–163. [CrossRef]
51. Schmidt, S.; Schumacher, N.; Schwarz, J.; Tangermann, S.; Kenner, L.; Schlederer, M.; Sibilia, M.; Linder, M.; Altendorf-Hofmann, A.; Knosel, T.; et al. ADAM17 is required for EGF-R-induced intestinal tumors via IL-6 trans-signaling. *J. Exp. Med.* **2018**, *215*, 1205–1225. [CrossRef] [PubMed]
52. Becker, C.; Fantini, M.C.; Wirtz, S.; Nikolaev, A.; Lehr, H.A.; Galle, P.R.; Rose-John, S.; Neurath, M.F. IL-6 signaling promotes tumor growth in colorectal cancer. *Cell Cycle* **2005**, *4*, 217–220. [CrossRef] [PubMed]
53. Matsumoto, S.; Hara, T.; Mitsuyama, K.; Yamamoto, M.; Tsuruta, O.; Sata, M.; Scheller, J.; Rose-John, S.; Kado, S.-i.; Takada, T. Essential Roles of IL-6 Trans-Signaling in Colonic Epithelial Cells, Induced by the IL-6/Soluble–IL-6 Receptor Derived from Lamina Propria Macrophages, on the Development of Colitis-Associated Premalignant Cancer in a Murine Model. *J. Immunol.* **2010**, *184*, 1543–1551. [CrossRef] [PubMed]
54. Srivatsa, S.; Paul, M.C.; Cardone, C.; Holcmann, M.; Amberg, N.; Pathria, P.; Diamanti, M.A.; Linder, M.; Timelthaler, G.; Dienes, H.P.; et al. EGFR in Tumor-Associated Myeloid Cells Promotes Development of Colorectal Cancer in Mice and Associates With Outcomes of Patients. *Gastroenterology* **2017**, *153*, 178–190.e110. [CrossRef] [PubMed]
55. Catalogue of Somatic Mutations in Cancer (COSMIC). Available online: cancer.sanger.ac.uk (accessed on 27 February 2017).
56. Tate, J.G.; Bamford, S.; Jubb, H.C.; Sondka, Z.; Beare, D.M.; Bindal, N.; Boutselakis, H.; Cole, C.G.; Creatore, C.; Dawson, E.; et al. COSMIC: the Catalogue Of Somatic Mutations In Cancer. *Nucleic Acids Res.* **2018**, *47*, D941–D947. [CrossRef]
57. Integrative OncoGenomics (IntOGen). Available online: www.intogen.org (accessed on 27 February 2017).
58. Gonzalez-Perez, A.; Perez-Llamas, C.; Deu-Pons, J.; Tamborero, D.; Schroeder, M.P.; Jene-Sanz, A.; Santos, A.; Lopez-Bigas, N. IntOGen-mutations identifies cancer drivers across tumor types. *Nat. Methods* **2013**, *10*, 1081–1082. [CrossRef] [PubMed]
59. The Cancer Genome Atlas Program (TCGA). Available online: https://www.cancer.gov/tcga (accessed on 27 February 2017).
60. International Cancer Genome, C.; Hudson, T.J.; Anderson, W.; Artez, A.; Barker, A.D.; Bell, C.; Bernabé, R.R.; Bhan, M.K.; Calvo, F.; Eerola, I.; et al. International network of cancer genome projects. *Nature* **2010**, *464*, 993–998. [CrossRef]
61. Pérez, L.; Kerrigan, J.E.; Li, X.; Fan, H. Substitution of methionine 435 with leucine, isoleucine, and serine in tumor necrosis factor alpha converting enzyme inactivates ectodomain shedding activity. *Biochem. Cell. Biol.* **2007**, *85*, 141–149. [CrossRef]

62. Pettersen, E.F.; Goddard, T.D.; Huang, C.C.; Couch, G.S.; Greenblatt, D.M.; Meng, E.C.; Ferrin, T.E. UCSF Chimera—A visualization system for exploratory research and analysis. *J. Comput. Chem.* **2004**, *25*, 1605–1612. [CrossRef]
63. Sanner, M.F.; Olson, A.J.; Spehner, J.C. Reduced surface: an efficient way to compute molecular surfaces. *Biopolymers* **1996**, *38*, 305–320. [CrossRef]
64. Cabron, A.-S.; El Azzouzi, K.; Boss, M.; Arnold, P.; Schwarz, J.; Rosas, M.; Dobert, J.P.; Pavlenko, E.; Schumacher, N.; Renné, T.; et al. Structural and Functional Analyses of the Shedding Protease ADAM17 in HoxB8-Immortalized Macrophages and Dendritic-like Cells. *J. Immunol.* **2018**, *201*, 3106–3118. [CrossRef]
65. Saad, M.I.; Rose-John, S.; Jenkins, B.J. ADAM17: An Emerging Therapeutic Target for Lung Cancer. *Cancers* **2019**, *11*, 1218. [CrossRef] [PubMed]
66. Hoseki, J.; Ushioda, R.; Nagata, K. Mechanism and components of endoplasmic reticulum-associated degradation. *J. Biochem.* **2009**, *147*, 19–25. [CrossRef] [PubMed]

Publisher's Note: MDPI stays neutral with regard to jurisdictional claims in published maps and institutional affiliations.

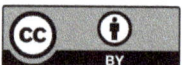

© 2020 by the authors. Licensee MDPI, Basel, Switzerland. This article is an open access article distributed under the terms and conditions of the Creative Commons Attribution (CC BY) license (http://creativecommons.org/licenses/by/4.0/).

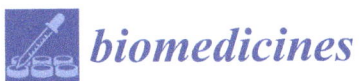

Review

The Liquid Biopsy in the Management of Colorectal Cancer: An Overview

Marco Vacante *, Roberto Ciuni, Francesco Basile and Antonio Biondi

Department of General Surgery and Medical-Surgical Specialties, University of Catania, Via S. Sofia 78, 95123 Catania, Italy; ciuni.r@gmail.com (R.C.); fbasile@unict.it (F.B.); abiondi@unict.it (A.B.)
* Correspondence: marcovacante@yahoo.it

Received: 4 August 2020; Accepted: 24 August 2020; Published: 26 August 2020

Abstract: Currently, there is a crucial need for novel diagnostic and prognostic biomarkers with high specificity and sensitivity in patients with colorectal cancer. A "liquid biopsy" is characterized by the isolation of cancer-derived components, such as circulating tumor cells, circulating tumor DNA, microRNAs, long non-coding RNAs, and proteins, from peripheral blood or other body fluids and their genomic or proteomic assessment. The liquid biopsy is a minimally invasive and repeatable technique that could play a significant role in screening and diagnosis, and predict relapse and metastasis, as well as monitoring minimal residual disease and chemotherapy resistance in colorectal cancer patients. However, there are still some practical issues that need to be addressed before liquid biopsy can be widely used in clinical practice. Potential challenges may include low amounts of circulating tumor cells and circulating tumor DNA in samples, lack of pre-analytical and analytical consensus, clinical validation, and regulatory endorsement. The aim of this review was to summarize the current knowledge of the role of liquid biopsy in the management of colorectal cancer.

Keywords: liquid biopsy; colorectal cancer; biomarkers; circulating tumor cells; circulating tumor DNA

1. Introduction

Colorectal cancer (CRC) is one of the most common solid cancers in developed countries, with approximately 1.8 million incident cases and 900,000 deaths every year worldwide [1,2]. The burden of CRC is growing in the majority of low- and middle-income countries, probably due to environmental risk factors, such as changes in diet and life-style (i.e., obesity, smoking, alcohol consumption, and suboptimal dietary habits) [3], aging, and urbanization [4,5]. According to the American Cancer Society (ACS), the 5-year survival rate ranges from 90% if CRC is diagnosed at a localized stage to 14% in patients presenting with metastatic disease [6]. Treatment decisions for CRC should take into account the stage of the disease, the general condition, and performance status of the patient, and the molecular characteristics of the tumor [7,8]. The diagnosis of CRC is frequently made using colonoscopy, and confirmed by histological examination of the tumor tissue biopsy. The TNM staging of CRC is based on the depth of invasion of the primary tumor, regional lymph node involvement, and distant metastases, which may contribute to the choice of the most appropriate therapeutic approach, including adjuvant chemotherapy [9]. Surgical resection with lymph node dissection represents the base of curative treatment for localized colon cancer. Patients with stage III colon cancer are treated with adjuvant therapy using the FOLFOX (leucovorin, 5-fluorouracil and oxaliplatin) regimen; however more data are needed to confirm the efficacy of such treatment for rectal cancer patients. Combination of doublet or triplet chemotherapy (i.e., 5-fluorouracil/leucovorin, capecitabine, oxaliplatin, irinotecan) and a targeted agent (i.e., cetuximab, bevacizumab, panitumumab) are routinely used for the treatment of metastatic CRC [10,11]. Histopathological tumor tissue analysis cannot be considered to be a reliable source of clinically helpful prognostic or predictive information for

CRC at the individual patient's level; thus, research is constantly moving towards the identification of more accurate and personalized biomarkers [12]. Indeed, there is a critical need for new diagnostic and prognostic biomarkers with high specificity and sensitivity in patients with CRC [13,14]. In this context, liquid biopsy could represent the new era for biomarkers detection: the term "liquid biopsy" refers to the isolation of cancer-derived components, such as circulating tumor cells (CTC), circulating tumor DNA (ctDNA), microRNAs (miRNAs), long non-coding RNAs (lncRNAs) and proteins, from peripheral blood or other body fluids (i.e., ascites, urine, pleural effusion, and cerebrospinal fluid), and their genomic or proteomic assessment [15,16]. Furthermore, exosomes (EXOs) which are membrane-bound extracellular vesicles containing proteins and nucleic acids released in the bloodstream by cancer cells, could represent potential biomarkers [17,18]. The aim of this review was to summarize the current knowledge of the role of liquid biopsy in the management of CRC.

2. Clinical Utility of Liquid Biopsies in Patients with Colorectal Cancer

Assessment of peripheral blood components, such as CTCs, ctDNA, miRNAs, and lncRNAs could improve CRC screening and diagnosis, and predict relapse and metastasis [19–22]. Blood-based liquid biopsies could also be effective in monitoring minimal residual disease (MRD) and drug resistance in CRC patients receiving chemotherapy [23,24] (Table 1).

Table 1. Potential clinical applications of liquid biopsy biomarkers in CRC.

Study (Year)	Biomarkers	Sample Size	Methods	Statistical Significance (p Value), Sensitivity/Specificity (%) and/or Hazard Ratio	Potential Clinical Applications
Tsai et al. (2018) [25]	CTC	$n = 620$ ($n = 438$ adenoma, polyps, or stage I–IV CRC, $n = 182$ healthy controls).	CellMax biomimetic platform (CMx)	All subjects: Sn 84.0/Sp 97.3 Precancerous lesions: Sn 76.6/Sp 97.3 CRC: Sn 86.9/Sp 97.3	Screening
Bork et al. (2015) [26]	CTC	Total $n = 287$ ($n = 239$ stage I–III CRC)	CellSearch	OS: HR 5.5 (95% CI 2.3–13.6, $p < 0.001$) PFS: HR 12.7 (95% CI 5.2–31.1, $p < 0.001$)	Prognostic in non-mCRC
Gazzaniga et al. (2013) [27]	CTC	$n = 37$ high-risk stage II or III CRC	CellSearch	The presence of CTC was detected in 8 of 37 patients (22%) 87.5% of CTC-positive patients had N1–2 disease and stage III CRC	Selection of high-risk stage II CRC patient candidates for adjuvant chemotherapy
Tsai et al. (2016) [28]	CTC	$n = 158$ ($n = 27$ healthy, $n = 21$ benign, $n = 95$ non-mCRC, $n = 15$ m-CRC)	CellMax biomimetic platform (CMx)	CRC: Sn 63.0/Sp 82.0 All colorectal neoplasms, including adenomatous polyps, dysplastic polyps, and CRC: Sn 61.0/Sp 94.0	Prognostic in non-mCRC at high risk of early recurrence
Musella et al. (2015) [29]	CTC	$n = 38$ advanced RAS-BRAF-wild-type CRC receiving third-line therapy with cetuximab-irinotecan or panitumumab.	AdnaTest ColonCancerSelect	OS: HR 8.06 (95% CI, 2.54–25.59, $p < 0.001$) PFS: HR 6.10 (95% CI, 2.49–14.96, $p < 0.001$)	Prognostic and predictive in CRC patients treated with anti-EGFR monoclonal antibodies
Krebs et al. (2014) [30]	CTC	$n = 48$ (CTC enumeration performed only in 42 patients)	CellSearch	ORR: 71% Median OS for high and low CTC count: 18.7 and 22.3 months (log-rank test, $p < 0.038$)	Prognostic in CRC patients treated with irinotecan, oxaliplatin, and tegafur-uracil with leucovorin and cetuximab
Tie et al. (2016) [31]	ctDNA	$n = 230$ resected stage II colon cancer	Safe-SeqS	Postoperative recurrence at 36 months: Sn 48.0/Sp 100.0	Monitoring of MRD and identification of CRC patients at very high risk of recurrence

Table 1. Cont.

Study (Year)	Biomarkers	Sample Size	Methods	Statistical Significance (p Value), Sensitivity/Specificity (%) and/or Hazard Ratio	Potential Clinical Applications
Sun et al. (2018) [32]	ctDNA	$n = 11$ CRC treated surgically	NGS	$n = 7$: decreased mutation rates in postoperative vs. preoperative period $n = 4$: no mutations $n = 1$ patient with metastatic rectal cancer: the rate of TP53 mutation increased from 8.95 (preoperative) to 71.4% (postoperative)	Prognostic and Predictive
Tie et al. (2015) [33]	ctDNA	$n = 53$ mCRC patients receiving standard first-line chemotherapy	Safe-SeqS	10-fold change ctDNA threshold: Sn 75.0/Sp 64.0	Predictive during first-line chemotherapy
Tie et al. (2018) [34]	ctDNA	$n = 95$ stage III colon cancer receiving adjuvant chemotherapy	Safe-SeqS	Inferior RFS: in case of positive ctDNA post-surgery (HR 3.52, $p = 0.004$). Superior RFS: when ctDNA became undetectable after chemotherapy (HR 5.11, $p = 0.02$). Inferior RFS: when ctDNA status changed from negative to positive after chemotherapy (HR 5.30, $p = 0.006$). Inferior RFS: positive ctDNA after adjuvant chemotherapy completion (HR 7.14, $p < 0.001$)	Prognostic and therapy monitoring in stage III colon cancer
Grasselli et al. (2017) [35]	ctDNA	$n = 146$ mCRC patients	SoC PCR and Digital PCR (BEAMing)	ctDNA BEAMing RAS testing showed 89.7% agreement with SoC (Kappa index 0.80, 95% CI 0.71–0.90) BEAMing in tissue showed 90.9% agreement with SoC (Kappa index 0.83, 95% CI 0.74–0.92)	Predictive and anti-EGFR treatment selection

Table 1. Cont.

Study (Year)	Biomarkers	Sample Size	Methods	Statistical Significance (p Value), Sensitivity/Specificity (%) and/or Hazard Ratio	Potential Clinical Applications
Khan et al. (2018) [36]	ctDNA	n = 27 RAS mutant mCRC	Digital-droplet PCR	PFS: HR 0.21 (95% CI 0.06–0.71, p = 0.01)	Predictive of duration of anti-angiogenic response to regorafenib
Flamini et al. (2006) [37]	ctDNA	n = 75 healthy subjects n = 75 CRC	qPCR	ctDNA alone: Sn 81.3/Sp 73.3 ctDNA + CEA: Sn 84.0/Sp 88.0	Diagnosis of early-stage CRC
Hao et al. (2014) [38]	ctDNA	n = 104 primary CRC, n = 85 operated CRC, n = 16 recurrent/mCRC, n = 63 intestinal polyps, n = 110 normal controls	ALU-qPCR	ALU115: Sn 69.23/Sp 99.09 ALU247/115: Sn 73.08/Sp 97.27	Early complementary diagnosis, monitoring of progression and prognosis of CRC
Sun et al. (2019) [39]	mSEPT9 DNA	n = 650	Epigenomics AG for Epi proColon 2.0	CRC: Sn 73.0/Sp 94.5 Polyps and adenoma: Sn 17.1/Sp 94.5	Screening and recurrence monitoring
Link et al. (2010) [40]	Fecal miRNAs	n = 8 healthy controls, n = 29 normal colonoscopies, colon adenomas, and CRCs	TaqMan qRT-PCR	Increased expression of miR-21 and miR-106a in CRC and adenomas vs. normal controls (p < 0.05)	Screening
Ya et al. (2017) [41]	Serum miR-129	n = 18 female patients with CRC	Real-time PCR	Contribution to carcinogenesis by targeting ERβ (p < 0.01)	Development of therapeutic agents
He et al. (2018) [42]	Serum miR-24-2	n = 68 healthy subjects, n = 228 CRC	Real-time qRT-PCR	Higher levels in CRC than healthy subjects (p < 0.05)	Negative biomarker in the diagnosis of the progression of CRC
Wang et al. (2017) [43]	Serum miR-31, miR-141, miR-224-3p, miR-576-5p, and miR-4669	n = 44 healthy subjects, n = 50 CRC. Double-blind validation using sera from 30 CRC, 30 colonic polyps, 30 healthy controls	Real-time PCR	AUC = 0.995 (microarrays) AUC = 0.964 (double-blind validation test)	Panel for diagnosis of CRC

Table 1. Cont.

Study (Year)	Biomarkers	Sample Size	Methods	Statistical Significance (p Value), Sensitivity/Specificity (%) and/or Hazard Ratio	Potential Clinical Applications
Toiyama et al. (2014) [44]	Serum miR-200c	Total $n = 446$ colorectal specimens. First phase: $n = 12$ stage I and IV CRC. Second phase: $n = 182$ CRC, $n = 24$ controls. Third phase: $n = 156$ tumor tissues from 182 CRC and an independent set of 20 matched primary CRC and corresponding liver mts	Real-time qRT-PCR	Correlation with lymph node mts ($p = 0.0026$), distant mts ($p = 0.0023$), and prognosis ($p = 0.0064$) Predictor for lymph node mts (OR 4.81, 95% CI 1.98–11.7, $p = 0.0005$) and tumor recurrence (HR 4.51, 95% CI 1.56–13.01, $p = 0.005$) Prognostic (HR 2.67, 95% CI 1.28–5.67, $p = 0.01$)	Prognostic and predictive of metastasis
Tang et al. (2019) [45]	Exosomal miR-320d	$n = 34$ mCRC, $n = 108$ non-mCRC	qPCR	miR-320d: AUC = 0.633, $p = 0.019$ miR-320d + CEA: AUC = 0.804	Predictive of metastasis
Koga et al. (2013) [46]	Fecal miR-106a	$n = 117$ CRC, $n = 107$ healthy subjects	Real-time RT-PCR	FmiRT: Sn 34.2/Sp 97.2. iFOBT + FmiRT: Sn 70.9/Sp 96.3	Screening
Sazanov et al. (2017) [47]	Plasma and saliva miR-21	Plasma: total $n = 65$ CRC ($n = 34$ controls, $n = 6$ stage II, $n = 16$ stage III, $n = 9$ stage IV) Saliva: total $n = 68$ CRC ($n = 34$ controls, $n = 6$ stage II, $n = 18$ stage III, $n = 10$ stage IV)	Real-time qRT-PCR	Plasma: Sn 65/Sp 85 Saliva: Sn 97/Sp 91	Screening
Fu et al. (2018) [48]	Exosomal miR-17-5p and miR-92a-3p	$n = 10$ normal controls, $n = 18$ CRC, $n = 11$ mCRC	Real-time qPCR	miR-17-5p: AUC = 0.897 (95% CI 0.800–0.994) for CRC, and 0.841 (95% CI 0.720–0.962) for mts miR-92a-3p: AUC = 0.845 (95% CI 0.724–0.966) for CRC and 0.854 (95% CI 0.735–0.973) for mts miR-17-5p + miR-92a-3p: AUC = 0.910 (95% CI 0.820–1) for CRC and 0.841 (95% CI 0.718–0.964) for mts	Prognostic

Table 1. Cont.

Study (Year)	Biomarkers	Sample Size	Methods	Statistical Significance (p Value), Sensitivity/Specificity (%) and/or Hazard Ratio	Potential Clinical Applications
Tsukamoto et al. (2017) [49]	Exosomal miR-21	Total $n = 326$ CRC ($n = 51$ stage I, $n = 110$ stage II, $n = 98$ stage III, $n = 67$ stage IV)	TaqMan miRNA assays	OS: HR 2.28 (95% CI 1.81–5.74, $p < 0.01$) DFS: HR 2.34 (95% CI 1.87–4.60, $p < 0.01$)	Prediction of recurrence and poor prognosis in CRC patients with TNM stage II, III, or IV
Liu et al. (2016) [50]	Exosomal miR-4772-3p	$n = 84$ stage II–III colon cancer	Real-time qRT-PCR	AUC = 0.72 (95% CI 0.59–0.85, $p = 0.001$)	Prognostic for tumor recurrence in stage II and III colon cancer patients
Yan et al. (2018) [51]	Exosomal miR-6803-5p	$n = 168$ CRC	qRT-PCR	OS: HR 2.93 (95% CI 1.35–6.37, $p < 0.007$) DFS: HR 3.26 (95% CI 1.56–6.81, $p < 0.002$) AUC = 0.7399	Diagnostic and prognostic
Liu et al. (2018) [52]	Exosomal miR-27a and miR-130a	Training phase: $n = 40$ healthy subjects $n = 40$ stage I CRC. Validation phase: $n = 40$ stage I, $n = 20$ stage II, $n = 14$ stage III, $n = 6$ stage IV CRC, $n = 40$ healthy subjects. External validation phase: 50 stage I CRC, 50 adenomas, 50 healthy subjects	qRT-PCR	miR-27a: AUC = 0.773 Sn 75/Sp 77.5 in the training phase, AUC = 0.82 Sn 80.0/Sp 77.5 in the validation phase, and AUC = 0.746 Sn 80.0/Sp 77.5 in the external validation phase miR-130a: AUC = 0.742 Sn 82.5/Sp 62.5 in the training phase, AUC = 0.787 Sn 70.0/Sp 80.0 in the validation phase, AUC = 0.697 Sn 70.0/Sp 80.0 in the external validation phase miR-27a + miR-130a: training phase AUC = 0.846 Sn 82.5/Sp 75, validation phase AUC = 0.898, Sn 80.0/Sp 90.0 and external validation phase AUC = 0.801 Sn 80.0/Sp 90.0	Diagnostic and prognostic

Table 1. Cont.

Study (Year)	Biomarkers	Sample Size	Methods	Statistical Significance (p Value), Sensitivity/Specificity (%) and/or Hazard Ratio	Potential Clinical Applications
Peng et al. (2018) [53]	Exosomal miR-548c-5p	$n = 108$ CRC	Real-time qPCR	OS: HR 3.40 (95% CI 1.02–11.27, $p = 0.046$)	Diagnostic and prognostic
Jin et al. (2019) [54]	Exosomal miR-21-5p, miR-1246, miR-1229-5p, and miR-96-5p	Drug-resistant CRC cell lines	qRT-PCR	AUC = 0.804, $p < 0.05$	Predictive for chemoresistance in advanced CRC
Yagi et al. (2019) [55]	Exosomal miR-125b	$n = 55$ patients with advanced/recurrent CRC treated with mFOLFOX6	qRT-PCR	PFS: HR 0.71 (95% CI 0.36–0.94, $p < 0.041$)	Predictive and detection of chemotherapy resistance
Wang et al. (2018) [56]	lncRNA H19	$n = 110$ paired CRC tissues and para-tumor tissues	qRT-PCR	RFS: log-rank test $p < 0.001$ High H19: HR 2.383 (95% CI 1.157–4.909, $p = 0.018$)	Predictive of 5-FU resistance
Li et al. (2017) [57]	lncRNA MEG3	$n = 316$ CRC	qRT-PCR	AUC = 0.784, Sn 72.86/Sp 61.43 OS: HR 1.390 (95% CI 0.324–2.089, $p = 0.007$)	Prognostic and promotion of chemosensitivity
Sun et al. (2019) [58]	lncRNAs CRNDE, H19, UCA1, and HOTAIR	CRC cell lines (HCT116, HT29, and LoVo)	Gene Expression Profiling Interactive Analysis	HOTAIR OS: HR 1.9, $p = 0.0066$ DFS: HR 1.8, $p = 0.012$	Predictive of treatment sensitivity
Tang et al. (2019) [59]	lncRNA GLCC1	In vitro: Human colorectal cancer cell lines SW1116, SW480, Caco2, LoVo, HT29, RKO, DLD-1, and HCT116 In vivo: BALB/c nude mice	Real-time qPCR	Stabilization of c-Myc after knockdown of lncGLCC1 ($p < 0.001$)	Prognostic
Liu et al. (2016) [60]	Exosomal lncRNA CRNDE-h	$n = 468$	qRT-PCR	AUC = 0.892 Sn 70.3/Sp 94.4	Diagnostic and prognostic
Liang et al. (2019) [61]	Exosomal lncRNA RPPH1	$n = 61$ CRC	qRT-PCR	OS: HR 2.145 (95% CI 1.450–3.174, $p < 0.001$) DFS: HR 1.820 (95% CI 1.257–2.637, $p = 0.001$)	Prognostic, therapeutic, and diagnostic target

CTC: circulating tumor cells; UICC: Union for International Cancer Control; HR: hazard ratio; Sn: sensitivity; Sp: Specificity; mCRC: metastatic colorectal cancer; ctDNA: circulating tumor DNA; OS: overall survival; PFS: progression-free survival; ORR: objective response rate; EGFR: epidermal growth factor receptor; MRD: minimal residual disease; RFS: recurrence-free survival; CI: confidence interval; CEA: carcinoembryonic antigen; NGS: next-generation sequencing; SoC: Standard of care; qPCR: quantitative polymerase chain reaction; qRT-PCR: quantitative reverse transcription polymerase chain reaction; mSeptin9: methylated septin9; ERβ: estrogen receptor β; AUC: area under the ROC (Receiver Operating Characteristic) curve; OR: odds ratio; iFOBT: immunochemical fecal occult blood test; FmiRT: fecal microRNA test; mts: metastasis; DFS: disease-free survival.

2.1. Screening and Early Diagnosis

Global CRC screening guidelines recommend colonoscopy (every ten years), or flexible sigmoidoscopy (every five years) or fecal occult blood test (FOBT; every one or two years) for average-risk subjects aged 50–75 [62]. Blood-based detection tests represent an appealing alternative to these methods, as they are non-invasive and low-risk tests that can be easily performed during a routine medical check-up.

2.1.1. Circulating Tumor Cells (CTC) and Circulating Endothelial Cell Clusters (ECC)

CTC detection is uncommon and rather difficult in early-stage CRC; thus, the utility of CTCs for CRC screening or early detection seems to be very poor [63]. However, a study by Tsai et al., carried out on 620 subjects (438 with adenoma, polyps, or stage I–IV CRC and 182 healthy controls) reported an overall accuracy of 88% for all tumor stages, including precancerous lesions, using a new CTC assay [25]. Tumor-derived circulating endothelial cell clusters (ECC) may represent a promising type of cell-based liquid biopsy for early detection of CRC. These circulating benign cell clusters are released directly from the tumor vasculature and their isolation and enumeration discriminated healthy subjects from treatment-naïve as well as pathological early-stage (≤IIA) CRC patients with high accuracy [64].

2.1.2. Circulating Tumor DNA (ctDNA)

A recent meta-analysis concluded that the diagnostic accuracy of ctDNA has insufficient sensitivity but satisfactory specificity for diagnosis of CRC [23]. Nonetheless, there is growing evidence that ctDNA detection could be used along with the traditional screening methods to improve diagnosis of early-stage CRC [63,65,66]. In particular, a study by Flamini et al. showed that ctDNA, particularly when combined with carcinoembryonic antigen (CEA), may represent a useful tool for early detection of CRC (area under the ROC curve 0.92, with 84% sensitivity and 88% specificity) [37]. Combined assessment of ALU115, DNA integrity index (ALU247/115) and CEA could increase the diagnostic efficiency for CRC. Of note, serum DNA integrity index was superior to the absolute DNA concentration in diagnostic accuracy of CRC [38]. ctDNA methylation showed higher sensitivity compared to traditional serum tumor markers in early-stage CRC and could represent a potential diagnostic biomarker. Sun et al. showed that circulating, cell-free, methylated Septin 9 (mSEPT9) DNA had higher specificity than FOBT for the screening of CRC in 650 subjects (73% of CRC patients were mSEPT9-positive at 94.5% specificity, and 17.1% of patients with intestinal polyps and adenoma were mSEPT9-positive at 94.5% specificity) [39]. Furthermore, a recent prospective cohort study carried out on a high-risk population of 1493 subjects, demonstrated that a single ctDNA methylation marker, cg10673833, had high sensitivity (89.7%) and specificity (86.8%) for detection of precancerous lesions and CRC [67]. A meta-analysis by Nian et al. pointed out the efficacy of Epipro Colon 2.0 with 2/3 algorithm (Epigenomics), a test used to screen the methylation status of the SEPT9 promoter in ctDNA, for CRC detection. Positive ratio of mSEPT9 was higher in advanced CRC stages (45% in I, 70% in II, 76% in III, 79% in IV) and low differentiation tissue (31% in high, 73% in moderate, 90% in low). However, according to previous research, mSEPT9 did not seem to identify effectively precancerous lesions [68]. Other potential blood tests include a multi-analyte test (CancerSEEK) that could detect eight common solid tumor types, including CRC, through assessment of the levels of circulating proteins and mutations in ctDNA. The median test sensitivity was 73% for stage II, 78% for stage III and 43% for stage I tumors, with a specificity greater than 99% [69].

2.1.3. Serum, Fecal, and Salivary MicroRNAs (miRNAs)

Alterations in miRNAs have been reported in blood or fecal samples from CRC patients, or even in subjects with precancerous advanced adenomas [40]. miRNAs can be observed in the circulation alone or combined with some proteins; also, they can be released directly into extracellular fluids and carried by microvesicles, mostly exosomes [70,71]. miR-129 is highly expressed in CRC plasma, while miR-24-2 levels are low in CRC serum, thus representing potential positive or negative biomarkers in the diagnosis of CRC patients [41,42]. A study showed that serum expression levels of five miRNAs (miR-31, miR-141, miR-224-3p, miR-576-5p and miR-4669) were significantly different between patients with colon cancer and healthy controls, suggesting their potential use as a miRNA panel for diagnosis of CRC [43]. miRNAs detection could be used to distinguish metastatic and non-mCRC patients. Indeed, high serum levels of miR-200c in CRC patients could potentially represent a predictive biomarker for local and distant metastasis [44]. A study demonstrated that exosomal miR-320d could significantly discriminate metastatic from non-mCRC patients with an AUC of 0.633 (95% CI: 0.526–0.740), the sensitivity of 62.0% and the specificity of 64.7%. The combination of miR-320d and CEA had an AUC of 0.804, with the sensitivity of 63.3% and the specificity of 91.3% [45]. Numerous miRNAs (i.e., miR-29a, miR-223, miR-224, miR-106a, and miR-135b) found in feces could represent useful biomarkers for screening and diagnosis of CRC [72]. Fecal miR-106a test combined with routine immunochemical FOBT have been reported to be effective in discriminating CRC patients from those with negative iFOBT results and could improve the sensitivity to identify CRC [46]. A study demonstrated that salivary miR-21 is significantly up-regulated in CRC patients with a very high sensitivity and specificity of 97 and 91% respectively, and could be an accurate biomarker for CRC screening [47]. More studies are needed to confirm if salivary miRNAs could represent reliable biomarker candidates for CRC detection [73].

2.2. Prognosis, Progression, and Response to Treatment

2.2.1. Circulating Tumor Cells (CTC)

Several studies demonstrated that CTC could potentially play an important role in monitoring treatment outcomes and for detection of resistance against chemotherapy in CRC patients [26–28]. A prospective study by Bork et al. carried out on 287 patients with potentially curable CRC (including 239 patients with stage I–III) showed that preoperative CTC identification represented a strong and independent prognostic marker in non-mCRC [26]. In a cohort of 37 high-risk stages II–III CRC patients, Gazzaniga et al. pointed out that CTCs detection could facilitate the selection of high-risk stage II CRC patient candidates for adjuvant chemotherapy [27]. A study by Tsai et al. showed that rising counts of CTC in peripheral blood was associated with tumor progression and poor prognosis in CRC patients: CTC counts in 2 mL of peripheral blood increased from 0, 1, 5, to 36 in healthy ($n = 27$), benign ($n = 21$), non-metastatic ($n = 95$), and mCRC ($n = 15$) patients, respectively. After 2-year follow-up, non-mCRC patients who had ≥5 CTCs showed an 8-fold increased risk to develop metastasis within one year after curable surgery than those who had <5 CTC [28]. Furthermore, CTC could be used as tool for assessment of chemotherapy resistance [29,74]. High-toxicity multidrug regimens used against advanced CRC, often require the use of biomarkers to select the patients who will receive the most benefit. Stratification by CTC count was effective in detecting patients with previously untreated KRAS wild-type advanced CRC who could benefit the most from an intensive 4-drug protocol (oxaliplatin, irinotecan, and tegafur-uracil with leucovorin and cetuximab), avoiding high-toxicity treatment in low CTC groups [30]. A meta-analysis of 13 studies showed significant differences between CTC-low and CTC-high levels in CRC patients treated with chemotherapy with regard to disease control [Relative Risk (RR) = 1.354, 95% CI 1.002–1.830, $p = 0.048$], progression-free survival [PFS; Hazard Ratio (HR) = 2.500, 95% CI 1.746–3.580, $p < 0.001$] and overall survival (OS; HR = 2.856, 95% CI 1.959–4.164, $p < 0.001$). These results confirmed the prognostic and predictive role of CTCs for the response to chemotherapy in CRC patients [75].

2.2.2. Circulating Tumor DNA (ctDNA)

The proportion of CRC patients in whom ctDNA can be identified depends on the tumor volume and ranges from 50% to 90% in those with non-metastatic or metastatic disease, respectively [76]. There is evidence that after CRC curative resection, the detection rate of ctDNA could range from

8–15% in stage II to 50% in stage IV [31,32,77]. Serum DNA concentrations and integrity index may play an important role not only in early complementary diagnosis but also in monitoring of progression and prognosis of CRC. A study showed that the median absolute serum ALU115 and ALU247/115 levels in patients with primary CRC were significantly higher than those in subjects with polyps or normal controls ($p < 0.0001$), in recurrent or metastatic CRC were significantly higher compared to primary CRC ($p = 0.0021$, $p = 0.0018$) or operated CRC ($p < 0.0001$, respectively) and during follow-up, ALU115 and ALU247/115 levels increased before surgery and reduced significantly after surgery [38]. A prospective study conducted on 53 metastatic colorectal cancer (mCRC) patients receiving standard first-line chemotherapy, showed that ctDNA is detectable in a high proportion of treatment-naïve mCRC patients, and early alterations in ctDNA during first-line chemotherapy could predict the later radiologic response. Significant decrease in ctDNA (median 5.7-fold; $p < 0.001$) levels were detected before cycle 2, which correlated with computerized tomography (CT) responses at 8–10 weeks [Odds Ratio (OR) = 5.25 with a 10-fold ctDNA reduction; $p = 0.016$]. Major decrease ($\geq$10-fold) versus minor decrease in ctDNA precycle 2 was correlated with a trend for raised PFS (median 14.7 vs. 8.1 months; HR = 1.87; $p = 0.266$) [33]. Another prospective cohort study of 230 patients showed that detection of ctDNA after resection of stage II colon cancer may detect patients at very high risk of recurrence, thus giving direct evidence of residual disease and helpful information on adjuvant treatment choices. ctDNA was detected after surgery in 7.9% of patients who did not receive any adjuvant chemotherapy, and among these, 79% had recurred at a median follow-up of 27 months; recurrence was observed in 9.8% of 164 patients with negative ctDNA [HR = 18; 95% confidence interval (CI), 7.9 to 40; $p < 0.001$]. In patients who completed chemotherapy, the presence of ctDNA was correlated with a lower recurrence-free survival (HR = 11; 95% CI, 1.8 to 68; $p = 0.001$) [31]. ctDNA could detect the presence of residual metastatic cancer cells not evident on CT also in stage III CRC patients. Indeed, serial assessment of ctDNA could characterize subsets of patients benefiting or not benefiting from chemotherapy and represent a marker of adjuvant treatment efficacy [34,78]. It is well known that anti-epidermal growth factor receptor (EGFR) treatment is unsuccessful in the case of RAS mutations [79]. ctDNA detection could represent an alternative tool for selection of anti-EGFR treatment due to its agreement with mutational status of RAS in CRC tissue. A prospective-retrospective cohort study carried out on 146 mCRC patients, showed that plasma RAS assessment had high overall concordance and identified a mCRC population responsive to EGFR therapy with the same predictive level as standard of care PCR techniques tissue testing [35]. A prospective phase II clinical trial of cetuximab in RAS wild-type patients with CRC, combined sequential profiling of ctDNA and matched tissue biopsies with imaging and mathematical modeling of tumor progression, and showed that liquid biopsies were able to detect spatial and temporal heterogeneity of the resistance to anti-EGFR monoclonal antibodies [80]. In a phase II trial, the levels of RAS mutated ctDNA were assessed in mCRC patients treated with the oral multi-kinase inhibitor regorafenib. The reduction of RAS mutations in plasma within 8 weeks of therapy was associated with improved PFS and OS. Combination of dynamic contrast-enhanced magnetic resonance imaging (DCE-MRI) and ctDNA predicted duration of anti-angiogenic response and could improve management of patient treated with regorafenib [36]. A recent study by Siravegna et al. showed that plasma HER-2 (ERBB2) copy number analysis based on ctDNA could predict beneficial effects from HER-2-targeted therapy with high accuracy (97%) in 28 out of 29 patients [81].

2.2.3. MicroRNAs (miRNAs)

Studies reported an association between high expression levels of specific miRNAs (including miR-21, miR-1290, miR-193a, miR-17-5p, miR-92a-3p, miR-203, miR-1229, and miR-17/92 cluster) and poor prognosis of CRC patients due to metastatic disease, post-treatment relapse, and poor OS [48,49,82–86]. On the other hand, low levels of serum exosomal miR-4772-3p and miR-6869-5p were associated with high risk of tumor recurrence in stage II and III and poor 3-year survival in CRC patients, respectively [50,51]. Furthermore, significantly higher expression of miR-6803-5p in CRC patients was associated with later TNM stage, lymph node or liver metastasis, and poor disease-free survival (DFS), thus representing a potential diagnostic and prognostic biomarker [51]. There is evidence that serum exosomal miR-21 could be a useful biomarker for the prediction of recurrence and poor prognosis at TNM stages II, III or IV in CRC patients [49]. Also, higher expression levels of serum exosomal miR-17-5p and miR-92a-3p predicted pathologic grades and stages of CRC [48]. A study reported that the exosomal miR-27a and miR-130a panel in plasma correlated with tumor grade and stage of CRC and could be effective for predicting poor OS (HR = 2.74; 95% CI, 1.25–6.01; p = 0.012; and HR = 2.36; 95% CI, 1.07–5.23; p = 0.034, respectively). Furthermore, both miRNAs could be used for detection of CRC: miR-27a showed a sensitivity of 82% and a specificity of 91%, while miR-130a showed a sensitivity of 70% and a specificity of 100% [52]. Serum exosomal miR-548c and miR-6803 could be important predictive biomarkers of DFS and OS in CRC patients. Indeed, studies showed that elevated levels of miR-6803 and decreased levels of miR-548c represented poor prognostic markers, particularly in later stages of CRC and in the presence of liver metastasis [51,53]. Specific miRNAs may be used for monitoring resistance or tolerance to chemotherapy and for selection of clinical therapeutic approach. A panel of serum exosomal miRNAs including miR-1246, miR-21-5p, miR-1229-5p, and miR-96-5p could significantly discriminate chemotherapy-resistant subjects to 5-FU and oxaliplatin from advanced CRC patients (AUC = 0.804; p < 0.05). Targeting these miRNAs could enhance chemosensitivity to oxaliplatin and 5-FU, thus representing a promising approach for CRC treatment [54]. A study by Yagi et al. suggested that increased plasma exosomal miR-125b levels could detect resistance to modified FOLFOX6-based first-line chemotherapy in patients with advanced or recurrent CRC. Furthermore, PFS was significantly inferior in patients with high miR-125b levels before chemotherapy than in those with low levels, thus confirming the utility of miR-125b as a predictive biomarker in advanced or recurrent CRC [55].

2.2.4. Long Non-Coding RNAs (lncRNAs)

lncRNAs interact with DNA, mRNA, proteins, and miRNAs, playing a role in multiple biological processes, such as epigenetic or gene expression regulation, and chromatin remodeling [87,88]. Several studies showed that lncRNAs were abnormally expressed in many cancers, including CRC, and therefore could have potential application in diagnosis, prognosis and potential treatment [89–92]. Indeed, lncRNAs could regulate drug function and chemoresistance through different mechanisms in many tumors, including CRC [56,57]. More than 70 CRC-related lncRNAs have been identified so far, including HOTAIR, MEG3, CRNDE, UCA1, CCAT1, CCAT2, MALAT-1 and H19 [93]. Alterations in the expression of these lncRNAs could lead to chemotherapy and radiotherapy resistance. Sun et al. identified four hub lncRNAs (CRNDE, H19, UCA1, and HOTAIR) involved in the process of resistance to oxaliplatin or irinotecan in patients with advanced CRC. In particular, high expression of HOTAIR was associated with advanced and metastatic disease and poor prognosis [58]. Decreased serum MEG3 levels were correlated with poor response to chemotherapy and OS in CRC patients treated with oxaliplatin. MEG3 increased oxaliplatin-induced cell apoptosis in CRC; therefore, overexpression of MEG3 could represent a promising therapeutic strategy to defeat oxaliplatin resistance in CRC patients [57]. Tang et al. demonstrated that up-regulation of a lncRNA, GLCC1, under glucose-limited conditions in CRC cells, promoted cell survival and proliferation by stabilizing c-Myc and stimulating glycolysis. From a clinical point of view, GLCC1 was associated with carcinogenesis, tumor volume and poor prognosis in CRC patients [59,94]. Levels of serum exosomal CRNDE-h were higher in CRC patients compared to those with benign colorectal disease or healthy controls. CRNDE-h expression could be related to the presence of lymph node metastasis and was associated with a low OS in CRC. Furthermore, the prognostic value of CRNDE was better than CEA, with a sensitivity of 70% vs. 37% and a specificity of 94% vs. 89% [60]. Liang et al. reported that high exosomal RPPH1 levels were associated with advanced TNM stages, promotion of metastasis, and poor prognosis in CRC patients, whereas lower RPPH1 levels were observed after tumor resection. Plasma exosomal RPPH1 levels showed a better diagnostic value (AUC = 0.86) compared to CEA and CA19.9 [61]. A study by

Barbagallo et al. demonstrated that UCA1 was down-regulated in serum of CRC patients compared to healthy subjects; UCA1 showed an AUC of 0.719 (95% CI, 0.533–0.863; $p = 0.01$) with 100% sensitivity and 43% specificity in discriminating between the cancer and control groups. These results suggested that the UCA1 regulatory axis could be a promising target to develop novel RNA-based therapies against CRC [95].

3. Current Issues and Limitations of Liquid Biopsy

Despite all the potential advantages of liquid biopsy in the management of CRC, there are still some practical issues that need to be addressed before it can be widely used in clinical practice [96]. Potential challenges may include low amounts of CTCs and ctDNA in samples, lack of pre-analytical and analytical consensus, clinical validation, regulatory endorsement and cost effectiveness [97,98]. Currently, the use of CTCs in routine diagnostics is limited, mainly due to methodological constraints, such as the lack of an established assessment practice, beyond enumeration [99,100]. The epithelial cell adhesion molecule (EpCAM)-dependent technique was approved by the U.S. Food and Drug Administration (FDA) in 2004, and represents the "gold standard" for CTC isolation in different cancers, including CRC [101]. However, only CTCs that maintain epithelial features can be detected by EpCAM, excluding CTCs with mesenchymal characteristics [102]. On the other hand, ctDNA analysis has been better optimized for routine diagnostic use [103]. The concentration of ctDNA in the peripheral blood depends on the site, volume, and vascularity of the tumor, which can also be responsible for the large variations frequently observed in ctDNA levels [104]. Analysis of ctDNA can be performed by either quantitative assessment of ctDNA in a blood sample or by the identification of mutations. The introduction of next-generation sequencing (NGS)-based technologies reduced the error rate and enhanced sensitivity in ctDNA detection [105]. NGS technology enables the analysis of thousands of DNA sequences in parallel followed by either sequence alignment to a reference genome or de novo sequence assembly [104,106]. Deep sequencing represents the first approach to identify mutations at a low allele frequency (<0.2%) by sequencing the target regions with high coverage (>10,000×) [107]. Therefore, the sensitivity of deep sequencing for detecting mutations in ctDNA can achieve 100%, even if the specificity can be lower, around 80% [108,109]. Advantages of NGS included detection of genomic rearrangements, new mutations or alterations in genes, and the possible evaluation of response to treatment [110]. However, NGS-based approaches are rather expensive and time-consuming. Furthermore, data should be analyzed and interpreted by experts in bioinformatics [111]. Data storage and the difficulty in interpreting massive quantity of information obtained with NGS may represent a computational challenge to researchers. Also, the selection of proper validation methods to detect clinically significant mutations among a large number of samples can represent a challenging task [112]. Clinical validation of NGS data is carried out by assessing various parameters such as analytical sensitivity (the ability of the test to identify true sequence variants e.g., false negative rate), and analytical specificity (the probability of the test to not identify mutations where none are present (e.g., false positive rate) [113]. Limitations of NGS, principally with regard to the overall clinical sensitivity, could be overtaken implementing NGS with mutant allele enrichment or using digital PCR to improve reliability [96,114]. Mass-spectrometry and Real-Time PCR are other promising techniques for ctDNA assessment, which are rapid and cheap, require small quantities of input material, and have high sensitivity and specificity [77,115]. If possible, ctDNA should be analyzed in combination with CTCs and exosomal miRNAs, to obtain as much data as possible from a single blood sample [116]. However, different blood collection tubes, changes in storage temperatures and centrifugation may affect DNA or cells stability [117–119]. ctDNA degradation due to DNase activity could be avoided by isolating plasma within an hour after blood draw [120]. Reduction of cell lysis and stabilization of the total ctDNA pool can be obtained by means of specific blood collection tubes containing preservatives and additives [121]. Furthermore, accuracy and reproducibility of the liquid biopsy represent a main issue for analytic validity [122]. A study by Vivancos et al. showed that two liquid biopsy platforms, OncoBEAM™ RAS CRC and Idylla™ ctKRAS Mutation Test, had different sensitivity for identifying KRAS mutations in plasma samples from mCRC patients. The European Molecular Genetics Quality Network (EMQN) evaluated ctDNA detection approaches, and underlined that multiple pre-analytical and analytical variants may produce variable results; the EMQN pilot external quality assessment (EQA) scheme showed that the existing variability in multiple phases of ctDNA processing and analysis (e.g., due to specimen volume, ctDNA quantification technique, and choice of genotyping platform), resulted in an overall error rate of 6.09% [123]. These results highlighted the critical need for better standardization and validation of liquid biopsy assessment [124].

4. Future Perspectives and Conclusions

The use of CTCs, ctDNA, miRNAs and lncRNAs as potential biomarkers is an emerging area with a great potential for the management of CRC. Currently, the clinical utility of liquid biopsies in CRC limited, but it is expected to achieve a clear consensus in the near future. Indeed, the liquid biopsy is a minimally invasive, cheap, and repeatable technique that can facilitate CRC screening and early diagnosis, providing more information for the clinical staging of CRC patients. Furthermore, blood-based liquid biopsies are useful for monitoring disease progression and treatment efficacy, prognosis, and acquired resistance to chemotherapy in CRC. It is reasonable to think that in the future, it will be possible to choose the most appropriate therapy based on real-time genetic information through a liquid biopsy, in the way of personalized medicine. In this context, performing prospective clinical trials is essential for clinical utility and development of practice changing protocols. Nevertheless, the transfer of liquid biopsies from bench to bedside necessitates larger-scale and multicenter trials to confirm its advantages. Also, optimization of pre-analytical and analytical processing is fundamental for clinical validity, and standardization of laboratory methods is firmly required to guarantee elevated reproducibility of the results. The lack of clinical applicability is currently due to large quantity of liquid biopsy assays. For example, many ctDNA assays are presently commercially available, but each assay shows specific detection limit, sensitivity, and specificity. Therefore, the results obtained from different liquid biopsy platforms cannot be easily compared, and EQA studies are needed before application in routine diagnostics. Further studies should be conducted on the effectiveness of liquid biopsy biomarkers, such as ctDNA, in combination with other blood tests and radiological monitoring, in order to better identify and stratify CRC patients and to choose the appropriate treatment. In the future, advances in liquid biopsy methodologies and their increased sensitivity should facilitate detection of MRD and early CRC diagnosis even in asymptomatic subjects. Only a few trials have investigated a specific intervention based on the results of liquid biopsies (i.e., CTC or ctDNA status), so far. Many of these studies did not include a control group, and therefore the results could not lead to significant changes in clinical practice. Further prospective studies are needed to establish future clinical applications of liquid biopsies and delineate their impact in the management of CRC.

Author Contributions: Conceptualization, M.V. and A.B.; writing—original draft preparation, M.V.; writing—review and editing, M.V., R.C., F.B. and A.B. All authors have read and agreed to the published version of the manuscript.

Funding: This research received no external funding.

Acknowledgments: The images used in the graphical abstract are distributed under Creative Commons License and can be freely available at the following link: https://smart.servier.com/.

Conflicts of Interest: The authors declare no conflict of interest.

References

1. GBD 2017 Colorectal Cancer Collaborators. The global, regional, and national burden of colorectal cancer and its attributable risk factors in 195 countries and territories, 1990–2017: A systematic analysis for the Global Burden of Disease Study 2017. *Lancet Gastroenterol. Hepatol.* **2019**, *4*, 913–933. [CrossRef]

2. Bray, F.; Ferlay, J.; Soerjomataram, I.; Siegel, R.L.; Torre, L.A.; Jemal, A. Global cancer statistics 2018: GLOBOCAN estimates of incidence and mortality worldwide for 36 cancers in 185 countries. *CA Cancer J. Clin.* **2018**, *68*, 394–424. [CrossRef] [PubMed]
3. Bishehsari, F.; Mahdavinia, M.; Vacca, M.; Malekzadeh, R.; Mariani-Costantini, R. Epidemiological transition of colorectal cancer in developing countries: Environmental factors, molecular pathways, and opportunities for prevention. *World J. Gastroenterol.* **2014**, *20*, 6055–6072. [CrossRef] [PubMed]
4. Hui, L. Quantifying the effects of aging and urbanization on major gastrointestinal diseases to guide preventative strategies. *BMC Gastroenterol.* **2018**, *18*. [CrossRef] [PubMed]
5. Valli, A.; Harris, A.L.; Kessler, B.M. Hypoxia metabolism in ageing. *Aging Albany N. Y.* **2015**, *7*, 465–466. [CrossRef]
6. Cancer Facts & Figures 2020|American Cancer Society. Available online: https://www.cancer.org/research/cancer-facts-statistics/all-cancer-facts-figures/cancer-facts-figures-2020.html (accessed on 14 July 2020).
7. Stintzing, S. Management of colorectal cancer. *F1000Prime Rep.* **2014**, *6*, 108. [CrossRef] [PubMed]
8. Nakayama, G.; Tanaka, C.; Kodera, Y. Current Options for the Diagnosis, Staging and Therapeutic Management of Colorectal Cancer. *Gastrointest. Tumors* **2013**, *1*, 25–32. [CrossRef]
9. Bender, U.; Rho, Y.S.; Barrera, I.; Aghajanyan, S.; Acoba, J.; Kavan, P. Adjuvant therapy for stages II and III colon cancer: Risk stratification, treatment duration, and future directions. *Curr. Oncol.* **2019**, *26*, S43–S52. [CrossRef]
10. Pfeiffer, P.; Köhne, C.-H.; Qvortrup, C. The changing face of treatment for metastatic colorectal cancer. *Expert Rev. Anticancer Ther.* **2019**, *19*, 61–70. [CrossRef]
11. Moriarity, A.; O'Sullivan, J.; Kennedy, J.; Mehigan, B.; McCormick, P. Current targeted therapies in the treatment of advanced colorectal cancer: A review. *Ther. Adv. Med. Oncol.* **2016**, *8*, 276–293. [CrossRef]
12. Norcic, G. Liquid biopsy in colorectal cancer-current status and potential clinical applications. *Micromachines* **2018**, *9*, 300. [CrossRef] [PubMed]
13. Vacante, M.; Borzì, A.M.; Basile, F.; Biondi, A. Biomarkers in colorectal cancer: Current clinical utility and future perspectives. *World J. Clin. Cases* **2018**, *6*, 869–881. [CrossRef] [PubMed]
14. Palmirotta, R.; Lovero, D.; Cafforio, P.; Felici, C.; Mannavola, F.; Pellè, E.; Quaresmini, D.; Tucci, M.; Silvestris, F. Liquid biopsy of cancer: A multimodal diagnostic tool in clinical oncology. *Ther. Adv. Med. Oncol.* **2018**, *10*. [CrossRef]
15. Crowley, E.; Di Nicolantonio, F.; Loupakis, F.; Bardelli, A. Liquid biopsy: Monitoring cancer-genetics in the blood. *Nat. Rev. Clin. Oncol.* **2013**, *10*, 472–484. [CrossRef] [PubMed]
16. Fernández-Lázaro, D.; García Hernández, J.L.; García, A.C.; Córdova Martínez, A.; Mielgo-Ayuso, J.; Cruz-Hernández, J.J. Liquid biopsy as novel tool in precision medicine: Origins, properties, identification and clinical perspective of cancer's biomarkers. *Diagnostics* **2020**, *10*, 215. [CrossRef] [PubMed]
17. Carretero-González, A.; Otero, I.; Carril-Ajuria, L.; de Velasco, G.; Manso, L. Exosomes: Definition, role in tumor development and clinical implications. *Cancer Microenviron.* **2018**, *11*, 13–21. [CrossRef] [PubMed]
18. Wong, C.-H.; Chen, Y.-C. Clinical significance of exosomes as potential biomarkers in cancer. *World J. Clin. Cases* **2019**, *7*, 171–190. [CrossRef] [PubMed]
19. Lampis, A.; Ghidini, M.; Ratti, M.; Mirchev, M.B.; Okuducu, A.F.; Valeri, N.; Hahne, J.C. Circulating tumour DNAs and Non-Coding RNAs as liquid biopsies for the management of colorectal cancer patients. *Gastrointest. Disord.* **2020**, *2*, 22. [CrossRef]
20. Osumi, H.; Shinozaki, E.; Yamaguchi, K.; Zembutsu, H. Clinical utility of circulating tumor DNA for colorectal cancer. *Cancer Sci.* **2019**, *110*, 1148–1155. [CrossRef]
21. Mathai, R.A.; Vidya, R.V.S.; Reddy, B.S.; Thomas, L.; Udupa, K.; Kolesar, J.; Rao, M. Potential utility of liquid biopsy as a diagnostic and prognostic tool for the assessment of solid tumors: Implications in the precision oncology. *J. Clin. Med.* **2019**, *8*, 373. [CrossRef]
22. Rubis, G.D.; Krishnan, S.R.; Bebawy, M. Liquid biopsies in cancer diagnosis, monitoring, and prognosis. *Trends Pharmacol. Sci.* **2019**, *40*, 172–186. [CrossRef] [PubMed]
23. Gold, B.; Cankovic, M.; Furtado, L.V.; Meier, F.; Gocke, C.D. Do circulating tumor cells, exosomes, and circulating tumor nucleic acids have clinical utility? A report of the association for molecular pathology. *J. Mol. Diagn.* **2015**, *17*, 209–224. [CrossRef] [PubMed]

24. Ding, Y.; Li, W.; Wang, K.; Xu, C.; Hao, M.; Ding, L. Perspectives of the Application of Liquid Biopsy in Colorectal Cancer. Available online: https://www.hindawi.com/journals/bmri/2020/6843180/ (accessed on 16 July 2020).
25. Tsai, W.-S.; Nimgaonkar, A.; Segurado, O.; Chang, Y.; Hsieh, B.; Shao, H.-J.; Wu, J.; Lai, J.-M.; Javey, M.; Watson, D.; et al. Prospective clinical study of circulating tumor cells for colorectal cancer screening. *J. Clin. Oncol.* **2018**, *36*, 556. [CrossRef]
26. Bork, U.; Rahbari, N.N.; Schölch, S.; Reissfelder, C.; Kahlert, C.; Büchler, M.W.; Weitz, J.; Koch, M. Circulating tumour cells and outcome in non-metastatic colorectal cancer: A prospective study. *Br. J. Cancer* **2015**, *112*, 1306–1313. [CrossRef]
27. Gazzaniga, P.; Gianni, W.; Raimondi, C.; Gradilone, A.; Lo Russo, G.; Longo, F.; Gandini, O.; Tomao, S.; Frati, L. Circulating tumor cells in high-risk nonmetastatic colorectal cancer. *Tumour Biol.* **2013**, *34*, 2507–2509. [CrossRef]
28. Tsai, W.-S.; Chen, J.-S.; Shao, H.-J.; Wu, J.-C.; Lai, J.-M.; Lu, S.-H.; Hung, T.-F.; Chiu, Y.-C.; You, J.-F.; Hsieh, P.-S.; et al. Circulating tumor cell count correlates with colorectal neoplasm progression and is a prognostic marker for distant metastasis in non-metastatic patients. *Sci. Rep.* **2016**, *6*. [CrossRef]
29. Musella, V.; Pietrantonio, F.; Di Buduo, E.; Iacovelli, R.; Martinetti, A.; Sottotetti, E.; Bossi, I.; Maggi, C.; Di Bartolomeo, M.; de Braud, F.; et al. Circulating tumor cells as a longitudinal biomarker in patients with advanced chemorefractory, RAS-BRAF wild-type colorectal cancer receiving cetuximab or panitumumab. *Int. J. Cancer* **2015**, *137*, 1467–1474. [CrossRef]
30. Krebs, M.G.; Renehan, A.G.; Backen, A.; Gollins, S.; Chau, I.; Hasan, J.; Valle, J.W.; Morris, K.; Beech, J.; Ashcroft, L.; et al. Circulating Tumor Cell Enumeration in a Phase II Trial of a Four-Drug Regimen in Advanced Colorectal Cancer. *Clin. Colorectal Cancer* **2015**, *14*, 115.e2–122.e2. [CrossRef]
31. Tie, J.; Wang, Y.; Tomasetti, C.; Li, L.; Springer, S.; Kinde, I.; Silliman, N.; Tacey, M.; Wong, H.-L.; Christie, M.; et al. Circulating tumor DNA analysis detects minimal residual disease and predicts recurrence in patients with stage II colon cancer. *Sci. Transl. Med.* **2016**, *8*, 346ra92. [CrossRef]
32. Sun, X.; Huang, T.; Cheng, F.; Huang, K.; Liu, M.; He, W.; Li, M.; Zhang, X.; Xu, M.; Chen, S.; et al. Monitoring colorectal cancer following surgery using plasma circulating tumor DNA. *Oncol. Lett.* **2018**, *15*, 4365–4375. [CrossRef]
33. Tie, J.; Kinde, I.; Wang, Y.; Wong, H.L.; Roebert, J.; Christie, M.; Tacey, M.; Wong, R.; Singh, M.; Karapetis, C.S.; et al. Circulating tumor DNA as an early marker of therapeutic response in patients with metastatic colorectal cancer. *Ann. Oncol.* **2015**, *26*, 1715–1722. [CrossRef] [PubMed]
34. Tie, J.; Cohen, J.; Wang, Y.; Lee, M.; Wong, R.; Kosmider, S.; Ananda, S.; Cho, J.H.; Faragher, I.; McKendrick, J.J.; et al. Serial circulating tumor DNA (ctDNA) analysis as a prognostic marker and a real-time indicator of adjuvant chemotherapy (CT) efficacy in stage III colon cancer (CC). *J. Clin. Oncol.* **2018**, *36*, 3516. [CrossRef]
35. Grasselli, J.; Elez, E.; Caratù, G.; Matito, J.; Santos, C.; Macarulla, T.; Vidal, J.; Garcia, M.; Viéitez, J.M.; Paéz, D.; et al. Concordance of blood- and tumor-based detection of RAS mutations to guide anti-EGFR therapy in metastatic colorectal cancer. *Ann. Oncol.* **2017**, *28*, 1294–1301. [CrossRef] [PubMed]
36. Khan, K.; Rata, M.; Cunningham, D.; Koh, D.-M.; Tunariu, N.; Hahne, J.C.; Vlachogiannis, G.; Hedayat, S.; Marchetti, S.; Lampis, A.; et al. Functional imaging and circulating biomarkers of response to regorafenib in treatment-refractory metastatic colorectal cancer patients in a prospective phase II study. *Gut* **2018**, *67*, 1484–1492. [CrossRef]
37. Flamini, E.; Mercatali, L.; Nanni, O.; Calistri, D.; Nunziatini, R.; Zoli, W.; Rosetti, P.; Gardini, N.; Lattuneddu, A.; Verdecchia, G.M.; et al. Free DNA and carcinoembryonic antigen serum levels: An important combination for diagnosis of colorectal cancer. *Clin. Cancer Res.* **2006**, *12*, 6985–6988. [CrossRef]
38. Hao, T.B.; Shi, W.; Shen, X.J.; Qi, J.; Wu, X.H.; Wu, Y.; Tang, Y.Y.; Ju, S.Q. Circulating cell-free DNA in serum as a biomarker for diagnosis and prognostic prediction of colorectal cancer. *Br. J. Cancer* **2014**, *111*, 1482–1489. [CrossRef]
39. Sun, J.; Fei, F.; Zhang, M.; Li, Y.; Zhang, X.; Zhu, S.; Zhang, S. The role of mSEPT9 in screening, diagnosis, and recurrence monitoring of colorectal cancer. *BMC Cancer* **2019**, *19*, 450. [CrossRef]
40. Link, A.; Balaguer, F.; Shen, Y.; Nagasaka, T.; Lozano, J.J.; Richard Boland, C.; Goel, A. Fecal microRNAs as novel biomarkers for colon cancer screening. *Cancer Epidemiol. Biomark. Prev.* **2010**, *19*, 1766–1774. [CrossRef]

41. Ya, G.; Wang, H.; Ma, Y.; Hu, A.; Ma, Y.; Hu, J.; Yu, Y. Serum miR-129 functions as a biomarker for colorectal cancer by targeting estrogen receptor (ER) β. *Pharmazie* **2017**, *72*, 107–112. [CrossRef]
42. He, H.W.; Wang, N.N.; Yi, X.M.; Tang, C.P.; Wang, D. Low-level serum miR-24-2 is associated with the progression of colorectal cancer. *Cancer Biomark.* **2018**, *21*, 261–267. [CrossRef]
43. Wang, Y.; Chen, Z.; Chen, W. Novel circulating microRNAs expression profile in colon cancer: A pilot study. *Eur. J. Med. Res.* **2017**, *22*. [CrossRef] [PubMed]
44. Toiyama, Y.; Hur, K.; Tanaka, K.; Inoue, Y.; Kusunoki, M.; Boland, C.R.; Goel, A. Serum miR-200c is a novel prognostic and metastasis-predictive biomarker in patients with colorectal cancer. *Ann. Surg.* **2014**, *259*, 735–743. [CrossRef] [PubMed]
45. Tang, Y.; Zhao, Y.; Song, X.; Song, X.; Niu, L.; Xie, L. Tumor-derived exosomal miRNA-320d as a biomarker for metastatic colorectal cancer. *J. Clin. Lab. Anal.* **2019**, *33*. [CrossRef]
46. Koga, Y.; Yamazaki, N.; Yamamoto, Y.; Yamamoto, S.; Saito, N.; Kakugawa, Y.; Otake, Y.; Matsumoto, M.; Matsumura, Y. Fecal miR-106a is a useful marker for colorectal cancer patients with false-negative results in immunochemical fecal occult blood test. *Cancer Epidemiol. Biomark. Prev.* **2013**, *22*, 1844–1852. [CrossRef] [PubMed]
47. Sazanov, A.A.; Kiselyova, E.V.; Zakharenko, A.A.; Romanov, M.N.; Zaraysky, M.I. Plasma and saliva miR-21 expression in colorectal cancer patients. *J. Appl. Genet.* **2017**, *58*, 231–237. [CrossRef] [PubMed]
48. Fu, F.; Jiang, W.; Zhou, L.; Chen, Z. Circulating exosomal miR-17-5p and miR-92a-3p predict pathologic stage and grade of colorectal cancer. *Transl. Oncol.* **2018**, *11*, 221–232. [CrossRef]
49. Tsukamoto, M.; Iinuma, H.; Yagi, T.; Matsuda, K.; Hashiguchi, Y. Circulating exosomal MicroRNA-21 as a biomarker in each tumor stage of colorectal cancer. *Oncology* **2017**, *92*, 360–370. [CrossRef]
50. Liu, C.; Eng, C.; Shen, J.; Lu, Y.; Takata, Y.; Mehdizadeh, A.; Chang, G.J.; Rodriguez-Bigas, M.A.; Li, Y.; Chang, P.; et al. Serum exosomal miR-4772-3p is a predictor of tumor recurrence in stage II and III colon cancer. *Oncotarget* **2016**, *7*, 76250–76260. [CrossRef]
51. Yan, S.; Jiang, Y.; Liang, C.; Cheng, M.; Jin, C.; Duan, Q.; Xu, D.; Yang, L.; Zhang, X.; Ren, B.; et al. Exosomal miR-6803-5p as potential diagnostic and prognostic marker in colorectal cancer. *J. Cell. Biochem.* **2018**, *119*, 4113–4119. [CrossRef]
52. Liu, X.; Pan, B.; Sun, L.; Chen, X.; Zeng, K.; Hu, X.; Xu, T.; Xu, M.; Wang, S. Circulating exosomal miR-27a and miR-130a act as novel diagnostic and prognostic biomarkers of colorectal cancer. *Cancer Epidemiol. Biomark. Prev.* **2018**, *27*, 746–754. [CrossRef]
53. Peng, Z.-Y.; Gu, R.-H.; Yan, B. Downregulation of exosome-encapsulated miR-548c-5p is associated with poor prognosis in colorectal cancer. *J. Cell. Biochem.* **2018**, *120*, 1457–1463. [CrossRef] [PubMed]
54. Jin, G.; Liu, Y.; Zhang, J.; Bian, Z.; Yao, S.; Fei, B.; Zhou, L.; Yin, Y.; Huang, Z. A panel of serum exosomal microRNAs as predictive markers for chemoresistance in advanced colorectal cancer. *Cancer Chemother. Pharmacol.* **2019**, *84*, 315–325. [CrossRef] [PubMed]
55. Yagi, T.; Iinuma, H.; Hayama, T.; Matsuda, K.; Nozawa, K.; Tsukamoto, M.; Shimada, R.; Akahane, T.; Tsuchiya, T.; Ozawa, T.; et al. Plasma exosomal microRNA-125b as a monitoring biomarker of resistance to mFOLFOX6-based chemotherapy in advanced and recurrent colorectal cancer patients. *Mol. Clin. Oncol.* **2019**, *11*, 416–424. [CrossRef] [PubMed]
56. Wang, M.; Han, D.; Yuan, Z.; Hu, H.; Zhao, Z.; Yang, R.; Jin, Y.; Zou, C.; Chen, Y.; Wang, G.; et al. Long non-coding RNA H19 confers 5-Fu resistance in colorectal cancer by promoting SIRT1-mediated autophagy. *Cell Death Dis.* **2018**, *9*, 1–14. [CrossRef] [PubMed]
57. Li, L.; Shang, J.; Zhang, Y.; Liu, S.; Peng, Y.; Zhou, Z.; Pan, H.; Wang, X.; Chen, L.; Zhao, Q. MEG3 is a prognostic factor for CRC and promotes chemosensitivity by enhancing oxaliplatin-induced cell apoptosis. *Oncol. Rep.* **2017**, *38*, 1383–1392. [CrossRef] [PubMed]
58. Sun, F.; Liang, W.; Qian, J. The identification of CRNDE, H19, UCA1 and HOTAIR as the key lncRNAs involved in oxaliplatin or irinotecan resistance in the chemotherapy of colorectal cancer based on integrative bioinformatics analysis. *Mol. Med. Rep.* **2019**, *20*, 3583–3596. [CrossRef]
59. Tang, J.; Yan, T.; Bao, Y.; Shen, C.; Yu, C.; Zhu, X.; Tian, X.; Guo, F.; Liang, Q.; Liu, Q.; et al. LncRNA GLCC1 promotes colorectal carcinogenesis and glucose metabolism by stabilizing c-Myc. *Nat. Commun.* **2019**, *10*, 3499. [CrossRef]

60. Liu, T.; Zhang, X.; Gao, S.; Jing, F.; Yang, Y.; Du, L.; Zheng, G.; Li, P.; Li, C.; Wang, C. Exosomal long noncoding RNA CRNDE-h as a novel serum-based biomarker for diagnosis and prognosis of colorectal cancer. *Oncotarget* **2016**, *7*, 85551–85563. [CrossRef]
61. Liang, Z.-X.; Liu, H.-S.; Wang, F.-W.; Xiong, L.; Zhou, C.; Hu, T.; He, X.-W.; Wu, X.-J.; Xie, D.; Wu, X.-R.; et al. LncRNA RPPH1 promotes colorectal cancer metastasis by interacting with TUBB3 and by promoting exosomes-mediated macrophage M2 polarization. *Cell Death Dis.* **2019**, *10*, 829. [CrossRef]
62. Bénard, F.; Barkun, A.N.; Martel, M.; von Renteln, D. Systematic review of colorectal cancer screening guidelines for average-risk adults: Summarizing the current global recommendations. *World J. Gastroenterol.* **2018**, *24*, 124–138. [CrossRef]
63. Marcuello, M.; Vymetalkova, V.; Neves, R.P.L.; Duran-Sanchon, S.; Vedeld, H.M.; Tham, E.; van Dalum, G.; Flügen, G.; Garcia-Barberan, V.; Fijneman, R.J.A.; et al. Circulating biomarkers for early detection and clinical management of colorectal cancer. *Mol. Asp. Med.* **2019**, *69*, 107–122. [CrossRef] [PubMed]
64. Cima, I.; Kong, S.L.; Sengupta, D.; Tan, I.B.; Phyo, W.M.; Lee, D.; Hu, M.; Iliescu, C.; Alexander, I.; Goh, W.L.; et al. Tumor-derived circulating endothelial cell clusters in colorectal cancer. *Sci. Transl. Med.* **2016**, *8*, 345ra89. [CrossRef] [PubMed]
65. Bi, F.; Wang, Q.; Dong, Q.; Wang, Y.; Zhang, L.; Zhang, J. Circulating tumor DNA in colorectal cancer: Opportunities and challenges. *Am. J. Transl. Res.* **2020**, *12*, 1044–1055.
66. Wang, X.; Shi, X.-Q.; Zeng, P.-W.; Mo, F.-M.; Chen, Z.-H. Circulating cell free DNA as the diagnostic marker for colorectal cancer: A systematic review and meta-analysis. *Oncotarget* **2018**, *9*, 24514–24524. [CrossRef] [PubMed]
67. Luo, H.; Zhao, Q.; Wei, W.; Zheng, L.; Yi, S.; Li, G.; Wang, W.; Sheng, H.; Pu, H.; Mo, H.; et al. Circulating tumor DNA methylation profiles enable early diagnosis, prognosis prediction, and screening for colorectal cancer. *Sci. Transl. Med.* **2020**, *12*. [CrossRef] [PubMed]
68. Nian, J.; Sun, X.; Ming, S.; Yan, C.; Ma, Y.; Feng, Y.; Yang, L.; Yu, M.; Zhang, G.; Wang, X. Diagnostic accuracy of methylated SEPT9 for blood-based colorectal cancer detection: A systematic review and meta-analysis. *Clin. Transl. Gastroenterol.* **2017**, *8*, e216. [CrossRef]
69. Cohen, J.D.; Li, L.; Wang, Y.; Thoburn, C.; Afsari, B.; Danilova, L.; Douville, C.; Javed, A.A.; Wong, F.; Mattox, A.; et al. Detection and localization of surgically resectable cancers with a multi-analyte blood test. *Science* **2018**, *359*, 926–930. [CrossRef]
70. O'Brien, J.; Hayder, H.; Zayed, Y.; Peng, C. Overview of MicroRNA Biogenesis, Mechanisms of Actions, and Circulation. *Front. Endocrinol. Lausanne* **2018**, *9*, 402. [CrossRef]
71. Ragusa, M.; Statello, L.; Maugeri, M.; Majorana, A.; Barbagallo, D.; Salito, L.; Sammito, M.; Santonocito, M.; Angelica, R.; Cavallaro, A.; et al. Specific alterations of the microRNA transcriptome and global network structure in colorectal cancer after treatment with MAPK/ERK inhibitors. *J. Mol. Med.* **2012**, *90*, 1421–1438. [CrossRef]
72. Chen, B.; Xia, Z.; Deng, Y.-N.; Yang, Y.; Zhang, P.; Zhu, H.; Xu, N.; Liang, S. Emerging microRNA biomarkers for colorectal cancer diagnosis and prognosis. *Open Biol.* **2019**, *9*, 180212. [CrossRef]
73. Rapado-González, Ó.; Majem, B.; Muinelo-Romay, L.; Álvarez-Castro, A.; Santamaría, A.; Gil-Moreno, A.; López-López, R.; Suárez-Cunqueiro, M.M. Human salivary microRNAs in Cancer. *J. Cancer* **2018**, *9*, 638–649. [CrossRef] [PubMed]
74. Tellez-Gabriel, M.; Heymann, M.-F.; Heymann, D. Circulating tumor cells as a tool for assessing tumor heterogeneity. *Theranostics* **2019**, *9*, 4580–4594. [CrossRef] [PubMed]
75. Huang, X.; Gao, P.; Song, Y.; Sun, J.; Chen, X.; Zhao, J.; Liu, J.; Xu, H.; Wang, Z. Relationship between circulating tumor cells and tumor response in colorectal cancer patients treated with chemotherapy: A meta-analysis. *BMC Cancer* **2014**, *14*, 976. [CrossRef] [PubMed]
76. Bettegowda, C.; Sausen, M.; Leary, R.J.; Kinde, I.; Wang, Y.; Agrawal, N.; Bartlett, B.R.; Wang, H.; Luber, B.; Alani, R.M.; et al. Detection of Circulating Tumor DNA in Early- and Late-Stage Human Malignancies. *Sci. Transl. Med.* **2014**, *6*, 224ra24. [CrossRef] [PubMed]
77. Dasari, A.; Morris, V.K.; Allegra, C.J.; Atreya, C.; Benson, A.B.; Boland, P.; Chung, K.; Copur, M.S.; Corcoran, R.B.; Deming, D.A.; et al. ctDNA applications and integration in colorectal cancer: An NCI Colon and Rectal–Anal Task Forces whitepaper. *Nat. Rev. Clin. Oncol.* **2020**, 1–14. [CrossRef]
78. Osumi, H.; Shinozaki, E.; Yamaguchi, K. Circulating tumor DNA as a novel biomarker optimizing chemotherapy for colorectal cancer. *Cancers* **2020**, *12*, 1566. [CrossRef]

79. Siravegna, G.; Mussolin, B.; Buscarino, M.; Corti, G.; Cassingena, A.; Crisafulli, G.; Ponzetti, A.; Cremolini, C.; Amatu, A.; Lauricella, C.; et al. Clonal evolution and resistance to EGFR blockade in the blood of colorectal cancer patients. *Nat. Med.* **2015**, *21*, 795–801. [CrossRef]
80. Khan, K.H.; Cunningham, D.; Werner, B.; Vlachogiannis, G.; Spiteri, I.; Heide, T.; Mateos, J.F.; Vatsiou, A.; Lampis, A.; Damavandi, M.D.; et al. longitudinal liquid biopsy and mathematical modeling of clonal evolution forecast time to treatment failure in the PROSPECT-C Phase II colorectal cancer clinical trial. *Cancer Discov.* **2018**, *8*, 1270–1285. [CrossRef]
81. Siravegna, G.; Sartore-Bianchi, A.; Nagy, R.J.; Raghav, K.; Odegaard, J.I.; Lanman, R.B.; Trusolino, L.; Marsoni, S.; Siena, S.; Bardelli, A. Plasma HER2 (ERBB2) Copy Number Predicts Response to HER2-targeted Therapy in Metastatic Colorectal Cancer. *Clin. Cancer Res.* **2019**, *25*, 3046–3053. [CrossRef]
82. To, K.K.; Tong, C.W.; Wu, M.; Cho, W.C. MicroRNAs in the prognosis and therapy of colorectal cancer: From bench to bedside. *World J. Gastroenterol.* **2018**, *24*, 2949–2973. [CrossRef]
83. Zhang, K.; Zhang, L.; Zhang, M.; Zhang, Y.; Fan, D.; Jiang, J.; Ye, L.; Fang, X.; Chen, X.; Fan, S.; et al. Prognostic value of high-expression of miR-17-92 cluster in various tumors: Evidence from a meta-analysis. *Sci. Rep.* **2017**, *7*, 8375. [CrossRef]
84. Ma, Q.; Wang, Y.; Zhang, H.; Wang, F. miR-1290 Contributes to Colorectal Cancer Cell Proliferation by Targeting INPP4B. *Oncol. Res.* **2018**, *26*, 1167–1174. [CrossRef] [PubMed]
85. Falzone, L.; Scola, L.; Zanghì, A.; Biondi, A.; Di Cataldo, A.; Libra, M.; Candido, S. Integrated analysis of colorectal cancer microRNA datasets: Identification of microRNAs associated with tumor development. *Aging Albany N. Y.* **2018**, *10*, 1000–1014. [CrossRef] [PubMed]
86. Ragusa, M.; Majorana, A.; Statello, L.; Maugeri, M.; Salito, L.; Barbagallo, D.; Guglielmino, M.R.; Duro, L.R.; Angelica, R.; Caltabiano, R.; et al. Specific alterations of microRNA transcriptome and global network structure in colorectal carcinoma after cetuximab treatment. *Mol. Cancer Ther.* **2010**, *9*, 3396–3409. [CrossRef] [PubMed]
87. Nagano, T.; Fraser, P. No-nonsense functions for long noncoding RNAs. *Cell* **2011**, *145*, 178–181. [CrossRef] [PubMed]
88. Zhang, X.; Wang, W.; Zhu, W.; Dong, J.; Cheng, Y.; Yin, Z.; Shen, F. Mechanisms and Functions of Long Non-Coding RNAs at Multiple Regulatory Levels. *Int. J. Mol. Sci.* **2019**, *20*, 5573. [CrossRef]
89. Xie, X.; Tang, B.; Xiao, Y.-F.; Xie, R.; Li, B.-S.; Dong, H.; Zhou, J.-Y.; Yang, S.-M. Long non-coding RNAs in colorectal cancer. *Oncotarget* **2015**, *7*, 5226–5239. [CrossRef]
90. Siddiqui, H.; Al-Ghafari, A.; Choudhry, H.; Al Doghaither, H. Roles of long non-coding RNAs in colorectal cancer tumorigenesis: A Review. *Mol. Clin. Oncol.* **2019**, *11*, 167–172. [CrossRef]
91. He, Q.; Long, J.; Yin, Y.; Li, Y.; Lei, X.; Li, Z.; Zhu, W. Emerging Roles of lncRNAs in the Formation and Progression of Colorectal Cancer. *Front. Oncol.* **2020**, *9*. [CrossRef]
92. Han, D.; Wang, M.; Ma, N.; Xu, Y.; Jiang, Y.; Gao, X. Long noncoding RNAs: Novel players in colorectal cancer. *Cancer Lett.* **2015**, *361*, 13–21. [CrossRef]
93. Luo, J.; Qu, J.; Wu, D.-K.; Lu, Z.-L.; Sun, Y.-S.; Qu, Q. Long non-coding RNAs: A rising biotarget in colorectal cancer. *Oncotarget* **2017**, *8*, 22187–22202. [CrossRef]
94. Valli, A.; Morotti, M.; Zois, C.E.; Albers, P.K.; Soga, T.; Feldinger, K.; Fischer, R.; Frejno, M.; McIntyre, A.; Bridges, E.; et al. Adaptation to HIF1α Deletion in Hypoxic Cancer Cells by Upregulation of GLUT14 and Creatine Metabolism. *Mol. Cancer Res.* **2019**, *17*, 1531–1544. [CrossRef]
95. Barbagallo, C.; Brex, D.; Caponnetto, A.; Cirnigliaro, M.; Scalia, M.; Magnano, A.; Caltabiano, R.; Barbagallo, D.; Biondi, A.; Cappellani, A.; et al. LncRNA UCA1, Upregulated in CRC Biopsies and Downregulated in Serum Exosomes, Controls mRNA Expression by RNA-RNA Interactions. *Mol. Ther. Nucleic Acids* **2018**, *12*, 229–241. [CrossRef]
96. Beije, N.; Martens, J.W.M.; Sleijfer, S. Incorporating liquid biopsies into treatment decision-making: Obstacles and possibilities. *Drug Discov. Today* **2019**, *24*, 1715–1719. [CrossRef]
97. Kolenčík, D.; Shishido, S.N.; Pitule, P.; Mason, J.; Hicks, J.; Kuhn, P. Liquid Biopsy in Colorectal Carcinoma: Clinical Applications and Challenges. *Cancers* **2020**, *12*, 1376. [CrossRef]
98. Leers, M.P.G. Circulating tumor DNA and their added value in molecular oncology. *Clin. Chem. Lab. Med. CCLM* **2020**, *58*, 152–161. [CrossRef]
99. Hong, B.; Zu, Y. Detecting circulating tumor cells: Current challenges and new trends. *Theranostics* **2013**, *3*, 377–394. [CrossRef]

100. Mamdouhi, T.; Twomey, J.D.; McSweeney, K.M.; Zhang, B. Fugitives on the run: Circulating tumor cells (CTCs) in metastatic diseases. *Cancer Metastasis Rev.* **2019**, *38*, 297–305. [CrossRef]
101. Millner, L.M.; Linder, M.W.; Valdes, R. Circulating tumor cells: A review of present methods and the need to identify heterogeneous phenotypes. *Ann. Clin. Lab. Sci.* **2013**, *43*, 295–304.
102. Barrière, G.; Tartary, M.; Rigaud, M. Epithelial mesenchymal transition: A new insight into the detection of circulating tumor cells. *ISRN Oncol.* **2012**, *2012*. [CrossRef]
103. Castro-Giner, F.; Gkountela, S.; Donato, C.; Alborelli, I.; Quagliata, L.; Ng, C.K.Y.; Piscuoglio, S.; Aceto, N. Cancer diagnosis using a liquid biopsy: Challenges and expectations. *Diagnostics* **2018**, *8*, 31. [CrossRef]
104. Elazezy, M.; Joosse, S.A. Techniques of using circulating tumor DNA as a liquid biopsy component in cancer management. *Comput. Struct. Biotechnol. J.* **2018**, *16*, 370–378. [CrossRef]
105. D'Haene, N.; Fontanges, Q.; De Nève, N.; Blanchard, O.; Melendez, B.; Delos, M.; Dehou, M.-F.; Maris, C.; Nagy, N.; Rousseau, E.; et al. Clinical application of targeted next-generation sequencing for colorectal cancer patients: A multicentric Belgian experience. *Oncotarget* **2018**, *9*, 20761–20768. [CrossRef]
106. Qin, D. Next-generation sequencing and its clinical application. *Cancer Biol. Med.* **2019**, *16*, 4–10. [CrossRef]
107. Narayan, A.; Carriero, N.J.; Gettinger, S.N.; Kluytenaar, J.; Kozak, K.R.; Yock, T.I.; Muscato, N.E.; Ugarelli, P.; Decker, R.H.; Patel, A.A. Ultrasensitive measurement of hotspot mutations in tumor DNA in blood using error-suppressed multiplexed deep sequencing. *Cancer Res.* **2012**, *72*, 3492–3498. [CrossRef]
108. Couraud, S.; Vaca-Paniagua, F.; Villar, S.; Oliver, J.; Schuster, T.; Blanché, H.; Girard, N.; Trédaniel, J.; Guilleminault, L.; Gervais, R.; et al. Noninvasive diagnosis of actionable mutations by deep sequencing of circulating free DNA in lung cancer from never-smokers: A proof-of-concept study from BioCAST/IFCT-1002. *Clin. Cancer Res.* **2014**, *20*, 4613–4624. [CrossRef]
109. Fontanges, Q.; De Mendonca, R.; Salmon, I.; Le Mercier, M.; D'Haene, N. Clinical application of targeted next generation sequencing for colorectal cancers. *Int. J. Mol. Sci.* **2016**, *17*, 2117. [CrossRef]
110. Grada, A.; Weinbrecht, K. Next-generation sequencing: Methodology and application. *J. Investig. Dermatol.* **2013**, *133*, e11. [CrossRef]
111. Ng, C.; Li, H.; Wu, W.K.K.; Wong, S.H.; Yu, J. Genomics and metagenomics of colorectal cancer. *J. Gastrointest. Oncol.* **2019**, *10*, 1164–1170. [CrossRef]
112. Kim, R.Y.; Xu, H.; Myllykangas, S.; Ji, H. Genetic-based biomarkers and next-generation sequencing: The future of personalized care in colorectal cancer. *Pers. Med.* **2011**, *8*, 331–345. [CrossRef]
113. Wadapurkar, R.M.; Vyas, R. Computational analysis of next generation sequencing data and its applications in clinical oncology. *Inform. Med. Unlocked* **2018**, *11*, 75–82. [CrossRef]
114. Rachiglio, A.M.; Abate, R.E.; Sacco, A.; Pasquale, R.; Fenizia, F.; Lambiase, M.; Morabito, A.; Montanino, A.; Rocco, G.; Romano, C.; et al. Limits and potential of targeted sequencing analysis of liquid biopsy in patients with lung and colon carcinoma. *Oncotarget* **2016**, *7*, 66595–66605. [CrossRef] [PubMed]
115. Del Vecchio, F.; Mastroiaco, V.; Di Marco, A.; Compagnoni, C.; Capece, D.; Zazzeroni, F.; Capalbo, C.; Alesse, E.; Tessitore, A. Next-generation sequencing: Recent applications to the analysis of colorectal cancer. *J. Transl. Med.* **2017**, *15*, 246. [CrossRef]
116. Soda, N.; Rehm, B.H.A.; Sonar, P.; Nguyen, N.-T.; Shiddiky, M.J.A. Advanced liquid biopsy technologies for circulating biomarker detection. *J. Mater. Chem. B* **2019**, *7*, 6670–6704. [CrossRef]
117. Risberg, B.; Tsui, D.W.Y.; Biggs, H.; Ruiz-Valdepenas Martin de Almagro, A.; Dawson, S.-J.; Hodgkin, C.; Jones, L.; Parkinson, C.; Piskorz, A.; Marass, F.; et al. Effects of Collection and Processing Procedures on Plasma Circulating Cell-Free DNA from Cancer Patients. *J. Mol. Diagn.* **2018**, *20*, 883–892. [CrossRef]
118. Grölz, D.; Hauch, S.; Schlumpberger, M.; Guenther, K.; Voss, T.; Sprenger-Haussels, M.; Oelmüller, U. Liquid Biopsy Preservation Solutions for Standardized Pre-Analytical Workflows—Venous Whole Blood and Plasma. *Curr. Pathobiol. Rep.* **2018**, *6*, 275–286. [CrossRef]
119. Harouaka, R.; Kang, Z.; Zheng, S.; Cao, L. Circulating tumor cells: Advances in isolation and analysis, and challenges for clinical applications. *Pharmacol. Ther.* **2014**, *141*, 209–221. [CrossRef]
120. Tamkovich, S.N.; Cherepanova, A.V.; Kolesnikova, E.V.; Rykova, E.Y.; Pyshnyi, D.V.; Vlassov, V.V.; Laktionov, P.P. Circulating DNA and DNase activity in human blood. *Ann. N. Y. Acad. Sci.* **2006**, *1075*, 191–196. [CrossRef]
121. Siravegna, G.; Mussolin, B.; Venesio, T.; Marsoni, S.; Seoane, J.; Dive, C.; Papadopoulos, N.; Kopetz, S.; Corcoran, R.B.; Siu, L.L.; et al. How liquid biopsies can change clinical practice in oncology. *Ann. Oncol.* **2019**, *30*, 1580–1590. [CrossRef]

122. Heitzer, E.; Haque, I.S.; Roberts, C.E.S.; Speicher, M.R. Current and future perspectives of liquid biopsies in genomics-driven oncology. *Nat. Rev. Genet.* **2019**, *20*, 71–88. [CrossRef]
123. Haselmann, V.; Ahmad-Nejad, P.; Geilenkeuser, W.J.; Duda, A.; Gabor, M.; Eichner, R.; Patton, S.; Neumaier, M. Results of the first external quality assessment scheme (EQA) for isolation and analysis of circulating tumour DNA (ctDNA). *Clin. Chem. Lab. Med.* **2018**, *56*, 220–228. [CrossRef]
124. Vivancos, A.; Aranda, E.; Benavides, M.; Élez, E.; Gómez-España, M.A.; Toledano, M.; Alvarez, M.; Parrado, M.R.C.; García-Barberán, V.; Diaz-Rubio, E. Comparison of the Clinical Sensitivity of the Idylla Platform and the OncoBEAM RAS CRC Assay for KRAS Mutation Detection in Liquid Biopsy Samples. *Sci. Rep.* **2019**, *9*. [CrossRef]

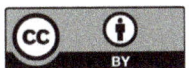

© 2020 by the authors. Licensee MDPI, Basel, Switzerland. This article is an open access article distributed under the terms and conditions of the Creative Commons Attribution (CC BY) license (http://creativecommons.org/licenses/by/4.0/).

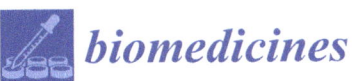

Review

What Is Known about Theragnostic Strategies in Colorectal Cancer

Alessandro Parisi [1,2], Giampiero Porzio [2,3], Fanny Pulcini [3], Katia Cannita [2,3], Corrado Ficorella [2,3], Vincenzo Mattei [4] and Simona Delle Monache [3,*]

1. Department of Life, Health and Environmental Sciences, University of L'Aquila, 67100 L'Aquila, Italy; alexparis@hotmail.it
2. Medical Oncology Unit, St. Salvatore Hospital, 67100 L'Aquila, Italy; porzio.giampiero@gmail.com (G.P.); kcannita@gmail.com (K.C.); corrado.ficorella@univaq.it (C.F.)
3. Department of Biotechnology and Applied Clinical Sciences, University of L'Aquila, 67100 L'Aquila, Italy; fanny.pulcini@graduate.univaq.it
4. Biomedicine and Advanced Technologies Rieti Center, Sabina Universitas, via Angelo Maria Ricci 35A, 02100 Rieti, Italy; v.mattei@sabinauniversitas.it
* Correspondence: simona.dellemonache@univaq.it; Tel.: +39-086-243-3569

Abstract: Despite the paradigmatic shift occurred in recent years for defined molecular subtypes in the metastatic setting treatment, colorectal cancer (CRC) still remains an incurable disease in most of the cases. Therefore, there is an urgent need for new tools and biomarkers for both early tumor diagnosis and to improve personalized treatment. Thus, liquid biopsy has emerged as a minimally invasive tool that is capable of detecting genomic alterations from primary or metastatic tumors, allowing the prognostic stratification of patients, the detection of the minimal residual disease after surgical or systemic treatments, the monitoring of therapeutic response, and the development of resistance, establishing an opportunity for early intervention before imaging detection or worsening of clinical symptoms. On the other hand, preclinical and clinical evidence demonstrated the role of gut microbiota dysbiosis in promoting inflammatory responses and cancer initiation. Altered gut microbiota is associated with resistance to chemo drugs and immune checkpoint inhibitors, whereas the use of microbe-targeted therapies including antibiotics, pre-probiotics, and fecal microbiota transplantation can restore response to anticancer drugs, promote immune response, and therefore support current treatment strategies in CRC. In this review, we aim to summarize preclinical and clinical evidence for the utilization of liquid biopsy and gut microbiota in CRC.

Keywords: CRC; liquid biopsy; CTC; ctDNA; mi-RNA; nc-RNA; gut microbiota

1. Introduction

Colorectal cancer (CRC) is the third leading cause of cancer-related death and morbidity worldwide according to the global cancer statistics (GLOBOCAN) presented in 2018. The 5-year survival rate ranges from 90% to 14% if CRC is diagnosed at a localized or metastatic stage, respectively, and approximately 25% of CRC patients present metastatic disease at diagnosis, while almost half of them will develop metastases [1].

If early diagnosis and treatment of CRC can significantly improve the cure rate, traditional biomarkers (Carcino Embryonic Antigen (CEA), Carbohydrate Antigen 19-9 (CA19-9), Fecal Occult Blood Test (FOBT)) as well as colon/sigmoidoscopy do not fully satisfy clinical needs in CRC screening due to their lack in sensitivity and specificity [2]. Furthermore, primary tumor resection is eventually associated to adjuvant chemotherapy with fluoropyrimidines with or without oxaliplatin according to TNM stage and pathological risk factors in early CRC [3], does not always seem sufficient to eliminate circulating tumor cells (CTCs) and other components involved in establishing pre-metastatic niche-promoting immune evasion and maintenance of stemness [4].

Circulating tumor DNA (ctDNA) and RNAs and non-coding RNAs (ncRNAs) released into the bloodstream via microvescicles or tumor cell lysis represent, together with CTCs, different sides of the same coin: liquid biopsy. Liquid biopsy has emerged as a promising minimally invasive tool for precision medicine due to its ability to provide multiple global snapshots of primary and metastatic tumors at different times and more representative images of the spatial and temporal tumor heterogeneity [5] compared to tissue biopsy. In fact, even though tissue biopsy remains the gold standard for the histopatological definition and the molecular stratification of tumors, it is often difficult to perform, especially in relapsed and metastatic settings, and it does not support intratumoral heterogeneity and clonal evolutions related to driver mutations, which may occur during tumor development or treatment.

Among other elements potentially involved in cancer initiation, development, recurrence, and metastasis, one that only recently received its due attention is the host microbiota—and for CRC, especially the gut microbiota. The host microbiota is composed of bacteria (≈99%), viruses, and mycetes, existing in a condition of eubosis with the human body conferring important benefits related to physical and mental health, and the development of the individual [6]. In turn, this dynamic balance is affected by host genetics, lifestyle [7], and dietary habits [8] and gut microbiota dysbiosis may play a role in promoting inflammatory responses and alterations of the immunosurveillance, which can led to cancer initiation and/or progression [9].

In this review, we summarize the state of the art regarding the potential role and the future perspectives of liquid biopsy and host microbiome as "theragnostic" tools in CRC (Figure 1).

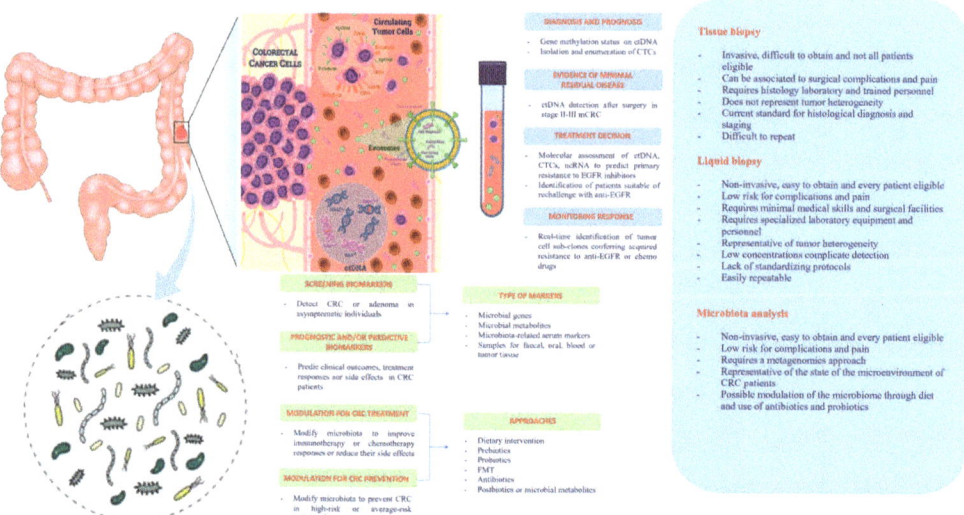

Figure 1. Potential clinical applications related to liquid biopsy and gut microbiota in colorectal cancer. Circulating tumor cells (CTCs), circulating tumor DNA (ctDNA), non-coding RNA (ncRNA), and exosomes are promising liquid biopsy markers for colorectal cancer with multiple potential advantages compared to tissue biopsy. CTCs from colorectal cancer (CRC) can be shed from the primary tumor into the bloodstream, which also contains ctDNA released from tumor tissue through apoptosis, necrosis, and secretion, as well as circulating normal DNA released from healthy tissue. NcRNAs (miRNAs and lncRNAs) encapsulated by exosomes can be actively secreted into the extracellular fluid by various types of cells in the tumor or passively released due to the apoptosis and necrosis of tumor cells and can eventually be found in the circulation. Besides liquid biopsy, several potential clinical applications for harnessing the gut microbiota in CRC include development of screening, prognostic and predictive biomarkers, and microbiota modulation for CRC prevention and treatment. FMT, fecal microbiota transplantation.

2. Liquid Biopsy

The term liquid biopsy refers to procedures of isolation of cancer-derived components such as CTCs, exosomes, ctDNA, ncRNAs, and proteins from peripheral blood or other body fluids, and their genomic or proteomic evaluation [10]. Assessment of such elements via non-invasive and low-risk blood-based detection tests could improve CRC screening, diagnosis, staging, and predict relapse and metastasis [11,12] and be effective in monitoring residual disease and drug resistance in CRC patients receiving systemic treatment [13,14].

2.1. Circulating Tumor Cells (CTCs)

CTCs are tumor cells released into the bloodstream from the primary tumor or metastases [15], which could escape from immune recognition and drug treatment, and subsequently form a niche in other tissues, promoting tumor recurrence and metastasis [16].

2.1.1. Screening and Early Diagnosis

Since counting CTCs reflects the patient's tumor burden and the CTCs detection rate is positively correlated to the TNM stages, it is rather difficult and quite uncommon to detect CTCs in early-stage CRC, and therefore, their utility in CRC screening and early detection seems to be very poor [17]. However, a recent prospective study involving 667 patients (including healthy control subjects, patients with adenomas, and those with stage I–IV CRC) showed a significant association between CTC counts (performed using a novel CTC assay) and worsening disease status with respect to the adenoma-carcinoma sequence. Furthermore, the assay showed high specificity (86%) and sensitivity across all CRC stages (95%) and adenomatous lesions (79%) [18].

2.1.2. Prognostic and Predictive Factor, Staging Tool and Guide for Systemic Treatment, Resistance Evaluation, and MRD Assessment

CTCs could potentially play a role as a prognostic marker, in monitoring treatment outcomes and follow-up, for modulating the intensity of systemic therapies and for detecting resistance against these. A meta-analysis of 15 studies including 3129 non-metastatic and metastatic CRC (non-mCRC and mCRC) patients showed significantly worse progression-free survival (PFS) and overall survival (OS) for CTC-positive with respect to CTC-negative CRC patients, regardless of sampling time (baseline or during treatment), detection methods (CellSearch, RT-PCR and others), and cut-off value of CTC (≥ 1, ≥ 2 and $\geq 3/7.5$ mL blood), thus providing strong evidence for the presence of CTCs as an independent prognostic factor of poor survival [19]. A study conducted on 158 patients showed that rising of CTCs counts in 2 mL of peripheral blood (0 for healthy, 1 for benign, 5 for non-mCRC, and 36 for mCRC patients) was associated with tumor progression and poor prognosis at baseline. Notably, after 2 year follow-up on the non-mCRC patients, those who had ≥ 5 CTCs were eight times more likely to develop distant metastasis within one year after curable surgery than those who had <5 [20], therefore providing a support to the possible application of CTC detection during the follow-up of early CRC patients. Intensive first-line regimens with a triplet chemotherapy backbone plus the antiangiogenic bevacizumab provided better survival outcome if compared with doublet regimens, especially in *RAS-BRAF* mutated mCRC [21,22], paying the price of a major incidence of adverse events. Patient stratification by CTC detection could help modulate the intensity of the systemic treatment by reserving a more aggressive therapy to patients with a worse prognosis. In the randomized phase III VISNÚ-1 trial, a first-line systemic treatment with FOLFOXIRI (oxaliplatin, irinotecan, 5-fluorouracil (5-FU), and leucovorin) plus bevacizumab significantly improved PFS compared with FOLFOX (association of oxaliplatin, 5-FU, and leucovorin) plus bevacizumab in mCRC patients with ≥ 3 CTCs/7.5 mL blood at baseline [22]. In *RAS-BRAF* wild-type mCRC, a standard first-line regimen includes a doublet chemotherapy backbone in association with an anti-EGFR antibody (panitumumab or cetuximab), usually followed at disease progression by the alternative doublet regimen in association with an antiangiogenic drug [23,24]. As showed by a prospective study on 38 *RAS-BRAF* wild-type mCRC patients who received a third-line treatment with irinotecan and cetuximab, early CTC-negative and CTC status changes assessment during treatment were significantly associated with tumor response and better PFS and OS, predicting treatment failure in advance compared to imaging-based tools [25].

2.2. Circulating Tumor DNA (ctDNA)

Circulating tumor DNA (CtDNA) is a kind of double-stranded DNA, a fragment of cell-free DNA (cfDNA), that originates from active, apoptotic, necrotic, or circulating tumor cells. CtDNA retains epigenetic characteristics and harbors tumor-specific mutations detectable in the bloodstream and other body fluids [10,26]. Importantly, ctDNA half-life varies from several minutes to a few hours, and as for CTCs, its plasma levels depend on tumor load, ranging from 50% to 90% in non-metastatic and metastatic cancer patients, respectively [4,10,25,27]. Furthermore, healthy people and cancer patients can be distinguished according to the fragment length distribution pattern of cfDNA [26]. These data suggest that ctDNA analysis may represent a real-time tumor burden assessment.

2.2.1. Screening and Early Diagnosis

Even if a recent meta-analysis concerning quantitative analysis of ctDNA for CRC screening, including 1258 CRC patients and 803 healthy individuals from 14 studies, concluded that the diagnostic accuracy of ctDNA has unsatisfactory sensitivity but acceptable specificity for CRC diagnosis [28], there is growing evidence that ctDNA detection could be used along with the traditional screening methods (i.e., colonscopy, FOBT, digital rectal examination, and serum tumor marker) to improve the diagnosis of early CRC [16,29]. In particular, ctDNA, especially when combined with carcinoembryonic antigen (CEA), showed higher diagnostic capacity (area under the ROC curve (AUC) 0.92, with 84% sensitivity and 88% specificity) [30]. Furthermore, epigenetic changes as DNA methylation and histone modifications are early events in carcinogenesis and clinical data that suggest that ctDNA methylation shows better sensitivity than traditional serum tumor markers in early-stage CRC [31,32]. Particularly, a meta-analysis of 25 studies assessing the diagnostic role of methylated Septin 9 (mSEPT9) promoter in ctDNA for CRC screening highlighted the efficacy of Epi proColon 2.0 with 2/3 algorithm (Epigenomics). A positive ratio of mSEPT9 was higher in advanced CRC stages (45%, 70%, 76%, 79% in I, III, III, and IV, respectively) and low-grade tumors (31%, 73% and 90% in high, moderate, and low grade, respectively), with a sensitivity, specificity, and AUC of 0.71, 0.92, and 0.88, respectively. Previous results confirmed the poor ability of mSEPT9 to identify precancerous lesions [31]. On the other hand, a recent prospective cohort study conducted on a high-risk population of 1493 individuals demonstrated that a particular single ctDNA methylation marker, cg10673833, could reach high sensitivity (89.7%) and specificity (86.8%) for the detection of CRC and precancerous lesions [32].

2.2.2. Prognostic and Predictive Factor, Staging Tool, and Guide for Systemic Treatment, Resistance Evaluation, and MRD Assessment

A systematic review and metanalysis including 1076 mCRC patients treated with chemotherapy and/or targeted agents showed that lower baseline levels of cfDNA correlated with better OS [33]. A more recent systematic review and meta-analysis including 1779 non-mCRC and mCRC patients found that the presence or high concentration of ctDNA with KRAS mutation was associated with poor disease-free survival (DFS), PFS, and OS [34]. Moreover, as anti-EGFR therapy with cetuximab and panitumumab is approved for wild-type *RAS* mCRC and *KRAS* and *BRAF* are considered effective predictors of anti-EGFR therapy [35,36], ctDNA detection could represent an alternative tool for the selection of anti-EGFR treatment due to its correlation with *RAS* mutational status of tumor tissue [37]. In particular, *RAS* clones raised in blood during EGFR blockade decline after the withdrawal of anti-EGFR antibodies, therefore restoring the drug sensitivity of cancer cells and providing a rationale for anti-EGFR retreatment [37]. Moreover, ctDNA has a great potential to supplement Response Evaluation Criteria in Solid Tumors (RECIST) evaluation.

As already discussed, ctDNA is strictly dependent by tumor load, and tumor burden can be monitored in real-time due to the short half-life of ctDNA [26,27]. Compared to radiological approaches, serial monitoring of ctDNA is able to track treatment response weeks to months earlier, allowing anticipating disease progression and modifying treatment consequently [37]. A prospective phase II clinical trial of cetuximab in *RAS* wild-type mCRC patients combined the sequential profiling of ctDNA and matched tissue biopsies with imaging and mathematical modeling of cancer evolution, showing that liquid biopsies were able to detect spatial and temporal heterogeneity of resistance to anti-EGFR monoclonal antibodies [38]. In another phase II trial that tested the multikinase inhibitor regorafenib in *RAS* mutated mCRC patients, combining dynamic contrast-enhanced (DCE), MRI, and ctDNA predicts the duration of antiangiogenic response to regorafenib, improving patient management with potential health and economic implications [39]. As for CTCs, ctDNA concentration is positively correlated with tumor size, resulting lower in stage I with respect to stage IV CRC patients [15,16,40]. As a result of the strong link between CTCs, ctDNA, primary tumor, and metastasis, it has been suggested to integrate the blood-based liquid biopsy into the actual TNM staging system, and the concept of "TNMB" (B as blood) has been proposed to improve the existing cancer staging system [2,4,41]. In this regard, the ability to optimize systemic treatments, especially in the adjuvant setting in stage II-III CRC patients, has been historically limited by the use of clinicopathologic characteristics, which are not always able to properly prognosticate the risk of recurrence [42], and by conventional surveillance modalities (CEA, computed tomography (CT), and colonoscopy), which are not perfectly able to identify MRD and early recurrence [2,4,11,12]. In a prospective cohort of 230 stage II CRC patients, 7.9% were postoperative ctDNA positive, 79% of whom relapsed, while disease relapse occurred only in 9.8% of ctDNA-negative patients. The presence of ctDNA after the completion of chemotherapy was also associated with worse recurrence-free survival [43]. In a recent prospective cohort of 130 stage I–III CRC patients, ctDNA was quantified pre- and postoperatively, and after adjuvant chemotherapy. CtDNA-positive patients after surgery, adjuvant chemotherapy, and during follow-up were respectively 7, 17, and 40 times more likely to relapse with respect to ctDNA-negative patients [44]. Some authors proposed that monitoring ctDNA levels every 3-6 months after surgery can be used to supplement serum markers, CT, endoscopy, and other conventional monitoring tools, emphasizing that positive ctDNA preceded radiological and clinical evidence of recurrence by a median of 3 months, even if 6% of patients with positive ctDNA never relapsed [45]. A great effort is ongoing to validate the clinical utility of ctDNA, particularly in the adjuvant setting of CRC (Table 1).

Table 1. List of major ongoing prospective trials investigating liquid biopsy in colorectal cancer.

Brief Study Title	NCT Number/Study Name	Country Study Period	Stage	N	Study Type/Phase/Endp	Target/Assay-Test (If Available)	Study Overview/Schematic Description
ctDNA Analysis Informing ACT in Stage III CRC	ACTRN12617001566325 (DYNAMIC-III)	Australia 2017–2024	III	1000	Int rand/2–3/DFS, OS, ctDNA clear	ctDNA	Surgery followed by ctDNA detection and clinician's choice ACT (no ACT > fluoropyrimidine > XELOX/FOLFOX) followed by randomization to: (1) SOC arm: SOC ACT (ctDNA blinded) or (2) EXP arm ctDNA+: escalated ACT (FOLFOXIRI allowed) or (3) EXP arm ctDNA-: de-escalated ACT
ctDNA Analysis Informing ACT in Stage II CRC	ACTRN12615000381583 (DYNAMIC II)	Australia 2015–2024	II	450	Int rand/2/DFS, OS, ctDNA clear	ctDNA	Surgery followed by ctDNA detection and randomization to: (1) SOC arm: SOC, (2) EXP arm ctDNA+: ACT (fluoropyrimidine or XELOX/FOLFOX according to clinician's choice), (3) EXP arm ctDNA-: follow-up
Tracking mutations in ctDNA to predict relapse in early CRC	NCT04050345 (TRACC)	UK 2016–2024	HR II-III	1000	Int rand/3/DFS, OS, QoL	ctDNA/RM NGS	Surgery followed by randomization to: (1) SOC arm: SOC ACT, (2) EXP arm: ctDNA guided de-escalated ACT—If ctDNA-: CAPOX × 3 months is reduced to cape × 6 months and CAPE × 6 months is reduced to observation—After 3 months if ctDNA+: switch to CAPOX
ctDNA Based Decision for ACT in CRC Stage II Evaluation	NCT04089631 (CIRCULATE)	Germany Austria Switzerland 2019–2026	II	4812	Int rand/3/DFS, OS, TT ctDNA clear	ctDNA/Dresden NGS	After radical surgery, ctDNA+ are randomized to: (1) CAPE × 6 months (or CAPOX × 3–6 months, investigator choice) or (2) follow-up and CtDNA- are randomized to: (1) follow-up inside the study or (2) follow-up outside the study (off-study)
Decision for ACT in stage II CRC based on ctDNA	NCT04120701 (CIRCULATE-PRODIGE 70)	France 2019–2026	II	1980	Int rand/3/DFS, TTR, OS, ctDNA clear	ctDNA/ddPCR of 2 methylated probes	After radical surgery, ctDNA+ are randomized to: (1) ACT (FOLFOX) or (2) surveillance inside the trial. CtDNA- are randomized to (1) surveillance inside the trial or (2) surveillance outside the trial

Table 1. Cont.

Brief Study Title	NCT Number/Study Name	Country Study Period	Stage	N	Study Type/Phase/Endp	Target/Assay-Test (If Available)	Study Overview/Schematic Description
Intervention Trial Implementing Non-invasive ctDNA Analysis to Optimize the Operative and Postoperative Treatment for CRC Patients	NCT03748680 (IMPROVE-IT)	Denmark 2018–2025	I–II	64	Int rand/2/DFS, LR, TTR, OS, ctDNA clear	ctDNA/NGS + ddPCR	After radical surgery, ctDNA+ patients with no indication to ACT according to DCCG guidelines are randomized to: (1) SOC arm: intensified follow-up or (2) EXP arm: CAPOX or FOLFOX followed by intensified follow-up
ctDNA Testing in Predicting Treatment for Patients With Stage IIA CRC After Surgery	NCT04068103 (COBRA)	USA Canada 2019–2024	IIA	1408	Int rand/2-3/ctDNA clear, RFS, OS, TTR	ctDNA	After radical surgery, patients are randomized to: (1) SOC arm: active surveillance (blood stored and tested for ctDNA later), (2) EXP arm ctDNA+: FOLFOX or XELOX × 6 months, (3) EXP arm ctDNA-: active surveillance
Early identification and treatment of occult metastatic disease in stage III CRC	NCT03803553	USA 2020–2023	III	500	Int/3/DFS, OS, ctDNA clear	ctDNA	Surgery followed by SOC ACT followed by ctDNA assessment for MRD: (1) ctDNA+ MSI-h: Nivolumab, (2) ctDNA+ BRAF V600E: Enco/Bini/Cet × 6 months, (3) ctDNA+ others: randomization to FOLFIRI × 6 months or SOC observation, (4) ctDNA-: SOC observation
Post-surgical Liquid Biopsy-guided Treatment of Stage III and HR Stage II CRC Patients	NCT04259944 (PEGASUS)	Italy Spain 2020–2023	HR II–III	140	Int/2/DFS, OS, TT, QoL, ctDNA clear	ctDNA/LUNAR1 test	After surgical surgery: (1) ctDNA+: CAPOX × 3 months, (2) ctDNA-: CAPOX × 6 months and early switch to CAPOX if ctDNA+ after first cycleAfter ACT: (3) ctDNA+/+: FOLFIRI × 6 months, 2 ctDNA-/+: CAPOX × 3 months, switch to FOLFIRI if still ctDNA-/+, 3ctDNA+/-: CAPE × 3 months, switch to FOLFIRI if ctDNA-/+ after 3 LB, (4) ctDNA-/-: follow-up, switch to CAPOX if ctDNA+ after 2 LB
Initial Attack on Latent Metastasis Using TAS-102 for ctDNA Identified CRC After Curative Resection	NCT04457297 (ALTAIR)	Japan 2020–2023	I–IV resected	240	Int rand/3/DFS, OS, TT	ctDNA/Signatera test	After radical surgery and SOC ACT, ctDNA+ patients are randomized to: (1) EXParm: TAS-102 × 6 months or (2) SOC arm: placebo × 6 months
ctDNA guided ACT in stage II CRC according the trials within cohorts design	Planning NTR6455 (MEDOCC CrEATE)	Netherland 2018–2022	LR II	1320	Int rand/3/DFS, OS, QoL	ctDNA/gene panel (PG Dx elio platform)	Surgery followed by randomization to: (1) EXP arm: if ctDNA+ FOLFOX/CAPOX × 6 months or follow-up (patient choice), (2) SOC arm: if ctDNA- follow-up, (3) SOC arm: follow up (ctDNA tested later)

Table 1. Cont.

Brief Study Title	NCT Number/Study Name	Country Study Period	Stage	N	Study Type/Phase/Endp	Target/Assay-Test (If Available)	Study Overview/Schematic Description
A Phase II Clinical Trial Comparing the Efficacy of RO7198457 Versus Watchful Waiting in Patients With ctDNA positive, Resected HR Stage II and Stage III CRC	NCT04486378 BNT122-01	USA 2020–2023	HR II-III	201	Int rand/2/DFS, OS, TTR, TTF, TT	ctDNA	After radical surgery, ctDNA+ patients receive SOC ACT and are then randomized to: (1) EXP arm: RO7198457 (a personalized cancer vaccine) or (2) SOC arm: watchful waiting
ctDNA Analysis to Optimize Treatment for Patients with CRC	NCT03637686 (IMPROVE)	Denmark 2018–2026	III	1800	Obs/DFS	ctDNA	Part 1—Surgery: ctDNA detection pre- and postoperative. Part II—Surveillance: ctDNA detection over 5 years follow-up
BESPOKE study of ctDNA guided therapy in CRC	NCT04264702	USA 2020–2024	II-III	1000	Obs/DFS	ctDNA/Signatera test	To examine the impact of SIGNATERA test on ACT decisions and clinical outcomes during a 2-year follow-up
Use of ctDNA for Monitoring of Stage III CRC	NCT02842203 (PRO1602037.4)	USA 2016–2021	III	150	Obs/OS, PFS	ctDNA	ctDNA serial assessment up to 5 years and correlation with CEA and clinical outcomes
The implication of ctDNA in the recurrence surveillance of stage II and III CRC	NCT03416478 FFJC2017-01	China 2018–2020	II-III	50	Obs/DFS, OS	ctDNA	ctDNA serial assessment before and after curative surgery up to 2 years of follow-up
A phase II Clinical Trial comparing Efficacy of RO7198457 vs. watchful waiting in ctDNA positive stage II-III resected CRC	NCT04486378	USA 2020–2027	II-III	201	Int rand/2/DFS, RFS, TTR, TTF, OS, TT, ctDNA clear	ctDNA	To compare the efficacy of RO7198457 vs. watchful waiting after surgery and SOC ACT in ctDNA positive stage II-III CRC
ctDNA as a Prognostic Marker for Postoperative Relapse in Early and Intermediate Stage CRC	NCT03312374	China 2017–2020	II-III	350	Obs/DFS	ctDNA/NGS	ctDNA serial assessment before and after curative surgery and ACT up to 2 years of follow-up
The Implication of Plasma ctDNA Methylation Haplotypes in Detecting CRC and Adenomas	NCT03737591	China 2018–2020	I-IV adenomas healthy	500	Obs	ctDNA/NGS	To evaluate the sensitivity and specificity of ctDNA methylation haplotypes in detecting CRC and adenomas

Table 1. *Cont.*

Brief Study Title	NCT Number/Study Name	Country Study Period	Stage	N	Study Type/Phase/Endp	Target/Assay-Test (If Available)	Study Overview/Schematic Description
Dynamic monitoring of ctDNA methylation to predict relapse in stage II-III CRC after radical resection	NCT03737539	China 2018–2022	II-III	300	Obs/DFS	ctDNA/NGS	To correlate and compare postoperative, pre- and post-ACT ctDNA methylation markers with radiological imaging and clinical outcomes
Ct-DNA Testing in Guiding Treatment for Patients With Advanced or Metastatic CRC	NCT03844620	USA 2019–2020	III (uncurable)-IV	100	Int/2/TT, ctDNA clean, QoL, ORR, OS	ctDNA	Monitoring and correlating ctDNA changes and radiological progression or TT incidence during third-line SOC (TAS-102/Regorafenib) (arm A) vs. third-line SOC alone (arm B)
Predictive and Prognostic Value of Inflammatory Markers and microRNA in Stage IV CRC	NCT04149613	USA 2018–2021	IV	100	Obs	miRNAs	To evaluate the expression of selected microRNAs and inflammatory markers in patients with stage IV CRC and assess their correlation with tumor location, dietary patterns, survival rates, response to systemic chemotherapy, and other clinic-pathological parameters
Molecular Pathology of CRC: Investigating the Role of Novel Molecular Profiles, microRNAs, and their Targets in CRC Progression	NCT03309722	UK 2008–2025	I-IV	1000	Obs/OS, DFS, LR, DR	miRNA	Single-center observational cohort study of prospectively recruited patients for biomarker evaluation and identification of novel biomarkers
Contents of Circulating Extracellular Vesicles: Biomarkers in CRC Patients	NCT04523389 (ExoColon)	France 2020–2021	I-IV	172	Obs/OS, PFS, LR, DR	Exosomes	To investigate the prognostic and predictive role of exosomes and their contents (miRNAs and others)
ColoCare Transdisciplinary Research in CRC Prognosis	NCT02328677	USA 2007–2030	I-IV	5000	Obs/OS, DFS, QoL, TT	ctDNA, MiRNAs	To investigate the prognostic and predictive role of liquid biopsy in CRC patients in a 5-year follow-up

Table 1. Cont.

Brief Study Title	NCT Number/Study Name	Country Study Period	Stage	N	Study Type/Phase/Endp	Target/Assay-Test (If Available)	Study Overview/Schematic Description
Timing To Minimally Invasive Surgery After Neoadjuvant Chemoradiotherapy For Rectal Cancer: A Multicenter Randomized Controlled Trial—Biomarkers SubStudy	NCT03962088 (TiMiSNAR)	Italy 2019–2023	II-III	200	Obs/pCR, DFS	miRNA/miRNeasy Mini kit by Qiagen	(1) To investigate the association between pre-neoadjuvant and post-neoadjuvant expression levels of miRNA with pCR. (2) To investigate the correlation between changes in expression levels of miRNA following complete surgical resection with DFS and the relation between changes in miRNA during surveillance and tumor relapse
microRNAs Tool for Stratifying Stage II CRC: a Perspective Study of ACT	NCT02635087	China 2015–2025	II	630	Obs/DFS, OS	miRNA	To investigate the predictive and prognostic role of miRNAs in stage II CRC, stratifying patients at "high risk" and at "low risk" of recurrence according to a six miRNAs tool
Assessment Of Long Noncoding RNA CCAT1 Using Real-Time Polymerase Chain Reaction In CRC patients	NCT04269746	Egypt 2020–2021	Diagnostic	100	Obs	lncRNA	To evaluate the clinical utility of detecting long non-coding RNA (CCAT1) expression in diagnosis of CRC patients and its relation to tumor staging

ctDNA: circulating tumor DNA; Endp: study endpoints if not reported in study description; N: planned enrollment; Obs: observational; Int: interventional; CT: chemotherapy; LB: liquid biopsy; dPCR: digital PCR; ddPCR: digital droplet PCR; SOC: standard of care; ACT: adjuvant chemotherapy; NA: not available; Enco/Bini/Cet: Encorafenib/Binimetinib/Cetuximab; HR: high risk according to histopathological factors; LR: low risk according to histopathological factors; ctDNA clear: ctDNA clearance or modification rate of every study arm and correlation with clinical outcome measures (according to the design of each study); OS: overall survival; DFS: disease-free survival; RFS: relapse-free survival; LR: local recurrence; DR: distant recurrence; QoL: quality of life; TT: treatment toxicity/treatment-related adverse events; pCR: pathologic complete response; TTF: time to treatment failure; TTR: time to recurrence.

2.3. MicroRNAs (miRNAs) and Long Non-Coding RNAs (lncRNAs)

MicroRNAs (miRNAs) and long non-coding RNAs (lncRNAs) are ncRNAs molecules involved in the regulation of protein-coding gene expression through mRNA degradation and silencing or activating and repressing genes via a variety of mechanisms at both transcriptional and translational levels. Both classes of ncRNAs regulate multiple cellular processes such as growth, development, and differentiation showing to be crucial for cancer initiation, progression, and dissemination and can be found in serum or other body fluids bound to protein or lipid complexes, or more frequently inside extracellular vesicles (i.e., exosomes) [46]. Furthermore, these elements seem to be strongly associated with the development of drug resistance in CRC [47–50]. For these reasons, miRNA and lncRNAs could have potential application in diagnosis, prognosis, and treatment of CRC.

2.3.1. Diagnosis and Prognosis

MiR-150 appears upregulated in CRC and its downregulation together with elevated Gli1 (glioma-associated oncogene homolog 1) expression seems to be involved in the process of epithelial–mesenchymal transition (EMT), which is a necessary step in promoting invasion and metastasis in CRC [51]. The results of a recent metanalysis suggest that miR-150 could be effective as a diagnostic biomarker for CRC patients, while no significant evidence was found concerning its prognostic role [52]. Mir-181 seems to be involved in multiple signaling pathways such as FOXO, PI3K-Akt, VEGF, HIF-1, mTOR, and cAMP, therefore representing a promising biomarker with potential predictive and prognostic significance in CRC [53]. MiR-21, miR-200a, miR-543, miR-32, miR92a, miR-26a, miR-1061, and miR-181a act as oncogenes downregulating the oncosuppressor PTEN (phosphatase and tensin homolog), which is a diagnostic factor for CRC patients, therefore representing potential targets for CRC therapy [54]. The upregulation of miR21, miR215, miR143-5p, and miR106a is associated with worse prognosis in stage II CRC patients [55]. A panel of miR-21, miR29a, and miR125b is able to carefully distinguish between early CRC and healthy controls (AUC = 0.827) [56]. Serum miR-203 upregulation seems to be related to worse prognosis (HR = 2.1) and higher risk of liver (OR = 6.2) or peritoneum (OR = 7.2) metastasis [57]. In a population of 400 CRC patients, a four-miRNA panel (miR-142-5p, miR-23a-3p, miR376c-3p, and miR271-3p) showed good diagnostic performance (AUC = 0.922), while a two-miRNA signature (miR-23a-3p and miR-376c-3p) proved to be a prognostic tool for 3-year OS (HR = 2.30) [58].

A study focusing on circulating serum exosomes showed that the levels of lncRNA HOTTIP could predict OS in CRC patients and discriminate between CRC and healthy controls (AUC = 0.75) [59].

A recent systematic review and meta-analysis of 111 articles including 13,103 gastrointestinal cancer patients (3123 with esophageal cancer, 4972 with gastric cancer, and 5008 with CRC) showed that 74 lncRNAs were closely associated with poor prognosis in gastrointestinal cancer, including 58 significantly upregulated and 16 significantly down-regulated lncRNA expression, and with a strong interaction with miRNAs for 12 of these lncRNAs [60].

2.3.2. Drug Resistance

Several oncogenic miRNAs can promote platinum and fluoropyrimidine resistance. Complex interactions between miRNAs (miR-181a-5p, miR-136, miR-363-3p, miR20b-5p, miR-218, miR-145, Let-7a, miR141) and lncRNAs (CRNDE, LUCAT1, MALAT1, GIHCG, CASC15, ANRIL, MEG3, CCAL) in the context of Wnt/β-catenin and MDM2-P53 signaling pathways are ultimately involved in oxaliplatin resistance [47]. Moreover, mir-153, miR19b-3p, miR-203, and miR-625-3p upregulation in the context of FOXO3a, SMAD4, and ATM pathways, respectively, is associated with oxaliplatin resistance [48]. The upregulation of LncRNA NEAT1 acts as an oncogene in CRC through the regulation of CPSF4 expression, sponging miR-150-5p. The upregulation of NEAT1 ultimately results in 5-FU resistance, suppressed apoptosis, and enhanced invasion of CRC [49]. A recent systematic review and meta-analysis of 39 studies including 2822 CRC patients consistently showed that multiple miRNAs (almost 60) could act as clinical predictors of chemoresistance and sensitivity for a combination of 14 drugs, including 5-FU and oxaliplatin. Particularly, 28 miRNAs were associated with chemosensitivity, 20 were associated with chemoresistance, 1 was associated with differential expression and radiosensitivity, while 10 were not associated with any impact on chemotherapy. These results outline the importance of almost 34 drug-regulatory pathways of chemoresistance and chemosensitivity in CRC that are potentially targetable [61].

3. Microbiota

The study of microbiota started several years ago, and multiple definitions have been conceived to explain its meaning [62]. In general, the terms "microbiota" and "microbiome" refer to the complex of organisms found within a specific environment and their genomic pool, respectively [63,64]. Thus, the human gut microbiota consists of a multitude of microorganisms colonizing the gut and existing in that complex state of dynamic equilibrium (i.e., eubiosis), which is made of reciprocal interactions and multiple networks between themselves and the host cells. This is an equilibrium with specific spatial and temporal characteristics, whose deregulation might lead to dysbiosis [63].

The human gut microbiota—with its thousands of different bacterial taxa, eucaryotic microbes, and virus together with the intestinal barrier—is a very selective and important filter for the well-being of the whole organism, and as a neuroendocrine structure today considered as a "second brain", it is a component of the complex gut ecosystem [65,66]. The gastrointestinal microbiota varies according to the anatomical location and among individuals [11], and it plays different roles, from the supply of nutrients to the control of inflammation and carcinogenesis [63]. Commensal bacteria instruct the immune and physiological systems throughout life and are responsible for the presence of inflammatory and immune cells in the healthy intestine: the so-called "physiological" or "controlled" inflammation [67]. For this purpose, numerous evidence has demonstrated that a direct relationship between modification in the gut microbiota composition and some pathologies exist [68,69]. Among these diseases, obesity and metabolic alterations induced by some nutrients and diet, or autoimmune diseases such as type 1 diabetes and inflammatory bowel disease, are characterized by changes in the microbiome and gut dysbiosis [70].

3.1. Microbiota and Cancer

Gut microbiota emerged as a critical player also in the development of cancer. Several studies support the idea that a disturbance of the gut microbiota composition could lead to the onset of CRC [71]. Moreover, several studies reported a deep association between microbiota and CRC, demonstrating that microbiota dysbiosis can affect cancer susceptibility and progression through the modulation of several mechanisms such as inflammation, or inducing DNA damage, and producing metabolites involved in oncogenesis or tumor suppression [72]. For example, various bacterial pathogens are linked with the DNA damage response (DDR) pathway activation, which can be caused by both a direct effect of microbe produced genotoxins or an indirect effect of ROS produced in response to an excessive activation of immune cells stimulated by certain microbes or their metabolic end-products [73,74].

In particular, fecal metagenomic samples from CRC patients identified a CRC-enriched microbiota including *Enterobacteriaceae* [75], *Escherichia coli* [76,77], Enterotoxigenic *Bacteroides fragilis* (ETBF) [78], and *Fusobacterium nucleatum (Fn)* [79]. These bacteria seem to act as "pro-oncogenic" agents in different ways: promoting inflammation, impairing antitumor activity, inducing DNA damage, and tumor cell proliferation via the activation of β-catenin and other oncogenic pathways [75]. Several studies reported an association between an abundance of *Fusobacterium nucleatum*, carcinogenetic risk factors, and gene mutations in CRC [80]. In addition, a high abundance of *Fusobacterium nucleatum* was associated with CIMP status, wild-type p53, and MSI in colon tumor tissue [81].

On the other hand, the *Firmicutes* phylum (particularly the *Ruminococcaceae* and *Lachnospiraceae* families) [82] as well as *Bifidobacteria, Lactobacilli* [83,84] and non-enterotoxigenic *Bacteroides fragilis* (NTBF) [84] are substantially underrepresented in CRC patients [85] and have shown "anti-oncogenic" activities, such as a reduction of pro-inflammatory citokines, enhancement of antitumor immunity, epithelial cell renewal, regulation of intestinal barrier integrity, and short-chain fatty acid (SCFA) production [82–86]. SCFAs, by modulating histone deacetylase inhibitory activity, promote the accumulation and differentiation of Treg cells controlling tumor progression [86].

Similarly, a deeper review on the role of gut microbiota in the carcinogenesis of humans and animals observed that some bacteria appeared often augmented (including Fusobacteria, *Alistipes*, Porphyromonadaceae, Coriobacteridae, Staphylococcaceae, *Akkermansia* spp., and Methanobacteriales), whereas others decreased in CRC (*Bifidobacterium, Lactobacillus, Ruminococcus, Faecalibacterium* spp., *Roseburia*, and *Treponema* [87]. In addition, some microbial metabolites (such as nitrogenous compounds) were consistently elevated, whereas others (such as butyrate) were decreased throughout colonic carcinogenesis [87].

3.2. Signaling Pathways Activated in Microbiota and Cancer

The gut microenvironment homeostasis requires an intricate balance between cell proliferation, differentiation, and apoptosis processes in which several regulatory pathways are involved such as the Wnt, Notch, BMP, and Hedgehog signaling pathways [88,89]. Deregulation of these main signaling pathways can potentially determine a disruption of intestinal homeostasis and contribute to CRC development. For example, the Wnt/β-catenin signaling pathway is supposed to be closely connected with cancer biology [90]. In particular, the *adenomatous polyposis coli (APC)* gene truncating mutations that stabilize β-catenin are highly prevalent in CRC, making *APC* one of the most mutated genes in human cancers [91].

Among the canonical and non-canonical Wnt signaling pathways, the first is certainly the most critical for its function as regulator of the transcriptional co-activator β-catenin, in turn regulating inflammatory, proliferative, and differentiation pathways [92,93]. As reported in several studies, the Wnt pathway has been frequently considered together with the *RAS* pathway one of the major drivers of CSC expansion [93].

The gut microbiome can be the trigger of the (EMT), a transition taking place through the involvement of WNT and TGF-β signaling, as previously reported, causing the invasion and metastasis of CRC cells [94].

Recently, preclinical evidence demonstrated that defects in the colon barrier integrity associated with dysbiosis and with an increased expression of several inflammatory factors such as IL-17, *Cxcl2, Tnf-α*, and IL-1 can be responsible for the development of benign (e.g., hyperplastic polyp), pre-malignant (e.g., tubular adenoma), or malignant (e.g., colorectal adenocarcinoma) neoformations [71,95].

Taken together, these data suggest that alterations of gene expression or modifications of microbiota composition can trigger the development of cancer involving the deregulation of proliferative and inflammatory signaling pathways even though a clear cause–effect relationship between microbiota composition and changes in gene expression have not been well elucidated.

In conclusion, not only a genetic but also an epigenetic role has been highlighted in CRC progression and metastatization, as recently reported by Wu et al. [96].

3.3. Microbiota and Efficacy of Anticancer Agents

An emergent approach is taking into consideration the influence of the microbiota on the activity and efficacy of chemotherapy and immunotherapy drugs. For example, the hypothesis that gut microbiota can be strictly related to the pharmacological effects of chemotherapy agents, such as 5-FU, is supported by a pioneer study conducted with a CRC mouse model and high-throughput sequencing. The authors compared the tumor size and profiled the gut microbiota of mice treated with 5-FU, combined with probiotics or

ABX (an antibiotic cocktail of antibiotics), demonstrating the importance of pre-existing gut microbiota communities in the host response to 5-FU treatment. In particular, they found that antibiotics-induced dysbiosis during CRC treatment determined a dramatic increase of Proteobacteria, which may interact with the host inducing systemic inflammation and abolishing the therapeutic efficacy of the drug [97].

Regarding human studies, Zhang and colleagues investigated the relationship between *Fn* infection and efficacy of a systemic treatment with 5-FU in 94 CRC patients. They initially hypothesized a mechanism of reduced chemo-sensitivity of CRC cells to 5-FU linked to the upregulation of BIRC3, which is a member of the inhibitor of apoptosis proteins (IAPs). Next, they demonstrated that *Fn*-induced BIRC3 expression could be mediated by the TLR4/NFkB pathway. Indeed, other scientists had recently reported that *Fn* may mediate chemoresistance by activating the autophagic pathway in CRC [98].

Immunotherapy has revolutionized cancer treatment, and immune checkpoint inhibitors (ICIs) are now a standard of care in microsatellite-instable (MSI) CRC patients [99].

Recently, Lang et al. in their study showed that ileal microbiota can orchestrate the immunogenic cell death of ileal intestinal epithelial cells (IECs). They registered an accumulation of follicular T-helper (TFH) cells in CRC patients and mice and the suppression of IEC apoptosis. This effect could be linked to the impairment of the immunosurveillance mechanisms by chemotherapy directed against CRC in mice [100]. Protective immune responses in the ileum were associated with the colonization of specific bacteria such as *Bacteroides fragilis* and *Erysipelotrichaceae* that stimulate the production of programmed cell death (PD-1) molecules +TFH by secretion of interleukin 1R1 and interleukin 12. Moreover, the demonstration of apoptosis in the ileum can be considered a prognostic factor for CRC patients [100].

As for the relationship between bacteria species infection and efficacy of treatments, it has been postulated that the richness and diversity of species could be influenced by the different stages of gastric carcinogenesis and progression. In particular, more relevant changes seem to occur at the stage of precancerous lesions of gastric carcinoma (PLGC), suggesting that it is a turning point during GC progression. Moreover, the depletion of some bacteria such as *Akkermansia* and an enrichment of pathogenic bacteria such as *Escherichia Shigella* can overlap with the tumor progression stage [100].

Moreover, researchers have reported a reduction in the efficacy of immunotherapy regimens in metastatic renal cell carcinoma (mRCC) patients when treated with antibiotic drugs. In particular, worse clinical outcomes in terms of PFS and OS were found in mRCC patients who received antibiotics within four weeks of treatment initiation with respect to non-users [101].

3.4. Recent Advances in Metagenomics Technology for Diagnosis and Prognosis

Currently, the study of microbiomes, also named metagenomics, is based on two main approaches, which consider different aspects of the microbial community in a given environment. The structural metagenomics approach takes into consideration the structure, composition, and dynamics in a specific ecosystem of the uncultivated microbial population. Instead, functional genomics aims to study a specific gene coding for a function of interest. This approach requires the generation of expression libraries with thousands of metagenomics clones and its subsequent screening [102].

Metagenomics, investigating the wide populations of microbial communities and analyzing all the DNA present within a sample, can provide comprehensive and useful data regarding the state of the microenvironment of CRC patients. In metagenomics, datasets acquired from recent studies of the taxonomic clades related to CRC have been discovered [103].

Moreover, Meyerson et al. by using whole-genome sequences established the configuration of microbiota in healthy and CRC patients [104]. By the way, thanks to the multi-omics approach based on the plethora of recent technologies including genomics, transcriptomics, proteomics, and metabolomics respectively able to analyze DNA markers,

RNA transcript, protein, and metabolites produced inside the colon, researchers have a remarkable opportunity for the discovery of novel prognostic, diagnostic, and therapeutic biomarkers [104], even though the question of whether the microbiota and its metabolites could be considered replicable and useful biomarkers across cohorts and populations remains unclear. So, the aim of this interesting approach tries to examine the differences in patients and healthy individuals for identifying biomarker patterns to work toward a personalized medicine therapeutic approach [105].

For example, in a large cohort study conducted on 616 participants undergoing colonoscopy, the presence of distinct patterns of the microbiome in cases of multiple polypoid adenomas has been demonstrated. *Fn* appeared significantly elevated from intramucosal carcinoma to more advanced stages. Moreover, *Atopobium parvulum* and *Actinomyces odontolyticus*, which co-occurred in intramucosal carcinomas, were significantly increased only in multiple polypoid adenomas and/or intramucosal carcinomas. In addition, metabolome analyses indicated a significant increase of metabolites such as branched-chain amino acids and bile acids in intramucosal carcinomas. Futhermore, the authors suggested that the shift in the microbiome and metabolome seemed to occur from the very early stages of CRC development, confirming the potential diagnostic and etiological role of multi-omics data. Therefore, the authors proposed metagenomic and metabolomic markers to discriminate cases of intramucosal carcinoma from the healthy controls, highlighting the possible etiological and diagnostic importance of large-cohort multi-omics data [106]. Indeed, the application of metagenomics to explore the gut microbiota profile has also been prospectively investigated in 60 CRC patients and 30 healthy controls. This study revealed the importance of data from the gut microbiome in association with known clinical risk factors of CRC to discriminate between adenoma and carcinoma clinical groups [107]. On the other hand, a similar conclusion has been reported by a European study based on fecal samples metagenomic sequencing and taxonomic classification of a mixed group of CRC, adenomas patients, and healthy subjects. Indeed, this study indicated that observed gene pool differences may reveal tumor-related host–microbe interactions [108].

An emerging approach to study the intersection of the gut–microbial communities and human health is based on the study of microbe-derived extracellular vesicles (EVs). EVs, separated into three different types, outer membrane vesicles (OMVs), shedding vesicles, and apoptotic bodies, are composed of different macromolecules including lipids, proteins, nucleic acids, and metabolites [109,110].

For example, via metagenomic and metabolomics analysis of gut EVs of CRC and healthy subjects, Kim et al. found an alteration of compositional bacteria and metabolites profile in CRC patients, suggesting a potential diagnostic role of EVs metabolites profiles in the identification of cooperation between microbiome and cancer development [109].

3.5. Organoids Engineering

Organoid engineering has become an important tool for cancer assessment but also in modeling host–microbe interactions. New insights are rapidly being gained on the role of the microbiome in CRC development, and it is clear that CRC patients have an altered gut microbe population compared to healthy ones. However, whether they play a direct or indirect role in cancer development is a topic of great discussion [111].

Research suggests a key role for microbes in developing an inflammatory environment in which cancer cells can grow; they can also influence cancer development by producing metabolites that influence the host metabolism [112].

From a practical point of view, microbes can be administered to cell culture media, allow basolateral exposure, or be microinjected into the lumen of the organoid to faithfully reproduce the microbial activity [113].

For example, Pleguezuelos-Manzano et al. focused on the abundance, in stool samples of CRC patients, of some bacteria including *E. coli* and pks + *E. coli*, which are capable of producing the genotoxin colibactin. This toxin has been shown to damage DNA and create a non-physiological base pairing in epithelial cells [77].

By the use of organoids constituted with *E. coli* pKs + obtained from the colon of CRC patients co-cultured with the epithelial cells, these researchers reproduced in vivo the intestinal situation and demonstrated that exposure to *E. coli* pKs + would appear to be a risk factor in the development of CRC [114]. Therefore, in conclusion, the specificity of colibactin-induced mutations supports the need for further investigations relating to its link with cellular DNA as well as representing a valid support in the identification of a preventive biomarker [77].

New knowledge is also rapidly gaining in the field of "nutrition and gut microbiota". Several studies have established that after the ingestion of phytochemicals and fibers, the intestinal microbiota initiates complex catabolism that releases important metabolites of the intestinal microbiome (GMMs). Moreover, thanks to the use of organoids derived from colorectal lesions, the impact of diet and metabolites on tumorigenesis has been also investigated [115].

Recently, Toden and colleagues identified evidence that metabolites produced by the microbial catabolism of flavan-3-ols in the distal gastrointestinal tract could induce programmed cell death, inhibiting cancer and promoting gut health [116]. They used intestinal organoids as a preclinical model system and noted that flavan-3-ols suppressed the formation and growth of both intestinal organoids—those derived from APCM in mouse models and those from human CRC tumors—by inhibiting the cell cycle and inducing apoptosis. The gene expression profile revealed the suppression of survival and self-renewal pathways in organoids treated with flavan-3-ols. Flavan-3-ols is a commercial grape seed extract, consisting of monomers, dimers, and trimers. These compounds include proanthocyanidins (PACs); they can reach the distal gastrointestinal tract almost intact and are effectively transformed into low molecular weight phenolic compounds by the colonic microbiota [117–119]. The flavan-3-ols monomers, dimers, and trimers that reach the colon become available for the gut microbiota. Then, microbial catabolism begins, producing hydroxy-phenyl-γ-valerolactones (PVLs) and, to a lesser extent, their derivative hydroxy-phenylvaleric acids (PVAs), with only a small percentage of non-metabolized PACs remaining [120].

3.6. Therapeutic Use of Antibiotics, Probiotics, and Fecal Microbiota Transplantation

Several approaches, which include dietary interventions, antibiotic treatments, pre- and probiotics, and fecal microbiota transplantation (FMT), have been explored to modulate gut microbiota composition, including its physiology and metabolites involved in CRC occurrence, progression, or drug resistance.

Diet plays a significant role in the modulation of the microbiome. A normal gut microbiota depends upon the fermentation of the indigestible fiber component of our diet for its energy supplement. The symbiotic gut microbiota ferments dietary fibers into short-chain fatty acids (SCFAs) such as propionate, acetate and, most importantly, butyrate [67]. In a prospective cohort study, a diet rich in whole grains and dietary fiber was associated with a lower risk to develop *F. nucleatum*-positive CRC but not *F. nucleatum*-negative CRC, supporting a potential role for intestinal microbiota in mediating the association between diet and colorectal neoplasms [121]. As no clear guideline regarding the type of nutrition and cancer incidence has been established, different forms of reduced caloric intake, such as fasting, demonstrated a wide range of beneficial effects in cancer prevention and anticancer drug efficacy [122], at least in part mediated by gut microbiota. Indeed, every-other-day fasting leads to an increase in fermentation products such as acetate and lactate altering gut microbiota composition, with enriched levels of Firmicutes, the production of SCFAs, and reduction in Bacteroides, Actinobacteria, and Tenericutes [123]. Since tumors are not able to metabolize ketone bodies due to deficiencies in key mitochondrial enzymes, a ketogenic diet with low-carbohydrate and high-fat intake, mimicking the metabolic state of fasting by inducing a physiological increase in acetoacetate and beta-hydroxybutyrate, might be a reliable therapeutic strategy to inhibit cancer progression [124]. Omega-3 polyunsatured fatty acids (PUFAs) are widely used as nutritional supplements and multiple benefits have been claimed, included anticancer activity. PUFAs seem to increase "anti-oncogenic" bacteria, including *Bifidobacterium* and *Lactobacillus* other than SCFA-producing genera such as *Blautia, Bacterioides, Roseburia,* and *Coprococcus* [125]. A randomized trial showed that omega-3 PUFA supplementation induces a reversible increase in several SCFA-producing bacteria [126].

Since antibiotic administration represents an aggressive and non-selective means of manipulation of gut microbiota composition, its role in CRC management seems to be controversial. Although preclinical evidence showed that gut microbiome depletion seems to inhibit cancer progression [127], multiple lines of evidence highlight how antibiotics can undermine immunotherapy efficacy or promote disease progression emphasizing microbial dysbiosis [128,129].

Of course, a potential strategy of CRC prevention and management is represented by probiotics and fecal microbiota transplantation (FMT). Probiotics are living microorganisms with the potential to positively influence resident microbiota, intestinal epithelium cells, and the immune system, and they are generally considered safe and well tolerated in healthy subjects [130]. A randomized trial with *Lactobacillus* and *Bifidobacterium* strains significantly reduced the levels of proinflammatory cytokines such as TNF-α, IL-6, IL-10, IL-12, IL-17, and IL-22 and prevented post-surgical complications.

FMT consists of the transplantation of gut microbiota from healthy donors to patients to restore intestinal dysbiosis and reduce the activation of inflammatory, proliferative, and procarcinogenic pathways. These specimens are prepared according to well-established protocols to avoid potential risk factors such as viruses and parasites and stored in banks of donated feces [131]. Treatment with chemotherapy and ICIs can result in adverse events including colitis. FMT treatment has been shown to improve ICI-induced colitis in cancer patients [132]. Additionally, FMT reduced the severity of intestinal mucositis and diarrhea following FOLFOX treatment in preclinical models by suppressing IL-6 levels, increasing the number of goblet cells and zonula occludens-1, decreasing apoptotic and NFkB-positive cells as well as the expression of Toll-like receptors and MYD88, leading to a restoration of gut microbiota composition without complications such as bacteremia [133]. Another study conducted in a mouse model to assess the efficacy of FMT to reverse antibiotic- and chemotherapy-induced gut dysbiosis suggests that FMT may effectively help in preventing acute intestinal inflammation and mucosal barrier dysfunction. In particular, the administration of FMT reduced the proportions of pathogenic species and an increase of the relative distribution of Clostridium scindens and Faecalibacterium prausnitzii, which are species that exhibited anti-inflammatory properties [134].

Finally, as demonstrated by Hefazi et al. in cancer patients treated with cytotoxic chemotherapy, FMT treatment determined a reduction of multiply recurrent Clostridium difficile infection (CDI) and diarrhea episodes remarking its highly therapeutic efficacy [135].

4. Future Perspectives and Conclusions

Despite the recent advances in the systemic treatment of molecularly selected CRC patients with advanced disease (i.e., pembrolizumab in MSI [99] or the association of the anti-BRAF encorafenib, the anti-MEK binimetinib and the anti-EGFR cetuximab in BRAF V600E mutated [136] tumors), the survival benefit is limited to a small percentage (10–20%) of patients harboring these alterations.

The use of CTCs, ctDNA, miRNAs, and lncRNA could help find new potentially targetable biomarkers for the management of CRC. Furthermore, as a minimally invasive and repeatable procedure, liquid biopsy can improve CRC screening, early diagnosis, clinical staging, and prognostic stratification, allowing a higher rate of cure. Moreover, liquid biopsy might be useful to monitor minimal residual disease after surgical treatment, possibly allowing a finer modulation of the adjuvant systemic therapy, integrating clinicopathological risk factors and ctDNA or CTC detection. Finally, if properly integrated with clinical and instrumental assessment, liquid biopsy might help monitor disease progression, treatment efficacy, and acquired resistance to chemotherapy and targeted agents in CRC.

Of course, there is urgent need to optimize pre-analytical and analytical processing for clinical validity, to standardize laboratory methods in ensuring the reproducibility of the results and to properly assess the cost-effectiveness [137]. Indeed, the lack of clinical applicability is currently due to the large quantity of liquid biopsy assays, with different detection limits, sensitivity, and specificity [138]. To solve the pitfalls for liquid biopsies due to the difficulty of CTC detection, the application of various microfluidic platforms based on CTC characteristics has been explored [139]. Recently, for the selection of CTC, a "negative depletion" microfluidic chip has been developed [140]. In this system, named leukapheresis, the leukocyte depletion strategy can enrich for untagged CTCs in a "tumor-independent" manner applicable to all tumor types, as demonstrated in several tumor types [141–144].

CTC analyses performed on leukapheresis products should improve the reach of liquid biopsies in metastatic cancer, and combined with CTC detection, they may play a critical role in screening high-risk patients for early cancer, identifying the tissue of origin, and reducing the need for invasive biopsies.

Therefore, once the multiple ongoing randomized phase II–III trials will define and validate the role of liquid biopsy especially in the adjuvant setting of early CRC (Table 1), a process of harmonization of procedures and data will be necessary to transfer from bench to bedside this important tool of personalized medicine.

On the other hand, it is clear that CRC carcinogenesis is also defined by gut microbiota metabolic activity and its dysbiotic composition. Therefore, the integrated analysis of the gut microbiome and its interactions with the host, anticancer drugs, and other exogenous factors [7,139] is essential to improve the outcomes of CRC patients. Recent findings support the potential of microbial markers in cancer diagnosis and prognosis and the potential of FMT or pre-probiotics in remodeling the tumor microenvironment or in potentiating antitumor immunity. Continuous monitoring of changes in microbiota profiles and biomarkers may help in the identification of dysplasia. In addition, in this context, an important collaborative effort is required to elucidate the role of the gut microbiota in modulating responses to cancer treatment, and this aspect is particularly clear in several ongoing clinical trials investigating the effect of FMT in patients with cancer who are refractory to ICI. These trials, along with further validations, will determine whether the selective modulation of gut microbiota, either by FMT, probiotic treatment, or other means, enables CRC patients to overcome resistance to chemotherapy or immunotherapy (Table 2). Of course, a more complete and holistic approach toward cancer treatment should include host–microbiota interactions as important screening and treatment factors.

Table 2. List of major ongoing prospective trials investigating the role of microbiota in colorectal cancer.

Brief Study Title	NCT Number/Study Name	Country Study Period	Stage	N	Study Type/Phase (If Applicable)	Intervention	Study Overview/Schematic Description
Gut Microbiome Dynamics in Metastasized or Irresectable CRC	NCT03941080 GIMICC	Netherlands 2020–2022	IV	300	Obs	Fecal and blood sample collection + behavioral questionnaire at baseline and every 3 months	To investigate characteristics and alterations of the gut microbiome and its predictive value for RR and TT during CT for mCRC
Gut Microbiome and Oral Fluoropyrimidine Study in Patients With CRC	NCT04054908 GO	USA 2018–2022	all	60	Obs	1 stool sample at baseline and at least 1 stool sample during treatment + questionnaires regarding bowel habits and dietary habits	To investigate the alterations of the gut microbiome occurring in three cohorts of CRC: Cohort A: patients treated with CAPE as SOC, Cohort B: patients treated with TAS-102 with or without Y-90 radioembolization in T, Cohort C: patients treated with CAPE + pembrolizumab + bevacizumab in T
Human Intestinal Microbiome and Surgical Outcomes in Patients Undergoing CRC Cancer Surgery	NCT04405118 Microbiota	France	all	50	Obs	2 fresh fecal samples for LM detection (1 pre- and 1 post-operatively) + 1 intraoperatively sample for MAM	To investigate the association between microbiome composition and occurrence of postoperative complications (anastomotic leakage, surgical site infection, prolonged postoperative ileus)
Bowel Preparation Impact on the Intestinal Microbiome: Oral Preparation vs. Enema	NCT04013841 BowelPrepMicrobiome	USA 2020–2022	Left-sided CRC	60	Int rand	Stool samples before and after bowel preparation and surgery	To investigate differences in microbiome composition according to oral and enema bowel preparation for left side colon surgery and its correlation with surgical outcomes
The Role of Microbiome in Cancer Therapy	NCT02960282	USA 2016–2021	IV	80	Obs	Fecal specimen collection at baseline, prior to each cycle and at PD or off-treatment	To investigate microbiome composition, its gene and protein expression profile and correlation with RR and TT in two cohorts: Cohort A: patients treated with FOLFOX or FOLFIRI CT backbone as first line regimen, Cohort B: patients treated with pembrolizumab
Colorectal Cancer Cohort Study	NCT04185779 COLO-COHORT	UK 2019–2024	diagnostic	15000	Obs	Blood and fecal tests + behavioral questionnaires	To develop a prediction model to stratify patients at risk of having adenomas or CRC (past medical history, family history, blood tests, FIT level, colonoscopy, and microbiome stool)
Stool and Blood Sample Bank for CRC Patients	NCT04638751 ARGONAUT	USA 2020–2024	III–IV	4000		2 blood and stool samples each over a 6-month period	To determine whether the microbiome composition can predict PFS and OS in different cohorts of cancer patients (NSCLC, CRC, TNBC, and PC) treated with CT or IT. To identify correlations between microbiome composition and immune markers

Table 2. Cont.

Brief Study Title	NCT Number/Study Name	Country Study Period	Stage	N	Study Type/Phase (If Applicable)	Intervention	Study Overview/Schematic Description
Omega-3 Fatty Acid for the Immune Modulation of Colorectal Cancer	NCT03661047 OMICC	USA 2019–2023	I-III, HR adenomas	36	Int rand/2/	Blood and stool samples + lifestyle nutritional survey between CRC/adenomas detection and surgery	To evaluate the effect of a 30-day administration of AMRI01 (VASCEPA, icosapent ethyl) on MO3PUFA composition, gut microbiome, and immune system elements concentration (CD8+ T cells, CD49b, CTLA-4, PD-L1, PD-1, LAG-3, IL10, FOXP3) in both normal and tumor tissue
Metagenomic Evaluation of the Gut Microbiome in Patients With Lynch Syndrome and Other Hereditary Colonic Polyposis Syndromes	NCT02371135	USA 2015–2021	High hereditary CRC risk	225	Obs	Stool sample + Brief Diet and Lifestyle Questionnaire before every colonoscopy	To investigate the association of the gut microbiome and dietary factors with risk of adenoma or cancer in Lynch syndrome and other hereditary colonic polyposis syndrome patients
Pilot Trial of Resistant Starch in Stage I-III CRC Survivors	NCT03781778	USA 2018–2020	I-III	24	Int rand/2	Stool samples + Diet questionnaire at beginning and at 8 weeks	To compare the effect of a 8-week consumption of foods made of resistant (experimental arm) or corn (control arm) starch in addition to usual daily diet in modifying markers of inflammation, insulin resistance, and gut microbiome composition of CRC patients
Development and Analysis of a Stool Bank for Cancer Patients	NCT04291755	USA 2019–2021	all	100	Obs	Five stool, blood, and urine samples each over a 12-month period	To investigate the impact of gut microbiota on the efficacy of immune checkpoint inhibitors in NSCLC and CRC patients
Microbiome and Rectal Cancer	NCT04223102	USA 2020–2027	II-III	40	Int	Serial rectal biopsy specimens in a 5-year follow-up	To investigate the association between microbiome and pathologic response to neoadjuvant therapy in rectal cancer
Fecal Microbiota Transplant (FMT) Capsule for Improving the Efficacy of Anti-PD-1	NCT04130763	China 2020–2021	IV	10	Int	Induction dose with FMT capsules one week before anti-PD-1 treatment beginning followed by maintenance dose	To determine whether the FMT capsule improves ORR of anti-PD-1 treatment in resistant/refractory gastrointestinal cancer patients

Obs: observational; RR: response rate; TT: treatment toxicity/treatment-related adverse events; SOC: standard of care; T: clinical trial; LM: luminal microbiota; MAM: mucosal associated microbiota; CT: chemotherapy; IT: immunotherapy; NSCLC: non-small cell lung cancer; TNBC: triple negative breast cancer; PC: pancreatic cancer; HR: high-risk; MO3UFA: marine omega-3 polyunsaturated fatty acid; FMT: fecal microbiota transplant.

Author Contributions: A.P. and S.D.M. conceptualized and organized the manuscript; A.P., S.D.M., F.P. have been involved in collection of bibliographic materials and writing—original draft preparation; A.P., S.D.M., F.P, V.M., K.C., G.P. have been involved in writing—review and editing, A.P., S.D.M., G.P and C.F. provided supervision and proofread the manuscript. All authors have read and agreed to the published version of the manuscript.

Funding: This research was funded by ALCLI "Giorgio e Silvia" ONLUS, a non-profit association.

Conflicts of Interest: The authors declare no conflict of interest.

Abbreviations

5-FU	5-Fluorouracil
ACT	Adjuvant Chemotherapy
Akt	Protein Kinase B
APC	Adenomatous Polyposis Coli
APCMin	Multiple Intestinal Neoplasia, a mutant allele of the Murine Adenomatous Polyposis Coli Locus
ATM	Ataxia Telangiectasia Mutated Serine/Threonine Kinase
AUC	Area Under the Curve
BIRC3	Baculoviral IAP Repeat Containing 3
BMP	Bone Morphogenetic Protein
CA19-9	Carbohydrate Antigen 19-9
cAMP	3'-5'-Cyclic Adenosine Monophosphate
CDI	Clostridium Difficile Infection
CEA	Carcino Embryonic Antigen
CEA	Carcinoembryonic Antigen
cf-DNA	Cell-Free DNA
CIMP	CpG Island Methylator Phenotype
CPSF4	Cleavage And Polyadenylation Specific Factor 4
CRC	Colorectal Cancer
CSC	Cancer Stem Cells
CT	Computed Tomography
CT	Chemotherapy
CTCs	Circulating Tumor Cells
ctDNA	Circulating Tumor DNA
ctDNA clear	ctDNA clearance or modification rate of every study arm and correlation with clinical outcome measures (according to the design of each study)
ctRNAs	Circulating Tumor RNAs
Cxcl2	C-X-C Motif Chemokine Ligand 2
DCE	Dynamic Contrast-Enhanced
ddPCR	Digital Droplet PCR
DDR	DNA Damage Response
DFS	Disease-free Survival
dPCR	Digital PCR
DR	Distant Recurrence
EGFR	Epidermal Growth Factor Receptor
EMT	Epithelial–Mesenchymal Transition
Enco/Bini/Cet	Encorafenib/Binimetinib/Cetuximab
Endp	Study Endpoints if not Reported in Study Description
ETBF	Enterotoxigenic Bacteroides Fragilis
EVs	Extracellular Vesicles
FMT	Fecal Microbiota Transplantation
Fn	*Fusobacterium Nucleatum*
FOBT	Fecal Occult Blood Test
FOXO	Forkhead Box O3
GC	Gastric Cancer
GI	Gastrointestinal

Gli1	Glioma-Associated Oncogene Homolog 1
GLOBOCAN	Global Cancer Statistics
GMMs	Metabolites of the Intestinal Microbiome
HIF-1	Hypoxia-Inducible Factor 1
HR	Hazard Ratio
HR	High-Risk According to Histopathological Factors
HR	High-Risk
IAPs	Inhibitor of Apoptosis Proteins
ICIs	Immune Checkpoint Inhibitors
IECs	Ileal Intestinal Epithelial Cells
IL-17	Interleukin-17
Int	Interventional
IT	Immunotherapy
LB	Liquid Biopsy
LM	Luminal Microbiota
lncRNAs	Long non-coding RNAs
LR	Low-Risk According to Histopatological Factors
LR	Local Recurrence
MAM	Mucosal Associated Microbiota
mCRC	Metastatic CRC
MDM2	Mouse Double Minute 2
MEK	Mitogen-Activated Protein Kinase
MIR	MicroRNA
miRNAs	MicroRNAs
MO3UFA	Marine Omega-3 Polyunsaturated Fatty Acid
mRCC	Metastatic Renal Cell Carcinoma
MRD	Minimal Residual Disease
MRI	Magnetic Resonance Imaging
mSEPT9	methylated Septin 9
MSI	Micro-Satellite Instability
mTOR	Mammalian Target of Rapamycin
MYD88	Myeloid Differentiation Primary Response 88
N	Planned Enrollment
NA	Not Available
ncRNAs	non-coding RNAs
NEAT1	Nuclear Enriched Abundant Transcript 1
NFkB	Nuclear Factor Kappa-Light-Chain-Enhancer of Activated B Cells
NSCLC	Non-Small Cell Lung Cancer
NTBF	Non-Enterotoxigenic Bacteroides Fragilis
Obs	Observational
OMVs	Outer Membrane Vesicles
OS	Overall Survival
PACs	Proanthocyanidins
PC	Pancreatic Cancer
pCR	Pathologic Complete Response
PD-1	Programmed Death-1
PFS	Progression-Free Survival
PI3K	Phosphatidylinositol 3-Kinase
PLGC	Precancerous lesions of gastric carcinoma
PTEN	Phosphatase and Tensin Homolog
PUFAs	Omega-3 Polyunsatured Fatty Acids
PVAs	Hydroxy-Phenylvaleric Acids
PVLs	Hydroxy-Phenyl-γ-Valerolactones
QoL	Quality of Life
RECIST	Response Evaluation Criteria in Solid Tumors
RFS	Relapse-Free Survival
ROC	Receiver Operating Characteristic Curve

ROS	Reactive Oxygen Species
RR	Response Rate
SCFA	Short-Chain Fatty Acid
SMAD4	Mothers Against Decapentaplegic Homolog 4
SOC	Standard of Care
T	Clinical Trial
TDEs	Tumor-Derived Exosomes
TFH	Follicular T-helper Cell
TGF-β	Transforming Growth Factor Beta
TLR4	Toll-like Receptor 4
TNBC	Triple Negative Breast Cancer
TNF-α	Tumor Necrosis Factor- alpha
TNM	Classification of Malignant Tumors (Tumor-Nodes-Metastasis)
TNMB	Tumor-Nodes-Metastasis-Blood
TT	Treatment Toxicity/Treatment-Related Adverse Events
TTF	Time to Treatment Failure
TTR	Time to Recurrence
VEGF	Vascular Endothelial Growth Factor

References

1. Ferlay, J.; Colombet, M.; Soerjomataram, I.; Mathers, C.; Parkin, D.M.; Pineros, M.; Znaor, A.; Bray, F. Estimating the global cancer incidence and mortality in 2018: GLOBOCAN sources and methods. *Int. J. Cancer* **2019**, *144*, 1941–1953. [CrossRef] [PubMed]
2. Ludwig, J.A.; Weinstein, J.N. Biomarkers in cancer staging, prognosis and treatment selection. *Nat. Rev. Cancer* **2005**, *5*, 845–856. [CrossRef] [PubMed]
3. van Zijl, F.; Krupitza, G.; Mikulits, W. Initial steps of metastasis: Cell invasion and endothelial transmigration. *Mutat. Res.* **2011**, *728*, 23–34. [CrossRef]
4. Corcoran, R.B.; Chabner, B.A. Application of Cell-free DNA Analysis to Cancer Treatment. *N. Engl. J. Med.* **2018**, *379*, 1754–1765. [CrossRef] [PubMed]
5. Backhed, F.; Ley, R.E.; Sonnenburg, J.L.; Peterson, D.A.; Gordon, J.I. Host-bacterial mutualism in the human intestine. *Science* **2005**, *307*, 1915–1920. [CrossRef]
6. Gomez, A.; Espinoza, J.L.; Harkins, D.M.; Leong, P.; Saffery, R.; Bockmann, M.; Torralba, M.; Kuelbs, C.; Kodukula, R.; Inman, J.; et al. Host Genetic Control of the Oral Microbiome in Health and Disease. *Cell Host Microbe* **2017**, *22*, 269–278.e263. [CrossRef]
7. David, L.A.; Materna, A.C.; Friedman, J.; Campos-Baptista, M.I.; Blackburn, M.C.; Perrotta, A.; Erdman, S.E.; Alm, E.J. Host lifestyle affects human microbiota on daily timescales. *Genome Biol.* **2014**, *15*, R89. [CrossRef]
8. Graf, D.; Di Cagno, R.; Fak, F.; Flint, H.J.; Nyman, M.; Saarela, M.; Watzl, B. Contribution of diet to the composition of the human gut microbiota. *Microb. Ecol. Health Dis.* **2015**, *26*, 26164. [CrossRef]
9. Wong, S.H.; Yu, J. Gut microbiota in colorectal cancer: Mechanisms of action and clinical applications. *Nat. Rev. Gastroenterol. Hepatol.* **2019**, *16*, 690–704. [CrossRef]
10. Crowley, E.; Di Nicolantonio, F.; Loupakis, F.; Bardelli, A. Liquid biopsy: Monitoring cancer-genetics in the blood. *Nat. Rev. Clin. Oncol.* **2013**, *10*, 472–484. [CrossRef]
11. Lampis, A.; Hahne, J.C.; Hedayat, S.; Valeri, N. MicroRNAs as mediators of drug resistance mechanisms. *Curr. Opin. Pharmacol.* **2020**, *54*, 44–50. [CrossRef] [PubMed]
12. Osumi, H.; Shinozaki, E.; Yamaguchi, K.; Zembutsu, H. Clinical utility of circulating tumor DNA for colorectal cancer. *Cancer Science* **2019**, *110*, 1148–1155. [CrossRef] [PubMed]
13. Kilgour, E.; Rothwell, D.G.; Brady, G.; Dive, C. Liquid Biopsy-Based Biomarkers of Treatment Response and Resistance. *Cancer Cell* **2020**, *37*, 485–495. [CrossRef] [PubMed]
14. Masuda, T.; Hayashi, N.; Iguchi, T.; Ito, S.; Eguchi, H.; Mimori, K. Clinical and biological significance of circulating tumor cells in cancer. *Mol. Oncol.* **2016**, *10*, 408–417. [CrossRef] [PubMed]
15. Romiti, A.; Raffa, S.; Di Rocco, R.; Roberto, M.; Milano, A.; Zullo, A.; Leone, L.; Ranieri, D.; Mazzetta, F.; Medda, E.; et al. Circulating tumor cells count predicts survival in colorectal cancer patients. *J. Gastrointest. Liver Dis. JGLD* **2014**, *23*, 279–284. [CrossRef] [PubMed]
16. Marcuello, M.; Vymetalkova, V.; Neves, R.P.L.; Duran-Sanchon, S.; Vedeld, H.M.; Tham, E.; van Dalum, G.; Flugen, G.; Garcia-Barberan, V.; Fijneman, R.J.; et al. Circulating biomarkers for early detection and clinical management of colorectal cancer. *Mol. As. Med.* **2019**, *69*, 107–122. [CrossRef]
17. Tsai, W.S.; You, J.F.; Hung, H.Y.; Hsieh, P.S.; Hsieh, B.; Lenz, H.J.; Idos, G.; Friedland, S.; Yi-Jiun Pan, J.; Shao, H.J.; et al. Novel Circulating Tumor Cell Assay for Detection of Colorectal Adenomas and Cancer. *Clin. Transl. Gastroenterol.* **2019**, *10*, e00088. [CrossRef]
18. Tan, Y.; Wu, H. The significant prognostic value of circulating tumor cells in colorectal cancer: A systematic review and meta-analysis. *Curr. Probl. Cancer* **2018**, *42*, 95–106. [CrossRef]

19. Tsai, W.S.; Chen, J.S.; Shao, H.J.; Wu, J.C.; Lai, J.M.; Lu, S.H.; Hung, T.F.; Chiu, Y.C.; You, J.F.; Hsieh, P.S.; et al. Circulating Tumor Cell Count Correlates with Colorectal Neoplasm Progression and Is a Prognostic Marker for Distant Metastasis in Non-Metastatic Patients. *Sci. Rep.* **2016**, *6*, 24517. [CrossRef]
20. Cremolini, C.; Schirripa, M.; Antoniotti, C.; Moretto, R.; Salvatore, L.; Masi, G.; Falcone, A.; Loupakis, F. First-line chemotherapy for mCRC-a review and evidence-based algorithm. *Nat. Rev. Clin. Oncol.* **2015**, *12*, 607–619. [CrossRef]
21. Cortellini, A.; Cannita, K.; Parisi, A.; Lanfiuti Baldi, P.; Venditti, O.; D'Orazio, C.; Dal Mas, A.; Calvisi, G.; Giordano, A.V.; Vicentini, V.; et al. Weekly alternate intensive regimen FIrB/FOx in metastatic colorectal cancer patients: An update from clinical practice. *OncoTargets Ther.* **2019**, *12*, 2159–2170. [CrossRef] [PubMed]
22. Aranda, E.; Vieitez, J.M.; Gomez-Espana, A.; Gil Calle, S.; Salud-Salvia, A.; Grana, B.; Garcia-Alfonso, P.; Rivera, F.; Quintero-Aldana, G.A.; Reina-Zoilo, J.J.; et al. FOLFOXIRI plus bevacizumab versus FOLFOX plus bevacizumab for patients with metastatic colorectal cancer and >/=3 circulating tumour cells: The randomised phase III VISNU-1 trial. *ESMO Open* **2020**, *5*. [CrossRef] [PubMed]
23. Van Cutsem, E.; Nordlinger, B.; Cervantes, A.; Group, E.G.W. Advanced colorectal cancer: ESMO Clinical Practice Guidelines for treatment. *Ann. Oncol. Off. J. Eur. Soc. Med. Oncol.* **2010**, *21* (Suppl. 5), v93–v97. [CrossRef] [PubMed]
24. Parisi, A.; Cortellini, A.; Cannita, K.; Venditti, O.; Camarda, F.; Calegari, M.A.; Salvatore, L.; Tortora, G.; Rossini, D.; Germani, M.M.; et al. Evaluation of Second-line Anti-VEGF after First-line Anti-EGFR Based Therapy in RAS Wild-Type Metastatic Colorectal Cancer: The Multicenter "SLAVE" Study. *Cancers* **2020**, *12*, 1259. [CrossRef]
25. Musella, V.; Pietrantonio, F.; Di Buduo, E.; Iacovelli, R.; Martinetti, A.; Sottotetti, E.; Bossi, I.; Maggi, C.; Di Bartolomeo, M.; de Braud, F.; et al. Circulating tumor cells as a longitudinal biomarker in patients with advanced chemorefractory, RAS-BRAF wild-type colorectal cancer receiving cetuximab or panitumumab. *Int. J. Cancer* **2015**, *137*, 1467–1474. [CrossRef]
26. Cristiano, S.; Leal, A.; Phallen, J.; Fiksel, J.; Adleff, V.; Bruhm, D.C.; Jensen, S.O.; Medina, J.E.; Hruban, C.; White, J.R.; et al. Genome-wide cell-free DNA fragmentation in patients with cancer. *Nature* **2019**, *570*, 385–389. [CrossRef]
27. Diehl, F.; Schmidt, K.; Choti, M.A.; Romans, K.; Goodman, S.; Li, M.; Thornton, K.; Agrawal, N.; Sokoll, L.; Szabo, S.A.; et al. Circulating mutant DNA to assess tumor dynamics. *Nat. Med.* **2008**, *14*, 985–990. [CrossRef]
28. Wang, X.; Shi, X.Q.; Zeng, P.W.; Mo, F.M.; Chen, Z.H. Circulating cell free DNA as the diagnostic marker for colorectal cancer: A systematic review and meta-analysis. *Oncotarget* **2018**, *9*, 24514–24524. [CrossRef]
29. Masuda, T.; Wang, X.; Maeda, M.; Canver, M.C.; Sher, F.; Funnell, A.P.; Fisher, C.; Suciu, M.; Martyn, G.E.; Norton, L.J.; et al. Transcription factors LRF and BCL11A independently repress expression of fetal hemoglobin. *Science* **2016**, *351*, 285–289. [CrossRef]
30. Flamini, E.; Mercatali, L.; Nanni, O.; Calistri, D.; Nunziatini, R.; Zoli, W.; Rosetti, P.; Gardini, N.; Lattuneddu, A.; Verdecchia, G.M.; et al. Free DNA and carcinoembryonic antigen serum levels: An important combination for diagnosis of colorectal cancer. *Clin. Cancer Res.* **2006**, *12*, 6985–6988. [CrossRef]
31. Nian, J.; Sun, X.; Ming, S.; Yan, C.; Ma, Y.; Feng, Y.; Yang, L.; Yu, M.; Zhang, G.; Wang, X. Diagnostic Accuracy of Methylated SEPT9 for Blood-based Colorectal Cancer Detection: A Systematic Review and Meta-Analysis. *Clin. Transl. Gastroenterol.* **2017**, *8*, e216. [CrossRef] [PubMed]
32. Luo, H.; Zhao, Q.; Wei, W.; Zheng, L.; Yi, S.; Li, G.; Wang, W.; Sheng, H.; Pu, H.; Mo, H.; et al. Circulating tumor DNA methylation profiles enable early diagnosis, prognosis prediction, and screening for colorectal cancer. *Sci. Translat. Med.* **2020**, *12*, eaax7533m. [CrossRef] [PubMed]
33. Spindler, K.G.; Boysen, A.K.; Pallisgard, N.; Johansen, J.S.; Tabernero, J.; Sorensen, M.M.; Jensen, B.V.; Hansen, T.F.; Sefrioui, D.; Andersen, R.F.; et al. Cell-Free DNA in Metastatic Colorectal Cancer: A Systematic Review and Meta-Analysis. *Oncologist* **2017**, *22*, 1049–1055. [CrossRef] [PubMed]
34. Perdyan, A.; Spychalski, P.; Kacperczyk, J.; Rostkowska, O.; Kobiela, J. Circulating Tumor DNA in KRAS positive colorectal cancer patients as a prognostic factor—A systematic review and meta-analysis. *Crit. Rev. Oncol. Hematol.* **2020**, *154*, 103065. [CrossRef]
35. Douillard, J.Y.; Oliner, K.S.; Siena, S.; Tabernero, J.; Burkes, R.; Barugel, M.; Humblet, Y.; Bodoky, G.; Cunningham, D.; Jassem, J.; et al. Panitumumab-FOLFOX4 treatment and RAS mutations in colorectal cancer. *N. Engl. J. Med.* **2013**, *369*, 1023–1034. [CrossRef]
36. Di Nicolantonio, F.; Martini, M.; Molinari, F.; Sartore-Bianchi, A.; Arena, S.; Saletti, P.; De Dosso, S.; Mazzucchelli, L.; Frattini, M.; Siena, S.; et al. Wild-type BRAF is required for response to panitumumab or cetuximab in metastatic colorectal cancer. *J. Clin. Oncol.* **2008**, *26*, 5705–5712. [CrossRef]
37. Siravegna, G.; Mussolin, B.; Buscarino, M.; Corti, G.; Cassingena, A.; Crisafulli, G.; Ponzetti, A.; Cremolini, C.; Amatu, A.; Lauricella, C.; et al. Clonal evolution and resistance to EGFR blockade in the blood of colorectal cancer patients. *Nat. Med.* **2015**, *21*, 827. [CrossRef]
38. Khan, K.H.; Cunningham, D.; Werner, B.; Vlachogiannis, G.; Spiteri, I.; Heide, T.; Mateos, J.F.; Vatsiou, A.; Lampis, A.; Damavandi, M.D.; et al. Longitudinal Liquid Biopsy and Mathematical Modeling of Clonal Evolution Forecast Time to Treatment Failure in the PROSPECT-C Phase II Colorectal Cancer Clinical Trial. *Cancer Dis.* **2018**, *8*, 1270–1285. [CrossRef]
39. Khan, K.; Rata, M.; Cunningham, D.; Koh, D.M.; Tunariu, N.; Hahne, J.C.; Vlachogiannis, G.; Hedayat, S.; Marchetti, S.; Lampis, A.; et al. Functional imaging and circulating biomarkers of response to regorafenib in treatment-refractory metastatic colorectal cancer patients in a prospective phase II study. *Gut* **2018**, *67*, 1484–1492. [CrossRef]

40. Yang, Y.C.; Wang, D.; Jin, L.; Yao, H.W.; Zhang, J.H.; Wang, J.; Zhao, X.M.; Shen, C.Y.; Chen, W.; Wang, X.L.; et al. Circulating tumor DNA detectable in early- and late-stage colorectal cancer patients. *Biosci. Rep.* **2018**, *38*. [CrossRef]
41. Yang, M.; Forbes, M.E.; Bitting, R.L.; O'Neill, S.S.; Chou, P.C.; Topaloglu, U.; Miller, L.D.; Hawkins, G.A.; Grant, S.C.; DeYoung, B.R.; et al. Incorporating blood-based liquid biopsy information into cancer staging: Time for a TNMB system? *Ann. Oncol.* **2018**, *29*, 311–323. [CrossRef] [PubMed]
42. Schrag, D.; Rifas-Shiman, S.; Saltz, L.; Bach, P.B.; Begg, C.B. Adjuvant chemotherapy use for Medicare beneficiaries with stage II colon cancer. *J. Clin. Oncol.* **2002**, *20*, 3999–4005. [CrossRef] [PubMed]
43. Tie, J.; Wang, Y.; Tomasetti, C.; Li, L.; Springer, S.; Kinde, I.; Silliman, N.; Tacey, M.; Wong, H.L.; Christie, M.; et al. Circulating tumor DNA analysis detects minimal residual disease and predicts recurrence in patients with stage II colon cancer. *Sci. Transl. Med.* **2016**, *8*, 346ra392. [CrossRef] [PubMed]
44. Reinert, T.; Henriksen, T.V.; Christensen, E.; Sharma, S.; Salari, R.; Sethi, H.; Knudsen, M.; Nordentoft, I.; Wu, H.T.; Tin, A.S.; et al. Analysis of Plasma Cell-Free DNA by Ultradeep Sequencing in Patients With Stages I to III Colorectal Cancer. *JAMA Oncol.* **2019**, *5*, 1124–1131. [CrossRef] [PubMed]
45. Wang, Y.; Li, L.; Cohen, J.D.; Kinde, I.; Ptak, J.; Popoli, M.; Schaefer, J.; Silliman, N.; Dobbyn, L.; Tie, J.; et al. Prognostic Potential of Circulating Tumor DNA Measurement in Postoperative Surveillance of Nonmetastatic Colorectal Cancer. *JAMA Oncol.* **2019**, *5*, 1118–1123. [CrossRef] [PubMed]
46. Tang, X.J.; Wang, W.; Hann, S.S. Interactions among lncRNAs, miRNAs and mRNA in colorectal cancer. *Biochimie* **2019**, *163*, 58–72. [CrossRef]
47. Qi, F.F.; Yang, Y.; Zhang, H.; Chen, H. Long non-coding RNAs: Key regulators in oxaliplatin resistance of colorectal cancer. *Biomed. Pharmacother.* **2020**, *128*, 110329. [CrossRef]
48. Wei, L.; Wang, X.; Lv, L.; Liu, J.; Xing, H.; Song, Y.; Xie, M.; Lei, T.; Zhang, N.; Yang, M. The emerging role of microRNAs and long noncoding RNAs in drug resistance of hepatocellular carcinoma. *Mol. Cancer* **2019**, *18*, 147. [CrossRef]
49. Wang, X.; Jiang, G.; Ren, W.; Wang, B.; Yang, C.; Li, M. LncRNA NEAT1 Regulates 5-Fu Sensitivity, Apoptosis and Invasion in Colorectal Cancer Through the MiR-150-5p/CPSF4 Axis. *OncoTargets Ther.* **2020**, *13*, 6373–6383. [CrossRef]
50. Xian, Z.; Hu, B.; Wang, T.; Zeng, J.; Cai, J.; Zou, Q.; Zhu, P. lncRNA UCA1 Contributes to 5-Fluorouracil Resistance of Colorectal Cancer Cells Through miR-23b-3p/ZNF281 Axis. *OncoTargets Ther.* **2020**, *13*, 7571–7583. [CrossRef]
51. He, Z.; Dang, J.; Song, A.; Cui, X.; Ma, Z.; Zhang, Y. The involvement of miR-150/beta-catenin axis in colorectal cancer progression. *Biomed. Pharmacother.* **2020**, *121*, 109495. [CrossRef] [PubMed]
52. Sur, D.; Burz, C.; Sabarimurugan, S.; Irimie, A. Diagnostic and Prognostic Significance of MiR-150 in Colorectal Cancer: A Systematic Review and Meta-Analysis. *J. Pers. Med.* **2020**, *10*, 99. [CrossRef]
53. Peng, Q.; Yao, W.; Yu, C.; Zou, L.; Shen, Y.; Zhu, Y.; Cheng, M.; Feng, Z.; Xu, B. Identification of microRNA-181 as a promising biomarker for predicting the poor survival in colorectal cancer. *Cancer Med.* **2019**, *8*, 5995–6009. [CrossRef] [PubMed]
54. Liu, J.; Ke, F.; Chen, T.; Zhou, Q.; Weng, L.; Tan, J.; Shen, W.; Li, L.; Zhou, J.; Xu, C.; et al. MicroRNAs that regulate PTEN as potential biomarkers in colorectal cancer: A systematic review. *J. Cancer Res. Clin. Oncol.* **2020**, *146*, 809–820. [CrossRef] [PubMed]
55. Sabarimurugan, S.; Madhav, M.R.; Kumarasamy, C.; Gupta, A.; Baxi, S.; Krishnan, S.; Jayaraj, R. Prognostic Value of MicroRNAs in Stage II Colorectal Cancer Patients: A Systematic Review and Meta-Analysis. *Mol. Diagn. Ther.* **2020**, *24*, 15–30. [CrossRef] [PubMed]
56. Yamada, A.; Horimatsu, T.; Okugawa, Y.; Nishida, N.; Honjo, H.; Ida, H.; Kou, T.; Kusaka, T.; Sasaki, Y.; Yagi, M.; et al. Serum miR-21, miR-29a, and miR-125b Are Promising Biomarkers for the Early Detection of Colorectal Neoplasia. *Clin. Cancer Res.* **2015**, *21*, 4234–4242. [CrossRef]
57. Hur, K.; Toiyama, Y.; Okugawa, Y.; Ide, S.; Imaoka, H.; Boland, C.R.; Goel, A. Circulating microRNA-203 predicts prognosis and metastasis in human colorectal cancer. *Gut* **2017**, *66*, 654–665. [CrossRef]
58. Vychytilova-Faltejskova, P.; Radova, L.; Sachlova, M.; Kosarova, Z.; Slaba, K.; Fabian, P.; Grolich, T.; Prochazka, V.; Kala, Z.; Svoboda, M.; et al. Serum-based microRNA signatures in early diagnosis and prognosis prediction of colon cancer. *Carcinogenesis* **2016**, *37*, 941–950. [CrossRef]
59. Oehme, F.; Krahl, S.; Gyorffy, B.; Muessle, B.; Rao, V.; Greif, H.; Ziegler, N.; Lin, K.; Thepkaysone, M.L.; Polster, H.; et al. Low level of exosomal long non-coding RNA HOTTIP is a prognostic biomarker in colorectal cancer. *RNA Biol.* **2019**, *16*, 1339–1345. [CrossRef]
60. Kang, W.; Zheng, Q.; Lei, J.; Chen, C.; Yu, C. Prognostic Value of Long Noncoding RNAs in Patients with Gastrointestinal Cancer: A Systematic Review and Meta-Analysis. *Dis. Markers* **2018**, *2018*, 5340894. [CrossRef]
61. Madurantakam Royam, M.; Kumarasamy, C.; Baxi, S.; Gupta, A.; Ramesh, N.; Kodiveri Muthukaliannan, G.; Jayaraj, R. Current Evidence on miRNAs as Potential Theranostic Markers for Detecting Chemoresistance in Colorectal Cancer: A Systematic Review and Meta-Analysis of Preclinical and Clinical Studies. *Mol. Diagn. Ther.* **2019**, *23*, 65–82. [CrossRef] [PubMed]
62. Brussow, H. Problems with the concept of gut microbiota dysbiosis. *Microb. Biotechnol.* **2020**, *13*, 423–434. [CrossRef] [PubMed]
63. Ursell, L.K.; Metcalf, J.L.; Parfrey, L.W.; Knight, R. Defining the human microbiome. *Nutr. Rev.* **2012**, *70* (Suppl. 1), S38–S44. [CrossRef] [PubMed]
64. Marchesi, J.R.; Ravel, J. The vocabulary of microbiome research: A proposal. *Microbiome* **2015**, *3*, 31. [CrossRef]
65. Human Microbiome Project Consortium. Structure, function and diversity of the healthy human microbiome. *Nature* **2012**, *486*, 207–214. [CrossRef]

66. Qin, J.; Li, R.; Raes, J.; Arumugam, M.; Burgdorf, K.S.; Manichanh, C.; Nielsen, T.; Pons, N.; Levenez, F.; Yamada, T.; et al. A human gut microbial gene catalogue established by metagenomic sequencing. *Nature* **2010**, *464*, 59–65. [CrossRef]
67. O'Keefe, S.J. Diet, microorganisms and their metabolites, and colon cancer. *Nat. Rev. Gastroenterol. Hepatol.* **2016**, *13*, 691–706. [CrossRef]
68. Tilg, H.; Adolph, T.E.; Gerner, R.R.; Moschen, A.R. The Intestinal Microbiota in Colorectal Cancer. *Cancer Cell* **2018**, *33*, 954–964. [CrossRef]
69. Garrett, W.S. Cancer and the microbiota. *Science* **2015**, *348*, 80–86. [CrossRef]
70. Gagniere, J.; Raisch, J.; Veziant, J.; Barnich, N.; Bonnet, R.; Buc, E.; Bringer, M.A.; Pezet, D.; Bonnet, M. Gut microbiota imbalance and colorectal cancer. *World J. Gastroenterol.* **2016**, *22*, 501–518. [CrossRef]
71. Sanchez-Alcoholado, L.; Ramos-Molina, B.; Otero, A.; Laborda-Illanes, A.; Ordonez, R.; Medina, J.A.; Gomez-Millan, J.; Queipo-Ortuno, M.I. The Role of the Gut Microbiome in Colorectal Cancer Development and Therapy Response. *Cancers* **2020**, *12*, 1406. [CrossRef] [PubMed]
72. Bhatt, A.P.; Redinbo, M.R.; Bultman, S.J. The role of the microbiome in cancer development and therapy. *CA A Cancer J. Clin.* **2017**, *67*, 326–344. [CrossRef] [PubMed]
73. Gagnaire, A.; Nadel, B.; Raoult, D.; Neefjes, J.; Gorvel, J.P. Collateral damage: Insights into bacterial mechanisms that predispose host cells to cancer. *Nat. Rev. Microbiol.* **2017**, *15*, 109–128. [CrossRef] [PubMed]
74. Fahrer, J.; Huelsenbeck, J.; Jaurich, H.; Dorsam, B.; Frisan, T.; Eich, M.; Roos, W.P.; Kaina, B.; Fritz, G. Cytolethal distending toxin (CDT) is a radiomimetic agent and induces persistent levels of DNA double-strand breaks in human fibroblasts. *DNA Repair* **2014**, *18*, 31–43. [CrossRef] [PubMed]
75. Levy, M.; Kolodziejczyk, A.A.; Thaiss, C.A.; Elinav, E. Dysbiosis and the immune system. *Nat. Rev. Immunol.* **2017**, *17*, 219–232. [CrossRef]
76. Dalmasso, G.; Cougnoux, A.; Delmas, J.; Darfeuille-Michaud, A.; Bonnet, R. The bacterial genotoxin colibactin promotes colon tumor growth by modifying the tumor microenvironment. *Gut Microbes* **2014**, *5*, 675–680. [CrossRef]
77. Pleguezuelos-Manzano, C.; Puschhof, J.; Rosendahl Huber, A.; van Hoeck, A.; Wood, H.M.; Nomburg, J.; Gurjao, C.; Manders, F.; Dalmasso, G.; Stege, P.B.; et al. Mutational signature in colorectal cancer caused by genotoxic pks(+) E. coli. *Nature* **2020**, *580*, 269–273. [CrossRef]
78. Zamani, S.; Taslimi, R.; Sarabi, A.; Jasemi, S.; Sechi, L.A.; Feizabadi, M.M. Enterotoxigenic Bacteroides fragilis: A Possible Etiological Candidate for Bacterially-Induced Colorectal Precancerous and Cancerous Lesions. *Front. Cell. Infect. Microbiol.* **2019**, *9*, 449. [CrossRef]
79. Brennan, C.A.; Garrett, W.S. Fusobacterium nucleatum—Symbiont, opportunist and oncobacterium. *Nat. Rev. Microbiol.* **2019**, *17*, 156–166. [CrossRef]
80. Sun, C.H.; Li, B.B.; Wang, B.; Zhao, J.; Zhang, X.Y.; Li, T.T.; Li, W.B.; Tang, D.; Qiu, M.J.; Wang, X.C.; et al. The role of Fusobacterium nucleatum in colorectal cancer: From carcinogenesis to clinical management. *Chronic Dis. Transl. Med.* **2019**, *5*, 178–187. [CrossRef]
81. Koi, M.; Okita, Y.; Carethers, J.M. Fusobacterium nucleatum Infection in Colorectal Cancer: Linking Inflammation, DNA Mismatch Repair and Genetic and Epigenetic Alterations. *J. Anus Rectum Colon* **2018**, *2*, 37–46. [CrossRef]
82. Zitvogel, L.; Daillere, R.; Roberti, M.P.; Routy, B.; Kroemer, G. Anticancer effects of the microbiome and its products. *Nat. Rev. Microbiol.* **2017**, *15*, 465–478. [CrossRef]
83. Feng, Q.; Liang, S.; Jia, H.; Stadlmayr, A.; Tang, L.; Lan, Z.; Zhang, D.; Xia, H.; Xu, X.; Jie, Z.; et al. Gut microbiome development along the colorectal adenoma-carcinoma sequence. *Nat. Commun.* **2015**, *6*, 6528. [CrossRef] [PubMed]
84. Lee, A.; Lee, Y.J.; Yoo, H.J.; Kim, M.; Chang, Y.; Lee, D.S.; Lee, J.H. Consumption of Dairy Yogurt Containing Lactobacillus paracasei ssp. paracasei, Bifidobacterium animalis ssp. lactis and Heat-Treated Lactobacillus plantarum Improves Immune Function Including Natural Killer Cell Activity. *Nutrients* **2017**, *9*, 558. [CrossRef] [PubMed]
85. Long, S.; Yang, Y.; Shen, C.; Wang, Y.; Deng, A.; Qin, Q.; Qiao, L. Metaproteomics characterizes human gut microbiome function in colorectal cancer. *NPJ Biofilms Microbiomes* **2020**, *6*, 14. [CrossRef] [PubMed]
86. Wang, G.; Yu, Y.; Wang, Y.Z.; Wang, J.J.; Guan, R.; Sun, Y.; Shi, F.; Gao, J.; Fu, X.L. Role of SCFAs in gut microbiome and glycolysis for colorectal cancer therapy. *J. Cell. Physiol.* **2019**, *234*, 17023–17049. [CrossRef]
87. Borges-Canha, M.; Portela-Cidade, J.P.; Dinis-Ribeiro, M.; Leite-Moreira, A.F.; Pimentel-Nunes, P. Role of colonic microbiota in colorectal carcinogenesis: A systematic review. *Rev. Esp. de Enferm. Dig.* **2015**, *107*, 659–671. [CrossRef]
88. Grazioso, T.P.; Brandt, M.; Djouder, N. Diet, Microbiota, and Colorectal Cancer. *iScience* **2019**, *21*, 168–187. [CrossRef]
89. Wan, M.L.; Wang, Y.; Zeng, Z.; Deng, B.; Zhu, B.S.; Cao, T.; Li, Y.K.; Xiao, J.; Han, Q.; Wu, Q. Colorectal cancer (CRC) as a multifactorial disease and its causal correlations with multiple signaling pathways. *Biosci. Rep.* **2020**, *40*. [CrossRef]
90. Duchartre, Y.; Kim, Y.M.; Kahn, M. The Wnt signaling pathway in cancer. *Crit. Rev. Oncol. Hematol.* **2016**, *99*, 141–149. [CrossRef]
91. Zhang, L.; Shay, J.W. Multiple Roles of APC and its Therapeutic Implications in Colorectal Cancer. *J. Natl. Cancer Inst.* **2017**, *109*. [CrossRef] [PubMed]
92. Wang, B.; Tian, T.; Kalland, K.H.; Ke, X.; Qu, Y. Targeting Wnt/beta-Catenin Signaling for Cancer Immunotherapy. *Trends Pharmacol. Sci.* **2018**, *39*, 648–658. [CrossRef] [PubMed]
93. Koni, M.; Pinnaro, V.; Brizzi, M.F. The Wnt Signalling Pathway: A Tailored Target in Cancer. *Int. J. Mol. Sci.* **2020**, *21*, 7697. [CrossRef] [PubMed]

94. Hofman, P.; Vouret-Craviari, V. Microbes-induced EMT at the crossroad of inflammation and cancer. *Gut Microbes* **2012**, *3*, 176–185. [CrossRef] [PubMed]
95. Vogelstein, B.; Fearon, E.R.; Hamilton, S.R.; Kern, S.E.; Preisinger, A.C.; Leppert, M.; Nakamura, Y.; White, R.; Smits, A.M.; Bos, J.L. Genetic alterations during colorectal-tumor development. *N. England J. Med.* **1988**, *319*, 525–532. [CrossRef] [PubMed]
96. Wu, R.; Wang, L.; Yin, R.; Hudlikar, R.; Li, S.; Kuo, H.D.; Peter, R.; Sargsyan, D.; Guo, Y.; Liu, X.; et al. Epigenetics/epigenomics and prevention by curcumin of early stages of inflammatory-driven colon cancer. *Mol. Carcinog.* **2020**, *59*, 227–236. [CrossRef]
97. Yuan, L.; Zhang, S.; Li, H.; Yang, F.; Mushtaq, N.; Ullah, S.; Shi, Y.; An, C.; Xu, J. The influence of gut microbiota dysbiosis to the efficacy of 5-Fluorouracil treatment on colorectal cancer. *Biomed. Pharmacother.* **2018**, *108*, 184–193. [CrossRef]
98. Zhang, S.; Yang, Y.; Weng, W.; Guo, B.; Cai, G.; Ma, Y.; Cai, S. Fusobacterium nucleatum promotes chemoresistance to 5-fluorouracil by upregulation of BIRC3 expression in colorectal cancer. *J. Exp. Clin. Cancer Res. CR* **2019**, *38*, 14. [CrossRef]
99. Andre, T.; Shiu, K.K.; Kim, T.W.; Jensen, B.V.; Jensen, L.H.; Punt, C.; Smith, D.; Garcia-Carbonero, R.; Benavides, M.; Gibbs, P.; et al. Pembrolizumab in Microsatellite-Instability-High Advanced Colorectal Cancer. *N. Engl. J. Med.* **2020**, *383*, 2207–2218. [CrossRef]
100. Lang, M.; Baumgartner, M.; Rozalska, A.; Frick, A.; Riva, A.; Jarek, M.; Berry, D.; Gasche, C. Crypt residing bacteria and proximal colonic carcinogenesis in a mouse model of Lynch syndrome. *Int. J. Cancer* **2020**, *147*, 2316–2326. [CrossRef]
101. Lalani, A.A.; Xie, W.; Braun, D.A.; Kaymakcalan, M.; Bosse, D.; Steinharter, J.A.; Martini, D.J.; Simantov, R.; Lin, X.; Wei, X.X.; et al. Effect of Antibiotic Use on Outcomes with Systemic Therapies in Metastatic Renal Cell Carcinoma. *Eur. Urol. Oncol.* **2020**, *3*, 372–381. [CrossRef] [PubMed]
102. Ngara, T.R.; Zhang, H. Recent Advances in Function-based Metagenomic Screening. *Genom. Proteom. Bioinform.* **2018**, *16*, 405–415. [CrossRef] [PubMed]
103. Dai, Z.; Coker, O.O.; Nakatsu, G.; Wu, W.K.K.; Zhao, L.; Chen, Z.; Chan, F.K.L.; Kristiansen, K.; Sung, J.J.Y.; Wong, S.H.; et al. Multi-cohort analysis of colorectal cancer metagenome identified altered bacteria across populations and universal bacterial markers. *Microbiome* **2018**, *6*, 70. [CrossRef] [PubMed]
104. Dalal, N.; Jalandra, R.; Sharma, M.; Prakash, H.; Makharia, G.K.; Solanki, P.R.; Singh, R.; Kumar, A. Omics technologies for improved diagnosis and treatment of colorectal cancer: Technical advancement and major perspectives. *Biomed. Pharmacother.* **2020**, *131*, 110648. [CrossRef]
105. Behrouzi, A.; Nafari, A.H.; Siadat, S.D. The significance of microbiome in personalized medicine. *Clin. Transl. Med.* **2019**, *8*, 16. [CrossRef]
106. Yachida, S.; Mizutani, S.; Shiroma, H.; Shiba, S.; Nakajima, T.; Sakamoto, T.; Watanabe, H.; Masuda, K.; Nishimoto, Y.; Kubo, M.; et al. Metagenomic and metabolomic analyses reveal distinct stage-specific phenotypes of the gut microbiota in colorectal cancer. *Nat. Med.* **2019**, *25*, 968–976. [CrossRef]
107. Gao, R.; Kong, C.; Huang, L.; Li, H.; Qu, X.; Liu, Z.; Lan, P.; Wang, J.; Qin, H. Mucosa-associated microbiota signature in colorectal cancer. *Eur. J. Clin. Microbiol. Infect. Dis.* **2017**, *36*, 2073–2083. [CrossRef]
108. Zeller, G.; Tap, J.; Voigt, A.Y.; Sunagawa, S.; Kultima, J.R.; Costea, P.I.; Amiot, A.; Bohm, J.; Brunetti, F.; Habermann, N.; et al. Potential of fecal microbiota for early-stage detection of colorectal cancer. *Mol. Syst. Biol.* **2014**, *10*, 766. [CrossRef]
109. Kim, D.J.; Yang, J.; Seo, H.; Lee, W.H.; Ho Lee, D.; Kym, S.; Park, Y.S.; Kim, J.G.; Jang, I.J.; Kim, Y.K.; et al. Colorectal cancer diagnostic model utilizing metagenomic and metabolomic data of stool microbial extracellular vesicles. *Sci. Rep.* **2020**, *10*, 2860. [CrossRef]
110. Ahmadi Badi, S.; Moshiri, A.; Fateh, A.; Rahimi Jamnani, F.; Sarshar, M.; Vaziri, F.; Siadat, S.D. Microbiota-Derived Extracellular Vesicles as New Systemic Regulators. *Front. Microbiol.* **2017**, *8*, 1610. [CrossRef]
111. Tjalsma, H.; Boleij, A.; Marchesi, J.R.; Dutilh, B.E. A bacterial driver-passenger model for colorectal cancer: Beyond the usual suspects. *Nat. Rev. Microbiol.* **2012**, *10*, 575–582. [CrossRef] [PubMed]
112. Oke, S.; Martin, A. Insights into the role of the intestinal microbiota in colon cancer. *Ther. Adv. Gastroenterol.* **2017**, *10*, 417–428. [CrossRef] [PubMed]
113. Farin, H.F.; Karthaus, W.R.; Kujala, P.; Rakhshandehroo, M.; Schwank, G.; Vries, R.G.; Kalkhoven, E.; Nieuwenhuis, E.E.; Clevers, H. Paneth cell extrusion and release of antimicrobial products is directly controlled by immune cell-derived IFN-gamma. *J. Exp. Med.* **2014**, *211*, 1393–1405. [CrossRef] [PubMed]
114. Sato, T.; Stange, D.E.; Ferrante, M.; Vries, R.G.; Van Es, J.H.; Van den Brink, S.; Van Houdt, W.J.; Pronk, A.; Van Gorp, J.; Siersema, P.D.; et al. Long-term expansion of epithelial organoids from human colon, adenoma, adenocarcinoma, and Barrett's epithelium. *Gastroenterology* **2011**, *141*, 1762–1772. [CrossRef]
115. Rubert, J.; Schweiger, P.J.; Mattivi, F.; Tuohy, K.; Jensen, K.B.; Lunardi, A. Intestinal Organoids: A Tool for Modelling Diet-Microbiome-Host Interactions. *Trends Endocrinol. Metab. TEM* **2020**, *31*, 848–858. [CrossRef]
116. Toden, S.; Ravindranathan, P.; Gu, J.; Cardenas, J.; Yuchang, M.; Goel, A. Oligomeric proanthocyanidins (OPCs) target cancer stem-like cells and suppress tumor organoid formation in colorectal cancer. *Sci. Rep.* **2018**, *8*, 3335. [CrossRef]
117. Ozdal, T.; Sela, D.A.; Xiao, J.; Boyacioglu, D.; Chen, F.; Capanoglu, E. The Reciprocal Interactions between Polyphenols and Gut Microbiota and Effects on Bioaccessibility. *Nutrients* **2016**, *8*, 78. [CrossRef]
118. Zhang, L.S.; Davies, S.S. Microbial metabolism of dietary components to bioactive metabolites: Opportunities for new therapeutic interventions. *Genome Med.* **2016**, *8*, 46. [CrossRef]

119. Trost, K.; Ulaszewska, M.M.; Stanstrup, J.; Albanese, D.; De Filippo, C.; Tuohy, K.M.; Natella, F.; Scaccini, C.; Mattivi, F. Host: Microbiome co-metabolic processing of dietary polyphenols—An acute, single blinded, cross-over study with different doses of apple polyphenols in healthy subjects. *Food Res. Int.* **2018**, *112*, 108–128. [CrossRef]
120. Mena, P.; Bresciani, L.; Brindani, N.; Ludwig, I.A.; Pereira-Caro, G.; Angelino, D.; Llorach, R.; Calani, L.; Brighenti, F.; Clifford, M.N.; et al. Phenyl-gamma-valerolactones and phenylvaleric acids, the main colonic metabolites of flavan-3-ols: Synthesis, analysis, bioavailability, and bioactivity. *Nat. Prod. Rep.* **2019**, *36*, 714–752. [CrossRef]
121. Mehta, R.S.; Nishihara, R.; Cao, Y.; Song, M.; Mima, K.; Qian, Z.R.; Nowak, J.A.; Kosumi, K.; Hamada, T.; Masugi, Y.; et al. Association of Dietary Patterns With Risk of Colorectal Cancer Subtypes Classified by Fusobacterium nucleatum in Tumor Tissue. *JAMA Oncol.* **2017**, *3*, 921–927. [CrossRef] [PubMed]
122. Nencioni, A.; Caffa, I.; Cortellino, S.; Longo, V.D. Fasting and cancer: Molecular mechanisms and clinical application. *Nat. Rev. Cancer* **2018**, *18*, 707–719. [CrossRef] [PubMed]
123. Li, G.; Xie, C.; Lu, S.; Nichols, R.G.; Tian, Y.; Li, L.; Patel, D.; Ma, Y.; Brocker, C.N.; Yan, T.; et al. Intermittent Fasting Promotes White Adipose Browning and Decreases Obesity by Shaping the Gut Microbiota. *Cell Metabo.* **2017**, *26*, 672–685.e674. [CrossRef] [PubMed]
124. Nakamura, K.; Tonouchi, H.; Sasayama, A.; Ashida, K. A Ketogenic Formula Prevents Tumor Progression and Cancer Cachexia by Attenuating Systemic Inflammation in Colon 26 Tumor-Bearing Mice. *Nutrients* **2018**, *10*, 206. [CrossRef] [PubMed]
125. Robertson, R.C.; Seira Oriach, C.; Murphy, K.; Moloney, G.M.; Cryan, J.F.; Dinan, T.G.; Paul Ross, R.; Stanton, C. Omega-3 polyunsaturated fatty acids critically regulate behaviour and gut microbiota development in adolescence and adulthood. *Brain Behav. Immun.* **2017**, *59*, 21–37. [CrossRef] [PubMed]
126. Watson, H.; Mitra, S.; Croden, F.C.; Taylor, M.; Wood, H.M.; Perry, S.L.; Spencer, J.A.; Quirke, P.; Toogood, G.J.; Lawton, C.L.; et al. A randomised trial of the effect of omega-3 polyunsaturated fatty acid supplements on the human intestinal microbiota. *Gut* **2018**, *67*, 1974–1983. [CrossRef]
127. Bullman, S.; Pedamallu, C.S.; Sicinska, E.; Clancy, T.E.; Zhang, X.; Cai, D.; Neuberg, D.; Huang, K.; Guevara, F.; Nelson, T.; et al. Analysis of Fusobacterium persistence and antibiotic response in colorectal cancer. *Science* **2017**, *358*, 1443–1448. [CrossRef]
128. Routy, B.; Le Chatelier, E.; Derosa, L.; Duong, C.P.M.; Alou, M.T.; Daillere, R.; Fluckiger, A.; Messaoudene, M.; Rauber, C.; Roberti, M.P.; et al. Gut microbiome influences efficacy of PD-1-based immunotherapy against epithelial tumors. *Science* **2018**, *359*, 91–97. [CrossRef]
129. Buti, S.; Bersanelli, M.; Perrone, F.; Tiseo, M.; Tucci, M.; Adamo, V.; Stucci, L.S.; Russo, A.; Tanda, E.T.; Spagnolo, F.; et al. Effect of concomitant medications with immune-modulatory properties on the outcomes of patients with advanced cancer treated with immune checkpoint inhibitors: Development and validation of a novel prognostic index. *Eur. J. Cancer* **2021**, *142*, 18–28. [CrossRef]
130. Sanchez, B.; Delgado, S.; Blanco-Miguez, A.; Lourenco, A.; Gueimonde, M.; Margolles, A. Probiotics, gut microbiota, and their influence on host health and disease. *Mol. Nutr. Food Res.* **2017**, *61*, 1600240. [CrossRef]
131. Chen, D.; Wu, J.; Jin, D.; Wang, B.; Cao, H. Fecal microbiota transplantation in cancer management: Current status and perspectives. *Int. J. Cancer* **2019**, *145*, 2021–2031. [CrossRef]
132. Wang, Y.; Wiesnoski, D.H.; Helmink, B.A.; Gopalakrishnan, V.; Choi, K.; DuPont, H.L.; Jiang, Z.D.; Abu-Sbeih, H.; Sanchez, C.A.; Chang, C.C.; et al. Fecal microbiota transplantation for refractory immune checkpoint inhibitor-associated colitis. *Nat. Med.* **2018**, *24*, 1804–1808. [CrossRef] [PubMed]
133. Chang, C.W.; Lee, H.C.; Li, L.H.; Chiang Chiau, J.S.; Wang, T.E.; Chuang, W.H.; Chen, M.J.; Wang, H.Y.; Shih, S.C.; Liu, C.Y.; et al. Fecal Microbiota Transplantation Prevents Intestinal Injury, Upregulation of Toll-Like Receptors, and 5-Fluorouracil/Oxaliplatin-Induced Toxicity in Colorectal Cancer. *Int. J. Mol. Sci.* **2020**, *21*, 386. [CrossRef] [PubMed]
134. Le Bastard, Q.; Ward, T.; Sidiropoulos, D.; Hillmann, B.M.; Chun, C.L.; Sadowsky, M.J.; Knights, D.; Montassier, E. Fecal microbiota transplantation reverses antibiotic and chemotherapy-induced gut dysbiosis in mice. *Sci. Rep.* **2018**, *8*, 6219. [CrossRef]
135. Hefazi, M.; Patnaik, M.M.; Hogan, W.J.; Litzow, M.R.; Pardi, D.S.; Khanna, S. Safety and Efficacy of Fecal Microbiota Transplant for Recurrent Clostridium difficile Infection in Patients With Cancer Treated With Cytotoxic Chemotherapy: A Single-Institution Retrospective Case Series. *Mayo Clin. Proc.* **2017**, *92*, 1617–1624. [CrossRef] [PubMed]
136. Kopetz, S.; Grothey, A.; Yaeger, R.; Van Cutsem, E.; Desai, J.; Yoshino, T.; Wasan, H.; Ciardiello, F.; Loupakis, F.; Hong, Y.S.; et al. Encorafenib, Binimetinib, and Cetuximab in BRAF V600E-Mutated Colorectal Cancer. *N. Engl. J. Med.* **2019**, *381*, 1632–1643. [CrossRef] [PubMed]
137. Kolencik, D.; Shishido, S.N.; Pitule, P.; Mason, J.; Hicks, J.; Kuhn, P. Liquid Biopsy in Colorectal Carcinoma: Clinical Applications and Challenges. *Cancers* **2020**, *12*, 1376. [CrossRef]
138. Castro-Giner, F.; Gkountela, S.; Donato, C.; Alborelli, I.; Quagliata, L.; Ng, C.K.Y.; Piscuoglio, S.; Aceto, N. Cancer Diagnosis Using a Liquid Biopsy: Challenges and Expectations. *Diagnostics* **2018**, *8*, 31. [CrossRef]
139. Blaser, M.J. Antibiotic use and its consequences for the normal microbiome. *Science* **2016**, *352*, 544–545. [CrossRef]
140. Nagrath, S.; Sequist, L.V.; Maheswaran, S.; Bell, D.W.; Irimia, D.; Ulkus, L.; Smith, M.R.; Kwak, E.L.; Digumarthy, S.; Muzikansky, A.; et al. Isolation of rare circulating tumour cells in cancer patients by microchip technology. *Nature* **2007**, *450*, 1235–1239. [CrossRef]

141. Mishra, A.; Dubash, T.D.; Edd, J.F.; Jewett, M.K.; Garre, S.G.; Karabacak, N.M.; Rabe, D.C.; Mutlu, B.R.; Walsh, J.R.; Kapur, R.; et al. Ultrahigh-throughput magnetic sorting of large blood volumes for epitope-agnostic isolation of circulating tumor cells. *Proc. Natl. Acad. Sci. USA* **2020**, *117*, 16839–16847. [CrossRef] [PubMed]
142. Kalinich, M.; Bhan, I.; Kwan, T.T.; Miyamoto, D.T.; Javaid, S.; LiCausi, J.A.; Milner, J.D.; Hong, X.; Goyal, L.; Sil, S.; et al. An RNA-based signature enables high specificity detection of circulating tumor cells in hepatocellular carcinoma. *Proc. Natl. Acad. Sci. USA* **2017**, *114*, 1123–1128. [CrossRef] [PubMed]
143. Yu, M.; Bardia, A.; Aceto, N.; Bersani, F.; Madden, M.W.; Donaldson, M.C.; Desai, R.; Zhu, H.; Comaills, V.; Zheng, Z.; et al. Cancer therapy. Ex vivo culture of circulating breast tumor cells for individualized testing of drug susceptibility. *Science* **2014**, *345*, 216–220. [CrossRef]
144. Fachin, F.; Spuhler, P.; Martel-Foley, J.M.; Edd, J.F.; Barber, T.A.; Walsh, J.; Karabacak, M.; Pai, V.; Yu, M.; Smith, K.; et al. Monolithic Chip for High-throughput Blood Cell Depletion to Sort Rare Circulating Tumor Cells. *Sci. Rep.* **2017**, *7*, 10936. [CrossRef] [PubMed]

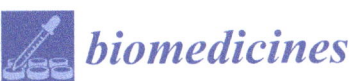

Article

Clinical Significance of Preoperative Inflammatory Markers in Prediction of Prognosis in Node-Negative Colon Cancer: Correlation between Neutrophil-to-Lymphocyte Ratio and Poorly Differentiated Clusters

Giulia Turri [1], Valeria Barresi [2], Alessandro Valdegamberi [1], Gabriele Gecchele [1], Cristian Conti [1], Serena Ammendola [2], Alfredo Guglielmi [1], Aldo Scarpa [2] and Corrado Pedrazzani [1,*,†]

[1] Unit of General and Hepatobiliary Surgery, Department of Surgical Sciences, Dentistry, Gynecology and Pediatrics, University of Verona, 37134 Verona, Italy; giulia.turri89@gmail.com (G.T.); alessandro.valdegamberi2@aovr.veneto.it (A.V.); gabrielegecchele11@gmail.com (G.G.); cristian.conti1988@gmail.com (C.C.); alfredo.guglielmi@univr.it (A.G.)
[2] Department of Diagnostics and Public Health, Section of Pathology, University of Verona, 37134 Verona, Italy; valeria.barresi@univr.it (V.B.); serena.ammendola88@gmail.com (S.A.); aldo.scarpa@univr.it (A.S.)
* Correspondence: corrado.pedrazzani@univr.it; Tel.: +39-(0)45-8124464-6719; Fax: +39-(0)45-8027426
† Current address: U.O.C. di Chirurgia Generale e Epatobiliare, Policlinico "G.B. Rossi", Piazzale "L. Scuro" 10, 37134 Verona, Italy.

Abstract: Although stage I and II colon cancers (CC) generally show a very good prognosis, a small proportion of these patients dies from recurrent disease. The identification of high-risk patients, who may benefit from adjuvant chemotherapy, becomes therefore essential. We retrospectively evaluated 107 cases of stage I ($n = 28$, 26.2%) and II ($n = 79$, 73.8%) CC for correlations among preoperative inflammatory markers, histopathological factors and long-term prognosis. A neutrophil-to-lymphocyte ratio greater than 3 (H-NLR) and a platelet-to-lymphocyte ratio greater than 150 (H-PLR) were significantly associated with the presence of poorly differentiated clusters (PDC) ($p = 0.007$ and $p = 0.039$, respectively). In addition, H-NLR and PDC proved to be significant and independent survival prognosticators for overall survival (OS; $p = 0.007$ and $p < 0.001$, respectively), while PDC was the only significant prognostic factor for cancer-specific survival (CSS; $p < 0.001$,). Finally, the combination of H-NLR and PDC allowed an optimal stratification of OS and CSS in our cohort, suggesting a potential role in clinical practice for the identification of high-risk patients with stage I and II CC.

Keywords: colon cancer; poorly differentiated clusters; prognostic factors; inflammatory markers; histopathological markers; immune system

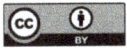

1. Introduction

Colorectal cancer (CRC) is one of the most frequent malignancies in the Western population [1]. Prognosis is mainly influenced by the completeness of surgical resection and pathological stage [2–4]. However, some histopathological and molecular features may play a relevant role in the definition of long-term outcomes [5] in patients affected by this neoplasia. The identification of additional prognostic factors, able to distinguish high-risk from low-risk patients, is particularly relevant in case of node-negative disease. Indeed, the use of adjuvant chemotherapy in these patients is controversial in view of the overall good prognosis [6].

In addition to tumor stage, the host immune system may play an important role in tumor development and progression [7–9]. Some inflammatory markers, expression of an imbalanced immune reaction, have been evaluated as prognostic factors in cancer patients [8,10,11]. In particular, neutrophil-to-lymphocyte ratio (NLR) has been tested in oncological patients [12–14], and its prognostic value was also suggested in patients with CRC. Various studies investigated the correlation between preoperative NLR and overall as well as disease-free survival in CRC, suggesting different threshold values and results. Most of the studies concluded that elevated NLR was associated with worse outcomes in patients with both localized and metastatic CRC [10,15–23]. Similarly, platelet-to-lymphocyte ratio (PLT) [23–25] and platelet count (PC) could predict long-term outcomes in patients with CRC [11,26,27].

Among the histopathological factors, the presence of lymphatic or vascular invasion, poor differentiation according to the World Health Organization (WHO) grading system and tumor budding are currently considered indicators of worse prognosis in stage II CRC [28–30]. More recently, the presence of poorly differentiated clusters (PDCs) [31] has gained attention in view of its significant correlation with higher recurrence risk and shorter overall survival in patients with stage II CRC [32–34]. Nevertheless, the assessment of PDC is rarely adopted for prognostic stratification in routine clinical practice, as conventional tumor grading system is still preferred in the AJCC guidelines [35].

This study aimed at evaluating the potential correlations between preoperative inflammatory biomarkers and histopathological characteristics in node negative colon cancer, as well as their impact on long-term prognosis.

2. Materials and Methods

2.1. Inclusion Criteria and Population under Study

The original population under study consisted of all patients undergoing surgery for CRC ($n = 1418$) at the Division of General and Hepatobiliary Surgery, University of Verona Hospital, between January 2005 and December 2015 The inclusion criteria were: age ≥ 18 years; histology-proven colon cancer; absence of nodal or distant metastasis (AJCC/UICC TNM Stage I and II); availability of histological slides or paraffin block of the primary tumor; data on preoperative NLR, PLR and PC; and absence of residual disease after surgery (R0 resection). Patients with rectal cancer were excluded from the analysis.

2.2. Assessment of Inflammatory Markers

Neutrophil count, lymphocyte count and PC were obtained from venous blood within 2 weeks before the date of surgery. NLR and PLR were calculated by dividing the absolute number of neutrophils or platelets by the absolute number of lymphocytes, respectively. Blood samples were drawn by an expert phlebotomist in vacuum blood tubes containing K2-EDTA (Terumo Europe NV, Leuven, Belgium). The complete blood cell count (CBC) was performed using Advia 2120 (Siemens Healthcare Diagnostics, Tarrytown NY, USA). The local reference ranges are 150–400 $\times 10^9$/L for platelets, 4.3–10.0 $\times 10^9$/L for total white blood cells (WBC), 2.0–7.0 $\times 10^9$/L for neutrophils and 0.95–4.5 $\times 10^9$/L for lymphocytes. The same analyzer was used throughout the study period. The quality and comparability of test results were validated by data of both internal quality control (IQC) and external quality assessment (EQA) [36].

2.3. Histological Evaluation

All cases included underwent histopathological revision as previously described in detail [32]. Briefly, hematoxylin–eosin-stained histological slides were revised to assess the depth of infiltration (pT1, pT2, pT3 and pT4) and histological grading according to the WHO criteria, lympho-vascular invasion (LVI), perineural invasion (PNI), tumor budding, presence of inflammation and PDC count. PDC were defined as clusters of at least 5 tumor cells lacking a glandular structure, at the invasive front or in the tumor stroma and counted in one hot spot under the microscopic field of $\times 20$ objective lens (i.e., a microscopic field with a major axis of 1 mm). The 8th Edition of the American Joint Committee on Cancer (AJCC) and the Union International Contre Le Cancer (UICC) criteria were used for reporting the pathology specimens [35].

2.4. Preoperative Work-Up and Surgical Technique

All patients were staged with preoperative colonoscopy, chest-abdomen-pelvis computed tomography (CT) and carcinoembryonic antigen (CEA) measurement. In the case of dubious hepatic lesions, magnetic resonance was used to clarify the preoperative staging.

The main goal of surgery was the complete excision of the cancer burden in order to obtain an R0 resection. The extent of the resection was planned according to cancer location, disease stage and patient's general conditions. Anatomical resections with ligation of vessels at their origin were the procedures of choice in order to achieve an adequate lymphadenectomy [37].

2.5. Data Collection and Statistical Analysis

Data were extracted from a prospectively maintained database. Demographic, clinical, surgical, hematological and histopathological variables were analyzed. All methods used in this study were performed in accordance with the relevant ethical guidelines and regulations of the University Hospital of Verona, where the investigation was carried out. The study was approved by the Verona University Hospital Ethics Committee (09/07/2016, ID number: 42763-CRINF-1034 CESC). Informed consent was obtained from all patients enrolled in the study. On preliminary analysis, preoperative NLR, PLR and PC were found to be normally distributed. The optimal cut-off values for NLR ($\geq$3) [19,20], PLR ($\geq$150) [25] and PC ($\geq 350 \times 10^9$/L) [10] as dichotomous predictors of survival were chosen based on previously published literature. The correlation between preoperative inflammatory markers and pathological features was investigated using independent t test or Mann–Whitney U test for continuous variables and chi-squared test or Fisher's exact test for categorical variables, as appropriate. Continuous data were reported as mean (+SD) or median (range) as appropriate according to distribution, while categorical data were reported as numbers and percentages.

Survival and follow-up data were obtained by collecting outpatient clinical records or by directly contacting the patient or their relatives. The median length (range) of follow up was 104 (3–160) months considering the whole population and 113 (76–160) months considering surviving patients only. At the time of analysis, 75 patients had completed their follow-up and 32 have died.

Survival analysis was computed using the Kaplan–Meier method and compared by the log-rank test, with time of overall survival (OS) measured from the date of surgery to the date of death from any cause or most recent follow-up and cancer-specific survival (CSS) as months from the date of surgery to the date of death from cancer. Multivariate analysis was performed by Cox regression model taking into account clinical and pathological characteristics and inflammatory markers that were found to significantly influence long-term survival on univariate analysis.

All statistical tests were two-sided, and association were considered statistically significant at a nominal level of 0.05 ($p < 0.05$). Statistical analysis was performed using SPSS (version 23, SPSS, Chicago, IL, USA).

3. Results

In total, 107 patients fulfilled the inclusion criteria and were included in the analysis (Figure 1). Twenty-eight (28) tumors (26.2%) were classified as TNM stage I and 79 (73.8%) as stage II. None of the patients received adjuvant chemotherapy.

Table 1 reports the correlation between inflammatory markers and clinical-pathological variables. Forty-five patients (42.1%) had an NLR value greater than 3 (H-NLR). H-NLR was significantly associated with serosal invasion (31% vs 11.3%; $p = 0.036$) and presence of PDC (51.1% vs 24.2%; $p = 0.007$). A PLR value greater than 150 (H-PLR) was associated with a significantly higher rate of mucinous histotype (18.8% vs 4.6%; $p = 0.042$) and presence of PDC (43.7% vs 23.2%; $p = 0.039$). Finally, a PC greater than 350×10^9/L (H-PC) was associated with a higher rate of right-sided CC (76.7% vs 39%; $p = 0.001$), mucinous histotype (30% vs 6.5%; $p = 0.003$) and poorly differentiated (G3) tumors (23.3%

vs 2.6%; $p = 0.002$). No significant associations were demonstrated between NLR, PLR and PC values and the amount of inflammatory reaction, nor with lympho-vascular, perineural invasion or tumor budding.

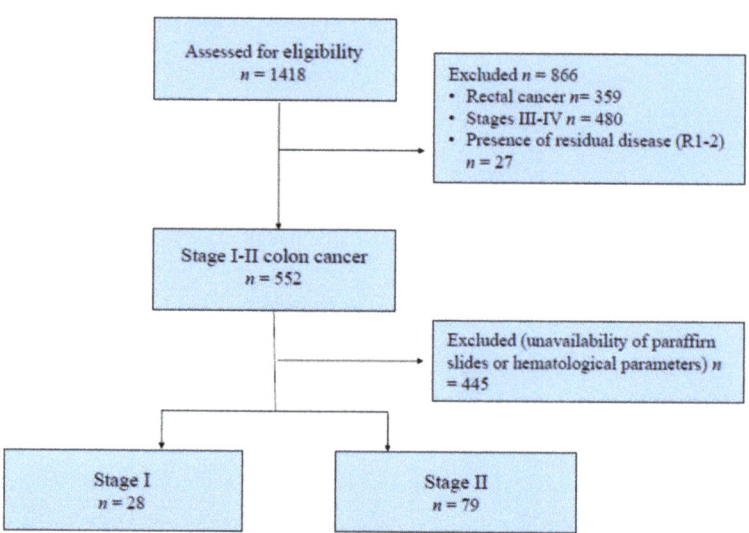

Figure 1. CONSORT diagram for patient inclusion.

Table 1. Correlations between NLR, PLR and PC and main clinical and pathological variables for the 107 patients under study.

Data		H-NLR (n = 45)	p Value	H-PLR (n = 64)	p Value	H-PC (n = 30)	p Value
Age, mean (SD)		70.5 (14.9)	0.238	70.8 (14.1)	0.294	68.5 (17.5)	0.846
Gender, male (%)		26 (57.7)	0.844	33 (51.6)	0.321	12 (40)	0.051
Tumor location (%)			0.331		0.238		0.001
	Right colon	25 (55.6)		35 (54.7)		23 (76.7)	
	Left colon	20 (44.4)		29 (45.3)		7 (23.3)	
Elective surgery (%)		42 (93.3)	0.307	61 (95.3)	0.647	29 (96.7)	1
CACI, mean (SD)		2.9 (1.5)	0.845	3.1 (1.6)	0.264	3.2 (2.0)	0.389
Mucinous carcinoma, n (%)		5 (11.1)	0.774	12 (18.8)	0.042	9 (30)	0.003
Depth of tumor invasion, n (%)			0.036		0.055		0.081
	pT1–2	11 (24.4)		12 (18.7)		6 (20)	
	pT3	20 (44.4)		36 (56.2)		14 (46.7)	
	pT4	14 (31.2)		16 (25.1)		10 (33.3)	
AJCC TNM Stage II, n (%)		34 (75.6)	0.825	51 (79.7)	0.118	23 (26.7)	0.808
Harvested lymph-nodes $\geq$ 12, n (%)		42 (93.3)	0.731	58 (90.6)	0.738	26 (86.7)	0.264
Tumor grading, high grade, n (%)		6 (13.3)	0.162	6 (9.4)	0.738	7 (23.3)	0.002
Inflammatory reaction, present, n (%)		36 (80)	0.602	52 (81.2)	0.604	25 (83.3)	1
Budding, high grade, n (%)		4 (8.9)	0.446	3 (4.7)	0.636	1 (3.3)	0.063
LVI present, n (%)		15 (33.3)	1	19 (29.7)	0.529	12 (40)	0.362
PNI present, n (%)		9 (20)	0.815	14 (21.9)	1	8 (26.7)	0.439
PDC present, n (%)		23 (51.1)	0.007	28 (43.7)	0.039	15 (50)	0.071

SD, standard deviation; CACI, Charlson Adjusted Comorbidity Index; LVI, Lymphovascular Invasion; PNI, Perineural Invasion; PDC, Poorly Differentiated Clusters. Number in parentheses are percentages, unless specified otherwise.

At survival analysis, NLR, among inflammatory markers and PDC, among histopathological factors, demonstrated to significantly and independently influence OS and CSS (Figure 2 and Table 2).

Accordingly, the combined effect on long-term outcomes of NLR and PDC was evaluated. As shown in Figure 3, excellent long-term outcomes were observed in PDC negative cases almost independently from NLR values. Conversely, long-term survival demonstrated to be negatively influenced by the presence of PDC, with a significantly worse prognosis in H-NLR cases, both considering OS ($p < 0.001$) and CSS ($p < 0.001$).

In the Cox regression multivariate analysis, age above the median ($p < 0.001$), TNM stage II ($p = 0.035$), H-NLR ($p = 0.007$) and the presence of PDC ($p < 0.001$) were independent predictors of shorter OS. Presence of PDC was the only independent prognostic factor for shorter CSS ($p < 0.001$), although H-NLR was nearly significantly associated ($p = 0.072$) (Table 3).

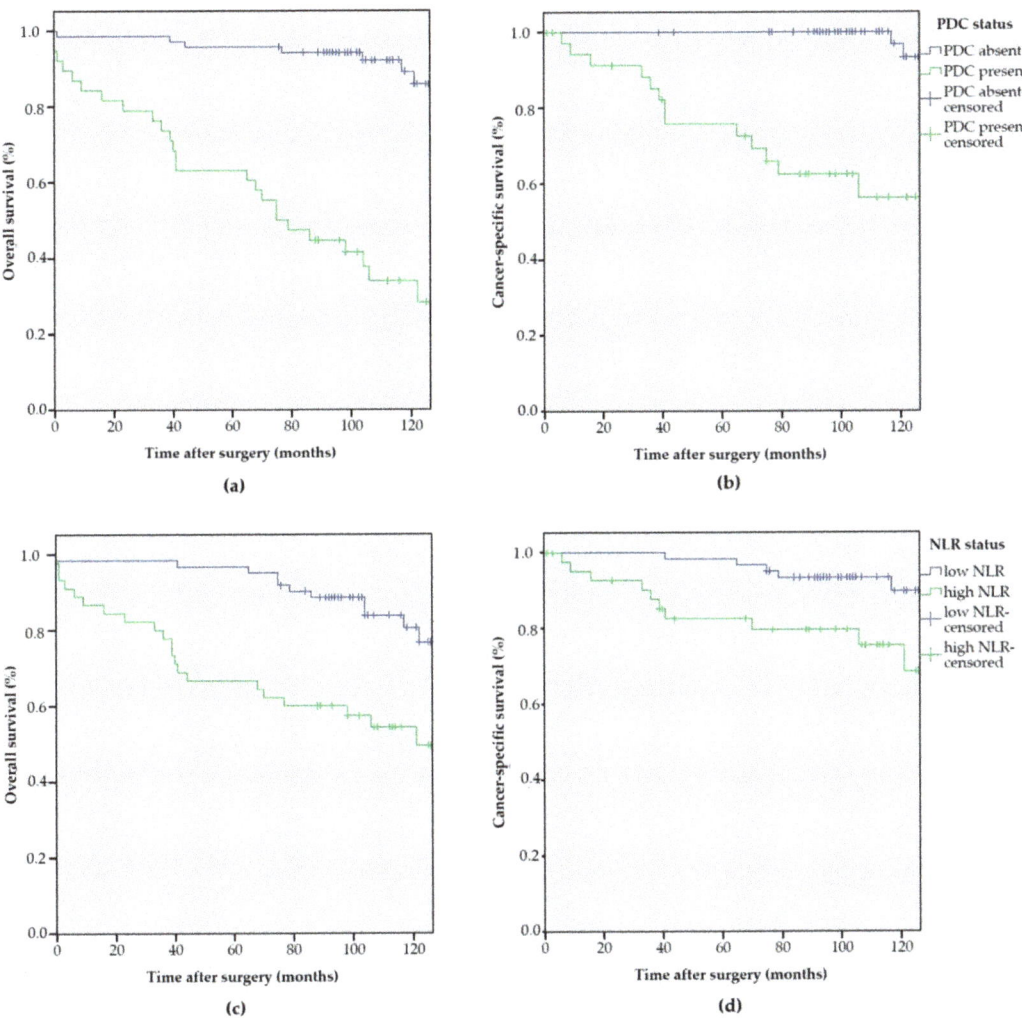

Figure 2. Kaplan–Meier estimates of overall survival (OS) and cancer-specific survival (CSS) according to PDC and NLR status: (**a**) OS according to PDC status ($p < 0.001$); (**b**) CSS according to PDC status ($p < 0.001$); (**c**) OS according to NLR status ($p < 0.001$); and (**d**) CSS according to NLR status ($p = 0.011$).

Table 2. Kaplan–Meier estimates of survival probability at 5 years according to main clinical–pathological variables for the 107 patients under study.

Data	Pts	OS	p	CSS	p
Age					
≤median	45 (42.1%)	95.6%	0.009	97.7%	0.521
>median	62 (57.9%)	75.8%		87.7%	
Gender					
Male	60 (56.1%)	91.7%	0.562	93%	0.862
Female	47 (43.9%)	78.7%		90.9%	
Tumor location					
Right colon	53 (49.5%)	88.7%	0.866	94%	0.533
Left colon	54 (50.5%)	79.6%		90.1%	
TNM Stage					
I	28 (26.2%)	82.1%	0.015	100%	0.868
II	79 (73.8%)	84.8%		89.5%	
Harvested lymph-nodes					
<12	9 (8.4%)	66.7%	0.269	87.5%	0.359
≥12	98 (91.6%)	85.7%		92.5%	
Lympho-vascular invasion					
LVI -	72 (67.3%)	88.9%	0.135	95.6%	0.109
LVI +	35 (32.7%)	74.3%		83.9%	
Perineural invasion					
PNI -	84 (78.5%)	84.5%	0.548	93.6%	0.576
PNI +	23 (21.5%)	82.6%		86.4%	
PDC					
Absent	69 (64.5%)	95.7%	<0.001	100%	<0.001
Present	38 (35.5%)	63.2%		75.7%	
NLR					
L-NLR	62 (57.9%)	96.8%	<0.001	98.4%	0.011
H-NLR	45 (42.1%)	66.7%		82.5%	
PLR			0.563		0.825
L-PLR	43 (40.2%)	90.7%		95.2%	
H-PLR	64 (59.8%)	79.7%		89.8%	
PC			0.457		0.894
L-PC	77 (72%)	88.3%		93.3%	
H-PC	30 (38%)	73.3%		88.6%	
Combined					
PDC absent/L-NLR	47 (43.9%)	100%	<0.001	100%	<0.001
PDC absent/H-NLR	22 (20.6%)	86.4%		100%	
PDC present/L-NLR	15 (14%)	86.7%		92.9%	
PDC present/H-NLR	23 (21.5%)	47.8%		63.3%	

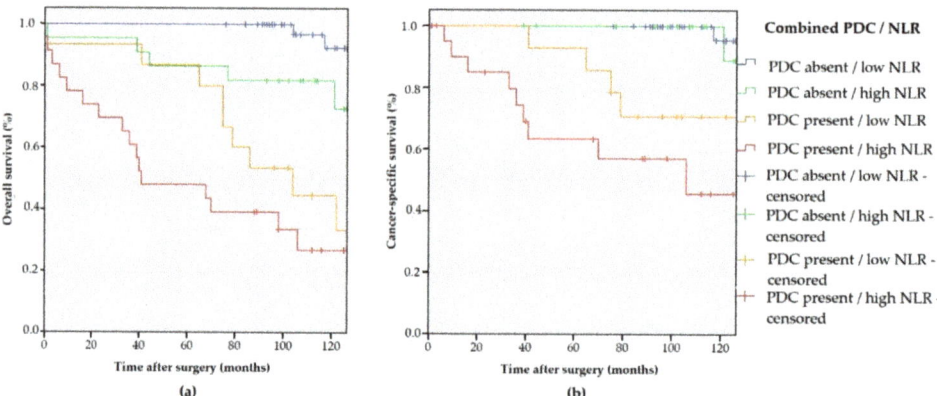

Figure 3. (a) Kaplan–Meier estimates of OS ($p < 0.001$) according to the combined PDC/NLR variable; and (b) Kaplan–Meier estimates of CSS ($p < 0.001$) according to the combined PDC/NLR variable.

Table 3. Multivariable analysis for overall- and cancer-specific survival.

Data	OS: HR (95% CI)	p Value	CSS: HR (95% CI)	p Value
Age		<0.001		0.169
≤median	-		-	
>median	5.0 (2.07–12.29)		2.27 (0.71–7.33)	
Gender		0.303		0.920
Male	-		-	
Female	0.67 (0.31–1.44)		0.94 (0.61–2.06)	
Tumor location		0.107		0.263
Right colon	-		-	
Left colon	2.05 (0.94–4.51)		1.95 (0.61–6.30)	
Stage		0.035		0.688
I	-		-	
II	0.43 (0.21–0.94)		1.30 (0.36–4.63)	
NLR		0.007		0.072
L-NLR	-		-	
H-NLR	4.25 (1.77–10.26)		4.38 (1.25–15.34)	
PDC		<0.001		<0.001
Absent	-		-	
Present	11.96 (4.70–30.40)		26.37 (5.30–131.28)	

The Cox regression multivariate analysis for OS and CSS was also conducted using the combination of PDC and NLR. The presence of both negative prognostic factors showed an additive effect; the HR for PDC-present/L-NLR was 19.91 (2.14–185.11) compared to an HR of 56.67 (95% CI 6.63–483.94) for PDC-present/H-NLR ($p < 0.001$) (Table 4).

Table 4. Multivariable analysis for overall- and cancer-specific survival conducted with the combination variable.

Data	OS: HR (95% CI)	p Value	CSS: HR (95% CI)	p Value
Age		0.001		0.196
≤ median	-		-	
> median	5.0 (2.07–12.29)		2.27 (0.71–7.33)	
Gender		0.170		0.572
Male	-		-	
Female	0.67 (0.31–1.44)		0.74 (0.61–2.06)	
Tumor location		0.107		0.263
Right colon	-		-	
Left colon	2.05 (0.94–4.51)		1.95 (0.61–6.30)	
Stage		0.04		0.688
I	-		-	
II	0.43 (0.21–0.94)		1.30 (0.36–4.63)	
Combined PDC/NLR		<0.001		<0.001
PDC absent/L-NLR	-		-	
PDC absent/H-NLR	5.78 (1.11–30.27)		2.52 (0.16–40.74)	
PDC present/L-NLR	19.13 (3.96–92.36)		19.91 (2.14–185.11)	
PDC present/H-NLR	43.58 (9.29–204.34)		56.67 (6.63–483.94)	

4. Discussion

In the current study, we analyzed the association and the prognostic role of preoperative inflammatory markers and the main histopathological features in surgically resected CCs in the absence of lymph node metastases. The main results of this study are: (1) H-NLR values are significantly associated with the presence of PDCs; (2) both H-NLR and

PDC confirmed to be significant and independent survival prognosticators; and (3) the combination of NLR and PDC allows a better stratification of OS and CSS in TNM Stage I and II colon cancer. To the best of our knowledge, this is the first study demonstrating a correlation between preoperative inflammatory markers and the presence of PDCs in patients with CC.

According to current guidelines [28–30], adjuvant chemotherapy in stage II CC is considered only for patients with specific risk factors, namely serosal infiltration (pT4), presence of lymphatic or vascular invasion and fewer than 12 analyzed nodes. However, among node-negative CCs, 5% of stage I and 12% of stage II tumors will develop a recurrence within five years from surgery [6]. Some molecular parameters, such as microsatellite instability and KRAS/BRAF mutations, have been associated with survival outcomes [5,38,39], however their assessment requires sophisticated and expensive techniques. Therefore, great interest has been directed towards the identification of some readily available and inexpensive markers which could be useful for the detection of patients who may benefit from systemic chemotherapy. Since neutrophils, platelets and lymphocytes are routinely measured as part of the preoperative work-up of patients undergoing surgery, their possible prognostic value could be very relevant in clinical practice.

The clinical impact of inflammatory markers has been partially confirmed in our study. Although NLR showed a significant association with increased risk of death from cancer (Table 2), and it was an independent prognostic variable for shorter OS at the multivariate analysis (Table 3), PLT and PC did not demonstrate any relevant association with long-term outcomes. This is in accordance with previously published studies [10,22,23,40]. Although other studies concluded that NLR is an important inflammatory biomarker in CRC, several issues should be remarked. In the study by Li and colleagues [21] on 5336 patients with CRC, which is largest published series, H-NLR was an independent prognostic factor for OS at multivariate analysis. However, the significance of NLR and other inflammatory markers in patients who did not undergo adjuvant chemotherapy was not demonstrated; this is in line with our results. Likewise, Haram at al. [22] conducted a systematic review to assess the prognostic role of NLR in metastatic and non-metastatic CRC. They concluded that preoperative NLR > 5 was associated with poorer overall survival in patients with CRC, but no association was found with the other chosen cut-offs. Malietzis et al. [20] did not identify an independent prognostic role of H-NLR (>3) in 506 patients with non-metastatic CRC who did not receive adjuvant chemotherapy. Finally, the systematic review and meta-analysis by Zhang et al. [23] found a significant association between NLR > 5, PLR > 150, PC > 400 and overall survival. However, none of the study evaluated cancer-specific survival. Furthermore, most of the studies included colon as well as rectal cancer [41,42], therefore producing results that may be biased because of the difference in treatment and prognosis of the two locations.

With regards to histopathological markers of poor prognosis, the presence of PDCs has recently gained attention as a promising prognostic factor in patients with CRC [33,34]. They reflect tumor de-differentiation, and their evaluation on hematoxylin and eosin-stained slides is more reproducible than WHO grading [32,43]. No previous study evaluated the association between PDC and inflammation-based scores in CC. This study is the first to show a significant association between H-NLR and PDC, and their cumulative negative effect on OS and CSS. The presence of an imbalanced inflammatory response measured on peripheral blood may reflect the presence of a more de-differentiated and aggressive disease. A previous study reported a significant correlation of tumor budding with preoperative neutrophil count, but not with NLR [44]. Although tumor budding and PDC have morphological and immunohistochemical similarities and might both represent tumor de-differentiation [45,46], there is not a clear evidence that they biologically overlap.

In patients with TNM stage I and II CC, inflammatory markers may permit preoperative identification of high-risk patients, whereas pathological markers lead to postoperative stratification of patients with a reduced survival probability and a higher risk of recurrence. Namely, patients with cT4 and one of these risk factors may be considered for neoadjuvant treatment, or patients with H-NLR and PDCs may receive adjuvant chemotherapy even in absence of node metastases and other risk factors. In fact, it should be noted that the association between NLR and PDC resulted to be a better prognosticator of CSS than TNM stage itself, suggesting than even TNM stage I patients with PDC (14 cases, 50%) or H-NLR (11 cases, 39.2%) may benefit from adjuvant chemotherapy. Similarly, PDC and NLR may assist in selecting endoscopically resected "early cancers" that should merit to undergo surgical resection.

The main limitation of this study relates to its retrospective nature and the limited sample size. Although we considered an initial large population, many patients were excluded due to the unavailability of all histological slides and/or hematological parameters. However, our study also has many strengths. First, the population includes homogeneous cases of node-negative CC who did not receive adjuvant chemotherapy. In fact, at their time of surgery, no adjuvant chemotherapy was indicated for TNM stage II cancers, even in the presence of pathological risk factors. This allows us to abolish the potential bias related to the administration of adjuvant chemotherapy. Second, the consistent follow-up time assured the identification of some late recurrences that may characterize the postoperative course of early stages CC.

5. Conclusions

Our study suggests that both NLR and PDC significantly affect survival even when limiting the analysis to stage I and II CCs. Noteworthy, we observed an increased rate of PDC positivity in patients with high values of NLR. In addition, NLR significantly and independently stratified OS and CSS in cases with PDC positivity. Further studies with a higher number of cases are required in order to confirm our observations and identify the effective clinical value of the association of H-NLR and PDC.

Author Contributions: Conceptualization, G.T., V.B., S.A. and C.P.; Data curation, G.T., A.V., G.G., C.C. and S.A.; Formal analysis, G.T., G.G. and C.C.; Investigation, G.T., V.B., A.V., G.G., C.C., S.A. and C.P.; Methodology, C.P.; Resources, V.B.; Software, G.G.; Supervision, V.B., A.V., A.G., A.S. and C.P.; Validation, V.B., A.V., G.G., C.C., A.G., A.S. and C.P.; Writing—original draft, G.T. and C.P.; and Writing—review and editing, G.T., V.B., C.C., A.G., A.S. and C.P. All authors have read and agreed to the published version of the manuscript.

Funding: FUR 2019: University of Verona, Italy, to VB.

Institutional Review Board Statement: The study was conducted according to the guidelines of the Declaration of Helsinki and approved by the local Ethics Committee (09/07/2016, ID number: 42763—CRINF-1034 CESC).

Informed Consent Statement: Informed consent was obtained from all subjects involved in the study.

Data Availability Statement: The data presented in this study are available on request from the corresponding author. The data are not publicly available due to privacy reasons.

Conflicts of Interest: The authors declare no conflict of interest.

References

1. Mattiuzzi, C.; Sanchis-Gomar, F.; Lippi, G. Concise update on colorectal cancer epidemiology. *Ann. Transl. Med.* **2019**, *7*, 609. [CrossRef]
2. Poornakala, S.; Prema, N. A study of morphological prognostic factors in colorectal cancer and survival analysis. *Indian J. Pathol. Microbiol.* **2019**, *62*, 36–42. [CrossRef]
3. Chi, Z.; Li, Z.; Cheng, L.; Wang, C. Comparison of long-term outcomes after laparoscopic-assisted and open colectomy for splenic flexure cancer. *J. BUON* **2018**, *23*, 322–328.
4. Micu, B.V.; Vesa, Ş.C.; Pop, T.R.; Micu, C.M. Evaluation of prognostic factors for 5 year-survival after surgery for colorectal cancer. *Ann. Ital. Chir.* **2020**, *91*, 41–48.
5. Guo, T.A.; Wu, Y.C.; Tan, C.; Jin, Y.T.; Sheng, W.Q.; Cai, S.J.; Liu, F.Q.; Xu, Y. Clinicopathologic features and prognostic value of KRAS, NRAS and BRAF mutations and DNA mismatch repair status: A single-center retrospective study of 1834 Chinese patients with Stage I–IV colorectal cancer. *Int. J. Cancer* **2019**, *145*, 1625–1634. [CrossRef]

6. Osterman, E.; Glimelius, B. Recurrence risk after up-to-date colon cancer staging, surgery, and pathology: Analysis of the entire Swedish population. *Dis. Colon Rectum* **2018**, *61*, 1016–1025. [CrossRef]
7. Mazaki, J.; Katsumata, K.; Kasahara, K.; Tago, T.; Wada, T.; Kuwabara, H.; Enomoto, M.; Ishizaki, T.; Nagakawa, Y.; Tsuchida, A. Neutrophil-to-lymphocyte ratio is a prognostic factor for colon cancer: A propensity score analysis. *BMC Cancer* **2020**, *20*, 1–8. [CrossRef]
8. Chen, J.H.; Zhai, E.T.; Yuan, Y.J.; Wu, K.M.; Xu, J.B.; Peng, J.J.; Chen, C.Q.; He, Y.L.; Cai, S.R. Systemic immune-inflammation index for predicting prognosis of colorectal cancer. *World J. Gastroenterol.* **2017**, *23*, 6261–6272. [CrossRef]
9. Shibutani, M.; Maeda, K.; Nagahara, H.; Ohtani, H.; Sakurai, K.; Yamazoe, S.; Kimura, K.; Toyokawa, T.; Amano, R.; Kubo, N.; et al. Significance of markers of systemic inflammation for predicting survival and chemotherapeutic outcomes and monitoring tumor progression in patients with unresectable metastatic colorectal cancer. *Anticancer Res.* **2015**, *35*, 5037–5046.
10. Pedrazzani, C.; Mantovani, G.; Fernandes, E.; Bagante, F.; Luca Salvagno, G.; Surci, N.; Campagnaro, T.; Ruzzenente, A.; Danese, E.; Lippi, G.; et al. Assessment of neutrophil-to-lymphocyte ratio, platelet-to-lymphocyte ratio and platelet count as predictors of long-term outcome after R0 resection for colorectal cancer. *Sci. Rep.* **2017**, *7*, 1–10. [CrossRef]
11. Pedrazzani, C.; Turri, G.; Mantovani, G.; Conti, C.; Ziello, R.; Conci, S.; Campagnaro, T.; Ruzzenente, A.; Guglielmi, A. Prognostic value of thrombocytosis in patients undergoing surgery for colorectal cancer with synchronous liver metastases. *Clin. Transl. Oncol.* **2019**, *21*, 1644–1653. [CrossRef]
12. Kosuga, T.; Konishi, T.; Kubota, T.; Shoda, K.; Konishi, H.; Shiozaki, A.; Okamoto, K.; Fujiwara, H.; Kudou, M.; Arita, T.; et al. Clinical significance of neutrophil-to-lymphocyte ratio as a predictor of lymph node metastasis in gastric cancer. *BMC Cancer* **2019**, *19*, 1187. [CrossRef]
13. Yin, X.; Wu, L.; Yang, H.; Yang, H.B. Prognostic significance of neutrophil-lymphocyte ratio (NLR) in patients with ovarian cancer: A systematic review and meta-analysis. *Medicine (Baltimore)* **2019**, *98*, e17475. [CrossRef]
14. Hasegawa, T.; Iga, T.; Takeda, D.; Amano, R.; Saito, I.; Kakei, Y.; Kusumoto, J.; Kimoto, A.; Sakakibara, A.; Akashi, M. Neutrophil-lymphocyte ratio associated with poor prognosis in oral cancer: A retrospective study. *BMC Cancer* **2020**, *20*, 1–9. [CrossRef]
15. Inamoto, S.; Kawada, K.; Okamura, R.; Hida, K.; Sakai, Y. Prognostic impact of the combination of neutrophil-to-lymphocyte ratio and Glasgow prognostic score in colorectal cancer: A retrospective cohort study. *Int. J. Colorectal Dis.* **2019**, *34*, 1303–1315. [CrossRef]
16. Silva, T.H.; Schilithz, A.O.C.; Peres, W.A.F.; Murad, L.B. Neutrophil-lymphocyte ratio and nutritional status are clinically useful in predicting prognosis in colorectal cancer patients. *Nutr. Cancer* **2020**, *72*, 1345–1354. [CrossRef]
17. Cruz-Ramos, M.; del Puerto-Nevado, L.; Zheng, B.; López-Bajo, R.; Cebrian, A.; Rodríguez-Remirez, M.; García-García, L.; Solanes-Casado, S.; García-Foncillas, J. Prognostic significance of neutrophil-to lymphocyte ratio and platelet-to lymphocyte ratio in older patients with metastatic colorectal cancer. *J. Geriatr. Oncol.* **2019**, *10*, 742–748. [CrossRef]
18. Xia, L.J.; Li, W.; Zhai, J.C.; Yan, C.W.; Chen, J.B.; Yang, H. Significance of neutrophil-to-lymphocyte ratio, platelet-to-lymphocyte ratio, lymphocyte-to-monocyte ratio and prognostic nutritional index for predicting clinical outcomes in T1-2 rectal cancer. *BMC Cancer* **2020**, *20*, 1–11. [CrossRef]
19. Dell'Aquila, E.; Cremolini, C.; Zeppola, T.; Lonardi, S.; Bergamo, F.; Masi, G.; Stellato, M.; Marmorino, F.; Schirripa, M.; Urbano, F.; et al. Prognostic and predictive role of neutrophil/lymphocytes ratio in metastatic colorectal cancer: A retrospective analysis of the TRIBE study by GONO. *Ann. Oncol.* **2018**, *29*, 924–930. [CrossRef]
20. Malietzis, G.; Giacometti, M.; Askari, A.; Nachiappan, S.; Kennedy, R.H.; Faiz, O.D.; Aziz, O.; Jenkins, J.T. A preoperative neutrophil to lymphocyte ratio of 3 predicts disease-free survival after curative elective colorectal cancer surgery. *Ann. Surg.* **2014**, *260*, 287–292. [CrossRef]
21. Li, Y.; Jia, H.; Yu, W.; Xu, Y.; Li, X.; Li, Q.; Cai, S. Nomograms for predicting prognostic value of inflammatory biomarkers in colorectal cancer patients after radical resection. *Int. J. Cancer* **2016**, *139*, 220–231. [CrossRef]
22. Haram, A.; Boland, M.R.; Kelly, M.E.; Bolger, J.C.; Waldron, R.M.; Kerin, M.J. The prognostic value of neutrophil-to-lymphocyte ratio in colorectal cancer: A systematic review. *J. Surg. Oncol.* **2017**, *115*, 470–479. [CrossRef]
23. Zhang, J.; Zhang, H.-Y.; Li, J.; Shao, X.-Y.; Zhang, C.-X. The elevated NLR, PLR and PLT may predict the prognosis of patients with colorectal cancer: A systematic review and meta-analysis. *Oncotarget* **2017**, *8*, 68837–68846. [CrossRef]
24. Huang, X.Z.; Chen, W.J.; Zhang, X.; Wu, C.C.; Zhang, C.Y.; Sun, S.S.; Wu, J. An Elevated Platelet-to-Lymphocyte Ratio Predicts Poor Prognosis and Clinicopathological Characteristics in Patients with Colorectal Cancer: A Meta-Analysis. *Dis. Markers* **2017**, *2017*, 1053125. [CrossRef]
25. Proctor, M.J.; Morrison, D.S.; Talwar, D.; Balmer, S.M.; Fletcher, C.D.; O'reilly, D.S.J.; Foulis, A.K.; Horgan, P.G.; Mcmillan, D.C. A comparison of inflammation-based prognostic scores in patients with cancer. A Glasgow Inflammation Outcome Study. *Eur. J. Cancer* **2011**, *47*, 2633–2641. [CrossRef]
26. Lee, Y.S.; Suh, K.W.; Oh, S.Y. Preoperative thrombocytosis predicts prognosis in stage II colorectal cancer patients. *Ann. Surg. Treat. Res.* **2016**, *90*, 322–327. [CrossRef]
27. Rao, X.-D.; Zhang, H.; Xu, Z.-S.; Cheng, H.; Shen, W.; Wang, X.-P. Poor prognostic role of the pretreatment platelet counts in colorectal cancer. *Medicine (Baltimore)* **2018**, *97*, e10831. [CrossRef]
28. Schmoll, H.J.; Van Cutsem, E.; Stein, A.; Valentini, V.; Glimelius, B.; Haustermans, K.; Nordlinger, B.; Van De Velde, C.J.; Cervantes, A. ESMO Consensus Guidelines for management of patients with colon and rectal cancer. A personalized approach to clinical decision making. *Ann. Oncol.* **2012**, *23*, 2479–2516. [CrossRef]

29. Benson, A.B.; Venook, A.P.; Al-Hawary, M.M.; Cederquist, L.; Chen, Y.J.; Ciombor, K.K.; Cohen, S.; Cooper, H.S.; Deming, D.; Engstrom, P.F.; et al. NCCN Guidelines® Insights Colon Cancer, Version 2.2018 Featured Updates to the NCCN Guidelines. *J. Natl. Compr. Cancer Netw.* **2018**, *16*, 359–369. [CrossRef]
30. Japanese Society for Cancer of the Colon and Rectum. Japanese Classification of Colorectal, Appendiceal, and Anal Carcinoma: The 3d English Edition [Secondary Publication]. *J. Anus Rectum Colon* **2019**, *3*, 175–195. [CrossRef]
31. Ryan, É.; Khaw, Y.L.; Creavin, B.; Geraghty, R.; Ryan, E.J.; Gibbons, D.; Hanly, A.; Martin, S.T.; O'Connell, P.R.; Winter, D.C.; et al. Tumor Budding and PDC Grade Are Stage Independent Predictors of Clinical Outcome in Mismatch Repair Deficient Colorectal Cancer. *Am. J. Surg. Pathol.* **2018**, *42*, 60–68. [CrossRef]
32. Ammendola, S.; Turri, G.; Marconi, I.; Burato, G.; Pecori, S.; Tomezzoli, A.; Conti, C.; Pedrazzani, C.; Barresi, V. The presence of poorly differentiated clusters predicts survival in stage II colorectal cancer. *Virchows Arch.* **2020**, 1–8. [CrossRef]
33. Shivji, S.; Conner, J.R.; Barresi, V.; Kirsch, R. Poorly differentiated clusters in colorectal cancer: A current review and implications for future practice. *Histopathology* **2020**, *77*, 351–368. [CrossRef]
34. Konishi, T.; Shimada, Y.; Lee, L.H.; Cavalcanti, M.S.; Hsu, M.; Smith, J.J.; Nash, G.M.; Temple, L.K.; Guillem, J.G.; Paty, P.B.; et al. Poorly Differentiated Clusters Predict Colon Cancer Recurrence. *Am. J. Surg. Pathol.* **2018**, *42*, 705–714. [CrossRef]
35. Amin, M.; Edge, S.B.; Greene, F. *AJCC Cancer Staging Manual*, 8th ed.; Springer: Berlin/Heidelberg, Germany, 2017; Volume 14.
36. Pedrazzani, C.; Tripepi, M.; Turri, G.; Fernandes, E.; Scotton, G.; Conci, S.; Campagnaro, T.; Ruzzenente, A.; Guglielmi, A. Prognostic value of red cell distribution width (RDW) in colorectal cancer. Results from a single-center cohort on 591 patients. *Sci. Rep.* **2020**, *10*, 1–9. [CrossRef]
37. Pedrazzani, C.; Lauka, L.; Sforza, S.; Ruzzenente, A.; Nifosì, F.; Delaini, G.G.; Guglielmi, A. Management of nodal disease from colon cancer in the laparoscopic era. *Int. J. Colorectal Dis.* **2015**, *30*, 303–314. [CrossRef]
38. Kim, C.G.; Ahn, J.B.; Jung, M.; Beom, S.H.; Kim, C.; Kim, J.H.; Heo, S.J.; Park, H.S.; Kim, J.H.; Kim, N.K.; et al. Effects of microsatellite instability on recurrence patterns and outcomes in colorectal cancers. *Br. J. Cancer* **2016**, *115*, 25–33. [CrossRef]
39. Domingo, E.; Camps, C.; Kaisaki, P.J.; Parsons, M.J.; Mouradov, D.; Pentony, M.M.; Makino, S.; Palmieri, M.; Ward, R.L.; Hawkins, N.J.; et al. Mutation burden and other molecular markers of prognosis in colorectal cancer treated with curative intent: Results from the QUASAR 2 clinical trial and an Australian community-based series. *Lancet Gastroenterol. Hepatol.* **2018**, *3*, 635–643. [CrossRef]
40. Rashtak, S.; Ruan, X.; Druliner, B.R.; Liu, H.; Therneau, T.; Mouchli, M.; Boardman, L.A. Peripheral Neutrophil to Lymphocyte Ratio Improves Prognostication in Colon Cancer. *Clin. Colorectal Cancer* **2017**, *16*, 115–123. [CrossRef]
41. Li, M.-X.; Liu, X.-M.; Zhang, X.-F.; Zhang, J.-F.; Wang, W.-L.; Zhu, Y.; Dong, J.; Cheng, J.-W.; Liu, Z.-W.; Ma, L.; et al. Prognostic role of neutrophil-to-lymphocyte ratio in colorectal cancer: A systematic review and meta-analysis. *Int. J. Cancer* **2014**, *134*, 2403–2413. [CrossRef]
42. Wu, Y.; Li, C.; Zhao, J.; Yang, L.; Liu, F.; Zheng, H.; Wang, Z.; Xu, Y. Neutrophil-to-lymphocyte and platelet-to-lymphocyte ratios predict chemotherapy outcomes and prognosis in patients with colorectal cancer and synchronous liver metastasis. *World J. Surg. Oncol.* **2016**, *14*, 289. [CrossRef]
43. Barresi, V.; Bonetti, L.R.; Branca, G.; Di Gregorio, C.; De Leon, M.P.; Tuccari, G. Colorectal carcinoma grading by quantifying poorly differentiated cell clusters is more reproducible and provides more robust prognostic information than conventional grading. *Virchows Arch.* **2012**, *461*, 621–628. [CrossRef]
44. Jakubowska, K.; Koda, M.; Kisielewski, W.; Kańczuga-Koda, L.; Grudzińska, M.; Famulski, W. Pre- and postoperative neutrophil and lymphocyte count and neutrophil-to-lymphocyte ratio in patients with colorectal cancer. *Mol. Clin. Oncol.* **2020**, *13*, 1–10. [CrossRef]
45. Barresi, V.; Branca, G.; Vitarelli, E.; Tuccari, G. Micropapillary Pattern and Poorly Differentiated Clusters Represent the Same Biological Phenomenon in Colorectal Cancer. *Am. J. Clin. Pathol.* **2014**, *142*, 375–383. [CrossRef]
46. Barresi, V.; Bonetti, L.R.; Leni, A.; Caruso, R.A.; Tuccari, G. Histological grading in colorectal cancer: New insights and perspectives. *Histol. Histopathol.* **2015**, *30*, 1059–1067.

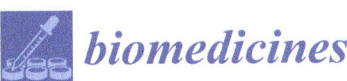

Review

Recent Advances in Monoclonal Antibody Therapy for Colorectal Cancers

Kyusang Hwang †, Jin Hwan Yoon †, Ji Hyun Lee † and Sukmook Lee *

Biopharmaceutical Chemistry Major, School of Applied Chemistry, Kookmin University, Seoul 02707, Korea; kyusang@kookmin.ac.kr (K.H.); yoonjinhwan8090@kookmin.ac.kr (J.H.Y.); 707jh@kookmin.ac.kr (J.H.L.)
* Correspondence: Lees2018@kookmin.ac.kr; Tel.: +82-2-910-6763
† These authors contributed equally to this work.

Abstract: Colorectal cancer (CRC) is one of the leading causes of cancer deaths worldwide. Recent advances in recombinant DNA technology have led to the development of numerous therapeutic antibodies as major sources of blockbuster drugs for CRC therapy. Simultaneously, increasing numbers of therapeutic targets in CRC have been identified. In this review, we first highlight the physiological and pathophysiological roles and signaling mechanisms of currently known and emerging therapeutic targets, including growth factors and their receptors as well as immune checkpoint proteins, in CRC. Additionally, we discuss the current status of monoclonal antibodies in clinical development and approved by US Food and Drug Administration for CRC therapy.

Keywords: colorectal cancer; monoclonal antibody; therapeutic target; therapy

1. Introduction

Monoclonal antibody therapy is an effective therapeutic intervention to treat patients with chronic (e.g., cancers and immunological disorders) as well as acute infectious diseases [1]. Since the discovery of hybridoma technology by Kohler and Milstein in 1975 [2], OKT3, the first US Food and Drug Administration (FDA)-approved mouse monoclonal antibody specific to CD3, was developed to prevent or reverse graft rejection by blocking T-cell activation [3]. However, it is not widely used in clinics because of the immunogenicity issue observed in OKT3 treatment [4]. Consequently, the remarkable development of recombinant DNA technology created many cutting-edge technologies for the development of therapeutic antibodies, including antibody library construction, phage display, high-throughput-based antibody selection, affinity maturation, humanization, and overproduction [5–10]. For example, phage display is the most common and practical technology for peptide or antibody selection that was initially developed by. Smith and Winter, the 2018 Nobel laureates in chemistry. Antibodies, such as antigen-binding fragments (Fab) or single-chain variable fragment (scFv), are displayed on a phage that confers antibodies with the key properties of replicability and mutability [11]. Furthermore, Gregory P. Winter and his team pioneered the humanization techniques to lower the immunogenicity elicited by nonhuman monoclonal antibodies [12]. Moreover, antibody humanization is a state-of-the-art technique to humanize the variable region of the antibodies obtained from nonhuman species including mice, rabbits, and chickens. Among several approaches, the complementarity-determining region (CDR) grafting method has been mostly used in antibody humanization for the development of therapeutic antibodies including cetuximab, rituximab, and infliximab. Humanized antibodies by CDR grafting are rendered by transferring the CDRs of a variable region to a human antibody scaffold [10,13–15]. As of December 2019, 79 therapeutic monoclonal antibodies have been approved by the US FDA. Furthermore, the global therapeutic monoclonal antibody market is the fastest-growing pharmaceutical industrial market and is expected to generate revenue of $300 billion by 2025 [14]. In addition, several antibody fragments such as Fab and scFv have also entered clinical trials [16]. Antibody fragments retain the targeting specificity of whole monoclonal antibodies and can be more economically produced. Furthermore, these fragments are smaller and easily penetrate tissues and tumors more rapidly and deeply than monoclonal antibodies having a higher molecular weight of 150 kDa. Antibody fragments have been also forged into multivalent and multispecific reagents, linked to therapeutic payloads (e.g., radionuclides, toxins, enzymes, liposomes, and viruses), and engineered for enhanced therapeutic efficacy [16–19].

Colorectal cancer (CRC) is the third most commonly occurring malignancy and second leading cause of cancer death worldwide. The increasing prevalence of CRC across the globe is one of the key factors driving the growth of the market [20]. According to statistics, the global CRC therapeutic market is expected to reach $18.5 billion by 2023 from $13.7 billion in 2018, at a compound annual growth rate of 6.1% from 2018 to 2023 [21]. Traditionally, 5-fluorouracil (5-FU)-based chemotherapeutic regimens, such as FOLFIRI (irinotecan-containing regimen) and FOLFOX (oxaliplatin-containing regimen), have been used clinically as standard therapies for treating CRC patients [22]. Recently, monoclonal antibodies have been used in combination with standard chemotherapy to improve the clinical outcomes of CRC patients. Compared with traditionally used chemotherapeutic agents, monoclonal antibodies have fewer side-effects because their target specificity and versatility are also being applied to next-generation antibody-based therapeutics, including bispecific/multispecific antibodies, antibody-drug conjugates, and chimeric antigen receptor T cells or natural killer cells [23–25].

Over several decades, extensive in vitro and in vivo biochemical and molecular biology studies have suggested many key signaling molecules closely associated with CRC progression and metastasis. Among them, several growth factors, including epidermal growth factor (EGF), vascular endothelial growth factor (VEGF), and hepatocyte growth factor (HGF) and their cognate receptors, are proven therapeutic targets in CRCs for monoclonal antibody therapy [26,27]. Further, human EGF receptor type 2 (HER2) is also known as a monoclonal antibody target in CRCs [28]. More recently, Alison and Honjo, the 2018 Nobel prize winners in physiology, discovered immune checkpoint proteins, such as programmed cell death protein-1 (PD-1) and cytotoxic T lymphocyte antigen 4 (CTLA-4), which are key negative regulators of the immune system and cancer growth [27]. Presently, these immune checkpoint proteins are drawing attention as the most promising therapeutic targets in other types of cancers as well as CRCs for monoclonal antibody therapy. In addition, with infrastructural and technical advancement in monoclonal antibody development, blockbuster humanized and fully human monoclonal antibodies, including cetuximab, bevacizumab, and pembrolizumab, have received FDA approval and are widely used to treat CRC patients [29].

In this review, we first highlight recent studies of the roles and relevance of therapeutic targets in CRCs for monoclonal antibody therapy to understand the pathological mechanism of CRCs governed by the target molecules. Simultaneously, presenting the current status of FDA approved monoclonal antibodies in clinical development for CRC therapy will provide insight into unmet medical needs in CRCs for monoclonal antibody-based therapy.

2. Physiological and Pathophysiological Roles of Therapeutic Targets in CRCs
2.1. EGF/EGFR

EGF is a 6 kDa growth factor with 53 amino acid residues; it binds to epidermal growth factor receptor (EGFR) that is a single transmembrane glycoprotein with 1186 amino acids. ErbB family members comprise ErbB1 (EGFR, HER1), ErbB2 (HER2), ErbB3 (HER3), and ErbB4 (HER4). EGF binding to EGFR occurs within the 622-amino acid extracellular domain (ECD), which is divided into four distinct domains: I–IV. Especially, domains I and III are responsible for ligand binding, whereas domains II and IV have two cysteine-rich regions that form disulfide bonds. Further, EGFR also has a 23-amino acid residue α-helical transmembrane domain, 250-amino acid tyrosine kinase domain, and 229-amino acid C-terminal tail with regulatory tyrosine residues [30–32].

Under physiological conditions, EGFR activation proceeds sequentially by two steps. First, prior to ligand binding, domain II is folded into domain IV via disulfide bonds in a tethered conformation. Second, once EGF binds to domains I and III of EGFR monomers, EGFRs promote domain rearrangement to expose dimerization arms in domain II, which leads to receptor dimerization via domain II [31,33]. In turn, the EGFR dimers induce trans-autophosphorylation by tyrosine kinase domains within the cytosolic parts of each EGFR, resulting in activation of their downstream signaling cascades, such as the rat sarcoma (RAS)/rapidly accelerated fibrosarcoma (RAF)/mitogen-activated protein kinase (MAPK) and phosphoinositide 3-kinase (PI3K)/Akt pathways [33–35]. The RAS–RAF–MAPK pathway is a major downstream signaling route of the ErbB family. EGF binding to EGFR and consecutive tyrosine phosphorylation in EGFRs leads to activation of RAS, a small GTP-binding protein, with the help of growth factor-bound protein 2 (GRB2), an adaptor protein, and son of sevenless (SOS), a guanine nucleotide exchange factor. In turn, activated RAS then activates downstream signaling molecules, including RAF and MAPK [36]. Activated MAPKs phosphorylate specific transcription factors and participate in regulation of cell migration and proliferation. EGFR activation also stimulates PI3K composed of separate regulatory (p85) and catalytic (p110) subunits. The p85 regulatory subunit directly binds to EGFR through the interaction of its Src homology domain 2 (SH2) with phosphotyrosine residues in activated EGFR. At the same time, the p110 catalytic subunit catalyzes phosphorylation of phosphatidylinositol 4,5-diphosphate to generate phosphatidylinositol 3,4,5-triphosphate (PIP_3), which in turn activates the protein serine/threonine kinase, Akt [37–40] (Figure 1).

Many previous reports have suggested the importance of EGFR as a therapeutic target in CRC. For example, immunohistochemical studies have shown that EGFR was highly overexpressed in 118 (80%) of 150 CRC patients, with a median follow-up of 40 months. In addition, *Balb/c* athymic nude mice subcutaneously injected with HCT116 or EGFR-knockout CT116 cells also revealed that depletion of EGFR in HCT116 cells was associated with reduced tumor growth [41]. Osimertinib (Tagrisso®, AstraZeneca, Cambridge, UK), a tyrosine kinase inhibitor of EGFR, was found to remarkably decrease the tumor size and growth rate in a DLD-1, a colorectal adenocarcinoma cell line, xenograft mouse model [42]. Administration of cetuximab, a human/mouse chimeric antibody, exhibited significant growth suppression and inhibited the EGFR/MAPK pathway in a HT29 xenograft mouse model [43]. Furthermore, another anti-EGFR antibody also showed similar growth inhibition of CRCs to cetuximab in preclinical settings. GC1118, a novel fully human anti-EGFR IgG1 antibody, exhibited potent inhibitory effects on EGFR signaling, enhanced antibody-mediated cytotoxicity, and significantly inhibited tumor growth in a CRC patient-derived xenograft (PDX) model [44]. Further, Ame55, an anti-EGFR IgG1 antibody, also inhibited tumor growth in a LoVo xenograft mouse model [45].

In addition, some reports show the interrelationship of EGFR with other biomarkers. Consequently, HER2 amplification has been implicated in therapeutic resistance to anti-EGFR antibody therapy in preclinical studies in metastatic CRC (mCRC) [46]. HER2 amplification is seen in a small subset of mCRC, predominantly in KRAS wild-type tumors, for which anti-EGFR antibodies are used as targeted therapies [47,48]. In these tumors, aberrant HER2 signaling results in the bypass of the activation of the RAS/MEK/MAPK signaling pathway, thereby blunting the effect of EGFR blockade [49,50]. Furthermore, the EGFR-MET interaction induced by transforming growth factor-α, a specific EGFR ligand, overexpression and concomitant phosphorylation of MET, and activation of MET downstream effectors have been proposed to be closely associated with the acquired resistance to cetuximab in CRC cells [51,52]. Thus, these pieces of evidence demonstrate that the combined inhibition of EGFR and other biomarkers can represent an effective strategy for overcoming cetuximab resistance in patients with CRCs [53].

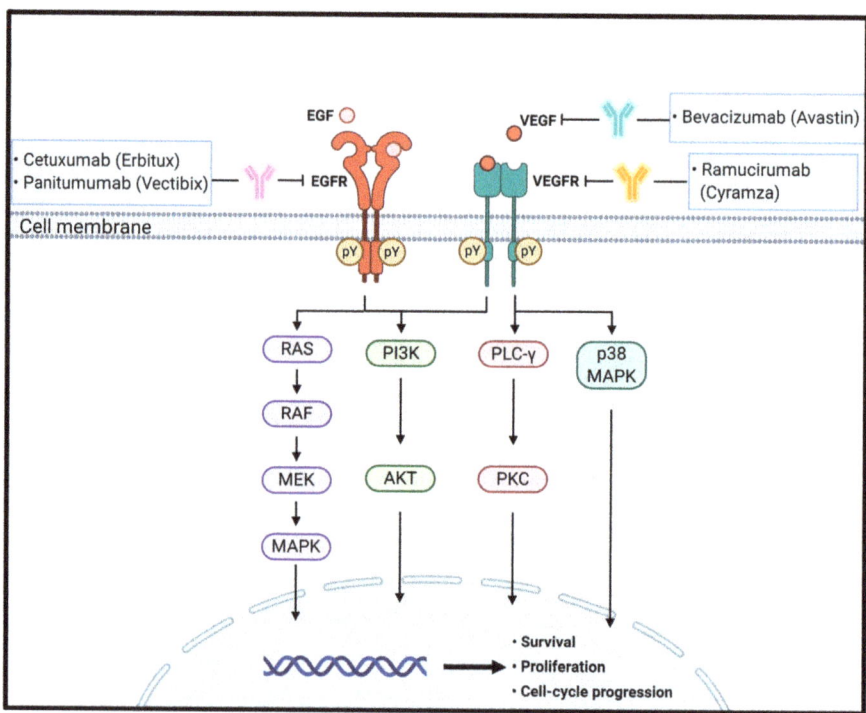

Figure 1. Schematic representation of the physiological roles and signaling pathways of EGF and VEGF and their cognate receptors and the effect of antibodies targeting these signaling molecules on CRC progression and metastasis. pY means phosphotyrosine residues.

2.2. VEGF/VEGFR

VEGF is a disulfide-bonded dimeric glycoprotein of 45 kDa. The VEGF family has five isotypes, including VEGF-A, placental growth factor, VEGF-B, VEGF-C, and VEGF-D [54]. Among them, VEGF-A is a glycosylated mitogen protein that is closely associated with regulation of numerous pro-angiogenic functions, including endothelial cell growth and migration, and vascular permeability in angiogenesis [55]. However, less is known about the function and regulation of VEGF-B, -C, and -D. VEGFR receptor (VEGFR) is a member of the receptor tyrosine kinase (RTK) family having multiple immunoglobulin-like ECDs and tyrosine kinase activity. VEGFRs are divided into three types: VEGFR1 (Flt-1), VEGFR2 (KDR or Flk-1), and VEGFR3 (Flt-4). Especially, VEGFR2, a 200–230 kDa protein, mostly interacts with VEGF-A and has a key role in angiogenesis at early embryogenesis and mostly at lymph angiogenesis [54,56].

Similar to that of other RTKs, the binding of VEGF to VEGFR forms a receptor dimer and induces trans-autophosphorylation. Specifically, signaling of VEGFRs is initiated upon binding of a covalently linked ligand dimer to the ECD of the receptor. This signaling promotes receptor homodimerization followed by phosphorylation of specific tyrosine residues located in the intracellular juxtamembrane domain, the kinase insert domain, and the carboxy terminal tail of the receptor. Subsequently, a variety of signaling molecules are recruited to VEGFR dimers [57,58]. These interactions next activate phospholipase C (PLC)γ and protein kinase C (PKC) to induce transcription of genes necessary for angiogenesis and cell proliferation [59]. Simultaneously, VEGFR-induced activation of PI3K results in accumulation of PIP3, which induces phosphorylation of Akt to increase endothelial cell survival and also induces systemic destruction of the entire basement membrane to increase vascular permeability [60,61]. Ligand binding to VEGFR-2 also triggers the activation of the RAS pathway, initiating signaling through the RAF–MEK–MAPK pathway known to be important in VEGF-induced cell proliferation [62]. In addition, VEGF stimulates p38 MAPK to regulate the rearrangements of the actin cytoskeleton in cell migration [63] (Figure 1).

It has been reported that 70% of patients with stage IV CRCs had positive VEGF expression, whereas 50% and 47% of patients with stage II and III CRCs, respectively, had positive VEGF expression. A statistically significant correlation was found between VEGF and 10-year disease-specific survival: VEGF-expressing tumors were more frequent in patients who died of the disease than in those who survived for 10 years [64]. Further, other reports have shown that the VEGF level also increased in CRC patients. In a prospective study by Anastasios et al. that included 67 consecutive colorectal patients, VEGF was detectable in all control subjects. Their median serum VEGF level was 186 pg/mL. Additionally, serum VEGF levels were higher in 67 patients with newly diagnosed and histologically confirmed primary CRC (492 pg/mL) than in the control subjects (186 pg/mL) [65].

An increasing number of reports have suggested VEGF/VEGFR signaling as a promising therapeutic target in CRCs. First, Foersch et al. generated a conditional knockout for VEGFR2 to investigate the functional role and underlying molecular mechanisms of the signaling. Specific deletion of VEGFR2 was confirmed by qPCR of cDNA. Immunofluorescence staining revealed a lack of receptor expression relative to that of VEGFR2-expressing control mice. Consequently, significantly fewer tumors developed in VEGFR2-knockout mice than in control mice [66]. Second, regorafenib, a novel small-molecule multi-kinase inhibitor, markedly slowed tumor growth in five of seven PDX models. The antitumor effects of regorafenib were evaluated in seven PD CRC xenografts [67]. Third, bevacizumab, a humanized antibody to VEGF, showed a significant delay in CRC tumor growth relative to that of the non-treated animals [68]. Fourth, intraperitoneal injection of DC101, an anti-VEGFR mouse monoclonal antibody, inhibited tumor growth and induced apoptosis in CRC in a KM12L4 xenograft model. Further, treatment with DC101 decreased tumor vascularity, growth, proliferation, and increased apoptosis [69]. Taken together, this large number of studies shows the importance of VEGF/VEGFR signaling for developing pharmaceutical anti-angiogenic drugs.

2.3. HGF/c-MET

HGF is synthesized as an inactive precursor (pro-HGF) that undergoes site-specific proteolytic cleavage by extracellular serine proteinases into an active 90-kDa heterodimer containing α and β chains. HGF is predominantly secreted by stromal cells and activates mesenchymal-epithelial transition factor (c-MET) on adjacent epithelial cells [70]. HGF contains two c-MET binding sites; a high affinity site in the N-terminal and first kringle regions that binds to the immunoglobulin-like fold shared by plexins and transcriptional factors (IPT) 3 and IPT4 domains in c-MET and a low-affinity site in the serine protease homology domain that interacts with the semaphorin domain in c-MET [71]. As a tyrosine-protein kinase Met or HGR receptor, c-MET is synthesized as a 170-kDa single-chain precursor protein (pro-c-MET) that undergoes furin-mediated post-translational cleavage, yielding a disulfide-linked heterodimer composed of an extracellular α-subunit and a single transmembrane β-subunit [70,72].

In the physiological state, HGF binding to c-MET induces c-MET dimerization and trans-autophosphorylation of the tyrosine residues Y1003 in the juxtamembrane domain and Y1234 and Y1235 within the kinase activation loop, resulting in phosphorylation of two tyrosine residues, Y1349 and Y1356, in the C-terminus. Tyrosine phosphorylation of Y1349 and Y1356 residues creates docking sites for recruitment of key intracellular adaptor proteins and signaling molecules through SH2-mediated interactions, including GRB2, GRB2-associated binding protein 1 (GAB1), signal transducer and activator of transcription 3 (STAT3), the p85 subunit of PI3K, SRC, PLC-γ, and Shc [73,74]. The potency, duration, and versatility of HGF/c-MET signaling are modulated by signaling amplifiers and co-receptors.

Recruitment and sustained phosphorylation of the multi-adaptor protein GAB1 is an important hallmark of sustained c-MET signaling that can either bind directly to c-MET through its unique 13-amino-acid c-MET binding site or indirectly by association with GRB2. The tyrosine-phosphorylated GAB1 protein serves as an auxiliary signal transduction platform through recruitment of various effector proteins, including PI3K. Cell survival response is related to the PI3K/Akt pathway activated by c-MET signaling [75,76]. Furthermore, HGF-induced c-MET-dependent RAS/RAF/MAPK activation has been found to require the co-receptor CD44v6, thus providing a platform for SOS recruitment to the complex and subsequently triggering proficient activation of RAS [32]. Invasion, branching morphogenesis, and tumorigenesis are mediated by STAT3 activation in a tissue-dependent manner. Typically, STAT3 activation is induced by phosphorylation on a critical tyrosine residue (Y705) that triggers STAT3 dimerization owing to reciprocal phosphotyrosine-SH2 domain interactions. In addition to tyrosine 705 phosphorylation, STAT3 is also activated through serine (S727) phosphorylation. Finally, the reversible acetylation of STAT3 by histone acetyltransferase on a single lysine residue (K685) represents a third mechanism of STAT3 activation. Acetylated STAT3 enhances the stability of STAT3 dimers, which are required for DNA-binding and transcriptional activity. Cellular migration and adhesion are mediated by a c-MET–SRC–focal adhesion kinase (FAK) interaction. Within the complex, Src phosphorylates Y576 and Y577 within the kinase domain activation loop and Y861 and Y925 within the C-terminal domain of FAK. The FAK–Src complex further binds to and phosphorylates various adaptor proteins, such as p130Cas and paxillin [77–79] (Figure 2).

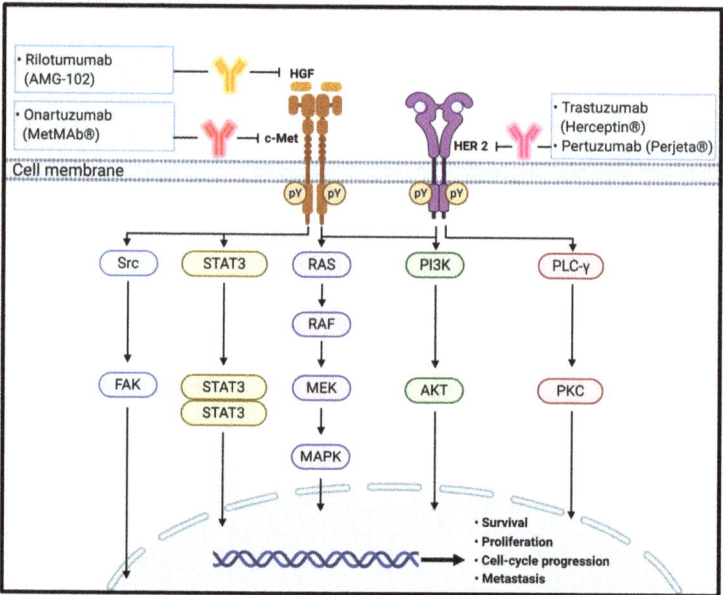

Figure 2. The schematic representation of the physiological roles and signaling pathways of HGF/c-MET and HER2 and effect of antibodies targeting these signaling molecules on CRC progression and metastasis. pY means phosphotyrosine residues.

c-MET is overexpressed in CRCs [80]. Specifically, immunohistochemistry with 23 cases of colorectal adenoma and 102 cases of primary colorectal carcinoma as well their corresponding metastases (44 lymph nodes, 21 peritoneal deposits, and 16 liver metastases) showed that normal tissues had a negative or weak c-MET expression, whereas c-MET was highly overexpressed in adenomas and primary CRC. Moreover, c-MET expression in metastatic tissues was significantly higher compared with the primary tumor [81].

Currently, HGF/c-MET signaling is one of the key therapeutic targets in CRC therapy. Small hairpin RNA-mediated c-MET knockdown dramatically suppressed tumor growth in a SW480 xenograft mouse model as well as SW480 cell proliferation in vitro [82]. SU11274, an ATP-competitive inhibitor of c-MET, significantly inhibited tumor growth in a LoVo xenograft mouse model. ARQ 197 (tivantinib), a non-ATP-competitive inhibitor of c-MET, decreased tumor growth in a HT29 xenograft mouse model [83]. Antibody-based targeting of c-MET also gave results similar to those of pre-existing chemical inhibitors. For example, YYB-101, a humanized neutralizing antibody specifically binding to HGF, inhibits c-MET activation and cell scattering in vitro and suppresses tumor growth in HCT116 xenograft mouse models [84]. R13 and R28, two fully human antibodies against c-MET, synergistically inhibit HGF binding to c-MET and elicit antibody-dependent cellular cytotoxicity. The combination of R13/28 significantly inhibited tumor growth in xenograft models of various colon tumors, including OMP-C12, 27, and 28. Inhibition of tumor growth was associated with induction of hypoxia. Moreover, in an experimental metastasis model, R13/28 increased survival by preventing recurrence of otherwise lethal lung metastases [85].

2.4. HER2

HER2 is an ErbB family member with a molecular weight of 185 kDa comprising a 632-amino acid ECD, 22-amino acid α-helical transmembrane domain, and a 580-amino acid tyrosine kinase domain. Despite the many intensive studies on HER2, a ligand of HER2 has not been clearly identified yet. It is known that HER2 forms complexes with HER2 or other ErbB family members, including EGFR, ErbB3, and ErbB4, to activate downstream signaling pathways [86,87].

Similar to EGF/EGFR signaling pathways, it has been suggested that in normal cells, the HER2 complex formation, such as through homodimerization or heterodimerization, leads to continuous trans-autophosphorylation on tyrosine residues of HER2 and activates downstream signaling pathways, including the RAS/RAF/MAPK pathway, PI3K/Akt pathway, and PLC/PKC pathway. HER2 activation ultimately promotes cell growth, proliferation, and survival. The RAS/RAF/MAPK and PI3K/Akt pathways are the two most important and extensively studied downstream signaling pathways upon activation of HER2 receptors. A third key signaling in the network is the PLC-γ/PKC pathway. Binding of PLC-γ to phosphorylated HER2 stimulates PLC-γ activity and results in hydrolytic cleavage of phosphatidylinositol-4,5-bisphosphate (PIP_2) to yield inositol 1,4,5-triphosphate (IP_3) and 1,2-diacylglycerol. These second messengers are important for intracellular calcium release and activation of PKC. As a result of these signaling pathways, different nuclear factors are recruited and modulate the transcription of different genes involved in cell-cycle progression, proliferation, and survival [32,33,88,89] (Figure 2).

In CRC, HER2 expression is varied because of many factors that influence the determination of HER2 expression, especially of the intracellular fraction of HER2. One report stated that HER2 overexpression was observed in 136 (11.4%) of 1195 CRC patients with moderately to poorly differentiated tubular adenocarcinomas. Further, HER2 overexpression correlated with shorter mean overall survival (OS) [90]. Other studies have also reported that membranous overexpression of HER2 occurs in only 5% of all CRC patients, whereas cytoplasmic HER2 overexpression is observed in a significant proportion (30%) of patients [91].

Several lines of evidence also support the idea that HER2 is a therapeutic target in CRCs. Tucatinib, a reversible inhibitor that binds to the ATP pocket of the internal domain of the HER2 receptor, prevents activation of HER2 signaling pathways [92]. Further, administration of tucatinib in a CRC PDX model significantly reduced tumor volume. Both H2Mab-19 and H2Mab-41, novel anti-HER2 IgG2 antibodies, significantly reduced tumor development in Caco-2 xenograft mouse models [93,94]. Treatment with Herceptin® (Genentech, San Francisco, CA, USA) caused a decrease in HER-2 protein levels in DLD-1, HT-29, Caco-2, and HCA-7 colon cancer cells in vitro. Treatment of athymic mice engrafted with EGFR-dependent colon cancers, including HCA-7, DLD-1, and HT-29 with Herceptin® showed tumor regression and decreased EGFR tyrosine phosphorylation in tumor cells [95].

2.5. Immune Checkpoint

2.5.1. CTLA-4

CTLA-4, also designated CD152, is a type I transmembrane T-cell inhibitory molecule that functions as an immune checkpoint, downregulates immune responses and is found as a covalent homodimer of 41–43 kDa [96]. CTLA-4 is a member of the IgG superfamily that is expressed by activated T cells. CTLA-4 contains an ECD with one Ig-like V-type domain, a transmembrane domain, and cytoplasmic tail. CTLA-4 is homologous to the T-cell co-stimulatory protein, CD28, and both molecules bind to B7-1/B7-2 on antigen-presenting cells [97]. CTLA-4 binds CD80 and CD86 with greater affinity and avidity than CD28, thus enabling it to outcompete CD28 for its ligands. CTLA-4 transmits an inhibitory signal to T cells, whereas CD28 transmits a stimulatory signal [98,99].

CTLA-4 is upregulated in a manner dependent on TCR stimulation. At the cell membrane, CTLA-4 undergoes dimerization, and each CTLA-4 dimer can bind two independent B7-1/B7-2 homodimers, forming a linear zipper-like structure between B7-1/B7-2 and CTLA-4 homodimers [100]. Activated CTLA-4 binds to PI3K, the tyrosine phosphatases (SHP1 and SHP2) and the serine/threonine phosphatase PP2A. SHP1 and SHP2 dephosphorylate TCR-signaling proteins, whereas PP2A targets phosphoserine/threonine residues and is known to interfere with the activation of Akt [101].

CTLA-4 can inhibit T-cell responses by several mechanisms. One mechanism involves antagonism of B7-CD28–mediated co-stimulatory signals by CTLA-4. The fact that CTLA-4 has a much higher affinity for B7 than CD28 supports the notion that the CTLA-4–mediated sequestration of B7 is closely associated with negative regulation of T-cell signaling [102]. Another mechanism for the inhibitory activity of CTLA-4 is related to direct interaction with the TCR–CD3 complex at the immunological synapse for negative regulation of downstream signaling after TCR activation [103]. When CTLA-4 interacts with the ITAMs present on the TCR–CD3 complex, the activated CTLA-4 binds to tyrosine phosphatases, including SHP1, SHP2, and PP2A, and eventually deactivates various downstream signaling molecules of activated T cells, including zeta-chain-associated protein kinase 70, spleen tyrosine kinase, and proto-oncogene tyrosine-protein kinase [104–106] (Figure 3).

Many previous reports have shown that CTLA-4 is a key therapeutic target in CRCs [107]. First, Long et al. used the CRISPR-Cas9 system to generate CTLA-4 knockout cytotoxic T lymphocytes (CTLs) and evaluated the effect on the antitumor activity of the CTLs [107]. The HCT-116 xenografted mice treated with CTLA-4 KO CTLs demonstrated repressed tumor growth and prolonged survival relative to those in the control group. All of the mice in the control group died from progressive tumors within 62 days. In contrast, only 10% of CTLA-4 KO CTLs treated mice died within that time [108]. Second, Fu et al. validated the efficacy of anti-CTLA-4 mouse monoclonal antibodies on tumor size in mice inoculated with CT26 cells. The tumor volumes were 2106 ± 205 mm^3 on day 17 in the control group treated with vehicle only but were 23 ± 4 mm^3 in the group treated with the anti-CTLA-4 antibodies on day 5, which indicated a statistically significant difference in antitumor activity between the treated and vehicle groups [109]. Third, Lute et al. also reported that anti-human CTLA-4 human monoclonal antibodies-treated mice survived longer than the control Ig-treated mice in a human peripheral blood leukocytes-SCID mouse model. Fourth, administration of 9H10, an anti-murine CTLA monoclonal antibody, as monotherapy moderately inhibited growth and metastatic spread of the colon cancer cells in an orthotropically implanted CT26 xenograft mouse model [110]. Further, the sole CTLA-4 inhibition significantly increased intratumoral CD8$^+$ and CD4$^+$ T cells and reduced FOXP3$^+$/CD4$^+$ Treg cells, which was associated with increased expression levels of the pro-inflammatory Th1/M1-related cytokines IFN-γ, IL-1α, IL-2, and IL-12 [111].

In summary, the evidence from the studies above shows that CTLA-4 blockade exerts inhibitory effects on growth and metastasis of CRCs.

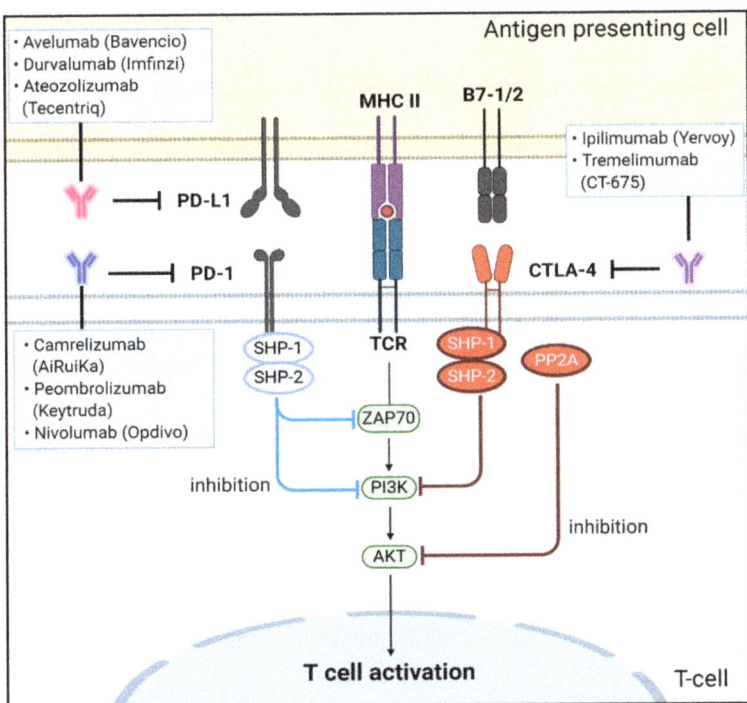

Figure 3. Schematic representation of the physiological roles and signaling pathways of immune checkpoint proteins of PD-1, PD-L1, CTLA-4, and B7-1/2 and effect of antibodies targeting these signaling molecules on CRC progression and metastasis.

2.5.2. PD-1/PD-L1

PD-1, also designated CD279, is a 55 kDa membrane protein consisting of an ECD followed by a transmembrane region and an intracellular tail containing two phosphorylation sites located in an immunoreceptor tyrosine-based inhibitory motif (ITIM) and an immunoreceptor tyrosine-based switch motif (ITSM). Programmed cell death-ligand 1 (PD-L1, designated CD274, B7-H1) is a 44 kDa transmembrane protein expressed on T cells, B cells, macrophages, and dendritic cells as well as on tumor cells, including CRCs [112,113].

Under physiological conditions, when T cells recognize antigens on major histocompatibility complex of the target cell, inflammatory cytokines, such as tumor necrosis factor alpha and interferon gamma (IFNγ) are produced to initiate inflammatory processes. These cytokines upregulate the expression of PD-L1 on tissues and PD-1 on T cells. In turn, PD-1 directly interacts with PD-L1 to negatively regulate T-cell receptor (TCR) signaling, inhibits interleukin-2 (IL-2) production in T cells, and increases T-cell apoptosis [114,115]. Specifically, this PD-1/PD-L1 interaction induces lymphocyte-specific protein tyrosine kinase-induced phosphorylation of two tyrosine-based motifs within ITIM and ITSM of the cytoplasmic tail of PD-1. The recruitment of Src homology 2 (SH2) domain-containing protein tyrosine phosphatase 1 (SHP1) and SHP-2 phosphatase then induces dephosphorylation of the TCR signalosome, including CD3ζ, ZAP70, and PI3K kinases, resulting in the deactivation of downstream signaling targets [116]. Moreover, the PD-1/PD-L1 interaction also downregulates the protein (casein) kinase 2 expression that phosphorylates the regulatory domain of phosphatase and tensin homolog (PTEN) and inhibits phosphatase activity to remove PIP3 produced by PI3K [112,117,118]. Thus, PTEN can terminate PI3K activities by dephosphorylating PIP3, which eventually leads to immune tolerance, a phenomenon in which the immune system loses the control to mount an inflammatory response even in the presence of actionable antigens [117,119] (Figure 3).

PD-L1 has been reported to be overexpressed in CRC. More specifically, among the 80 tumor specimens, 22 (27.5%) showed high PD-L1 expression, 24 (30.0%) showed moderate expression, and 34 (42.5%) showed weak or no PD-L1 staining. Furthermore, the high PD-L1 expression in normal tissues was observed in four (6.3%) cases [120].

Many studies have suggested PD-1 and PD-L1 as promising therapeutic targets in CRCs. First, in *BALB/c Rag2−/−γc−/−* mice engrafted with PD-L1-overexpressing and PD-L1-knockout CT26 murine colon cancer cells, Gordon et al. found that after 3 weeks, tumors were significantly smaller in the PD-L1-knockout group than in the PD-L1 over-expression group [121]. Second, Cai et al. examined the efficacy of anti-mouse PD-1 rat immunoglobulin (Ig) G2 antibodies on tumor growth in a CT26 colon cancer xenograft mouse model. The antibody treatment showed significant inhibition of transplanted-tumor growth in mice [122]. Third, in a humanized CRC PDX model established by Capasso et al., treatment with nivolumab, a fully human IgG4 (S228P) monoclonal antibody to PD-1, led to significant tumor growth inhibition coupled with increased numbers of IFNγ-producing human CD8$^+$ tumor-infiltrating lymphocytes [123]. Fourth, Stewart et al. reported that MEDI4736, a human IgG1 monoclonal antibody that binds with high affinity and specificity to PD-L1, significantly inhibited the growth of human tumors in a novel CT26 xenograft model containing co-implanted human T cells. This activity is entirely dependent on the presence of transplanted T cells. Further, anti-mouse PD-L1 significantly improved survival of mice implanted with CT26 CRC cells [124]. The antitumor activity of anti-PD-L1 was enhanced by combination with oxaliplatin, which resulted in increased release of high-motility group box 1 within CT26 tumors [125].

3. Current Status of Monoclonal Antibodies for CRC Therapy

3.1. Cetuximab

Cetuximab (Erbitux®), developed jointly by Merck KGaA (Darmstadt, Germany) and Imclone Systems (New York City, NY, USA), is a monoclonal antibody that binds to the ECD of the EGFR. It is a human/mouse chimeric IgG1 antibody that consists of the variable fragments (Fvs) of a murine anti-EGFR antibody and human constant heavy and kappa light chains [126,127].

Cetuximab was originally known as a blockade for inhibiting interactions between EGFR and all known EGFR ligands by specifically binding to domain III of the EGFR ECD [128]. Furthermore, its binding to EGFR is also able to promote receptor internalization and concomitantly downregulate EGFR protein levels expressed on the cell surface, resulting in suppression of EGFR-dependent downstream signaling pathways and transcription. In addition to these specific modes of action, cetuximab indirectly attacks cancer cells through antibody-dependent cell-mediated cytotoxicity (ADCC). After its binding to EGFR, the IgG1 portion of cetuximab may be recognized by Fcγ receptors (FcγR) on immune effector cells, such as natural killer cells and T cells, and participates in cancer cell death. In general, FcγRs bind effectively to IgG1 and IgG3 antibodies. Thus, cetuximab is speculated to more likely stimulate ADCC than panitumumab having IgG2. Consequently, cetuximab reduces tumor angiogenesis, invasiveness, and metastatic spread [129–132].

In 2004, cetuximab received FDA approval for metastatic CRCs and head and neck cancers, and its use is recommended in combination with standard chemotherapy for treatment of patients with metastatic CRCs having EGFR-positive and wild-type KRAS (Table 1). According to the CRYSTAL clinical trial (NCT00154102), compared with FOLFIRI alone, cetuximab plus FOLFIRI improved progression-free survival (PFS) from 8.0 to 9.0 months and OS from 20 to 23.5 months for treatment of patients with KRAS wild-type [133].

Table 1. Antibody therapeutics currently in clinical trials or approved by the US FDA.

Name	Trade Name	Company	Target	Format	Clinical Stage
Cetuximab	Erbitux®	Imclone Systems	EGFR	Chimeric IgG1	FDA approval in 2004
Panitumumab	Vectibix®	Abgenix Inc.	EGFR	Human IgG2	FDA approval 2006
Bevacizumab	Avastin®	Genentech	VEGF-A	Humanized IgG1	FDA approval in 2004
Ramucirumab	Cyramza®	ImClone Systems	VEGFR2	Human IgG1	FDA approval in 2015
Rilotumumab	AMG-102	Amgen Inc.	HGF	Human IgG1	P II
Onartuzumab	MetMab	Genentech	c-MET	Humanized IgG1, monovalent	P II, failure
Trastuzumab	Herceptin®	Genentech	HER2	Humanized IgG1	P II
Pertuzumab	Perjeta®	Genentech	HER2	Humanized IgG1	P II
Ipilimumab	Yervoy®	BMS	CTLA4	Human IgG1	FDA approval in 2018
Tremelimumab	CT-675	Medimmune	CTLA4	Human IgG2	P II
Pembrolizumab	Keytruda®	LifeArc	PD-1	Humanized IgG4	FDA approval in 2020
Nivolumab	Opdivo®	Ono Phar. & Medarex	PD-1	Humanized IgG4	P II
Camrelizumab	AiRuiKa	Jiangsu HengRui	PD-1	Humanized IgG4	P II
Atezolizumab	Tecentriq®	Genentech	PD-L1	Human IgG1	P II
Avelumab	Bavencio®	Merck KGaA	PD-L1	Human IgG1	P III
Durvalumab	Imfinzi®	Medimmune	PD-L1	Human IgG1	P II

Antibody information was obtained from the FDA Label database and the Drug Approval and Databases site maintained by the US FDA (https://www.fda.gov/drugs/development-approval-process-drugs/drug-approvals-and-databases) or Clinical Trial Information Site (https://clinicaltrials.gov).

3.2. Panitumumab

Panitumumab (Vectibix™) originally developed by Abgenix Inc. (Freemont, CA, USA) is a fully human IgG2 monoclonal antibody that specifically binds to the ECD of EGFR. Especially and different from cetuximab, it can also bind to a single-point mutation in domain III of EGFR (S468R) that confers acquired or secondary resistance only to cetuximab-treated patients [134].

In 2006, panitumumab was approved by the US FDA for treatment of patients with EGFR-expressing metastatic CRCs with disease progression or following fluoropyrimidine-, oxaliplatin-, and irinotecan-containing regimens (Table 1). Later, it was also approved for treatment of patients with refractory metastatic CRCs having EGFR-positive and wild-type KRAS. Currently, panitumumab was the first monoclonal antibody to use KRAS as a predictive biomarker [135].

Panitumumab is being used in combination with chemotherapy in the first- and second-line treatment of metastatic CRCs [136]. In the PRIME (NCT00364013) clinical trial, compared with chemotherapy alone, a first-line treatment of panitumumab plus FOLFOX improved PFS from 8.0 to 9.6 months and OS from 12 to 14 months. Further, in the 20,050,181 clinical trial (NCT00339183), compared with chemotherapy, a second-line treatment of panitumumab plus FOLFIRI improved PFS from 4 to 6 months and OS from 19 to 24 months [137,138].

3.3. Bevacizumab

Bevacizumab (Avastin®) developed by Genentech (South San Francisco, CA, USA) is a humanized IgG1 monoclonal antibody that binds to segment β5–β6 of VEGF165, known as VEGF-A; its binding to VEGF-A inhibits angiogenesis by specifically inhibiting the interaction between VEGF-A and VEGFR2. Thus, bevacizumab inhibits angiogenic signaling caused by the interaction of VEGF-A and VEGFR2 [139–141].

In 2004, bevacizumab received FDA approval for first- or second-line treatment with 5-FU-based therapy for patients with mCRCs (Table 1). As the first anti-angiogenic antibody drug, bevacizumab is currently being used in clinics for treatment of patients with NSCLC, mRCC, epithelial ovarian cancer, and recurrent glioblastoma as well as metastatic CRCs. In the clinical trial ECOG3200 (NCT00069095) for treatment of patients with mCRCs, compared with FOLFOX4 alone, bevacizumab plus FOLFOX4 improved OS from 10.8 to 12.9 months and PFS from 4.7 to 7.3 months [142–144].

3.4. Ramucirumab

Ramucirumab (Cyramza®) developed jointly by ImClone Systems (New York City, NY, USA) and Dyax (Cambridge, MA, USA) is a fully human monoclonal IgG1 antibody that binds to the ECD of human VEGFR2, which is a key receptor that mediates angiogenesis and is highly expressed in not only tumor microvessels but also malignant tumors. Bevacizumab strongly neutralizes VEGF and blocks binding to VEGFR1/VEGFR2, whereas ramucirumab specifically blocks the VEGF/VEGFR2 interaction by binding to VEGFR2 [145–147].

Ramucirumab was isolated from a Dyax's phage antibody library and developed as a therapeutic antibody for treatment of solid tumors. In 2014, ramucirumab first received FDA approval as a single-agent treatment for advanced gastric or gastro-esophageal junction adenocarcinoma after prior treatment with fluoropyrimidine- or platinum-containing chemotherapy. In 2015, ramucirumab in combination with FOLFIRI was also approved by the US FDA for the treatment of patients with mCRC with disease progression on or after prior therapy with bevacizumab, oxaliplatin, and fluoropyrimidine (Table 1). In the RAISE clinical trial (NCT01183780) for treatment of mCRC patients, compared with FOLFIRI alone, ramucirumab plus FOLFIRI improved OS from 11.7 to 13.3 months and PFS from 4.5 to 5.7 months [148,149].

3.5. Rilotumumab

Rilotumumab (AMG-102) developed by Amgen Inc. (Thousand Oaks, CA, USA) is a fully human monoclonal IgG2 antibody that binds to the beta chain of HGF. HGF, a scattering factor, influences cancer cell proliferation, survival, invasion, and metastasis through interaction with c-MET. Therefore, specific binding of rilotumumab to HGF neutralizes the interaction between HGF and c-MET and inhibits c-MET phosphorylation and downstream signaling, resulting in inhibition of cancer cell proliferation, survival, and invasion through partial antagonism of c-MET phosphorylation [150,151].

It has been reported that in the phase II clinical trial (NCT00788957) for treatment of patients with wild-type KRAS metastatic CRCs, compared with panitumumab alone, rilotumumab plus panitumumab combination therapy improved OS from 8.6 to 9.6 months and PFS from 3.7 to 5.2 months [152] (Table 1).

3.6. Onartuzumab

Onartuzumab (MetMAb) developed by Genentech (South San Francisco, CA, USA) is a humanized monoclonal antibody that binds to the semaphorin domain of c-MET; it is a human IgG1 with a monovalent arm. c-MET is an RTK through which downstream signals are transduced after dimerization or oligomerization by HGF binding. HGF/c-MET signaling has also been implicated in the metastatic growth of multiple cancers, making it an attractive target for various therapeutic agents [153]. When onartuzumab binds to c-MET, it inhibits cell proliferation and survival, cell motility, migration, and invasion [154]. In a clinical trial (NCT01418222) of the MET inhibitor onartuzumab in combination with mFOLFOX-6 plus bevacizumab for treatment of mCRC patients, no significant differences existed in PFS or OS between onartuzumab combination therapy with mFOLFOX-6 plus bevacizumab and bevacizumab plus mFOLPOX-6 therapy. Therefore, the phase II clinical trial of onartuzumab failed because it did not show any clinical improvement [155] (Table 1).

3.7. Trastuzumab

Trastuzumab (Herceptin®) developed by Genentech (South San Francisco, CA, USA) is a humanized IgG1 monoclonal antibody that binds to domain IV in the ECD of the HER2. This antibody is composed of humanized Fvs of murine anti-HER2 antibody and human constant heavy and kappa light chains. The antibody suppresses cancer growth and proliferation [156].

Trastzumab binds to HER2 on the cell surface of CRCs and inhibits downstream signaling pathways, such as RAS/RAF/MEK and PI3K/Akt pathways, thereby inhibiting the proliferation and survival of CRCs. This demonstrates that trastuzumab can be used as a therapeutic agent in HER2-overexpressed CRCs. In addition, trastuzumab indirectly attacks cancer cells through Fc effect functions, such as ADCC and complement-dependent cytotoxicity (CDC) [157,158].

In 1998, trastuzumab first received US FDA approval for the treatment of patients with metastatic HER2-overexpressing breast cancers, and its indications for numerous cancer treatments have expanded [159,160]. Despite the low-expression pattern observed in CRC patients, intriguingly, recent preclinical trials have shown that trastuzumab or pertuzumab in combination with lapatinib significantly suppressed tumor growth in HER2-amplified CRC tumor xenograft animal models. According to the HERACLES clinical trial (NCT03365882), compared with chemotherapy alone, trastuzumab plus lapatinib therapy in patients with HER2-positive, wild-type KRAS metastatic CRC improved PFS by 2.9 months and OS by 11.5 months [161] (Table 1).

3.8. Pertuzumab

Pertuzumab (Perjeta®) developed by Genentech (South San Francisco, CA, USA) is a humanized IgG1 monoclonal antibody that binds to HER2. The antibodies act as a blockade to inhibit dimerization of HER2 with other HER receptors, especially HER3, by specifically binding to domain II in the ECD of HER2, a different epitope for trastuzumab, resulting in inhibition of cell growth and initiation of apoptosis [162]. In 2012, the US FDA approved pertuzumab use in combination with trastuzumab and docetaxel for treatment of patients with metastatic HER2-positive metastatic breast cancers. According to the HERACLES study (NCT03365882), the randomized phase II trial studies is ongoing by evaluating the efficacy of pertuzumab and tratuzumab in patients with HER-amplified mCRCs, compared with cetuximab and irinotecan hydrochloride [163] (Table 1).

3.9. Ipilimumab

Ipilimumab (Yervoy®) developed by Medarex (Princeton, NJ, USA), is a fully humanized monoclonal antibody that binds to the ECD of CTLA-4, specifically blocks the interaction between CTLA-4 and B7-1 or B7-2, and eventually maintains T-cell cytotoxicity to attack cancer cells [164,165].

In 2011, ipilimumab first received FDA approval for melanoma treatment. Furthermore, it underwent clinical trials for the treatment of NSCLC, SCLC, and bladder cancer. Moreover, it was approved by the FDA for the treatment of mCRC in 2018 [166] (Table 1). This antibody is currently being evaluated in the CheckMate-142 clinical trial (NCT02060188) for treatment of patients with dMMR/MSI-H mCRC. The CheckMate-142 trial that is evaluating the combination therapy of ipilimumab plus nivolumab is the same clinical trial that is evaluating nivolumab [167].

3.10. Tremelimumab

Tremelimumab (CP-675) developed by AstraZeneca (Cambridge, UK) is a fully human monoclonal IgG2-kappa antibody that binds to the ECD of CTLA-4 and has an epitope similar to that for tremelimumab and ipilimumab. Its binding to CTLA-4 specifically blocks the interaction between CTLA-4 and B7-H1 and B7-H2 and downregulates the immune system. The function of tremelimumab is similar to that of ipilimumab, which maintains T-cell cytotoxicity against cancer cells [166,168].

In 2015, tremelimumab first received US FDA approval as an orphan drug for the treatment of patients with malignant mesothelioma. Currently, the indications that can be treated through clinical trials are expanding. In clinical trials, tremelimumab has been administered in various combination therapies with durvalumab and anti-cancer drugs. In a phase II clinical trial (NCT02870920) that compared the combination therapy of tremelizumab plus durvalumab with best supportive care for treatment of patients with advanced mCRC, the PFS was estimated to have improved to 1.8 months and the OS to have improved to 6.6 months after a median follow-up of 15.2 months (Table 1). This clinical trial is ongoing until December, 2020 [169,170].

3.11. Pembrolizumab

Pembrolizumab (Keytruda®) developed by LifeArc (London, UK) is a humanized monoclonal antibody that binds to PD-1. This antibody was generated by grafting the variable region sequences of a high affinity mouse anti-human PD-1 antibody onto a human IgG4-kappa isotype framework containing a stabilizing S228P Fc mutation for preventing Fab-arm exchange. The antibody specifically binds the PD-1 C'D-loop and antagonizes the interaction between PD-1 and its known ligands, PD-L1 and PD-L2 [171,172].

In 2014, pembrolizumab received FDA approval as the first PD-1/PD-L1 blockade drug for the treatment of metastatic melanoma [173]. In 2020, the FDA also approved pembrolizumab as the first-line treatment for patients with unresectable or metastatic microsatellite high-instability or mismatch repair-deficient CRCs [174] (Table 1). According to the KEYNOTE-177 clinical trial (NCT02563002) for treatment of MSI-H/dMMR CRCs, pembrolizumab improved PFS from 8.2 to 16.5 months compared with the standard chemotherapy [175].

3.12. Nivolumab

Nivolumab (Opdivo®) developed by Medarex (Princeton, NJ, USA) is a fully human monoclonal antibody that binds to the IgV domain of PD-1. The antibody has a variable region grafted into the human kappa and IgG4-constant region containing an S228P mutation in the hinge region. Especially, nivolumab specifically binds to the N-terminal loop of PD-1 different from an epitope for pembrolizumab. Nivolumab is also an immune checkpoint inhibitor that potentiates the cytotoxicity of T cells to kill malignant tumors [176,177].

In 2014, nivolumab first received US FDA approval for treatment of patients with advanced melanoma and was then approved to treat lung cancer in 2015. Currently, immunotherapy using nivolumab is widely used to treat mCRC [178]. In the CheckMate-142 phase II clinical trial (NCT02060188) for treatment of patients with dMMR/MSI-H mCRC, the PFS was estimated to be 12 months and the OS rate improved from 73% to 85% compared with that of nivolumab monotherapy as the primary endpoint after a median follow-up of 13.4 months (Table 1). This CheckMate-142 clinical trial is ongoing until primary completion in July 2022 [179,180].

3.13. Camrelizumab

Camrelizumab (AiRuiKa) developed by Jiangsu HengRui Medicine Co. Ltd. (Lianyungang, Jiangsu, China) is a humanized monoclonal antibody that binds to the flexible N- and C'D-loops of PD-1 and specifically blocks the interaction between PD-L1 and PD-1. It has epitopes partly overlapped with epitopes that bind to nivolumab and pembrolizumab. The cancer cell-killing mechanism of camrelizumab in immunotherapy is similar to that of pembrolizumab and nivolumab [181,182].

In 2019, camrelizumab first received China Food & Drug Administration approval for treatment of patients with classical Hodgkin's lymphoma. The indications for camrelizumab are expanding through multiple ongoing clinical trials. A phase II clinical trial (NCT03912857) for treatment of patients with advanced mCRC, the combination of camrelizumab plus apatinib, a VEGFR2 inhibitor, is expected to increase the overall response rate of advanced mCRC after standard chemotherapy [183,184] (Table 1).

3.14. Atezolizumab

Atezolizumab (Tecentriq®) developed by Genentech (South San Francisco, CA, USA) is a monoclonal antibody that binds to the IgV domain of PD-L1, a ligand of the PD-1 receptor expressed on the surface of T cells. It is a humanized antibody in which the variable region of atezolizumab is changed to a human germline sequence and Fc region of atezolizumab engineered to reduce the Fc-mediated effector functions. PD-L1 acts as a

T-cell suppressor through interaction with PD-1. Atezolizumab specifically binds to PD-L1 and blocks the interaction between PD-1 and PD-L1, thereby maintaining the anti-cancer effect of T cells [185,186].

In 2016, atezolizumab received FDA approval as an immune checkpoint PD-L1 inhibitor for the treatment of patients with locally advanced or metastatic urothelial carcinoma [10,16]. In 2019, the FDA also approved atezolizumab for the first-line treatment of adult patients with extensive-stage small-cell lung cancer in combination with carboplatin and etoposide, (NCT02763579) [19]. According to a clinical trial (NCT02873195) for treatment of refractory mCRC, compared with bevacizumab plus capecitabine therapy, bevacizumab and capecitabine combination therapy improved PFS from 3.3 to 4.3 months. Additionally, OS was maintained for 20 months, a result similar to that for bevacizumab and capecitabine combination therapy [155] (Table 1).

3.15. Avelumab

Avelumab (Bavencio®) developed by Merck KGaA (Darmstadt, Germany) is a fully human IgG1 antibody that binds to the IgV domain of PD-L1 in a manner similar to atezolizumab and blocks the interaction between PD-L1 and PD-1. Avelumab consists of human antibody sequences in both the variable and constant lambda light-chain and IgG1 heavy-chain regions [187].

In 2017, avelumab first received US FDA approval for the treatment of metastatic Merkel cell carcinoma [17]. Clinical trials for treatment of CRC patients ongoing. Specifically, avelumab was administered in clinical trials for CRC patients with POLE mutation observed in 3% of total CRC patients. One trial is a phase II clinical trial of avelumab monotherapy (NCT03150706) being conducted at Asan Medical Center (AMC) in South Korea. The other trial is a phase III clinical trial of avelumab plus 5-FU combination therapy (NCT03827044) being conducted at Royal Marsden Hospital in the UK that is expected to end in 2024 [188] (Table 1).

3.16. Durvalumab

Durvalumab (Imfinzi®) developed by Medimmune (Gaithersburg, MD, USA) is a fully human monoclonal antibody that binds to the ECD of PD-L1 and blocks the interaction between PD-L1 and PD-1. However, it has been reported that an epitope of PD-L1 for durvalumab is different from that of avelumab. It was engineered to prevent cytotoxic effector functions (ADCC or CDC) against PD-L1-positive immune cells [189]. Durvalumab is an immune checkpoint inhibitor used to promote immune responses for cancer therapy [189,190].

In 2017, durvalumab first received FDA approval for the treatment of metastatic urothelial carcinoma and is currently expanding indications through combination therapy [191]. The clinical trials using durvalumab are for refractory mCRC or mutated mCRC. The ILOC-EORTC phase II clinical trial (NCT030101475) for treatment of patients with refractory mCRC is ongoing with duvalumab plus tremelimumab combination therapy after radiation therapy as a primary completion in August 2021. Another phase II clinical trial (NCT03435107) for treatment of patients with POLE-mutated mCRC is ongoing to compare duvalumab monotherapy with chemotherapy. That trial has a primary completion date of March 2022 [192,193] (Table 1).

4. Conclusions

CRC is a highly complex and molecularly heterogeneous disease harboring frequent mutations that are resistant to common treatment. Despite recent advances in identification of therapeutic targets in CRCs and concomitant development of their therapeutic antibodies, several medical needs remain unmet in CRC therapy. As indicated by cetuximab treatment, antibody-drug resistance is one of the major hurdles for treating CRC patients. Cetuximab is only responsive to wild-type EGFR- and KRAS-expressing CRC patients who represent 10–20% of all CRC patients, whereas cetuximab is not responsive to approximately 80–90% of CRC patients harboring gene mutations in downstream EGFR effectors, including KRAS, PI3K catalytic subunit alpha (PI3KCA), PTEN, and BRAF. Furthermore, the 5-year survival rate of approximately 13% for stage IV CRC patients highlights the importance of basic studies for understanding CRC progression and metastasis. Therefore, to improve CRC patient clinical outcomes, understanding the pathological mechanisms and identification of novel therapeutic targets in CRC remain important for developing novel monoclonal antibodies for effective CRC therapy. Although this current review focused on discussing the roles and mechanisms of monoclonal antibodies in clinical development and approved by US FDA and their cognate therapeutic targets in CRC, the therapeutic potentials of bispecific antibodies and antibody-drug conjugates have also been validated for CRC therapy based on recent increasing studies. Lastly, scientific cooperation to create scientific knowledge and successful partnership between the industry and the academia will accelerate the development of an innovative new drug for effective CRC therapy.

Author Contributions: K.H., J.H.Y., J.H.L., and S.L. collected and analyzed the information, discussed and commented on the manuscript, and wrote the paper. S.L. supervised the project. All authors have read and agreed to the published version of the manuscript.

Funding: This research was supported by a grant from the Bio & Medical Technology Development Program of the National Research Foundation funded by the Korean government (NRF-2019M3E5D5065844, 2020M3A9I2107093).

Data Availability Statement: The data presented in this study are available on request form the corresponding author.

Acknowledgments: The authors acknowledge the contribution of the investigators whose experimental work has been cited in this article. We also acknowledge that images were created with Biorender.com.

Conflicts of Interest: The authors declare no conflict of interest. The funders have no role in the design of the study; in the collection, analyses, or interpretation of data; in the writing of the manuscript; or in the decision to publish the results.

Abbreviations

CRC	Colorectal cancer
FDA	Food and Drug Administration
OKT3	Muromonab-CD3
5-FU	5-fluorouracil
EGF	Epidermal growth factor
VEGF	Vascular endothelial growth factor
HGF	Hepatocyte growth factor
PD-1	Programmed cell death protein-1
CTLA-4	Cytotoxic T lymphocyte antigen 4
EGFR	Epidermal growth factor receptor
STAT	Signal transducer and activator of transcription
ADCC	Antibody-dependent cellular cytotoxicity
OS	Overall survival
PFS	Progression-free survival
CR	Complete remission
CHO cell	Chinese hamster ovary cell
AMC	Asan Medical Center
CDC	Complement-dependent cytotoxicity
DOI	Digital object identifier
ECD	Extracellular domain
FAK	Focal adhesion kinase
ITSM	Immunoreceptor tyrosine-based switch motif
KO	Knock out
MAPK	Mitogen-activated protein kinase
MCC	Merkel cell carcinoma
MHC	Major histocompatibility complex

PDX	Patient-derived xenograft
PFS	Progression-free survival
RAF	Rapidly accelerated fibrosarcoma
RAS	Rat sarcoma
RTK	Receptor tyrosine kinase
SOS	Son of sevenless
TCR	T-cell receptor
TIL	Tumor-infiltrating lymphocytes
VEGFR	VEGFR receptor

References

1. Mould, D.R.; Meibohm, B. Drug Development of Therapeutic Monoclonal Antibodies. *Biodrugs* **2016**, *30*, 275–293. [CrossRef] [PubMed]
2. Köhler, G.; Milstein, C. Continuous cultures of fused cells secreting antibody of predefined specificity. *Nature* **1975**, *256*, 495–497. [CrossRef] [PubMed]
3. Singh, S.; Kumar, N.K.; Dwiwedi, P.; Charan, J.; Kaur, R.; Sidhu, P.; Chugh, V.K. Monoclonal Antibodies: A Review. *Curr. Clin. Pharmacol.* **2018**, *13*, 85–99. [CrossRef] [PubMed]
4. Wilde, M.I.; Goa, K.L. Muromonab CD3. *Drugs* **1996**, *51*, 865–894. [CrossRef] [PubMed]
5. Ahmadzadeh, V.; Farajnia, S.; Feizi, M.A.H.; Nejad, R.A.K. Antibody Humanization Methods for Development of Therapeutic Applications. *Monoclon. Antib. Immunodiagn. Immunother.* **2014**, *33*, 67–73. [CrossRef]
6. Hoogenboom, H.R.; de Bruıne, A.P.; Hufton, S.E.; Hoet, R.M.; Arends, J.-W.; Roovers, R.C. Antibody phage display technology and its applications. *Immunotechnology* **1998**, *4*, 1–20. [CrossRef]
7. Shim, H. Therapeutic Antibodies by Phage Display. *Curr. Pharm. Des.* **2016**, *22*, 6538–6559. [CrossRef]
8. Tabasinezhad, M.; Talebkhan, Y.; Wenzel, W.; Rahimi, H.; Omidinia, E.; Mahboudi, F. Trends in therapeutic antibody affinity maturation: From in-vitro towards next-generation sequencing approaches. *Immunol. Lett.* **2019**, *212*, 106–113. [CrossRef]
9. De Wildt, R.M.T.; Mundy, C.R.; Gorick, B.D.; Tomlinson, I.M. Antibody arrays for high-throughput screening of antibody–antigen interactions. *Nat. Biotechnol.* **2000**, *18*, 989–994. [CrossRef]
10. Lu, R.-M.; Hwang, Y.-C.; Liu, I.J.; Lee, C.-C.; Tsai, H.-Z.; Li, H.-J.; Wu, H.-C. Development of therapeutic antibodies for the treatment of diseases. *J. Biomed. Sci.* **2020**, *27*, 1. [CrossRef]
11. Barderas, R.; Benito-Peña, E. The 2018 Nobel Prize in Chemistry: Phage display of peptides and antibodies. *Anal. Bioanal. Chem.* **2019**, *411*, 2475–2479. [CrossRef] [PubMed]
12. Riechmann, L.; Clark, M.; Waldmann, H.; Winter, G. Reshaping human antibodies for therapy. *Nature* **1988**, *332*, 323–327. [CrossRef] [PubMed]
13. Waldmann, H. Human Monoclonal Antibodies: The Benefits of Humanization. In *Human Monoclonal Antibodies: Methods and Protocols*; Steinitz, M., Ed.; Springer: New York, NY, USA, 2019; pp. 1–10.
14. Ling, W.-L.; Lua, W.-H.; Gan, S.K.-E. Sagacity in antibody humanization for therapeutics, diagnostics and research purposes: Considerations of antibody elements and their roles. *Antib. Ther.* **2020**, *3*, 71–79. [CrossRef]
15. Lua, W.-H.; Ling, W.-L.; Yeo, J.Y.; Poh, J.-J.; Lane, D.P.; Gan, S.K.-E. The effects of Antibody Engineering CH and CL in Trastuzumab and Pertuzumab recombinant models: Impact on antibody production and antigen-binding. *Sci. Rep.* **2018**, *8*, 718. [CrossRef] [PubMed]
16. Xenaki, K.T.; Oliveira, S.; van Bergen en Henegouwen, P.M.P. Antibody or Antibody Fragments: Implications for Molecular Imaging and Targeted Therapy of Solid Tumors. *Front. Immunol.* **2017**, *8*, 1287. [CrossRef]
17. Jain, R.K. Physiological barriers to delivery of monoclonal antibodies and other macromolecules in tumors. *Cancer Res.* **1990**, *50*, 814s–819s. [PubMed]
18. Nelson, A.L.; Reichert, J.M. Development trends for therapeutic antibody fragments. *Nat. Biotechnol.* **2009**, *27*, 331–337. [CrossRef]
19. Yokota, T.; Milenic, D.E.; Whitlow, M.; Schlom, J. Rapid tumor penetration of a single-chain Fv and comparison with other immunoglobulin forms. *Cancer Res.* **1992**, *52*, 3402–3408.
20. Haggar, F.A.; Boushey, R.P. Colorectal cancer epidemiology: Incidence, mortality, survival, and risk factors. *Clin. Colon. Rectal. Surg.* **2009**, *22*, 191–197. [CrossRef]
21. Taylor, P. *Global Cancer Therapeutics Market: Emphasis on Recurrent and Metastatic Divisions*; BCC Research Report Code: PHM177A; BCC Research: Wellesley, MA, USA, 2019.
22. Peinert, S.; Grothe, W.; Stein, A.; Müller, L.P.; Ruessel, J.; Voigt, W.; Schmoll, H.J.; Arnold, D. Safety and efficacy of weekly 5-fluorouracil/folinic acid/oxaliplatin/irinotecan in the first-line treatment of gastrointestinal cancer. *Ther. Adv. Med. Oncol.* **2010**, *2*, 161–174. [CrossRef]
23. Weiner, L.M.; Surana, R.; Wang, S. Antibodies and cancer therapy: Versatile platforms for cancer immunotherapy. *Nat. Rev. Immunol.* **2010**, *10*, 317–327. [CrossRef]
24. Hurwitz, H. Integrating the anti-VEGF-A humanized monoclonal antibody bevacizumab with chemotherapy in advanced colorectal cancer. *Clin. Colorectal. Cancer* **2004**, *4*, S62–S68. [CrossRef] [PubMed]

25. Rosa, B.; de Jesus, J.P.; de Mello, E.L.; Cesar, D.; Correia, M.M. Effectiveness and safety of monoclonal antibodies for metastatic colorectal cancer treatment: Systematic review and meta-analysis. *Ecancermedicalscience* **2015**, *9*, 582. [CrossRef]
26. Kong, D.H.; Kim, M.R.; Jang, J.H.; Na, H.J.; Lee, S. A Review of Anti-Angiogenic Targets for Monoclonal Antibody Cancer Therapy. *Int. J. Mol. Sci.* **2017**, *18*, 1786. [CrossRef] [PubMed]
27. Smyth, M.J.; Teng, M.W. 2018 Nobel Prize in physiology or medicine. *Clin. Transl. Immunol.* **2018**, *7*, e1041. [CrossRef] [PubMed]
28. Siena, S.; Sartore-Bianchi, A.; Marsoni, S.; Hurwitz, H.I.; McCall, S.J.; Penault-Llorca, F.; Srock, S.; Bardelli, A.; Trusolino, L. Targeting the human epidermal growth factor receptor 2 (HER2) oncogene in colorectal cancer. *Ann. Oncol.* **2018**, *29*, 1108–1119. [CrossRef]
29. Choi, E.; Yang, J.W. Updates to Clinical Information on Anticancer Immunotherapy. *Korean J. Clin. Pharm.* **2018**, *28*, 65–75. [CrossRef]
30. Beerli, R.R.; Hynes, N.E. Epidermal growth factor-related peptides activate distinct subsets of ErbB receptors and differ in their biological activities. *J. Biol. Chem.* **1996**, *271*, 6071–6076. [CrossRef]
31. Coussens, L.; Yang-Feng, T.L.; Liao, Y.C.; Chen, E.; Gray, A.; McGrath, J.; Seeburg, P.H.; Libermann, T.A.; Schlessinger, J.; Francke, U.; et al. Tyrosine kinase receptor with extensive homology to EGF receptor shares chromosomal location with neu oncogene. *Science* **1985**, *230*, 1132–1139. [CrossRef] [PubMed]
32. Wang, Z. ErbB Receptors and Cancer. *Methods Mol. Biol.* **2017**, *1652*, 3–35. [PubMed]
33. Yarden, Y.; Sliwkowski, M.X. Untangling the ErbB signalling network. *Nat. Rev. Mol. Cell Biol.* **2001**, *2*, 127–137. [CrossRef] [PubMed]
34. Schlessinger, J.; Ullrich, A. Growth factor signaling by receptor tyrosine kinases. *Neuron* **1992**, *9*, 383–391. [CrossRef]
35. Pawson, T. Protein modules and signalling networks. *Nature* **1995**, *373*, 573–580. [CrossRef] [PubMed]
36. Dickson, R.B.; Lippman, M.E. Estrogenic regulation of growth and polypeptide growth factor secretion in human breast carcinoma. *Endocr. Rev.* **1987**, *8*, 29–43. [CrossRef] [PubMed]
37. Mimeault, M.; Pommery, N.; Hénichart, J.P. New advances on prostate carcinogenesis and therapies: Involvement of EGF-EGFR transduction system. *Growth Factors* **2003**, *21*, 1–14. [CrossRef]
38. Prenzel, N.; Zwick, E.; Leserer, M.; Ullrich, A. Tyrosine kinase signalling in breast cancer. Epidermal growth factor receptor: Convergence point for signal integration and diversification. *Breast Cancer Res.* **2000**, *2*, 184–190. [CrossRef]
39. Ferguson, K.M.; Berger, M.B.; Mendrola, J.M.; Cho, H.S.; Leahy, D.J.; Lemmon, M.A. EGF activates its receptor by removing interactions that autoinhibit ectodomain dimerization. *Mol. Cell* **2003**, *11*, 507–517. [CrossRef]
40. Dawson, J.P.; Berger, M.B.; Lin, C.C.; Schlessinger, J.; Lemmon, M.A.; Ferguson, K.M. Epidermal growth factor receptor dimerization and activation require ligand-induced conformational changes in the dimer interface. *Mol. Cell. Biol.* **2005**, *25*, 7734–7742. [CrossRef]
41. Zhang, W.; Chen, L.; Ma, K.; Zhao, Y.; Liu, X.; Wang, Y.; Liu, M.; Liang, S.; Zhu, H.; Xu, N. Polarization of macrophages in the tumor microenvironment is influenced by EGFR signaling within colon cancer cells. *Oncotarget* **2016**, *7*, 75366–75378. [CrossRef]
42. Jin, P.; Jiang, J.; Xie, N.; Zhou, L.; Huang, Z.; Zhang, L.; Qin, S.; Fu, S.; Peng, L.; Gao, W.; et al. MCT1 relieves osimertinib-induced CRC suppression by promoting autophagy through the LKB1/AMPK signaling. *Cell Death Dis.* **2019**, *10*, 615. [CrossRef]
43. Matsuo, T.; Nishizuka, S.S.; Ishida, K.; Iwaya, T.; Ikeda, M.; Wakabayashi, G. Analysis of the anti-tumor effect of cetuximab using protein kinetics and mouse xenograft models. *BMC Res. Notes* **2011**, *4*, 140. [CrossRef] [PubMed]
44. Lee, H.W.; Son, E.; Lee, K.; Lee, Y.; Kim, Y.; Lee, J.C.; Lim, Y.; Hur, M.; Kim, D.; Nam, D.H. Promising Therapeutic Efficacy of GC1118, an Anti-EGFR Antibody, against KRAS Mutation-Driven Colorectal Cancer Patient-Derived Xenografts. *Int. J. Mol. Sci.* **2019**, *20*, 5894. [CrossRef] [PubMed]
45. Qiu, W.; Zhang, C.; Wang, S.; Yu, X.; Wang, Q.; Zeng, D.; Du, P.; Ma, J.; Zheng, Y.; Pang, B.; et al. A Novel Anti-EGFR mAb Ame55 with Lower Toxicity and Better Efficacy than Cetuximab When Combined with Irinotecan. *J. Immunol. Res.* **2019**, *2019*, 3017360. [CrossRef]
46. Bertotti, A.; Migliardi, G.; Galimi, F.; Sassi, F.; Torti, D.; Isella, C.; Corà, D.; di Nicolantonio, F.; Buscarino, M.; Petti, C.; et al. A Molecularly Annotated Platform of Patient-Derived Xenografts ("Xenopatients") Identifies HER2 as an Effective Therapeutic Target in Cetuximab-Resistant Colorectal Cancer. *Cancer Discov.* **2011**, *1*, 508–523. [CrossRef] [PubMed]
47. Richman, S.D.; Southward, K.; Chambers, P.; Cross, D.; Barrett, J.; Hemmings, G.; Taylor, M.; Wood, H.; Hutchins, G.; Foster, J.M.; et al. HER2 overexpression and amplification as a potential therapeutic target in colorectal cancer: Analysis of 3256 patients enrolled in the QUASAR, FOCUS and PICCOLO colorectal cancer trials. *J. Pathol.* **2016**, *238*, 562–570. [CrossRef]
48. Muzny, D.M.; Bainbridge, M.N.; Chang, K.; Dinh, H.H.; Drummond, J.A.; Fowler, G.; Kovar, C.L.; Lewis, L.R.; Morgan, M.B.; Newsham, I.F.; et al. Comprehensive molecular characterization of human colon and rectal cancer. *Nature* **2012**, *487*, 330–337.
49. Raghav, K.; Loree, J.M.; Morris, J.S.; Overman, M.J.; Yu, R.; Meric-Bernstam, F.; Menter, D.; Korphaisarn, K.; Kee, B.; Muranyi, A.; et al. Validation of HER2 Amplification as a Predictive Biomarker for Anti–Epidermal Growth Factor Receptor Antibody Therapy in Metastatic Colorectal Cancer. *JCO Precis. Oncol.* **2019**, *3*, 1–13. [CrossRef]
50. Yonesaka, K.; Zejnullahu, K.; Okamoto, I.; Satoh, T.; Cappuzzo, F.; Souglakos, J.; Ercan, D.; Rogers, A.; Roncalli, M.; Takeda, M.; et al. Activation of ERBB2 signaling causes resistance to the EGFR-directed therapeutic antibody cetuximab. *Sci. Transl. Med.* **2011**, *3*, 99ra86. [CrossRef]

51. Troiani, T.; Martinelli, E.; Napolitano, S.; Vitagliano, D.; Ciuffreda, L.P.; Costantino, S.; Morgillo, F.; Capasso, A.; Sforza, V.; Nappi, A.; et al. Increased TGF-α as a mechanism of acquired resistance to the anti-EGFR inhibitor cetuximab through EGFR-MET interaction and activation of MET signaling in colon cancer cells. *Clin. Cancer Res.* **2013**, *19*, 6751–6765. [CrossRef]
52. Liska, D.; Chen, C.T.; Bachleitner-Hofmann, T.; Christensen, J.G.; Weiser, M.R. HGF rescues colorectal cancer cells from EGFR inhibition via MET activation. *Clin. Cancer Res.* **2011**, *17*, 472–482. [CrossRef]
53. Zhao, B.; Wang, L.; Qiu, H.; Zhang, M.; Sun, L.; Peng, P.; Yu, Q.; Yuan, X. Mechanisms of resistance to anti-EGFR therapy in colorectal cancer. *Oncotarget* **2017**, *8*, 3980–4000. [CrossRef] [PubMed]
54. Peach, C.J.; Mignone, V.W.; Arruda, M.A.; Alcobia, D.C.; Hill, S.J.; Kilpatrick, L.E.; Woolard, J. Molecular Pharmacology of VEGF-A Isoforms: Binding and Signalling at VEGFR2. *Int. J. Mol. Sci.* **2018**, *19*, 1264. [CrossRef] [PubMed]
55. Woolard, J.; Bevan, H.S.; Harper, S.J.; Bates, D.O. Molecular diversity of VEGF-A as a regulator of its biological activity. *Microcirculation* **2009**, *16*, 572–592. [CrossRef] [PubMed]
56. Holmes, D.I.; Zachary, I. The vascular endothelial growth factor (VEGF) family: Angiogenic factors in health and disease. *Genome. Biol.* **2005**, *6*, 209. [CrossRef] [PubMed]
57. Koch, S.; Claesson-Welsh, L. Signal transduction by vascular endothelial growth factor receptors. *Cold. Spring Harb. Perspect. Med.* **2012**, *2*, a006502. [CrossRef] [PubMed]
58. Shaik, F.; Cuthbert, G.A.; Homer-Vanniasinkam, S.; Muench, S.P.; Ponnambalam, S.; Harrison, M.A. Structural Basis for Vascular Endothelial Growth Factor Receptor Activation and Implications for Disease Therapy. *Biomolecules* **2020**, *10*, 1673. [CrossRef] [PubMed]
59. Disatnik, M.H.; Hernandez-Sotomayor, S.M.; Jones, G.; Carpenter, G.; Mochly-Rosen, D. Phospholipase C-gamma 1 binding to intracellular receptors for activated protein kinase C. *Proc. Natl. Acad. Sci. USA* **1994**, *91*, 559–563. [CrossRef]
60. Napione, L.; Alvaro, M.; Bussolino, F. VEGF-Mediated Signal transduction in Tumor Angiogenesis. In *Physiologic and Pathologic Angiogenesis—Signaling Mechanisms and Targeted Therapy*; IntechOpen Limited: London, UK, 2017; Volume 227. [CrossRef]
61. Wu, H.M.; Yuan, Y.; Zawieja, D.C.; Tinsley, J.; Granger, H.J. Role of phospholipase C, protein kinase C, and calcium in VEGF-induced venular hyperpermeability. *Am. J. Physiol.* **1999**, *276*, H535–H542. [CrossRef]
62. Simons, M.; Gordon, E.; Claesson-Welsh, L. Mechanisms and regulation of endothelial VEGF receptor signalling. *Nat. Rev. Mol. Cell Biol.* **2016**, *17*, 611–625. [CrossRef]
63. Sawada, J.; Li, F.; Komatsu, M. R-Ras Inhibits VEGF-Induced p38MAPK Activation and HSP27 Phosphorylation in Endothelial Cells. *J. Vasc. Res.* **2015**, *52*, 347–359. [CrossRef]
64. Bendardaf, R.; Buhmeida, A.; Hilska, M.; Laato, M.; Syrjänen, S.; Syrjänen, K.; Collan, Y.; Pyrhönen, S. VEGF-1 expression in colorectal cancer is associated with disease localization, stage, and long-term disease-specific survival. *Anticancer Res.* **2008**, *28*, 3865–3870. [PubMed]
65. Karayiannakis, A.J.; Syrigos, K.N.; Zbar, A.; Baibas, N.; Polychronidis, A.; Simopoulos, C.; Karatzas, G. Clinical significance of preoperative serum vascular endothelial growth factor levels in patients with colorectal cancer and the effect of tumor surgery. *Surgery* **2002**, *131*, 548–555. [CrossRef] [PubMed]
66. Foersch, S.; Sperka, T.; Lindner, C.; Taut, A.; Rudolph, K.L.; Breier, G.; Boxberger, F.; Rau, T.T.; Hartmann, A.; Stürzl, M.; et al. VEGFR2 Signaling Prevents Colorectal Cancer Cell. Senescence to Promote Tumorigenesis in Mice with Colitis. *Gastroenterology* **2015**, *149*, 177–189. [CrossRef] [PubMed]
67. Schmieder, R.; Hoffmann, J.; Becker, M.; Bhargava, A.; Müller, T.; Kahmann, N.; Ellinghaus, P.; Adams, R.; Rosenthal, A.; Thierauch, K.-H.; et al. Regorafenib (BAY. 73-4506): Antitumor and antimetastatic activities in preclinical models of colorectal cancer. *Int. J. Cancer* **2014**, *135*, 1487–1496. [CrossRef] [PubMed]
68. Becherirat, S.; Valamanesh, F.; Karimi, M.; Faussat, A.M.; Launay, J.M.; Pimpie, C.; Therwath, A.; Pocard, M. Discontinuou Schedule of Bevacizumab in Colorectal Cancer Induces Accelerated Tumor Growth and Phenotypic Changes. *Transl. Oncol.* **2018**, *11*, 406–415. [CrossRef]
69. Shaheen, R.M.; Ahmad, S.A.; Liu, W.; Reinmuth, N.; Jung, Y.D.; Tseng, W.W.; Drazan, K.E.; Bucana, C.D.; Hicklin, D.J.; Ellis, L.M. Inhibited growth of colon cancer carcinomatosis by antibodies to vascular endothelial and epidermal growth factor receptors. *Br. J. Cancer* **2001**, *85*, 584–589. [CrossRef]
70. Frisch, R.N.; Curtis, K.M.; Aenlle, K.K.; Howard, G.A. Hepatocyte growth factor and alternativ splice. variants—Expression, regulation and implications in osteogenesis and bone health and repair. *Expert Opin. Ther. Targets* **2016**, *20*, 1087–1098. [CrossRef]
71. Christensen, J.G.; Burrows, J.; Salgia, R. c-Met as a target for human cancer and characterization of inhibitors for therapeutic intervention. *Cancer Lett.* **2005**, *225*, 1–26. [CrossRef]
72. Ma, P.C.; Maulik, G.; Christensen, J.; Salgia, R. c-Met: Structure, functions and potential for therapeutic inhibition. *Cancer Metastasis Rev.* **2003**, *22*, 309–325. [CrossRef]
73. Organ, S.L.; Tsao, M.S. An overview of the c-MET signaling pathway. *Adv. Med. Oncol.* **2011**, *3*, S7–S19. [CrossRef]
74. Comoglio, P.M.; Giordano, S.; Trusolino, L. Drug development of MET inhibitors: Targeting oncogene addiction and expedience. *Nat. Rev. Drug Discov.* **2008**, *7*, 504–516. [CrossRef] [PubMed]
75. Maulik, G.; Shrikhande, A.; Kijima, T.; Ma, P.C.; Morrison, P.T.; Salgia, R. Role of the hepatocyte growth factor receptor, c-Met, in oncogenesis and potential for therapeutic inhibition. *Cytokine Growth Factor Rev.* **2002**, *13*, 41–59. [CrossRef]
76. Furge, K.A.; Zhang, Y.W.; Woude, G.F.V. Met receptor tyrosine kinase: Enhanced signaling through adapter proteins. *Oncogene* **2000**, *19*, 5582–5589. [CrossRef] [PubMed]

77. Bradley, C.A.; Salto-Tellez, M.; Laurent-Puig, P.; Bardelli, A.; Rolfo, C.; Tabernero, J.; Khawaja, H.A.; Lawler, M.; Johnston, P.G.; van Schaeybroeck, S. Targeting c-MET in gastrointestinal tumours: Rationale, opportunities and challenges. *Nat. Rev. Clin. Oncol.* **2017**, *14*, 562–576. [CrossRef]
78. Gentile, A.; Trusolino, L.; Comoglio, P.M. The Met tyrosine kinase receptor in development and cancer. *Cancer Metastasis Rev.* **2008**, *27*, 85–94. [CrossRef] [PubMed]
79. Parizadeh, S.M.; Jafarzadeh-Esfehani, R.; Fazilat-Panah, D.; Hassanian, S.M.; Shahidsales, S.; Khazaei, M.; Parizadeh, S.M.R.; Ghayour-Mobarhan, M.; Ferns, G.A.; Avan, A. The potential therapeutic and prognostic impacts of the c-MET/HGF signaling pathway in colorectal cancer. *Iubmb Life* **2019**, *71*, 802–811. [CrossRef]
80. Lee, S.J.; Lee, J.; Park, S.H.; Park, J.O.; Lim, H.Y.; Kang, W.K.; Park, Y.S.; Kim, S.T. c-MET Overexpression in Colorectal Cancer: A Poor Prognostic Factor for Survival. *Clin. Colorectal Cancer* **2018**, *17*, 165–169. [CrossRef]
81. Gayyed, M.F.; El-Maqsoud, N.M.A.; El-Heeny, A.A.E.; Mohammed, M.F. c-MET expression in colorectal adenomas and primary carcinomas with its corresponding metastases. *J. Gastrointest. Oncol.* **2015**, *6*, 618–627.
82. Wang, S.; Ma, H.; Yan, Y.; Chen, Y.; Fu, S.; Wang, J.; Wang, Y.; Chen, H.; Liu, J. cMET promotes metastasis and epithelial-mesenchymal transition in colorectal carcinoma by repressing. *RKIP. J. Cell. Physiol.* **2020**. [CrossRef]
83. Gao, W.; Bing, X.; Li, M.; Yang, Z.; Li, Y.; Chen, H. Study of critical role of c-Met and its inhibitor SU11274 in colorectal carcinoma. *Med. Oncol.* **2013**, *30*, 546. [CrossRef]
84. Woo, J.K.; Kang, J.H.; Kim, B.; Park, B.H.; Shin, K.J.; Song, S.W.; Kim, J.J.; Kim, H.M.; Lee, S.J.; Oh, S.H. Humanized anti-hepatocyte growth factor (HGF) antibody suppresses innate irinotecan (CPT-11) resistance induced by fibroblast-derived HGF. *Oncotarget* **2015**, *6*, 24047–24060. [CrossRef] [PubMed]
85. Van der Horst, E.H.; Chinn, L.; Wang, M.; Velilla, T.; Tran, H.; Madrona, Y.; Lam, A.; Ji, M.; Hoey, T.C.; Sato, A.K. Discovery of fully human anti-MET monoclonal antibodies with antitumor activity against colon cancer tumor models in vivo. *Neoplasia* **2009**, *11*, 355–664. [CrossRef] [PubMed]
86. Rubin, I.; Yarden, Y. The basic biology of HER2. *Ann. Oncol.* **2001**, *12*, S3–S8. [CrossRef] [PubMed]
87. Cho, H.S.; Mason, K.; Ramyar, K.X.; Stanley, A.M.; Gabelli, S.B.; Denney, D.W., Jr.; Leahy, D.J. Structure of the extracellular region of HER2 alone and in complex with the Herceptin Fab. *Nature* **2003**, *421*, 756–760. [CrossRef] [PubMed]
88. Iqbal, N. Trastuzumab: Human Epidermal Growth Factor Receptor 2 (HER2) in Cancers: Overexpression and Therapeutic Implications. *Mol. Biol. Int.* **2014**, *2014*, 852748. [CrossRef]
89. Vu, T.; Claret, F.X. Trastuzumab: Updated mechanisms of action and resistance in breast cancer. *Front. Oncol.* **2012**, *2*, 62. [CrossRef]
90. Wang, X.Y.; Zheng, Z.X.; Sun, Y.; Bai, Y.H.; Shi, Y.F.; Zhou, L.X.; Yao, Y.F.; Wu, A.W.; Cao, D.F. Significance of HER2 protein expression and HER2 gene amplification in colorectal adenocarcinomas. *World J. Gastrointest. Oncol.* **2019**, *11*, 335–347. [CrossRef]
91. Blok, E.J.; Kuppen, P.J.; van Leeuwen, J.E.; Sier, C.F. Cytoplasmic Overexpression of HER2: A Key Factor in Colorectal Cancer. *Clin. Med. Insights Oncol.* **2013**, *7*, 41–51. [CrossRef]
92. Kulukian, A.; Lee, P.; Taylor, J.; Rosler, R.; de Vries, P.; Watson, D.; Forero-Torres, A.; Peterson, S. Preclinical Activity of HER2-Selective Tyrosine Kinase Inhibitor Tucatinib as a Single Agent or in Combination with Trastuzumab or Docetaxel in Solid Tumor Models. *Mol. Cancer* **2020**, *19*, 976–987. [CrossRef]
93. Kato, Y.; Ohishi, T.; Yamada, S.; Itai, S.; Takei, J.; Sano, M.; Nakamura, T.; Harada, H.; Kawada, M.; Kaneko, M.K. Anti-Human Epidermal Growth Factor Receptor 2 Monoclonal Antibody H(2)Mab-41 Exerts Antitumor Activity in a Mouse Xenograft Model of Colon Cancer. *Monoclon. Antib. Immunodiagn. Immunother.* **2019**, *38*, 157–161. [CrossRef]
94. Kato, Y.; Ohishi, T.; Takei, J.; Nakamura, T.; Sano, M.; Asano, T.; Sayama, Y.; Hosono, H.; Kawada, M.; Kaneko, M.K. An Anti-Human Epidermal Growth Factor Receptor 2 Monoclonal Antibody H2Mab-19 Exerts Antitumor Activity in Mouse Colon Cancer Xenografts. *Monoclon. Antib. Immunodiagn. Immunother.* **2020**, *39*, 123–128. [CrossRef] [PubMed]
95. Kuwada, S.K.; Scaife, C.L.; Kuang, J.; Li, X.; Wong, R.F.; Florell, S.R.; Coffey, R.J., Jr.; Gray, P.D. Effects of trastuzumab on epidermal growth factor receptor-dependent and -independent human colon cancer cells. *Int. J. Cancer* **2004**, *109*, 291–301. [CrossRef] [PubMed]
96. Lindsten, T.; Lee, K.P.; Harris, E.S.; Petryniak, B.; Craighead, N.; Reynolds, P.J.; Lombard, D.B.; Freeman, G.J.; Nadler, L.M.; Gray, G.S.; et al. Characterization of CTLA-4 structure and expression on human T cells. *J. Immunol.* **1993**, *151*, 3489–3499. [PubMed]
97. Linsley, P.S.; Brady, W.; Urnes, M.; Grosmaire, L.S.; Damle, N.K.; Ledbetter, J.A. CTLA-4 is a second receptor for the B cell activation antigen B7. *J. Exp. Med.* **1991**, *174*, 561–569. [CrossRef] [PubMed]
98. Wang, X.-Y.; Zuo, D.; Sarkar, D.; Fisher, P.B. Blockade of cytotoxic T-lymphocyte antigen-4 as a new therapeutic approach for advanced melanoma. *Expert Opin. Pharmacother.* **2011**, *12*, 2695–2706. [CrossRef]
99. McCoy, K.D.; Hermans, I.F.; Fraser, J.H.; le Gros, G.; Ronchese, F. Cytotoxic T lymphocyte-associated antigen 4 (CTLA-4) can regulate dendritic cell-induced activation and cytotoxicity of CD8(+) T cells independently of CD4(+) T cell help. *J. Exp. Med.* **1999**, *189*, 1157–1162. [CrossRef]
100. Rudd, C.E.; Taylor, A.; Schneider, H. CD28 and CTLA-4 coreceptor expression and signal transduction. *Immunol. Rev.* **2009**, *229*, 12–26. [CrossRef]
101. Teft, W.A.; Kirchhof, M.G.; Madrenas, J. A Molecular Perspective of Ctla-4 Function. *Annu. Rev. Immunol.* **2006**, *24*, 65–97. [CrossRef]

102. Sansom, D.M. CD28, CTLA-4 and their ligands: Who does what and to whom? *Immunology* **2000**, *101*, 169–177. [CrossRef]
103. Rowshanravan, B.; Halliday, N.; Sansom, D.M. CTLA-4: A moving target in immunotherapy. *Blood* **2018**, *131*, 58–67. [CrossRef]
104. Schneider, H.; Rudd, C.E. Diverse mechanisms regulate the surface expression of immunotherapeutic target ctla-4. *Front. Immunol.* **2014**, *5*, 619. [CrossRef] [PubMed]
105. Dempke, W.C.M.; Uciechowski, P.; Fenchel, K.; Chevassut, T. Targeting SHP-1, 2 and SHIP Pathways: A Novel Strategy for Cancer Treatment? *Oncology* **2018**, *95*, 257–269. [CrossRef] [PubMed]
106. Lorenz, U. SHP-1 and SHP-2 in T cells: Two phosphatases functioning at many levels. *Immunol. Rev.* **2009**, *228*, 342–359. [CrossRef] [PubMed]
107. Grosso, J.F.; Jure-Kunkel, M.N. CTLA-4 blockade in tumor models: An overview of preclinical and translational research. *Cancer Immunity* **2013**, *13*, 5. [PubMed]
108. Shi, L.; Meng, T.; Zhao, Z.; Han, J.; Zhang, W.; Gao, F.; Cai, J. CRISPR knock out CTLA-4 enhances the anti-tumor activity of cytotoxic T lymphocytes. *Gene* **2017**, *636*, 36–41. [CrossRef] [PubMed]
109. Fu, X.; Luo, H.; Zheng, Y.; Wang, S.; Zhong, Z.; Wang, Y.; Yang, Y. CTLA-4 immunotherapy exposes differences in immune response along with different tumor progression in colorectal cancer. *Aging* **2020**, *12*, 15656–15669. [CrossRef]
110. Lute, K.D.; May, K.F., Jr.; Lu, P.; Zhang, H.; Kocak, E.; Mosinger, B.; Wolford, C.; Phillips, G.; Caligiuri, M.A.; Zheng, P.; et al. Human CTLA4 knock-in mice unravel the quantitative link between tumor immunity and autoimmunity induced by anti-CTLA-4 antibodies. *Blood* **2005**, *106*, 3127–3133. [CrossRef]
111. Fiegle, E.; Doleschel, D.; Koletnik, S.; Rix, A.; Weiskirchen, R.; Borkham-Kamphorst, E.; Kiessling, F.; Lederle, W. Dual CTLA-4 and PD-L1 Blockade Inhibits Tumor Growth and Liver Metastasis in a Highly Aggressive Orthotopic Mouse Model of Colon Cancer. *Neoplasia* **2019**, *21*, 932–944. [CrossRef]
112. Boussiotis, V.A.; Chatterjee, P.; Li, L. Biochemical signaling of PD-1 on T cells and its functional implications. *Cancer J.* **2014**, *20*, 265–271. [CrossRef]
113. Zak, K.M.; Grudnik, P.; Magiera, K.; Dömling, A.; Dubin, G.; Holak, T.A. Structural Biology of the Immune Checkpoint Receptor PD-1 and Its Ligands PD-L1/PD-L2. *Structure* **2017**, *25*, 1163–1174. [CrossRef]
114. Jiang, X.; Wang, J.; Deng, X.; Xiong, F.; Ge, J.; Xiang, B.; Wu, X.; Ma, J.; Zhou, M.; Li, X.; et al. Role of the tumor microenvironment in PD-L1/PD-1-mediated tumor immune escape. *Mol. Cancer* **2019**, *18*, 10. [CrossRef] [PubMed]
115. Johansson, S.; Price, J.; Modo, M. Effect of inflammatory cytokines on major histocompatibility complex expression and differentiation of human neural stem/progenitor cells. *Stem Cells* **2008**, *26*, 2444–2454. [CrossRef] [PubMed]
116. Patsoukis, N.; Duke-Cohan, J.S.; Chaudhri, A.; Aksoylar, H.-I.; Wang, Q.; Council, A.; Berg, A.; Freeman, G.J.; Boussiotis, V.A. Interaction of SHP-2 SH2 domains with PD-1 ITSM induces PD-1 dimerization and SHP-2 activation. *Commun. Biol.* **2020**, *3*, 128. [CrossRef] [PubMed]
117. Sheppard, K.-A.; Fitz, L.J.; Lee, J.M.; Benander, C.; George, J.A.; Wooters, J.; Qiu, Y.; Jussif, J.M.; Carter, L.L.; Wood, C.R.; et al. PD-1 inhibits T-cell receptor induced phosphorylation of the ZAP70/CD3ζ signalosome and downstream signaling to PKCθ. *FEBS Lett.* **2004**, *574*, 37–41. [CrossRef] [PubMed]
118. Riley, J.L. PD-1 signaling in primary T cells. *Immunol. Rev.* **2009**, *229*, 114–125. [CrossRef] [PubMed]
119. Okkenhaug, K.; Turner, M.; Gold, M.R. PI3K Signaling in B Cell and T Cell Biology. *Front. Immunol.* **2014**, *5*, 557. [CrossRef] [PubMed]
120. Shan, T.; Chen, S.; Wu, T.; Yang, Y.; Li, S.; Chen, X. PD-L1 expression in colon cancer and its relationship with clinical prognosis. *Int. J. Clin. Exp. Pathol.* **2019**, *12*, 1764–1769.
121. Gordon, S.R.; Maute, R.L.; Dulken, B.W.; Hutter, G.; George, B.M.; McCracken, M.N.; Gupta, R.; Tsai, J.M.; Sinha, R.; Corey, D.; et al. PD-1 expression by tumour-associated macrophages inhibits phagocytosis and tumour immunity. *Nature* **2017**, *545*, 495–499. [CrossRef] [PubMed]
122. Cai, X.; Wei, B.; Li, L.; Chen, X.; Liu, W.; Cui, J.; Lin, Y.; Sun, Y.; Xu, Q.; Guo, W.; et al. Apatinib enhanced anti-PD-1 therapy for colon cancer in mice via promoting PD-L1 expression. *Int. Immunopharmacol.* **2020**, *88*, 106858. [CrossRef]
123. Capasso, A.; Lang, J.; Pitts, T.M.; Jordan, K.R.; Lieu, C.H.; Davis, S.L.; Diamond, J.R.; Kopetz, S.; Barbee, J.; Peterson, J.; et al. Characterization of immune responses to anti-PD-1 mono and combination immunotherapy in hematopoietic humanized mice implanted with tumor xenografts. *J. Immunother. Cancer* **2019**, *7*, 37. [CrossRef]
124. Stewart, R.; Morrow, M.; Hammond, S.A.; Mulgrew, K.; Marcus, D.; Poon, E.; Watkins, A.; Mullins, S.; Chodorge, M.; Andrews, J.; et al. Identification and Characterization of MEDI4736, an Antagonistic Anti-PD-L1 Monoclonal Antibody. *Cancer Immunol. Res.* **2015**, *3*, 1052–1062. [CrossRef] [PubMed]
125. Golchin, S.; Alimohammadi, R.; Nejad, M.R.; Jalali, S.A. Synergistic antitumor effect of anti-PD-L1 combined with oxaliplatin on a mouse tumor model. *J. Cell. Physiol.* **2019**, *234*, 19866–19874. [CrossRef]
126. U.S. Drug and Food. FDA Approved Drug Products: Herceptin (Trastuzumab) for Intravenous Injection. Available online: https://www.fda.gov/drugs/drug-approvals-and-databases/fda-approves-new-formulation-herceptin-subcutaneous-use (accessed on 28 February 2019).
127. Breece, T.N.; Fahrner, R.L.; Gorrell, J.R.; Lazzareschi, K.P.; Lester, P.M.; Peng, D. Protein Purification. U.S. Patent 6,870,034B2, 22 March 2005.
128. Li, S.; Schmitz, K.R.; Jeffrey, P.D.; Wiltzius, J.J.; Kussie, P.; Ferguson, K.M. Structural basis for inhibition of the epidermal growth factor receptor by cetuximab. *Cancer Cell* **2005**, *7*, 301–311. [CrossRef]

129. Kawaguchi, Y.; Kono, K.; Mimura, K.; Sugai, H.; Akaike, H.; Fujii, H. Cetuximab induce antibody-dependent cellular cytotoxicity against EGFR-expressing esophageal squamous cell carcinoma. *Int. J. Cancer* **2007**, *120*, 781–787. [CrossRef] [PubMed]
130. Chen, S.; Li, X.; Chen, R.; Yin, M.; Zheng, Q. Cetuximab intensifies the ADCC activity of adoptive NK cells in a nude mouse colorectal cancer xenograft model. *Oncol. Lett.* **2016**, *12*, 1868–1876. [CrossRef] [PubMed]
131. de Taeye, S.W.; Rispens, T.; Vidarsson, G. The Ligands for Human IgG and Their Effector Functions. *Antibodies* **2019**, *8*, 30. [CrossRef]
132. Okada, Y.; Kimura, T.; Nakagawa, T.; Okamoto, K.; Fukuya, A.; Goji, T.; Fujimoto, S.; Sogabe, M.; Miyamoto, H.; Muguruma, N.; et al. EGFR Downregulation after Anti-EGFR Therapy Predicts the Antitumor Effect in Colorectal Cancer. *Mol. Cancer Res.* **2017**, *15*, 1445–1454. [CrossRef]
133. Van Cutsem, E.; Köhne, C.H.; Hitre, E.; Zaluski, J.; Chien, C.R.C.; Makhson, A.; D'Haens, G.; Pintér, T.; Lim, R.; Bodoky, G.; et al. Cetuximab and chemotherapy as initial treatment for metastatic colorectal cancer. *N. Engl. J. Med.* **2009**, *360*, 1408–1417. [CrossRef]
134. Sickmier, E.A.; Kurzeja, R.J.; Michelsen, K.; Vazir, M.; Yang, E.; Tasker, A.S. The Panitumumab EGFR Complex Reveals a Binding Mechanism That Overcomes Cetuximab Induced Resistance. *PLoS ONE* **2016**, *11*, e0163366. [CrossRef]
135. Highlights of prescribing information of Vectibix. Available online: https://www.accessdata.fda.gov/drugsatfda_docs/label/2009/125147s080lbl.pdf (accessed on 5 November 2020).
136. Keating, G.M. Panitumumab: A review of its use in metastatic colorectal cancer. *Drugs* **2010**, *70*, 1059–1078. [CrossRef]
137. Muro, K.; Yoshino, T.; Doi, T.; Shirao, K.; Takiuchi, H.; Hamamoto, Y.; Watanabe, H.; Yang, B.B.; Asahi, D. A phase 2 clinical trial of panitumumab monotherapy in Japanese patients with metastatic colorectal cancer. *Jpn. J. Clin. Oncol.* **2009**, *39*, 321–326. [CrossRef] [PubMed]
138. Wadlow, R.C.; Hezel, A.F.; Abrams, T.A.; Blaszkowsky, L.S.; Fuchs, C.S.; Kulke, M.H.; Kwak, E.L.; Meyerhardt, J.A.; Ryan, D.P.; Szymonifka, J.; et al. Panitumumab in patients with KRAS wild-type colorectal cancer after progression on cetuximab. *Oncologist* **2012**, *17*, 14. [CrossRef] [PubMed]
139. Kazazi-Hyseni, F.; Beijnen, J.H.; Schellens, J.H. Bevacizumab. *Oncologist* **2010**, *15*, 819–825. [CrossRef] [PubMed]
140. Stacker, S.A.; Achen, M.G. The VEGF signaling pathway in cancer: The road ahead. *Chin. J. Cancer* **2013**, *32*, 297–302.
141. Verheul, H.M.; Lolkema, M.P.; Qian, D.Z.; Hilkes, Y.H.; Liapi, E.; Akkerman, J.W.; Pili, R.; Voest, E.E. Platelets take up the monoclonal antibody bevacizumab. *Clin. Cancer Res.* **2007**, *13*, 5341–5347. [CrossRef]
142. Lee, B.; Wong, H.L.; Tacey, M.; Tie, J.; Wong, R.; Lee, M.; Nott, L.; Shapiro, J.; Jennens, R.; Turner, N.; et al. The impact of bevacizumab in metastatic colorectal cancer with an intact primary tumor: Results from a large prospective cohort study. *Asia Pac. J. Clin. Oncol.* **2017**, *13*, 314–321. [CrossRef]
143. Wang, Z.; Liang, L.; Yu, Y.; Wang, Y.; Zhuang, R.; Chen, Y.; Cui, Y.; Zhou, Y.; Liu, T. Primary Tumour Resection Could Improve the Survival of Unresectable Metastatic Colorectal Cancer Patients Receiving -Containing Chemotherapy. *Cell. Physiol. Biochem.* **2016**, *39*, 1239–1246. [CrossRef]
144. Giantonio, B.J.; Catalano, P.J.; Meropol, N.J.; O'Dwyer, P.J.; Mitchell, E.P.; Alberts, S.R.; Schwartz, M.A.; Benson, A.B., III. Bevacizumab in Combination with Oxaliplatin, Fluorouracil, and Leucovorin (FOLFOX4) for Previously Treated Metastatic Colorectal Cancer: Results From the Eastern Cooperative Oncology Group Study E3200. *J. Clin. Oncol.* **2007**, *25*, 1539–1544. [CrossRef]
145. Clarke, J.M.; Hurwitz, H.I. Targeted inhibition of VEGF receptor 2: An update on ramucirumab. *Expert Opin. Biol.* **2013**, *13*, 1187–1196. [CrossRef]
146. Kowanetz, M.; Ferrara, N. Vascular endothelial growth factor signaling pathways: Therapeutic perspective. *Clin. Cancer Res.* **2006**, *12*, 5018–5022. [CrossRef]
147. Falcon, B.L.; Chintharlapalli, S.; Uhlik, M.T.; Pytowski, B. Antagonist antibodies to vascular endothelial growth factor receptor 2 (VEGFR-2) as anti-angiogenic agents. *Pharmacol. Ther.* **2016**, *164*, 204–225. [CrossRef] [PubMed]
148. Verdaguer, H.; Tabernero, J.; Macarulla, T. Ramucirumab in metastatic colorectal cancer: Evidence to date and place in therapy. *Adv. Med. Oncol.* **2016**, *8*, 230–242. [CrossRef] [PubMed]
149. Tabernero, J.; Yoshino, T.; Cohn, A.L.; Obermannova, R.; Bodoky, G.; Garcia-Carbonero, R.; Ciuleanu, T.E.; Portnoy, D.C.; van Cutsem, E.; Grothey, A.; et al. Ramucirumab versus placebo in combination with second-line FOLFIRI in patients with metastatic colorectal carcinoma that progressed during or after first-line therapy with bevacizumab, oxaliplatin, and a fluoropyrimidine (RAISE): A randomised, double-blind, multicentre, phase 3 study. *Lancet Oncol.* **2015**, *16*, 499–508. [PubMed]
150. Doshi, S.; Gisleskog, P.O.; Zhang, Y.; Zhu, M.; Oliner, K.S.; Loh, E.; Ruixo, J.J.P. Rilotumumab Exposure–Response Relationship in Patients with Advanced or Metastatic Gastric Cancer. *Clin. Cancer Res.* **2015**, *21*, 2453–2461. [CrossRef] [PubMed]
151. Giordano, S. Rilotumumab, a mAb against human hepatocyte growth factor for the treatment of cancer. *Curr. Opin. Mol.* **2009**, *11*, 448–455.
152. Van Cutsem, E.; Eng, C.; Nowara, E.; Swieboda-Sadlej, A.; Tebbutt, N.C.; Mitchell, E.; Davidenko, I.; Stephenson, J.; Elez, E.; Prenen, H.; et al. Randomized phase Ib/II trial of rilotumumab or ganitumab with panitumumab versus panitumumab alone in patients with wild-type KRAS metastatic colorectal cancer. *Clin. Cancer Res.* **2014**, *20*, 4240–4250. [CrossRef] [PubMed]
153. Kim, K.H.; Kim, H. Progress of antibody-based inhibitors of the HGF-cMET axis in cancer therapy. *Exp. Mol. Med.* **2017**, *49*, e307. [CrossRef] [PubMed]

154. Merchant, M.; Ma, X.; Maun, H.R.; Zheng, Z.; Peng, J.; Romero, M.; Huang, A.; Yang, N.Y.; Nishimura, M.; Greve, J.; et al. Monovalent antibody design and mechanism of action of onartuzumab, a MET antagonist with anti-tumor activity as a therapeutic agent. *Proc. Natl. Acad. Sci. USA* **2013**, *110*, E2987–E2996. [CrossRef]
155. Bendell, J.C.; Hochster, H.; Hart, L.L.; Firdaus, I.; Mace, J.R.; McFarlane, J.J.; Kozloff, M.; Catenacci, D.; Hsu, J.J.; Hack, S.P.; et al. A Phase II Randomized Trial (GO27827) of First-Line FOLFOX Plus with or Without the MET Inhibitor Onartuzumab in Patients with Metastatic Colorectal Cancer. *Oncologist* **2017**, *22*, 264–271. [CrossRef]
156. Zhang, X.; Chen, J.; Weng, Z.; Li, Q.; Zhao, L.; Yu, N.; Deng, L.; Xu, W.; Yang, Y.; Zhu, Z.; et al. A new anti-HER2 antibody that enhances the anti-tumor efficacy of trastuzumab and pertuzumab with a distinct mechanism of action. *Mol. Immunol.* **2020**, *119*, 48–58. [CrossRef]
157. Belli, V.; Matrone, N.; Napolitano, S.; Migliardi, G.; Cottino, F.; Bertotti, A.; Trusolino, L.; Martinelli, E.; Morgillo, F.; Ciardiello, D.; et al. Combined blockade of MEK and PI3KCA as an effective antitumor strategy in HER2 gene amplified human colorectal cancer models. *J. Exp. Clin. Cancer Res.* **2019**, *38*, 236. [CrossRef] [PubMed]
158. Xie, Y.H.; Chen, Y.X.; Fang, J.Y. Comprehensive review of targeted therapy for colorectal cancer. *Signal. Transduct Target. Ther.* **2020**, *5*, 22. [CrossRef] [PubMed]
159. Albanell, J.; Baselga, J. Trastuzumab, a humanized anti-HER2 monoclonal antibody, for the treatment of breast cancer. *Drugs Today* **1999**, *35*, 931–946.
160. Chen, S.; Liang, Y.; Feng, Z.; Wang, M. Efficacy and safety of HER2 inhibitors in combination with or without pertuzumab for HER2-positive breast cancer: A systematic review and meta-analysis. *BMC Cancer* **2019**, *19*, 973. [CrossRef]
161. Sartore-Bianchi, A.; Trusolino, L.; Martino, C.; Bencardino, K.; Lonardi, S.; Bergamo, F.; Zagonel, V.; Leone, F.; Depetris, I.; Martinelli, E.; et al. Dual-targeted therapy with trastuzumab and lapatinib in treatment-refractory, KRAS codon 12/13 wild-type, HER2-positive metastatic colorectal cancer (HERACLES): A proof-of-concept, multicentre, open-label, phase 2 trial. *Lancet Oncol.* **2016**, *17*, 738–746. [CrossRef]
162. Taieb, J.; Jung, A.; Sartore-Bianchi, A.; Peeters, M.; Seligmann, J.; Zaanan, A.; Burdon, P.; Montagut, C.; Laurent-Puig, P. The Evolving Biomarker Landscape for Treatment Selection in Metastatic Colorectal Cancer. *Drugs* **2019**, *79*, 1375–1394. [CrossRef]
163. Raghav, K.P.S.; McDonough, S.L.; Tan, B.R.; Denlinger, C.S.; Magliocco, A.M.; Choong, N.W.; Sommer, N.; Scappaticci, F.A.; Campos, D.; Guthrie, K.A.; et al. A randomized phase II study of trastuzumab and pertuzumab (TP) compared to cetuximab and irinotecan (CETIRI) in advanced/metastatic colorectal cancer (mCRC) with HER2 amplification: S1613. *J. Clin. Oncol.* **2018**, *36*, TPS3620. [CrossRef]
164. Highlights of Prescribing Information of YERVOY. Available online: https://www.accessdata.fda.gov/drugsatfda_docs/label/2020/125377s108lbl.pdf (accessed on 5 November 2020).
165. Weber, J.S.; Hamid, O.; Chasalow, S.D.; Wu, D.Y.; Parker, S.M.; Galbraith, S.; Gnjatic, S.; Berman, D. Ipilimumab increases activated T cells and enhances humoral immunity in patients with advanced melanoma. *J. Immunother.* **2012**, *35*, 89–97. [CrossRef]
166. Tarhini, A.A.; Kirkwood, J.M. Tremelimumab (CP-675,206): A fully human anticytotoxic T lymphocyte-associated antigen 4 monoclonal antibody for treatment of patients with advanced cancers. *Expert Opin. Biol.* **2008**, *8*, 1583–1593. [CrossRef]
167. Overman, M.J.; McDermott, R.; Leach, J.L.; Lonardi, S.; Lenz, H.J.; Morse, M.A.; Desai, J.; Hill, A.; Axelson, M.; Moss, R.A.; et al. Nivolumab in patients with metastatic DNA mismatch repair-deficient or microsatellite instability-high colorectal cancer (CheckMate 142): An open-label, multicentre, phase 2 study. *Lancet Oncol.* **2017**, *18*, 1182–1191. [CrossRef]
168. McKee, S. Tremelimumab Fails Mesothelioma Drug Trial. *PhamrTimes Online*, 1 March 2016.
169. Ribas, A.; Kefford, R.; Marshall, M.A.; Punt, C.J.; Haanen, J.B.; Marmol, M.; Garbe, C.; Gogas, H.; Schachter, J.; Linette, G.; et al. Phase III randomized clinical trial comparing tremelimumab with standard-of-care chemotherapy in patients with advanced melanoma. *J. Clin. Oncol.* **2013**, *31*, 616–622. [CrossRef]
170. Lee, H.T.; Lee, S.H.; Heo, Y.S. Molecular Interactions of Antibody Drugs Targeting PD-1, PD-L1, and CTLA-4 in Immuno-Oncology. *Molecules* **2019**, *24*, 1190. [CrossRef] [PubMed]
171. Poole, R.M. Pembrolizumab: First Global Approval. *Drugs* **2014**, *74*, 1973–1981. [CrossRef] [PubMed]
172. Scapin, G.; Yang, X.; Prosise, W.W.; McCoy, M.; Reichert, P.; Johnston, J.M.; Kashi, R.S.; Strickland, C. Structure of full-length human anti-PD1 therapeutic IgG4 antibody pembrolizumab. *Nat. Struct. Mol. Biol.* **2015**, *22*, 953–958. [CrossRef] [PubMed]
173. Raedler, L.A. Keytruda (Pembrolizumab): First PD-1 Inhibitor Approved for Previously Treated Unresectable or Metastatic Melanoma. *Am. Health Drug Benefits* **2015**, *8*, 96–100.
174. Kim, J.H.; Hong, H.J. Humanization by CDR grafting and specificity-determining residue grafting. *Methods Mol. Biol.* **2012**, *907*, 237–245.
175. Marcus, L.; Lemery, S.J.; Keegan, P.; Pazdur, R. FDA Approval Summary: Pembrolizumab for the Treatment of Microsatellite Instability-High Solid Tumors. *Clin. Cancer Res.* **2019**, *25*, 3753–3758. [CrossRef]
176. Sekhon, N.; Kumbla, R.A.; Mita, M. *Current Trends in Cancer Therapy, in Cardio-Oncology*; Chapter, 1; Gottlieb, R.A., Mehta, P.K., Eds.; Academic Press: Boston, MA, USA, 2017; pp. 1–24.
177. Wang, C.; Thudium, K.B.; Han, M.; Wang, X.T.; Huang, H.; Feingersh, D.; Garcia, C.; Wu, Y.; Kuhne, M.; Srinivasan, M.; et al. In vitro characterization of the anti-PD-1 antibody nivolumab, BMS-936558, and in vivo toxicology in non-human primates. *Cancer Immunol. Res.* **2014**, *2*, 846–856. [CrossRef]
178. Deeks, E.D. Nivolumab: A review of its use in patients with malignant melanoma. *Drugs* **2014**, *74*, 1233–1239. [CrossRef]

179. Golshani, G.; Zhang, Y. Advances in immunotherapy for colorectal cancer: A review. *Therap. Adv. Gastroenterol.* **2020**, *13*, 1756284820917527. [CrossRef]
180. Tan, S.; Zhang, H.; Chai, Y.; Song, H.; Tong, Z.; Wang, Q.; Qi, J.; Wong, G.; Zhu, X.; Liu, W.J.; et al. An unexpected N-terminal loop in PD-1 dominates binding by nivolumab. *Nat. Commun.* **2017**, *8*, 14369. [CrossRef] [PubMed]
181. Markham, A.; Keam, S.J. Camrelizumab: First Global Approval. *Drugs* **2019**, *79*, 1355–1361. [CrossRef] [PubMed]
182. Finlay, W.J.J.; Coleman, J.E.; Edwards, J.S.; Johnson, K.S. Anti-PD1 'SHR-1210' aberrantly targets pro-angiogenic receptors and this polyspecificity can be ablated by paratope refinement. *MAbs* **2019**, *11*, 26–44. [CrossRef] [PubMed]
183. Lickliter, J.D.; Gan, H.K.; Voskoboynik, M.; Arulananda, S.; Gao, B.; Nagrial, A.; Grimison, P.; Harrison, M.; Zou, J.; Zhang, L.; et al. A First-in-Human Dose Finding Study of Camrelizumab in Patients with Advanced or Metastatic Cancer in Australia. *Drug Des. Dev. Ther.* **2020**, *14*, 1177–1189. [CrossRef] [PubMed]
184. Wang, M.; Wang, J.; Wang, R.; Jiao, S.; Wang, S.; Zhang, J.; Zhang, M. Identification of a monoclonal antibody that targets PD-1 in a manner requiring PD-1 Asn58 glycosylation. *Commun. Biol.* **2019**, *2*, 392. [CrossRef]
185. Zhang, F.; Qi, X.; Wang, X.; Wei, D.; Wu, J.; Feng, L.; Cai, H.; Wang, Y.; Zeng, N.; Xu, T.; et al. Structural basis of the therapeutic anti-PD-L1 antibody atezolizumab. *Oncotarget* **2017**, *8*, 90215–90224. [CrossRef]
186. Lee, H.T.; Lee, J.Y.; Lim, H.; Lee, S.H.; Moon, Y.J.; Pyo, H.J.; Ryu, S.E.; Shin, W.; Heo, Y.S. Molecular mechanism of PD-1/PD-L1 blockade via anti-PD-L1 antibodies atezolizumab and durvalumab. *Sci. Rep.* **2017**, *7*, 5532. [CrossRef]
187. Juliá, E.P.; Amante, A.; Pampena, M.B.; Mordoh, J.; Levy, E.M. Avelumab, an IgG1 anti-PD-L1 Immune Checkpoint Inhibitor, Triggers NK Cell-Mediated Cytotoxicity and Cytokine Production Against Triple Negative Breast Cancer Cells. *Front. Immunol.* **2018**, *9*, 2140. [CrossRef]
188. Kim, J.H.; Kim, S.Y.; Baek, J.Y.; Cha, Y.J.; Ahn, J.B.; Kim, H.S.; Lee, K.-W.; Kim, J.-W.; Kim, T.-Y.; Chang, W.J.; et al. A Phase II Study of Avelumab Monotherapy in Patients with Mismatch Repair–Deficient/Microsatellite Instability–High or POLE-Mutated Metastatic or Unresectable Colorectal Cancer. *Cancer Res. Treat.* **2020**, *52*, 1135–1144. [CrossRef]
189. Tan, S.; Liu, K.; Chai, Y.; Zhang, C.W.; Gao, S.; Gao, G.F.; Qi, J. Distinct PD-L1 binding characteristics of therapeutic monoclonal antibody durvalumab. *Protein Cell* **2018**, *9*, 135–139. [CrossRef]
190. Syed, Y.Y. Durvalumab: First Global Approval. *Drugs* **2017**, *77*, 1369–1376. [CrossRef] [PubMed]
191. Highlights of Prescribing Information of Durvalumab. Available online: https://www.accessdata.fda.gov/drugsatfda_docs/label/2018/761069s002lbl.pdf (accessed on 5 November 2020).
192. Corcoran, R.B.; Grothey, A. Efficacy of Immunotherapy in Microsatellite-Stable or Mismatch Repair Proficient Colorectal Cancer-Fact or Fiction? *JAMA Oncol.* **2020**, *6*, 823–824. [CrossRef] [PubMed]
193. Tintelnot, J.; Stein, A. Immunotherapy in colorectal cancer: Available clinical evidence, challenges and novel approaches. *World J. Gastroenterol.* **2019**, *25*, 3920–3928. [CrossRef] [PubMed]

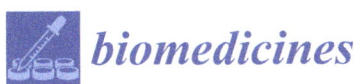

Review

Genetic Alterations of Metastatic Colorectal Cancer

Ugo Testa *, Germana Castelli and Elvira Pelosi

Department of Oncology, Istituto Superiore di Sanità, Viale Regina Elena 299, 00161 Rome, Italy; germana.castelli@iss.it (G.C.); elvira.pelosi@iss.it (E.P.)
* Correspondence: ugo.testa@iss.it; Tel.: +39-649902422

Received: 20 August 2020; Accepted: 9 October 2020; Published: 13 October 2020

Abstract: Genome sequencing studies have characterized the genetic alterations of different tumor types, highlighting the diversity of the molecular processes driving tumor development. Comprehensive sequencing studies have defined molecular subtypes of colorectal cancers (CRCs) through the identification of genetic events associated with microsatellite stability (MSS), microsatellite-instability-high (MSI-H), and hypermutation. Most of these studies characterized primary tumors. Only recent studies have addressed the characterization of the genetic and clinical heterogeneity of metastatic CRC. Metastatic CRC genomes were found to be not fundamentally different from primary CRCs in terms of the mutational landscape or of genes that drive tumorigenesis, and a genomic heterogeneity associated with tumor location of primary tumors helps to define different clinical behaviors of metastatic CRCs. Although CRC metastatic spreading was traditionally seen as a late-occurring event, growing evidence suggests that this process can begin early during tumor development and the clonal architecture of these tumors is consistently influenced by cancer treatment. Although the survival rate of patients with metastatic CRC patients improved in the last years, the response to current treatments and prognosis of many of these patients remain still poor, indicating the need to discover new improvements for therapeutic vulnerabilities and to formulate a rational prospective of personalized therapies.

Keywords: colorectal cancer; genomic alterations; metastasis; tumor heterogeneity; tumor evolution

1. Introduction

Colorectal cancer (CRC) is one of the most frequent cancers worldwide, corresponding to the second in males and third in females most frequent tumor. CRC is the second most common cause of cancer death in Europe [1].

Colorectal cancer is a highly heterogeneous disease that comprises different tumor phenotypes, characterized by specific molecular and morphological alterations. CRC is caused by genetic alterations that target tumor suppressor genes, oncogenes, and genes related to DNA repair mechanisms. Depending on the origin of these mutations, CRC can be classified as sporadic (70–75%), hereditary (5%), and familial (20–25%). Three major pathways are involved in CRC origin and progression: (a) chromosomal instability (CIN); (b) microsatellite instability (MSI); (c) CpG island methylation phenotype (CIMP). Each of these three different groups displays peculiar pathological, genetic, and clinical characteristics [2].

CIN is the most common (85% of total CRCs) genetic mechanism occurring in CRC. CIN is characterized by the acquisition of a consistent karyotypic variability, aneuploidy, chromosomal and subchromosomal aberrations, gene amplifications and loss of heterozygosity. Allelic losses at the level of chromosome arms 1p, 5q, 17p, 18p, 18q, 20p, and 22q are highly recurrent. A major pathogenic consequence of this CIN consists in the loss of heterozygosity at tumor suppressor gene loci. Furthermore, CIN tumors are associated with the accumulation of mutations at the level of several oncogenes, including *KRAS* and *BRAF* and of tumor suppressor genes such as *APC* and *TP53*.

The meta-analysis of the outcome of more than 10,000 CRC patients clearly indicated that CIN is associated with a worse prognosis [3].

MSI involves several recurrent alterations in the microsatellite zone, without apparent structural and numerical changes in the genome; approximately 15% of all CRCs have a high frequency of MSI due to germline mutations in mismatch repair (MMR) system or somatic inactivation by promoter hypermethylation of MLH1 gene [4].

CIMP pathway is responsible for 20–30% of total CRCs and is predominantly observed in the proximal colon (30–40%) and more rarely in distal colon (3–12%) [4].

The Cancer Genome Atlas provided in 2002 the first genome-scale analysis of a large set (276) of CRC samples, performing a comprehensive study involving exome sequencing, DNA copy number, promoter methylation, messenger RNA and micro RNA expression evaluation [4]. This analysis showed that CRCs can be classified according to their mutation pattern: (i) 16% of CRCs were found to be hypermutated (75% displayed high MSI, usually associated with hypermethylation and silencing of the *MLH1* gene, whereas the remaining 25% exhibited mismatch-repair gene and polymerase ε (POLE) gene mutations); (ii) the non-hypermutated CRCs that formed the most consistent group of tumors showed the recurrent mutations of *APC*, *TP53*, *KRAS*, *PIK3CA*, *FBXW7*, *SMAD4*, *TCF7L2*, and *NRAS* genes; (iii) in hypermutated CRCs, the most frequently mutated genes were *ACVR2A* (63%), *APC* (51%), *TGFBR2* (51%), *BRAF* (49%), *MSH3* (46%), *MSH6* (40%), *MYO18* (31%), *TCF7L2* (31%), and *CASP8* (29%); (iv) *APC* (81% vs. 51%) and *TP53* (60% vs. 20%) were significantly more mutated in the non-hypermutated cancers compared to hypermutated cancers. Integrated analysis of the genetic profiling showed that some pathways are recurrently altered in CRCs: (i) WNT pathway is altered in 93% of all tumors (in 80% of cases due to biallelic inactivation of *APC* or activating mutations of *CTNNB1*); (ii) PI3K signaling pathway is altered in 50% of non-hypermutated and 53% of hypermutated CRCs; (iii) RTK-RAS signaling pathway is more frequently altered in hypermutated (80%) than in non-hypermutated (59%); (iv) finally, TGF-β signaling pathway was much more frequently altered in hypermutated (87%) than in non-hypermutated (27%) CRCs [4].

The study by TCGA showed the existence of three subtypes of CRC according to their transcriptomic profile: microsatellite instability/CpG island methylator phenotype (MSI/CIMP); invasive; chromosome instability (CIN). In a subsequent study, Zhang et al. carried out a proteogenomic analysis on the CRCs previously characterized by TCGA [5]. This analysis showed the existence of a limited correlation between mRNA and protein levels. Five CRC subtypes (from A to E) were identified according to proteomic data: (i) B and C subtypes included all CRCs characterized by hypermutation, MSI-H, *POLE* and *BRAF* mutations: B subtype was associated with the CIMP-H methylation subtype of the TCGA study, absence of *TP53* mutations and chromosome 18 loss; C subtype was associated with a non-CIMP TCGA subtype. (ii) The A, D, and E subtypes were associated with the TCGA CIN subtype. (iii) The E subtype displayed several remarkable features, such as the presence of *TP53* mutations and chromosome 18q loss (both genomic alterations frequently associated with CIN CRCs) and with *HNF4A* amplification and HNF4α protein abundance [5]. CRCs display frequent copy number alterations (CNAs), particularly those characterized by CIN. However, only few CNAs are associated with significant changes at protein level. Among the various CNAs, the chromosome 20 amplicon was associated with the largest changes at both mRNA and protein level and is associated with HNF4 (hepatocyte nuclear factor 4, alpha), TOMM34 (translocase of outer mitochondrial membrane 34) and SRC (SRC proto-oncogene, non-receptor tyrosine kinase) overexpression [5].

Copy number alterations (CNAs) show significant changes during the progression of colorectal carcinogenesis from benign adenoma to CRC. Thus, chromosomal aneuploidies affecting chromosomes 7, 13, and 20q (all chromosomal gains) cooperate with APC mutations in the progression from adenoma with low-grade dysplasia to adenoma with high-grade dysplasia. Losses of chromosomes 8p, 15q, 17p, and 18q and gain of 8q are involved in tumor progression to infiltrating adenocarcinoma [6].

The analysis of gene expression profiles obtained through the study of thousands cases of colorectal cancers supported a classification of colon cancer, based on four major consensus molecular subtypes (CMS), CMS1 to CMS4 (Table 1) [7]. CMS1 group (MSI immune subtype, including 14% of all CRCs) is characterized at genetic level by hypermutation, hypermethylation, enrichment for $BRAF^{V600E}$ mutations (observed in 40% of these tumors) and by pronounced infiltration of the tumor microenvironment by immune cells, particularly represented by T lymphocytes (both Cytotoxic CD8$^+$ and CD4$^+$ T helper) and natural killer lymphocytes; frequent in these tumors are mutations at the level of *APC* (35%), *TP53* (30%) and *KRAS* (25%) genes. Frequent in these tumors are mutations in *MSH6*, *RNF43*, *ATM*, *TGFBR2*, *BRAF*, and *PTEN* genes. Predominantly, these tumors originate from precursor lesions with a serrated histology, with preferential location at the level of proximal regions of the colon; their prognostic outcome is intermediate but poor after relapse. The CMS2 subtype corresponds to the canonical subtype (37% of CRCs) and is characterized by CIN-high, microsatellite stability (MSS) and low levels of gene hypermethylation; a mutational profile typically observed in CIN-high CRCs, including recurrent *APC* (75%), *TP53* (70%), and *KRAS* (30%) mutations, whereas *BRAF* mutations were absent; pronounced upregulation of WNT and MYC downstream targets, elevated expression of EGFR, HER2, IGF2, IRS2, HNF4A, and cyclin; complex tubular histological structure, predominantly located in the distal region of the colon. The CMS3 subtype corresponds to the metabolic subtype (10% of CRCs) that is characterized by activation of glutaminolysis and lipidogenesis and by the presence of a distinctive genomic and epigenomic profile compared with other CIN tumors, for the presence of a mixed CIMP-H (20% of cases), MSI-H (15% of cases), hypermutation (30% of cases), and CIN-H (54% of cases); at mutational level, frequent *KRAS* and *APC* mutations but less frequent *TP53* and *BRAF* mutations are observed; these tumors predominantly display papillary morphology and are located at the level of both proximal and distal regions of colon. CMS4 corresponds to the mesenchymal subtype (25% of all cases) and is characterized by the presence of tumors exhibiting activation of the pathways related to epithelial-mesenchymal transition (EMT) and stemness (TGF-β signaling and integrins) and overexpression of genes involved in extracellular matrix remodeling, complement-associated inflammation, stromal invasion and angiogenesis; marked stromal cell infiltration at the level of peritumoral microenvironment is a typical histological feature of these tumors; these tumors are frequently CIN-H but rarely hypermutated, CIMP-H and MSI-H; at mutational level, frequent are the mutations of *APC*, *TP53* and *KRAS*, associated with rare *BRAF* mutations; at histological level, these tumors are characterized by a desmoplastic reaction with high stroma; these tumors are associated with a poor outcome compared with the other CMS subtypes [7].

Finally, there is a residual unclassified group representing 10–15% of all tumors with mixed features, that seemingly represents a transitional phenotype or reflects an intra-tumoral heterogeneity [7].

Importantly, the CMS classification was predictive of chemotherapy and targeted-therapy response in CRC patients with advanced/metastatic disease [8–10].

The CMS transcriptional classification was implemented through the analysis of microenvironment signatures, showing consistent correlation between these two classification systems: CMS1 subgroup was characterized by elevated expression of genes specific to cytotoxic T lymphocytes; CMS4 subgroup was characterized by several microenvironmental features, including expression of monocytic markers and a combined angiogenesis, inflammatory and immunosuppressive signature; at pathologic level, CMS4 tumors display numerous infiltrating fibroblasts, producing cytokines and chemokines inducing the angiogenetic and inflammatory phenotypes; CMS2 and CMS3 subgroups exhibit low inflammatory and immune signatures [11].

Isella and coworkers have proposed a new transcriptional classification of CRC, allowing the identification of five CRC intrinsic (CRIS) subtypes, displaying distinctive molecular, phenotypic and functional features [12]. This classification was based on a methodological approach to limit the impact of tumor stromal cells on the transcriptional classification of CRC. CRIS-A identifies a subgroup of CRCs enriched for MSI-H, *BRAF* or *KRAS*-mutated tumors, with secretory mucinous histology, with sustained glycolytic metabolism and inflammatory traits; CRIS-A englobes CRCs mainly corresponding to CMS1 and, at a minor extent, CMS4. CRIS-B identifies a subset of CRCs characterized by an impaired differentiation, activation of TGF-β signaling and epithelial to mesenchymal transition;

these tumors are mainly MSS and only in part MSI-H; these tumors are characterized by a poor prognosis and by an elevated infiltration of fibroblasts; CRIS-B englobes both CMS4 and CMS1 tumors. CRIS-C identifies a group of CRCs, CIN-H, and MSS, with absent *KRAS* mutations and exhibiting elevated EGFR activity and *MYC* copy number gains; these tumors are particularly sensitive to EGFR inhibitors; CRIS-C englobes CMS2 tumors and in part CMS4 tumors. CRIS-D tumors display a number of typical features mainly represented by a stem-like phenotype associated with high WNT signaling, a MSS status, strong enrichment of IGF2 overexpression/amplification and FGFR autocrine stimulation; CRIS-D englobes both CMS2 and CMS4 tumors. CRIS-E is characterized by a Paneth cell-like phenotype, an MSS status, numerous WNT-related features, and frequent *TP53* mutations; CRIS-E englobes both CMS2 and CMS4 CRCs [12].

Table 1. The gene expression-based consensus molecular classification of colorectal cancer.

Tumor Subtype	Frequency	Gene Expression Signature	Genetic Abnormalities	Tumor Location	Prognosis
CMS1 Hypermutated	14%	Immune infiltration and activation High PD-1 activation Low stromal cell infiltration	SCNA low Hypermutated MSI high CIMP high KRAS (25%) BRAF (40%) APC (35%) TP53 (30%)	Predominantly proximal (74%)	Intermediate Poor prognosis after relapse
CMS2 Canonical	40%	WNT and MYC activation Elevated expression of EGFR, HER2, IGF2, IRS2 and HNF4A Low immune infiltration and activation	SCNA high No hypermutated MSI low CIMP negative KRAS (30%) BRAF (0%) APC (80%) TP53 (70%)	Predominantly distal (80%)	Good
CMS3 Metabolic	10%	Metabolic deregulation, with upregulation of several metabolic signatures (glutaminolysis and lipidogenesis) Low immune and stromal cell infiltration.	SCNA mixed Hypermutated (30%) MSI low; MSI high (15%) CIMP mixed KRAS (70%) BRAF (10%) APC (75%) TP53 (30%)	Equally proximal and distal	Intermediate
CMS4 Mesenchymal	25%	Stromal infiltration TGF-β activation Angiogenesis Matrix-remodelling pathways Complement-mediated inflammation	SCNA high No hypermutated MSI low CIMP negative KRAS (40%) BRAF (5%) APC (65%) TP53 (55%)	Mainly distal (66%)	Negative Usually diagnosed at advanced stage

SCNA: somatic copy-nucleotide alteration.

The complex, variable and potentially confounding role of microenvironment in the evaluation of the transcriptomic expression of CRC, highlights the need of performing analyses at single-cell level as a tool to better define and understand intratumoral heterogeneity [13]. Only few studies have explored single-cell transcriptomic in CRC samples. In this context, particularly relevant was the study carried out by Li and coworkers investigating single-cell RNA sequencing on 969 tumor cells derived from primary tumors of 11 different CRC patients and 622 normal mucosal intestinal cells located near the CRC [14]. This analysis identified seven different cell clusters, corresponding to epithelial cells, endothelial cells, fibroblasts, T lymphocytes, B lymphocytes, mast cells, and myeloid cells [14]. The single-cell analysis allowed the identification of a larger set of differentially expressed genes compared with normal mucosa than the bulk analysis of gene expression [14]. Importantly, EMT (epithelial-mesenchymal transition)-related genes resulted to be upregulated only at the level of the cell population of cancer-associated fibroblasts but not at the level of epithelial cells [14]. The data obtained from single-cell transcriptomic allowed to define six different signatures of six tumor cell types: epithelial differentiated; epithelial stem, fibroblast, T cell, B cell, macrophages [14]. The integration of the six cell type signatures together with the data of bulk signatures obtained through the analysis of various cohorts of CRC patients allowed to define three tumor groups, defined as S1,

S2 and S3: S1 CRCs display a weak epithelial, an elevated myeloid and a strong fibroblast signature; S2 CRCs exhibit intermediate level of all signatures; S3 CRCs show a strong epithelial signature, associated with weak myeloid and fibroblast signatures [14]. In all the cohorts of CRC patients studied, S3 CRCs display a better survival than the two other groups [14]. A more recent study based on the analysis of >50,000 single cells from CRCs and matched normal tissues provided evidence that CRC development is associated in all cases analyzed with changes at the level of epithelial, immune and stromal cell compartments [15]. Interestingly, in the epithelium, five different tumor-specific stem and progenitor-like cell populations were identified [15]. This single-cell analysis showed also that epithelial tumor cells and cancer-associated fibroblasts are fundamental and essential for the assignment of each CRC to a given CMS subtype [15].

Although single-cell transcriptomic techniques cannot be proposed for the clinical classification of CRCs, their use may be of considerable support in the study of CRC patients undergoing immunotherapy treatments or myeloid-targeted therapies [16,17].

Very few studies have explored the gene expression profile observed at the level of metastatic CRC lesions. Kamal et al. reported the comparative analysis of the transcriptomic profile of primary tumors and corresponding metastases (liver and lung metastases) in some CRC patients [13]. According to the gene expression profile, two types of distant metastases were identified: M1 and M2 [13]. The M1 metastatic group is characterized by strong activation of inflammatory and immune response pathways (including immune evasion pathways, such as those involving PD-1/-L1 signaling) and enrichment in EMT activity. The M2 metastatic group exhibits MYC activation and cell proliferation [18]. Importantly, treatment modifies the gene expression profile of metastatic lesions: the immune phenotype of M1 metastases is lost in post-treatment metastases; treatment induces an enrichment of EMT activity [18]. The analysis of CMS groups in metastases showed the absence of CMS3 and the presence of CMS1 in only few cases; the majority of metastases were classified as CMS2 (37%) or CMS4 (45%); 86% of metastases were CMS4 in the M1 cluster, while 60% of metastases were CMS2 in the M2 cluster [18]. The comparison of gene expression in paired primary tumors and corresponding metastases showed that *FBN2* and *MMP3* were the most differentially expressed genes [18].

The incidence of CRC increases with the age. In a recent study, Lieu et al. on a large panel of CRC samples reported the occurrence of CRCs in 7.8% of patients under the age of 40, 17.6% in the age comprised between 40 and 49 years and 74.6% in patients with an age of 50 or older [19]. Overall genomic alterations were similar in the majority of genes currently mutated, with some notable differences: in MSS CRC patients, *TP53* and *CTNNB1* alterations were more common in younger patients with CRC [19]; in the MSI-H cohort, most of genes displayed a similar frequency of alterations in the two age groups, but significant differences were observed at the level of *APC* and *KRAS* alterations more frequent among younger than older patients and *BRAF* alterations markedly more recurrent among older than younger CRC patients [19].

The progresses made in primary and adjuvant treatments of CRC patients have led to an improvement of the survival times of these patients. The optimal treatment of CRC patients would imply complete surgical ablation of primary tumor and metastases. However, 25–30% of CRC patients display at diagnosis an advanced disease stage with metastatic diffusion; furthermore, a remaining 20% of patients develop metachronous metastases after standard treatments. Therefore, a significant proportion of CRC patients need an efficacious medical treatment to induce the regression of tumor cells that cannot be removed by surgery. The current medical treatment implies first line chemotherapy or radiotherapy that can be performed either before surgery in a neoadjuvant setting or after surgery in an adjuvant setting. Current chemotherapy treatment implies either single-drug treatment involving fluoropyrimidine (5-FU) and multiple-drug regimens, based on the use of irinotecan (IRI), capecitabine (CAP) or oxaliplatin (OX), such as FOLFOX (5-FU + OX), FOXFIRI (5-FU + IRI), CAPIRI (CAP + IRI) or CAPOX (CAP + OX) [1].

The studies carried out in the last years have shown that CRC exhibits a clinically relevant molecular heterogeneity related to various genetic and non-genetic mechanisms. The identification of molecular subtypes of CRCs helped to identify new strategies of treatment for selected groups of patients (targeted therapy): (i) the presence of *KRAS* or *NRAS* mutations allowed the identification of a group of CRC patients refractory to EGFR inhibitors; (ii) the absence of *KRAS*, *NRAS*, *BRAF*, and *PIK3CA/PTEN* mutations (CRC "wild-type") identifies a group of CRC patients responsive to EGFR inhibitors; (iii) CRCs bearing $BRAF^{V600E}$ mutations have a poor prognosis and are responsive to targeted inhibition in combination; (iv) CRCs with *HER2* amplifications display sensitivity to dual HER2 blockade; (v) CRCs bearing rare kinase fusion events are targetable with specific kinase inhibitors; (vi) MSI-H and *POLE* hypermutant CRCs are particularly sensitive to treatment with immune checkpoint inhibitors; (vii) CRCs with a mesenchymal phenotype display immunosuppressive mechanisms that could be removed through combined immunotherapy treatments [20].

The strategy recommended by the National Comprehensive Cancer Network (NCCN) for the targeted therapy of metastatic CRC patients implies a differential treatment according to the *RAS* mutational status and to the colon location of the primary tumor: (i) for patients with left colon mCRC, *RAS*-WT it is recommended an initial therapy based on EGFR inhibitors, and a subsequent therapy based on mutational status for *BRAF* mutations (BRAF inhibitors), *HER2* amplifications (HER2 inhibitors) *BRAF/HER2*-WT (anti-PD-1/L1 if deficient in mismatch repair (MMR); anti-VEGF if proficient in MMR); for patients with right colon mCRC it is recommended a therapeutic approach similar to that adopted for *RAS*-mutant patients; for patients with mCRC, RAS-mutant it is recommended a differential therapy according to the MMR status: for patients deficient in MMR it is recommended a first-line of therapy based on anti-PD-1/L1 and a second line based on anti-VEGF inhibitors, whereas for patients proficient in MMR, a first line based on anti-VEGF inhibitors and a second line of therapy based on best supportive care therapy are recommended [21].

A large body of molecular data on the genomic abnormalities observed in CRC has been generated; the majority of these studies focused on primary tumors. However, recent studies have characterized the molecular abnormalities observed in metastatic CRC. Some studies have molecularly characterized metastatic lesions with their corresponding primaries. The present review paper reports a detailed analysis of these recent studies on the characterization of metastatic CRCs, supporting the view that a better understanding of the molecular alterations and of their heterogeneity may improve the treatment outcome of these patients.

2. Genetic Abnormalities in Metastatic CRC

Few studies have explored the frequency of recurrent genetic alterations in metastatic CRC patients.

In 2017, Zehir and coworkers reported the mutational landscape of 10,945 metastatic tumors, including 975 metastatic CRCs, as encountered in clinical practice [22]. This study showed the presence of four recurrently mutated genes, represented by *APC*, *TP53*, *KRAS*, and *PIK3CA*. Furthermore, according to the somatic tumor burden, metastatic CRCs can be distinguished into three groups: normal, hypermutated, ultramutated. The metastatic CRCs with a high mutational burden displayed a dominant MMR signature. Finally, 35% of metastatic CRCs showed actionable somatic alterations [22].

The study carried out by Zehir et al. was based on targeted gene analysis [22]. A more recent study by Priestley et al. involved deep whole-genome sequencing of 2399 metastatic solid tumors, including 372 CRCs [23]. Metastatic CRCs are among the tumors displaying the highest levels of single-nucleotide variants (SNVs), with only urinary tract, esophagus, lung cancers and melanoma exhibiting higher levels among 20 different types of metastatic cancers [23]. Only 4% of metastatic CRCs displayed an MSI genotype/phenotype, a frequency that is lower than that reported for primary CRC, a finding that can be explained by the lower tendency of these tumors to metastasize [13]. Copy number alterations are frequent in metastatic CRC; an extreme form of CNA can be caused by whole genome duplication (WGD), an event frequent (>60% of cases) in metastatic CRCs, among the metastatic tumors most frequently showing WGD [23]. Metastatic CRCs displayed a mean number of total candidate driver events (6.5 per patient) only slightly higher than the mean number (5.7 per patient) observed in 20 different metastatic cancers [23]. The whole-genome sequencing (WGS) approach allowed to accurately define the frequency of genetic alterations occurring in mCRC at the level of genes possessing oncogenic activity when mutated or of tumor suppressor genes (Figure 1). The analysis of the co-mutation pattern of driver genes showed negative associations within the same transduction pathway for *KRAS-BRAF* and *KRAS-NRAS*, for *APC-CTNNB1*, for *APC* with *BRAF* and *RNF43* [23]. Interestingly, this study showed in 9 CRC patients with absent *APC* driver mutations, the occurrence of in-frame deletion of the complete exon 3, leading to activation of the WNT and β-catenin pathway [23]. Furthermore, 5.4% of mCRC samples displayed an amplification of *CDX2*, acting as a survival oncogene for these tumor cells [23]. The exploration of the mutational spectrum of metastatic CRC indicates that only 30% of these tumors possess biomarkers with either an approved therapy or with strong biological evidence or clinical trials that are actionable [23].

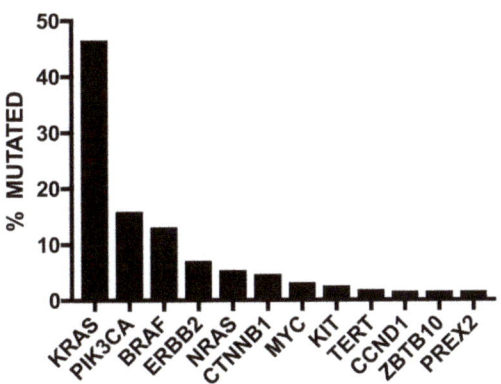

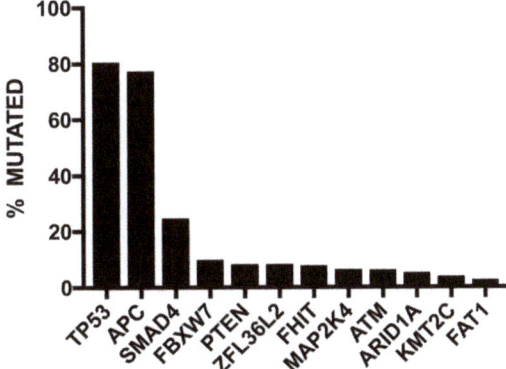

Figure 1. Frequency of the most recurrent gene alterations observed in metastatic CRC patients. The data on the frequency of the major genetic alterations were reported by Priestly et al. [23] and were based on the wide-genome sequencing analysis of 372 metastatic CRC patients.

Particularly relevant was the study carried out by Yaeger et al. [24] who reported the sequencing analysis of most 1134 CRCs, including 979 patients with metastatic disease. These tumors corresponded to three different molecular groups: POLE mutant (0.7%), MSI-H/hypermutated (8.7%) and MSS (90.5%), with predominant left colon localization of MSS tumors and predominant right colon localization of

POLE and MSI-H tumors [24]. The WNT pathway resulted to be altered in 85% of MSS tumors and in 93% of MSI-H tumors: *APC* gene alterations were more frequent in MSS CRCs than in MSI-H CRCs (81% vs. 61%), while *CTNNB1* and *RNF43* gene alterations were less frequent in MSS CRCs than in MSI-H CRCs (6% vs. 25% and 4% vs. 53%, respectively) [24] (Figure 2). Other remarkable differences in the rates of several genetic alterations between these two types of metastatic CRCs are represented by the more frequent alterations of *ERBB3*, *PIK3CA*, *PIK3R1*, *PTEN*, *NF1*, *BRAF*, *BRCA1*, and *BRCA2* gene alterations in MSI-H CRCs than in MSS CRCs [24]. (Figure 2) The analysis of mostly recurrently mutated genes in MSS CRCs showed a mutational frequency of 79% for *APC*, 78% for *TP53*, 44% for *KRAS*, 18% for *PIK3CA*, 16% for *SMAD4*, 10% for *TCF7L2* and 10% for *FBXW7* [24]. The analysis of the frequencies of some gene mutations in early-stage tumors, primary metastatic CRC and metastases from metastatic CRCs showed that most of these mutations do not display significant differences, but a minority of them are stage-related: the frequency of *TP53* mutations progressively increases from early-stage to primary mCRC and to metastases of mCRC; *FBXW7* mutations are more frequent in early-stage and primary mCRCs than in metastases of mCRC; *ERBB2* mutations are more frequent in early-stage than in metastatic CRCs [24]. *BRAF* mutations display a tendency to be more frequent in metastatic CRC than in early-stage CRC [24]. This study also showed some remarkable differences between primary tumor sites, i.e., right colon or left colon. Right-sided primary mCRC displayed fewer DNA copy-number alterations than left-sided mCRC; furthermore, an enrichment of genetic alterations in *KRAS*, *BRAF*, *PIK3CA*, *PTEN*, *AKT1*, *RNF43*, *SMAD2*, and *SMAD4* was observed in right-sided primary mCRC and in *APC* and *TP53* in left-sided primary mCRC [24]. Left-located mCRC had a significantly better overall survival than right-located mCRC [24]. The analysis of the overall survival in various molecular subgroups of mCRCs showed a poor survival for patients bearing *KRAS* mutations alone or in combination with PI3K pathway mutations. These CRCs showed also a greater tendency to have multiple first sites of metastases [24].

Using a multigene panel sequencing, Belardinilli and coworkers have explored the co-mutational profile of metastatic CRC; this study involved the analysis of 779 metastatic CRC primary tumors [25]. The results of this analysis showed the existence of positive associations between *EGFR* and *KRAS*, *EGFR* and *SMAD4*, *BRAF* and *PTEN*, and *NRAS* and *TP53* mutations, whose biological and clinical significance is at the moment unknown [25]. Importantly, according to the presence of *TP53* and *KRAS* mutations, metastatic CRCs can be subdivided into four different groups: MAP1, characterized by the co-mutation of *TP53* and *KRAS* and subdivided into a less frequent MAP1.1 subgroup, in which *TP53* and *KRAS* mutations are associated with other recurrent mutations, such as *PIK3CA*, *FBXW7*, *SMAD4* and *PTEN* mutations and a more frequent MAP 1.2 subgroup in which *TP53* and *KRAS* mutations are not associated with other recurrent mutations; MAP 2, characterized by the mutation of the *KRAS* gene and subdivided into a MAP 2.1 subgroup in which *KRAS* mutation is associated with highly recurrent *PIK3CA* mutations and a MAP 2.2 subgroup in which KRAS mutations are not associated with other recurrent mutations; MAP 3, characterized by *TP53* mutations, subdivided into a MAP 3.1 subgroup in which *TP53* mutations are associated with recurrent *PIK3CA*, *BRAF*, *NRAS*, and *SMAD4* recurrent mutations and a MAP 3.2 subgroup in which *TP53* mutations are not associated with other recurrent mutations; MAP 4, characterized by the absence of *TP53* and *KRAS* mutations, subdivided into a less frequent 4.1 subgroup, characterized by highly recurrent *BRAF* mutations and recurrent *PIK3CA*, *NRAS* and *FBXW7* mutations and a more frequent 4.2 subgroup, characterized by absence of recurrent mutations [25].

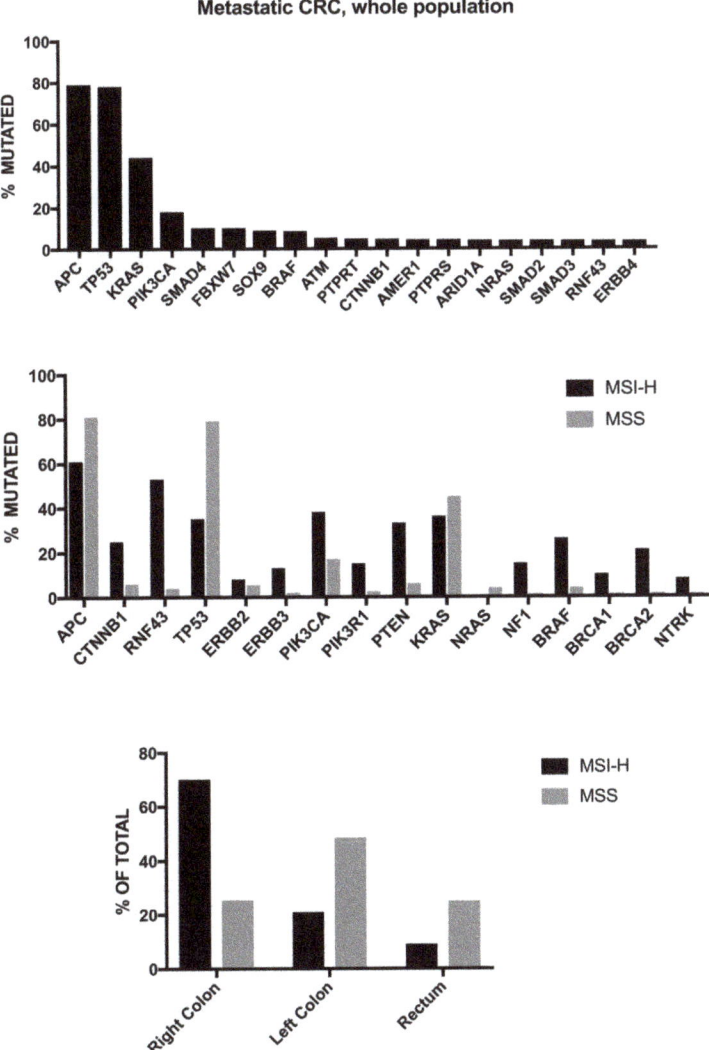

Figure 2. Frequency of the most recurrent genetic alterations observed in metastatic CRC patients (data reported by Yaeger et al., 2018) [24]. Top Panel: most recurrent genetic alterations observed in the whole population of metastatic CRC patients; Middle Panel: most recurrent genetic alterations observed in the population of metastatic CRC patients subdivided into MSI-H and MSS; Bottom Panel: tumor location in metastatic CRC patients exhibiting either MSI-H or MSS.

BRAF-mutant CRC represent a peculiar subgroup of mCRCs. In the metastatic setting, $^{600E}BRAF$ mutation occurs in 10% of cases and is associated with a poor prognosis [4]. Among $^{V600E}BRAF$-mutated CRCs, two subgroups have been distinguished according either to the activation of KRAS/mTOR/AKT/4EBP1 pathway (BM1 subtype) or to the deregulation in the cell cycle (BM2 subtype) [26]. In addition to $^{V600E}BRAF$-mutated CRCs, there is a rarer (occurring in 2% of metastatic CRC patients) subgroup of $^{nonV600E}BRAF$-mutated CRCs; these $^{nonV600E}BRAF$-mutated CRCs involve mutation at the level of 19 different codons [27,28]. Patients bearing mutations at the level of codons 594 and 596 seem to form a distinct subgroup with longer overall survival compared with $^{V600E}BRAF$-mutated patients [27,29]. A recent study reported the classification of *BRAF*-mutated CRCs into three sub groups: *BRAF* mutations activating RAS-independent as monomers (Class1 V600E); *BRAF* mutations activating RAS-independent signaling as dimers (class 2 codons 597/601); *BRAF* mutations activating RAS-dependent signaling with impaired kinase activity (class 3 codons 594/596) [30]. Class 3 *BRAF*-mutated metastatic CRCs were more frequently left sided and without peritoneal metastases compared to class 1; class 3 tumors have an overall survival comparable to that of *BRAF* wt tumors; while class 1 and 2 tumors have a poorer overall survival than *BRAF* wt tumors [30].

3. Comparative Analysis of the Genetic Abnormalities of Primary Metastatic CRCs and of Metastases

Several studies have performed comparative lesion sequencing of paired primary metastatic CRCs and of corresponding metastases.

About 20% of patients with CRC already have metastases at diagnosis [24]. The patterns of metastasis of colon and rectal cancer were recently explored in a very large cohort of patients (49,096, 31,285 with colon cancer and 17,811 with rectal cancer: 30% of colon cancer and 31% of rectal cancer patients had metastases) [31]. Of all patients with metastatic cancer, the most common sites of metastasis were the liver (70% in both colon and rectal cancer) and the thorax (32% in colon cancer and 47% in rectal cancer), followed by the peritoneum for colon cancer (21%) and the bone for rectal cancer (12%); nervous system metastases were more rare, being observed in 5% of colon cancer and 8% in rectal cancer [31]; thoracic metastases were more frequent in lower tumor stages, particularly in rectal cancer, whereas the relative frequency of liver metastases increased with tumor stages; liver metastases were most frequently solitary metastases (in 48% of colon and 45% of rectal cancer); lung metastases were frequently observed in association with liver metastases (73% in colon cancer and 63% in rectal cancer) [31].

Several comparative sequencing studies have shown a high concordance in the genomic profile between primary and metastatic CRCs. Jones and coworkers through a comparative sequencing analysis of a small number of patients observed a high degree of concordance between primary tumors and metastases [32]. Vakiani et al. reported the analysis for *KRAS, NRAS, BRAF, PIK3CA,* and *TP53* genes of 84 CRCs in whom tumor tissue from both primary and metastatic sites was available [33]. The results of this analysis showed that: the frequency of *KRAS, NRAS,* and *PIK3CA* mutations was similar in metastatic versus primary tumors; *TP53* mutations were more frequent in metastatic versus primary tumors (53% vs. 30%, respectively), whereas *BRAF* mutations were significantly less frequent (1.9% vs. 7.7%, respectively) [33]. In a subsequent analysis, 69 CRC patients were explored for their mutational profile by NGS in primary and metastatic tumor tissues [33]. The results of this study showed that 79% of the mutations were shared between primary and metastatic tumors. Particularly, a high degree of concordance at the level of early occurring and recurrent mutations was observed [33]. No discordant mutations in *KRAS/NRAS* and *BRAF* were observed; the only private mutations, defined as mutations observed only in the primary or the metastatic tumor, were observed at the level of *APC, PIK3CA, SMAD4* and *TP53* genes [34]. These findings have supported the view that genetic alterations occurring early during colorectal cancer genesis, such as *APC, KRAS, NRAS,* and *BRAF* mutations are maintained during the process of tumor evolution up to the final level of tumor metastases [34].

In some contrast with these studies, Vermaat et al., using next generation sequencing, showed a high degree of mutational discordance between primary and metastatic samples, with 52% and 86% of dissimilarities of *KRAS* and *EGFR* mutational status between paired primary and metastatic tumor samples. Modest variability was reported for *HRAS* (34%), *PIK3CA* (19%), *FLT1* (10%), *NRAS* (10%) and *BRAF* (14%) [35].

Lim et al [36] performed an analysis of 34 CRC patients with liver metastases by sequencing (whole exome and RNA sequencing) both primary tumors and metastases and showed in these patients frequent mutations of *APC* (65%), *TP53* (68%), *KRAS* (24%), *TCF7L2* (21%), *PIK3CA* (18%), *NRG1* (18%),

FBXW7 (15%), *SMAD4* (15%), *CARD11* (12%), and *BMI1* (9%) [36]. Based on the absence or presence of mutations in liver metastases, the mutations occurring in these patients were classified into three different classes: class 1, mutations shared between primary tumors and liver metastases (57.6% of all mutations); class 2 mutations present only in primary tumors (20.9% of all mutations); class 3 mutations, detected in only liver metastases (21.5% of all metastases) [36]. Importantly, the frequency of class 1 mutations was highly variable across individual patients (ranging from 25% to 92%), thus suggesting that the presence of a clonal selection during metastasis formation is an event highly variable among patients; a decreased clonality during metastasis formation was usually associated with a high-mutational concordance between primary tumors and metastases, whereas an increased clonality during metastasis formation was usually linked with low mutational concordance between primary tumors and liver metastases [36].

Vignot et al. reported a mutational analysis by targeted NGS on surgical samples from primary and matched metastatic tissues from 13 CRC patients [37]. A global concordance rate for mutations of 78% was observed between primary and metastatic tumors; this concordance raised to 90% for the 12 most recurrent mutations occurring in CRC [37]. On 17 pathways explored, only two pathways were upregulated in metastatic tissues compared to primary tumors [37].

Tan and coworkers reported a detailed analysis of the mutational profile and of CNAs of 18 matched primary and metastatic tumor tissues by high-depth sequencing of over 750 cancer-associated genes and copy number profiling, supporting a high concordance of primary tumor and metastases [38]. Particularly, their results showed a median of 79.3% of somatic gene mutations present both in the primary and metastasis and 81.7% of all alterations present in both primary tumors and metastases [38]. Private alterations, primary-specific or metastasis-specific are observed at lower allelic frequencies [38]. The mutations most frequently occurring only at the level of metastases are represented by *MLL3*, *FAT1*, and *GNAS* gene mutations [38]. Interestingly, distinct mutational signatures are observed in shared variants and private variants [38]. The analysis of copy number alterations similarly showed a conserved pattern between primary tumors and metastases: chromosomal regions of allelic imbalance were similar in the matched primary tumor and metastasis; focal gains and losses of genes commonly amplified or deleted in cancer were similar in the primary tumors and metastases [38]. These findings supported a model of linear evolution in most CRC patients with liver-limited metastatic disease.

Several studies reported a concordant mutation profile for the main CRC driver genes, including *KRAS*, *TP53*, *APC*, *PIK3CA*, *BRAF*, and *NRAS* between primary tumors and metastatic lesions regardless of the temporal relationship between metastases (synchronous or metachronous) [39,40]. Only in a minority of cases (7–15%) metastases differed from paired primary tumors [39,40]. Similarly, Jesinghaus and coworkers have explored the mutational landscape of 24 primary MSS CRCs and of their respective metastases: A high degree of genetic concordance of the mutations affecting the driver genes *APC*, *KRAS*, *FBXW7*, *PIK3CA*, *BRAF*, *SMAD4*, and *ACVR2A* was observed; only 16% of cases displayed the acquisition of new mutations in metastatic lesions involving the *TP53*, *CTNNB1*, *PTEN* and *SYNE1*, all the remaining cases sharing the genetic lesions of the primary tumor with metastases, for all types of metastases, lymph node and distant metastases [41].

Isaque and coworkers have performed a comprehensive whole-genome analysis of differences between metastatic lesions and their corresponding primary tumors in 12 MSS CRC patients [42]. This detailed analysis showed that 65% (range from 36% to 92%) of all mutation events were shared between primary tumors and corresponding metastases, suggesting the existence of a common truncal clone; 15% (range from 1% to 29%) were tumor-specific and 19% (ranging from 3 to 42%) were metastasis-specific; recurrent driver mutations were equally present in primary tumors and their matched metastases, with the exception of only metastatic TP53 mutation, absent in the corresponding primary tumor; a number of metastasis-specific mutations were identified, including non-silent mutations of *FAT1*, *FGF1*, *BRCA2*, *TP53*, and *KDR*, splice site mutations of *JAK2* and 3'-UTR mutations in *KDR*, *PDGFRA*, and *AKT2* genes [42].

Several studies have explored copy number profiles of paired primary and metastatic CRC. Kawamata et al. have analyzed CNAs in paired primary and metastatic tumor samples derived from 16 patients; the CNA profile was explored and was correlated with the timing of primary and metastatic tissue resection and with the exposure to chemotherapy [43]. An average copy number difference of 22% was observed when comparing primary and paired liver metastases; the differences observed between metastases and corresponding primary tumors increased when considering in this analysis post-therapy metastases; some loss of heterozygosity (LOH) events were unique either to primary tumor samples or to metastases: those unique to primary tumors occurred more frequently in those treatment naive, while LOH events unique to metastases occurred most frequently post-therapy [43]. Interestingly, events of amplification of clinically actionable genes *ERBB2*, *FGFR1*, *PIK3CA*, or *CDK8* were observed in some patients at the level of metastases but not in the corresponding primary CRCs [43].

Smeets and coworkers investigated the pattern of CNAs in 409 metastatic CRC patients undergoing treatment with chemotherapy alone or chemotherapy plus bevacizumab in the context of the phase II MoMa study [44]. mCRCs were clustered into three different subgroups according to increasing degrees of chromosomal instability: tumors belonging to the intermediate-to-high instability subgroups have improved outcome following treatment with chemotherapy plus bevacizumab versus chemotherapy alone; low instability tumors, including POLE-mutated and MSI tumors, derive no further benefit from bevacizumab [44].

The targeted therapy of metastatic CRC patients implies the exploration of the targeted biomarker and its presence in both primary and metastatic tumors. The introduction of EGFR inhibitors for treatment of metastatic CRC patients allowed the unique opportunity to obtain, through the analysis of numerous clinical studies, data on the concordance of the mutational status for *KRAS*, *NRAS*, *BRAF* and *PIK3CA* between primary tumors and metastases in more than 3500 patients [45]. This metanalysis involving 61 clinical studies and data on 3565 metastatic CRCs showed: (i) a very high median biomarker concordance for *KRAS* (93%), *NRAS* (100%), *BRAF* (99.4%), *PIK3CA* (93%); (ii) a pooled discordance of 8% for *KRAS*, 8% for *BRAF*, and 7% for *PIK3CA* [35]. These observations further support the maintenance of the main driver mutations in CRCs undergoing metastatic spreading [45].

4. Tumor Heterogeneity and Metastatic Evolution

Study of intratumor heterogeneity (ITH) is fundamental from both a biological and clinical perspective, to understand the genomic changes driving the evolution of the malignant process up to metastasis generation. Several studies have shown that CRCs display a consistent degree of spatial intratumor heterogeneity; particularly, three types of spatial heterogeneity of CRCs have been described: (i) ITH related to the existence of genetic differences at the level of tumor cells within the primary tumor; (ii) ITH related to differences at the level of various metastatic lesions within a single patient; (iii) ITH related to the existence of genetic differences within the cells of a single metastatic lesion (intrametastatic heterogeneity) [46].

An initial study by Baisse and coworkers provided evidence through multiregional sequencing analysis of 15–20 areas within a tumor, that 67% of advanced CRCs displayed significant ITH at the level of gene alterations and CNAs [47]. Jeantet and coworkers performed the analysis of the distribution of *RAS* mutations in different areas of primary tumor, metastatic lymph nodes and distant metastases: primary tumors displayed an intra-tumoral heterogeneity for *RAS* mutations in 33% of cases; the comparative analysis of primary tumors and metastatic tumors showed an inter-tumoral heterogeneity in 36% of cases; multiple *RAS* mutated subclones were observed in 28% of cases in the same tumor [48].

Kim and coworkers have performed a multiregion analysis of the mutational spectrum and CNAs at the level of both primary and metastatic colorectal cancer lesions from five CRC patients [49]. This study showed a substantial level of ITH in both primary and matched liver metastases, with 46% to 80% subclonal mutation fractions. The spatial localization of the mutations allowed their classification into three types: the universal mutations are those observed in all the regional biopsies, are enriched in genes such as *APC*, *KRAS*, and *TP53* and represent events occurring early during tumor evolution; metastasis-clonal mutations are those that are regionally clonal only in the metastatic regions and may represent genetic events involved in the development of distant metastases; primary-private mutations are those present in primary but absent at the level of metastases; metastasis-private mutations are those present in primary but absent in only a part of metastatic lesions and may represent events that are acquired during the expansion of metastatic clones [49]. It was estimated that 20–54% of mutations in a given sample were universal, whereas from 46% to 80% of mutations were subclonal; among the subclonal lesions, 1–15% were metastasis-clonal, 2–41% metastasis-private, and 14–56% primary-private [49]. Most CNAs containing genes involved in CRC development, such as *APC*, *PTEN* and *SMAD4* were observed in both primary and metastatic lesions, thus representing early or universal genomic events [49]. In contrast, copy number changes such as chromosomal gains of *c-MYC* and chromotripsis can be region-specific and may represent the source of genetic intra-tumor heterogeneity. Finally, the inferred evolution pattern of cancer progression was as a branched evolution, rather than as linear evolution [49].

Sveen et al [50] have reported high-resolution DNA copy number analysis of metastatic lesions from 45 CRC patients; this analysis showed a pronounced variation in the level of intra-patient inter-metastatic heterogeneity [50]. Interestingly, the level of intra-patient inter-metastatic heterogeneity resulted to be a strong prognostic determinant, stronger than commonly adopted clinico-pathological prognostic markers: patients with a high-level of heterogeneity had a three-year overall survival of 18%, compared to 66% for patients with a low-level of tumor heterogeneity [50].

Uchi and coworkers have investigated intratumor heterogeneity in CRC by analyzing samples from distinct areas of 9 different primary tumors [51]. Multiregional exome sequencing provided evidence about the existence of extensive intratumor heterogeneity and branched evolution. Particularly, the analysis of the various mutations showed that they can be classified as founder, shared and unique mutations: parental clones acquire mutations in driver genes, such as *APC*, *KRAS* and *FBWX7* as founder mutations during tumor development, whereas subclones acquire mutations in *PIK3CA* mutations as progressor mutations [41]. The age of patients correlated with the number of founder mutations. Similar to gene mutations, some copy number alterations occurred as founder events (such as amplifications of 7p, 13q, 10q, 20p, and 20q), while other CNAs, such as several focal deletions, predominantly occur as progressor CNAs [51]. The analysis of epigenetic intratumoral heterogeneity showed that CIMP-H occurs early in tumor evolution [51]. Similar to the other genetic alterations, some epigenomic modifications occurred as founder events, such as hypermethylation of *SFRPs*, *GATA4* and *GATA5* genes, whereas other epigenomic modifications occurred as progressor events [51]. An integrated view of the various parameters of intratumor genetic/epigenetic heterogeneity allowed the reconstruction of each CRC's life history. A typical example is given by one of these nine patients: in this patient, the initial founder mutations, *APC*, *KRAS* and *FBWX7* mutations, were observed at the level of the parental clone; this initial parental clone subdivided into two subclones, one characterized by the acquisition of a focal *MYC* amplification and the other one by several shared CNAs, such as 20p amplification and 1p deletion. At the subsequent steps of tumor evolution, the two subclones branched into minor subclones, a process accompanied by accumulation of progressor mutations and methylation alterations. These events caused the development of a consistent degree of intratumor heterogeneity, extended also at the level of transcriptome heterogeneity [51]. Interestingly, these authors have performed a comparative analysis of ITH in early and advanced CRCs, providing evidence that early tumors acquire more subclonal driver mutations compared to advanced tumors: in early CRCs 50% of driver mutations were branch mutations, while only 22% mutations were branch mutations in advanced colorectal cancers [52].

Some studies have explored ITH of CRCs using deep sequencing techniques. Thus, Wei et al. performed a high depth multiregional wide exome sequencing in 28 tissues from four CRC patients with matched primary and metastatic tumors. This study provided several interesting findings to better understand the process of CRC metastasization: metastatic tumors exhibited less intratumor heterogeneity than primary tumors; primary and metastatic tumors differ significantly based on the analysis of allelic frequency of the various mutations; all metastatic tumors inherited multiple genetically distinct subclones from primary tumors, thus suggesting a possible polyclonal seeding mechanism for metastasis [53]. In one of these patients, both lymph nodes and lung metastases were analyzed, showing a completely different genetic landscape in these two different metastatic sites; according to this finding, it was suggested that parallel metastatic dissemination to distant organs is independent of lymph nodes [53]. Suzuki et al. have shown a variable level of ITH using deep-targeted NGS followed by ultra-deep amplicon sequencing through the analysis of 4 different CRC patients investigated at the level of various tumor regions; different tumor regions shared mutations in driver genes, such as *APC*, *KRAS* and *TP53*. However, in addition, many mutations were observed only at subclonal levels and in many instances their detection was only revealed by an ultra-high-depth sequencing approach [54].

Very interestingly, Oh and coworkers performed a study of intratumor heterogeneity on a large set of patients across 8 different tumor types by targeted deep sequencing; using this technique, a ITH index was determined showing that CRCs are among the tumors with the highest ITH index [55]. In this study, CRC patients of all tumor stages were included showing that ITH index was already high in 40% of stage I patients and moderately increased with tumor stage progression, with a high ITH index in 55% of stage IV CRCs [55]. The presence of high ITH index was clearly associated with a decreased progression-free survival (PFS) in stage I-III patients, but not in stage IV patients [55].

It is important to note that intratumor heterogeneity is not dictated only by genetic mechanisms, but also by phenotypic heterogeneity/plasticity apparently unrelated to genetic determinants. A notable example is provided by a study by Kreso et al., based on the analysis of serially expanded CRC clones from patient samples, remaining genetically stable during serial transplantation; in spite this stability, reproducible differences in the functional fates and response to chemotherapy of individual CRC cells, suggesting that in vivo dynamic changes of CRCs are not dictated by genomic changes [56]. These observations support the view that, in addition to the well-known mechanisms of tumor heterogeneity driven by genetic diversity, other diversity-generating processes exist within a genetic clone, seemingly related to epigenetic diversity, variability of tumor microenvironment and multiple external factors affecting gene expression [56].

5. Liver Metastases

The liver is the most frequent metastatic site for CRC, with 60% of CRC patients developing colorectal liver metastases (CLMs). CLMs can be surgically removed or therapeutically ablated and these procedures may significantly improve the survival of these patients. Recent studies have explored a possible link between genomic features and outcomes of metastatic CRC undergoing CLM resection. Initial studies have suggested that mutations in *KRAS* and *BRAF* are associated with a poor outcome after CLM resection, whereas mutations in *NRAS*, *TP53*, *PIK3CA*, and *SMAD4* were shown to be potential prognostic factors after CLM resection [57].

More recent studies have shown that the analysis of co-mutation status is more predictive of outcome after CLM removal [57]. Thus, it was shown that *RAS/TP53* double-mutant metastatic CRC with predominant location in right colon of primary tumors, corresponding to 31% of patients, displayed a shorter five-year overall survival (12%), compared with 55% overall survival of *TP53* wild-type [57].

The presence of *V600E BRAF* mutations observed in 5.1% of metastatic CRC patients, but not non-*V600E BRAF* mutations was associated with worse prognosis (reduced survival and frequent and rapid recurrence) after resection of CLMs [58]. Interestingly, *V600E BRAF* mutations had a stronger association with overall and disease-free survival than *KRAS* mutations [58].

Datta and coworkers explored a large group of 935 patients with metastatic CRC and showed that co-alteration of oncogenic *TP53* with either *KRAS*, *NRAS*, or *BRAF* mutations was associated with significantly worse survival compared to alterations in either gene group alone [59]. Interestingly, *RAS/BRAF-TP53* co-mutated CRCs were associated with worse survival in patients with liver and lung, but not with peritoneal surface metastases Moreover, co-altered *BRAF/RAS-TP53* were significantly associated with the development of extra-hepatic metastatic sites [59]. Similar conclusions were reached by Kawaguchi et al. who analyzed the possible relationship between somatic gene mutation profile and outcome in 507 metastatic CRC patients who underwent CLM resection: *BRAF*, *RAS*, *TP53*, and *SMAD4* mutations were significantly associated with overall survival, coexisting mutations in *RAS*, *TP53*, and *SMAD4* were associated with negative outcome (reduced OS and RFS) than coexisting mutations in any two of these genes and mutations in one or more of these genes [60].

Smith et al. recently reported the results of a retrospective study on 370 metastatic CRC patients who underwent either colorectal liver hepatectomy followed by hepatic arterial infusion (HAI) chemotherapy or HAI and systematic therapy (patients with unresectable metastases); 34.8% of these patients have extrahepatic disease and 65.2% have liver-restricted disease [60]. Concurrently mutated *RAS/BRAF* and *SMAD4* were associated with negative survival in resectable patients, while concurrent *RAS/BRAF* and *TP53* mutations were associated with worse survival in unresectable patients [61].

Leung et al. have developed a highly multiplexed single-cell DNA sequencing to trace the metastatic lineage of two CRC patients with matched liver metastases [62]. In the first patient, a monoclonal seeding was observed, in which a single clone of tumor cells acquired a large number of mutations before developing the capacity to migrate to the liver and to develop an advanced, metastatic tumor; in the second patient, a polyclonal mechanism of seeding was observed, in which two clones that have diverged from the primary tumor metastasize to the liver [62]. Interestingly, the single-cell sequencing approach allowed to show the existence in one of the two patients of a rare subpopulation of diploid cells that carried a heterozygous mutation in *APC* gene, but not associated with other somatic mutations; these cells were diploid and seemingly represent the initial tumorigenic cells and remained present in the advanced tumor representing 2.6% of tumor cells [62]. A second unexpected finding was observed in the second patient and consisted in the detection of a small independent subpopulation of diploid tumor cells that harbored a completely different set of mutations than the main tumor lineage [62].

6. Lymphatic Metastases

Other studies have explored the process of CRC metastasization, focusing on the mechanisms of spreading of cancer cells from the primary tumors to regional lymph nodes. Lymph node metastasis associates with negative outcomes in CRCs and the presence of tumor cells in regional lymph nodes defines stage III disease and the need for adjuvant chemotherapy and lowers the 5-year survival compared to stage II disease without lymphatic lymph nodes metastasis [63].

Naxerova et al. have explored the evolutionary relationship between primary tumor, lymph node and distant metastases in CRC: through the study of 213 biopsy samples from 17 patients, these authors have used somatic variants in hypermutable DNA regions to reconstruct phylogenetic trees of tumor metastatic evolution [64]. This analysis provided evidence about the existence of two different pathways of lymph node and distant metastases generation in CRC patients. In fact, the genetic distances between lymph node metastases, distant metastases and corresponding primary tumors were measured showing that for the majority (73%) of lymph node metastases the distance with respect to the primary tumor was shorter than the distance with respect to distant metastases; distant metastases (69% of cases) had shorter distance to the primary tumor than to lymph nodes metastases [64]. In line with these observations, reconstruction of phylogenetic evolutionary tumor trees allowed to establish that in 35% of cases lymphatic and distant metastases have a common origin from the same subclone of the primary tumor (either they originate both from the primary tumor or, alternatively, distant metastases originate from lymph node metastases). In contrast, in 65% of cases, there is evidence of a distinct origin of lymphatic and distant metastases, as supported by the evidence of genetically different alterations, thus indicating that in these patients primary tumors harboring multiple subclones at different stages of evolution have seeded genetically distinct metastases [64].

Ulintz and coworkers have explored the clonal origin of lymph node metastasis in CRC. Thus, they have investigated multiple tumor regions and cancer-containing lymph nodes from 7 CRC patients, providing evidence that: (i) for each patient, the primary tumor regions and matched lymph node metastases were polyclonal and the clonal populations differed from one node to another; (ii) in a part of CRC patients, the cancer cells present in a given lymph node originated from multiple distinct regions of a primary tumor, while in other cases these metastatic cells originate from a single geographic region of the primary tumor; (iii) lymph node metastases contain subclones originated early or late during tumor development [65]. According to these findings, a model of lymph node metastatic spreading in CRCs involving multiple waves of seeding from the primary tumor over time was proposed [65].

Hu et al. have recently characterized the evolutionary dynamics of metastatic seeding by analyzing exome sequencing profiles from 118 biopsies derived from 23 patients with CRC with metastases to liver or brain [66]. Particularly, these authors performed multi-region sequencing on the primary tumor and paired metastasis to build phylogenetic trees. The results of this study indicate that the genomic divergence between the primary tumor and paired metastases is low: mutations in *KRAS*, *TP53*, *SMAD4*, *TCF7L2*, *FN1*, *ERLF3*, and *ATM* were highly concordant between primary tumors and metastases and 70% of highly frequent gene mutations were shared by both lesions, a finding similarly observed in liver and brain metastases; among the genes that tended to be private to the primary tumors or to metastases the most frequent were *SYNE1* and *APOB*. Somatic copy number alterations were generally concordant. Some putative oncogenes, such as *PIK3CA*, *GNAS*, *SRC*, *FXR1*, *MUCA*, *GPC6*, and *MECOM* were more recurrently amplified in metastases than in primary tumors [56]. Interestingly, the analysis of genetic data relative to large sets of CRC patients allowed to define the existence of metastasis-associated early driver gene modules present in early tumors and characterized by modules of tumor cells exhibiting CRC drivers (combinations of *APC*, *KRAS*, *TP53*, or *SMAD4*) associated with potential metastasis-associated genes, such as *TCF7L2*, *AMER1*, or *PTPRT* [56]. Interestingly, *PTPRT* mutations in combination with canonical CRC drivers are almost exclusively found in metastatic CRC patients [66]. The simulation of spatial tumor growth under selective or neutral growth evolutionary modes, coupled with the evaluation of the patterns of subclonal divergence at the level of different tumor regions allowed to establish whether a given tumor is driven by positive selective selection (either strong or weak) or by neutral evolution. The development of a spatial computational model of tumor progression and statistical inference framework to time dissemination in a patient-specific fashion, allowed to suggest that the capacity to seed metastasis is a property inherent to cancer cells originated early during tumor development (81% of cases), when the tumor bulk is clinically undetectable [66]. The analysis of a large set of public databases provided evidence that the large majority (90%) of metastatic primary CRCs displayed subclonal selection, thus suggesting that the metastatic clone possesses a consistent selective growth advantage. However, only a lower proportion (33%) of stage I-III CRCs displayed patterns of tumor evolution compatible with subclonal selection. Importantly, this observation suggests that type of tumor evolution may be dependent on disease stage or disease aggressiveness [66]. As mentioned above, driver mutations were usually not enriched in metastases; however, the stratification of CRC patients according to the profile of tumor evolution (early dissemination vs. late dissemination) showed a higher frequency of private driver mutations in metastases evolving under selection conditions compared to those evolving neutrally, thus suggesting that in these patients additional subclonal driver mutations may occur during the development of some metastases [66].

The same authors very recently reported the analysis of whole-exome sequencing data from 457 paired primary tumors and metastases derived from 136 patients with colorectal, breast and lung cancer: this study involved the analysis of 39 metastatic CRC patients, including both untreated and treated metastases [67]. The results of this study provided several interesting findings: (i) the mutational burden (single nucleotide variation and CNAs) was highly concordant between primary and metastatic tumors; (ii) metastases displayed a slight increase in the number of clonal single nucleotide mutations and fewer subclonal nucleotide variants, supporting the existence of an evolutionary bottleneck during metastasis; (iii) a high percentage (84%) of clonal drivers in each primary CRC tumor and metastasis was shared, while the fraction of subclonal drivers was 20%; (iv) among the three cancers investigated, CRC had the highest prevalence of primary tumor-private subclonal drivers; (v) driver mutations present in metastases are enriched in the trunk of the phylogenetic mutational tree; (vi) treatment induced a dramatic increase of the frequency of private clonal drivers across all the three cancers, including CRC (78% of metastasis-private clonal driver mutations), thus suggesting that therapy selects a minor micro metastatic subclone; (vii) a small number of driver genes that were more frequently amplified or deleted in metastases compared to primary tumors (such as amplification of *RAC1* or deletion of *FAT1* and *ALB* genes); (viii) polyclonal seeding was common in untreated lymph node metastases and distant metastases, but was less frequent in treated distant metastases [67]. The low number of metastasis-private clonal mutations is consistent with early metastatic seeding [67].

7. Effect of Therapy on Mutational Landscape of Metastatic CRC

The targeted therapy of metastatic CRC patients implies the exploration of the targeted biomarker and its presence in both the primary and the metastatic tumors. The introduction of EGFR inhibitors for treatment of metastatic CRC patients allowed the unique opportunity to obtain, through the analysis of numerous clinical studies, data on the concordance of the mutational status for *KRAS*, *NRAS*, *BRAF* and *PIK3CA* between primary tumors and metastases in more than 3500 patients [45]. This meta-analysis involving 61 clinical studies and data on 3565 metastatic CRCs, showed: (i) a median biomarker concordance for *KRAS* (93.7%), *NRAS* (100%), *BRAF* (99.4%), and *PIK3CA* (93%); (ii) a pooled discordance of 8% for *KRAS*, 8% for *BRAF*, and 7% for *PIK3CA* [45]. These observations further support the maintenance of the main driver gene alterations in CRCs undergoing metastatic spreading [45]. The detection of *KRAS* mutations in metastatic CRC is important because implies a negative prognosis and a poor response to standard chemotherapy [68].

An important example of the therapy-driven effects on the genomic alterations of metastatic CRC derives from the analysis of patients developing resistance to therapies based on EGFR inhibitors. EGFR inhibitors are effective in a subset of *KRAS* wild-type metastatic CRCs; however, after an initial response, the development of secondary resistance mechanisms cause disease relapse, thus limiting the clinical benefit of this treatment: The analyses of metastases of patients who developed resistance to EGFR inhibitors showed more rarely the emergence of *KRAS* amplification and more frequently the acquisition of secondary *KRAS* mutations; in these patients, *KRAS* mutant alleles were detectable in the blood circulating tumor DNA 10 months before the radiographic documentation of disease progression [69]. These observations suggest that EGFR-targeted therapy exerts a selective effect on CRCs either inducing the expansion of pre-existing *KRAS*-mutant subclones or favoring the development of new *KRAS* alterations [69]. Another mechanism of secondary resistance to EGFR blockade is represented by novel alterations of ectodomain of EGFR [70]. The study of individual patients has shown that different metastatic biopsies from the same patient with CRC display genetically distinct mechanisms of resistance to EGFR blockade: thus, in some patients, it was documented that distinct resistance mechanisms emerge in different metastases in the same patient and can drive lesion-specific responses to different targeted therapies [70].

Genetic mechanisms of primary resistance to EGFR inhibitors among *KRAS* wild-type CRC patients are represented by *NRAS* mutations, ^{V600E}*BRAF* mutations, *MET* amplification, *ERBB2* amplification, *PIK3CA* mutations at the level of exon 20, mutations in *FGFR1*, *PDGFRA*, and *MAP2K1*, and homozygous deletions of *PTEN* [71].

Using xenografts derived from hepatic metastases of CRC patients, amplification of *ERBB2* was identified as a potential therapeutic target in cetuximab-resistant CRCs [72]. These preclinical observations supported a clinical study (HERACLES) evaluating trastuzumab and lapatinib in metastatic CRC patients with amplified *ERBB2* refractory to standard cares: in 33 patients,

24.2% objective responses were observed with durable clinical benefit lasting >24 months in responding patients [72]. Although ERBB2 blockade was effective, most of responding patients relapse [73]. A recent study explored the mechanisms of tumor evolution responsible for relapse to HER2 blockade. In fact, the analysis of circulating tumor DNA allowed to define organ and metastases-private evolutionary patterns and high-levels in intra-patient molecular heterogeneity, defining lesion-specific evolutionary trees and potential pharmacologic vulnerabilities [74].

8. Models of CRC Progression and Evolution

The study of tumor heterogeneity is a fundamental tool to analyze and to define the molecular and cellular mechanisms responsible for the development of CRC and have provided a consistent contribution to the development of current theories to explain CRC development.

Two different models have been proposed in the time to explain the origin and development of CRC metastasis: one suggesting a common origin for both the primary tumor and metastases and the other hypothesizing a completely independent genesis of metastases and of the primary tumor. The sequencing data of matched primary tumors and metastases have strongly supported the existence of a common ancestor of both the primary tumor and of the corresponding metastases.

The development of CRC from a common ancestor implies two different models to explain metastasis evolution: the parallel progression model suggests that the dissemination of metastasizing tumor cells occurs during early stages of primary tumor and the primary tumor and metastases evolve separately thereafter. The linear progression model implies the occurrence of metastases as a sequential event occurring during primary tumor development.

8.1. Somatic Mutations in Normal Colonic Epithelium

Colon epithelium is organized in crypts, composed by about 2000 cells, representing the tissutal units. The main function of crypts consists in providing an efficient system of renewing of the short-lived colonic epithelium, through the differentiation of intestinal stem cells, located at the base of the crypts; these stem cells stochastically replace one another through a biologic process of neutral drift, thus ensuring that all stem cells and differentiated cells present in a crypt derive from a single ancestral stem cell. As a consequence of this hierarchical organization of the intestinal crypt, somatic mutations in these ancestor stem cells are present in all the stem cells composing the crypt; these stem cells are considered the cells of origin of CRCs [75]. A recent study explored somatic mutational landscape in normal colorectal epithelium through whole-genome sequencing of normal colorectal crypts from 42 individuals [76]. Signatures of multiple mutational processes were detected, with some signatures being ubiquitous, while other ones observed in some individuals, in some crypts. Driver mutations were observed in about 1% of normal colorectal crypts in middle-aged individuals [76]. Among the driver mutations detected in normal crypts there are *AXIN2, STAG2, PIK3CA, ERBB2, ERBB3, FBXW7* mutations [66]. A different pattern of mutations was observed in normal crypts compared to those observed in CRCs: *ERBB2* and *ERBB3* mutations are common in normal colon but rare in CRCs (1%), whereas mutations in driver genes mutations in *APC, KRAS* and *TP53* are common in CRCs, but are rare among normal crypts (one in 14) [66]. These observations strongly suggest a major oncogenic potential to *APC, KRAS,* and *TP53* mutations promoting the conversion to colorectal adenoma (CRA) and CRC, whereas mutations in *ERBB2* and *ERBB3* confer higher like hoods of crypt colonization by stem cells [76]. No significant difference was observed in the frequency of driver mutations between individuals who had CRC and those who did not [76]. According to these findings, it was concluded that CRAs and CRCs are rare outcomes of a pervasive process of neoplastic change occurring at the level of morphologically normal colorectal epithelium [76].

The investigation of individuals with inflammatory bowel disease provided evidence that the repeated inflammatory cycles affecting the colonic epithelium induce a 2.4-fold increase of the average rate of colonic crypts affected; the mutations observed in IBD non-neoplastic epithelium mostly involve *ARID1A, FBXW7, PIGR,* and *ZC3H12A* genes in the IL17 and Toll-like receptor pathways [77].

Mutations in *KRAS*, *APC* and *TP53* are rare in non-dysplastic tissues from IBD patients. At variance with the normal colon, where clonal expansions are limited to the crypts, in IBD epithelium, frequent widespread millimeter-scale clonal expansions were observed [77]. The differences in driver landscape of IBD colon, suggest that there are different selection mechanisms in the colitis-affected colon and that somatic mutations potentially play a causal role in IBD pathogenesis [77].

Nicholson and colleagues have analyzed stem cell dynamics in normal human colon to define the efficiency of clone fixation within the epithelium and the rate of subsequent lateral expansion [78]. The process of mutant clone fixation within colonic crypts takes years, due to the time required for the mutated intestinal stem cells to replace neighbors cells to populate the entire crypt; crypt fission allows the lateral expansion of mutant clones: this process is rare for neutral mutations (0.7% per year); biases in both fixation and expansion of stem cells increases age-related pro-oncogenic burden; pro-oncogenic mutations modify the stem cell turnover and accelerate fixation and clonal expansion by crypt fission to generate high mutant allelic frequencies with age [78].

8.2. Mutational Landscape in the Progression from Colorectal Adenomas to Colorectal Cancers

Several studies have compared the spectrum of genetic alterations in CRAs and in CRCs.

In an initial study, Jones et al. have performed an analysis of the mutations observed in benign, invasive and metastatic colorectal tumors and reached the conclusion that more selective mutational events are required for the transition of a benign adenoma into a CRC than those required for the acquisition of metastasizing properties by a CRC [32]. The results of this study supported a classical model of colorectal tumorigenesis, characterized by the progressive acquisition of mutational events through various clinical stages of tumor progression: the tumor process is initiated by the acquisition of a mutation into a gene of the Wnt pathway (mostly *APC* mutations) with consequent formation of a small adenoma; mutations constitutively activating *KRAS/BRAF* pathway are required for the proliferation of the small adenoma and for its transformation into a large adenoma; subsequent acquisition of mutations at the level of genes controlling the PIK3CA, TGF-β and TP53 pathways is required for the transformation of a benign adenoma into a CRC; only few metastasis-specific mutations are acquired during the transition of a CRC from an invasive condition to a metastatic status [32].

APC loss of function is a key event in the colon carcinogenesis and represents the first event in the tumor initiation. This conclusion was directly supported through sequencing studies on colon adenomas. Nikolaev and coworkers have performed an exome sequencing analysis of 24 human colon polyps, derived from 22 individuals with no family history of predisposition to cancer. The mutational profiles observed at the level of the cancer-driver genes *APC*, *CTNNB1* and *BRAF* genes allowed to subdivide polyps into three different groups: the group 1 with *APC* mutations, included the majority of polyps, mostly corresponding to colon adenomas: All the observed mutations introduced premature stop codon and none of these polyps retained a normal *APC* allele, due to the presence of two *APC* mutations or a single *APC* mutation associated with loss of heterozygosity; the group 2 with *CTNNB1* mutations included only a few minority of polyps: the *CTNNB1* mutation was homozygous, due to concomitant LOH; the group 3 with *BRAF* mutations included polyps with serrated histology: *BRAF* mutations were heterozygous [79]. Adenomas with *CTNNB1* or *BRAF* mutations did not display mutations in other cancer-driver genes, whereas adenomas with *APC* mutations showed additional cancer-driver mutations (at the level of *KRAS*, *NRAS*, *GNAS*, *AKT1*, *SOX9* and *TP53* genes), whose number correlated with the degree of dysplasia and invasiveness [79]. In addition to cancer-driver gene mutations, many passenger mutations were observed in colon adenomas [69]. According to the rate of single nucleotide substitutions, it was suggested the existence of a mutator phenotype in colon adenomas [79].

Lin and coworkers have reported the results of a whole-exome sequencing and targeted sequencing study on 149 colon adenocarcinoma samples, corresponding to 134 conventional adenomas (CADs) (104 non-advanced and 30 advanced) and 14 serrated adenomas (SSAs). No significant differences in the mutation rates were found between CNADs and SSAs (1.5 and 1.7 mutations/Mb, respectively) [80].

As it is expected, the gene most frequently mutated in CNADs was *APC*, while *BRAF* was the gene most recurrently mutated in SSAs [70]. In addition to *APC*, four genes were frequently mutated in CADs: *CTNNB1* (catenin beta 1), *KRTAP4-5* (keratin-associated protein 4-5), *GOLGA8B* (golgin A8 family member B) and TMPRSS13 (transmembrane protease, serine 13) [80]. The biological role of *GOLGA8B*, *TMPRSS13* and *KRTAP4-5* in the development of colon adenomas and in their progression to CRC remains largely unknown. The comparison of the mutational profile observed in non-advanced CADs, advanced CADs and CRCs showed that: *PIK3CA* and *SMAD* mutations are absent in CADs; *APC* mutations are increasing from non-advanced to advanced CADs; *KRAS* and *TP53* mutations are progressively increasing in the progression from non-advanced to advanced CADs and then to CRCs [80]. The identification of some CRC-specific mutated genes, absent in CADs, provides a tool for distinguishing between adenomas and CRCs and supports the view that some mutational events are essential for the transition from benign adenomas to CRCs [80].

Lee and coworkers reported the mutational profiling by whole-exome sequencing of 12 high-grade colon adenomas (HGCAs, 11 non-hypermutated and 1 hypermutated). This analysis showed that total numbers and spectrum of somatic mutations detected in HGCAs were not consistently different from those observed in CRCs [81]. The most recurrent gene alterations observed in these tumors consisted in mutations of *APC*, *KRAS*, *SMAD4*, *ERBB4*, *AMER1*, and *TP53* genes, copy number loss of *SMAD4*, and copy number gain of *GNAS* and *ARID2* genes [81]. The peculiar finding of this study was related to the observation that mono-allelic inactivation of *SMAD4* may occur in HGCAs.

Druliner and coworkers have recently reported the analysis of cancer-adjacent polyps (CAPs) and cancer-free polyps (CFPs): CAP cases included matched, distant normal colon epithelium, the polyp (residual polyp of origin) and the corresponding cancer that arose from the polyp, whereas CFP cases include matched, distant normal colonic epithelium and colon adenoma (polyp) [82]. The mutational spectrum of CAPs and CFPs was explored by wide exome sequencing; the majority of the top 10 genes involved in CRC tumorigenesis had a mutational frequency higher in CAPs than in CFPs: *TP53*, *FBXW7*, *PIK3CA*, *KIAA1804*, *SMAD2*, and *SMAD4* were almost exclusively mutated in CAPs [82]. Thus, the CAPs displayed an increased number of genetic variants as compared to the CFPs and the genes preferentially or exclusively mutated in the CAPs were enriched for cancer pathways [82]. Some genes, *GREM1*, *IGF2*, *CTGF*, and *PLAU* displayed significant changes between CFPs and CAPs [82].

In a recent study, Cross and coworkers have mapped the evolutionary landscape of CRAs and CRCs through the study of multi-targeted whole genome sequencing on 2–16 regions from 9 CRAs and 15 CRCs [83]. The mutational frequency (single nucleotide alterations) was similar in CRAs and CRCs; the burden of driver mutations was similar in CRAs and CRCs. Individual driver gene mutations were detected at similar frequencies across CRAs and CRCs, with the exception of TP53, which was more commonly mutated in CRCs than in CRAs [83]. Intra-tumor heterogeneity and phylogenetic analyses suggest that CRCs occupy sharper fitness peaks that CRAs: 56% of CRA single nucleotide alterations (SNAs) were subclonal, while only 45% of CRC SNAs were subclonal. The phylogenetic trees of CRAs have shorter trunks and longer branches/leaves than those of CRCs; CRAs were more heterogeneous than CRCs, suggesting that the former occupy a broader fitness peak than the latter ones [83]. The analysis of non-synonymous mutations to synonymous mutations on the branches/leaves of CRCs relative to their trunks, but not of CRAs, possibly suggesting a possible positive subclonal selection in CRAs; these findings suggest that subclonal selection is absent/weak at the level of established CRC [83]. The driver gene alterations can be subdivided into tier 1 mutations (mutations or gene alterations playing a defined role in CRC pathogenesis) and tier 2 mutations (gene alterations of uncertain pathogenic role or pan-cancer genes): tier 1 driver mutations were very frequently clonal in both CRAs (80%) and CRCs (89%); tier 2 driver mutations were less frequently clonal in CRAs (47%), compared to CRC (80%) [83]. The analysis of copy number alterations showed some remarkable differences between CRAs and CRCs: Adenomas had fewer CNAs than CRCs and the overall average proportion of the genome disrupted by CNAs was lower in adenomas (40%) than in CRCs (72%) [83]. Driver CNAs in CRC involve losses of chromosomes 5q (*APC*), 17p (*TP53*) and 18q (*SMAD4*): 17p loss occurred more frequently in CRCs than in CRAs, whereas loss of 5q and 18q occurred at similar frequencies in CRAs and CRCs [83]. 78% of CN gains were subclonal in CRAs compared to 48% in CRCs; 57% and 27% of CN losses were subclonal in CRAs and CRCs, respectively [83]. The evolution of CRC involves either a punctuated or a more gradual CNA acquisition [83]. Finally, the analysis of few MSI$^+$ CRCs indicate that these tumors evolve in a similar way to MSS CRCs, with a higher mutational burden and with a more limited evidence of subclonal selection [83]. The ensemble of these observations suggests that CRAs can harbor mutations in any CRC driver gene and driver acquisition does not necessarily involves selective sweeps, inducing stepwise evolution of the tumors, as supported by the finding that subclones with additional driver mutations do not replace subclones lacking these driver mutations, but co-exist in different areas of the tumors [84].

8.3. The Classical Linear Progression Model and the Big Bang Model

The classical linear progression model implies that a CRA is initiated by two genetic alterations at the level of the *APC* gene and progresses to invasive CRC through a progressive, stepwise acquisition of additional genetic alterations involving driver gene mutations such as *KRAS* and *TP53* and deletion of chromosome 18q4 [74]. The evolutionary dynamics of this process is governed by a series of progressive selective sweeps to fixation, each involving the progressive development of subclones exhibiting increasing fitness, due to the acquisition of new driver mutations [32].

Using early index-lesion sequencing and a mathematical model helping to translate the mutational events into distance of time, it was estimated a shorter time required for the development of metastases from advanced CRC (1.8 yeas) than for the development of an advanced CRC from a colon adenoma (17 years) [32].

In 2015, Sottoriva and coworkers proposed the "Big Bang" model of human colorectal tumor evolution, based on the assumption that these tumors are genetically heterogeneous from their initiation and subsequent genetic alterations are changes of their original ancestral cancer-driving alterations [85]. Several observations support the Big Band model: (i) Intratumor heterogeneity is a "constitutive" property of CRCs arising from their initiation and increasing with their progressive growth, not significantly influenced by events of clonal selection; this spontaneous propensity to intra-tumor heterogeneity predisposes the CRCs to a branched phylogeny pattern of growth. (ii) Marked clonal expansions or selective sweeps are rare events at the level of CRCs at an advanced stage of tumor development. (iii) Both universal and private genetic alterations originate early during tumor development a become widespread during tumor progression, thus becoming the dominating elements in the genetic structure of developed CRCs. (iv) Aggressive subclones are present in the primary tumor and remain rare; however, these subclones have a relative fitness advantage that contributes to fuel resistance to drug treatments and may become dominant under these circumstances [85].

Several observations directly support this theory. In fact, Kang et al [86] have explored the mutational heterogeneity of colorectal adenomas and reached the conclusion that these tumors display the presence of private mutations in different parts of the same tumor. This consistent intratumor heterogeneity originates from the first tumor divisions [86]. Sievers have investigated the mutational landscape of small colorectal polyps and showed that these tumors carried 0–3 driver pathogenic mutations, the most frequent being *APC, KRAS, TP53, BRAF, FBXW7*, and *BRAF* mutations [87]. About 31% of small polyps display two or more pathogenic mutations, with variable allelic frequencies, a finding supporting the presence of multiple tumor cell populations [87].

The large majority of driver mutations are clonal and arise before the start of tumor expansion, thus explaining the existence of only a minimal driver gene heterogeneity among untreated CRC metastases [88]. The rarity of subclonal driver mutations supports the view that subclones may differ by the selective presence of passenger mutations progressively accumulating during growth: these subclones have similar fitness and occupy different tumor regions, thus generating ITH and their size is mainly dependent on the timing of their generation during the process of tumor evolution [89].

Additional evidence in favor of the "Big Bang" model tumor growth comes from additional recent studies. Thus, Williams et al [90] have explored whether the subclonal mutant allele frequencies of a part of cancers of different origin follow a model of tumor evolution based on simple power-law distribution, as predicted by neutral growth. This analysis provided evidence that other cancers, such as stomach, bladder, lung and cervical cancers, as well as CRCs, follow a model of tumor evolution bye neutral growth [90]. In these malignancies, after an initial single tumor expansion, characterized by the formation of multiple heterogeneous subclones that, in spite their genetic heterogeneity, initially grow at comparable rates, without overtaking one another; thus, in these tumors, all clonal selection events occur at a very early stage of tumor development and not in late-developing subclones, thus resulting in the generation of numerous passenger mutations, involved in the generation of intra-tumor heterogeneity [90].

It is commonly believed that passenger mutations have no role in cancer development. However, many passenger mutations fall within protein-coding genes and, although individually weak, these mutations tend to accumulate during tumor progression evading negative selection mechanisms, and in their collective burden, alter the course of tumor progression [91,92].

Lineage tracing experiments in human colorectal adenomas further support the "Bing Bang" theory of colony cancer development [93]. These experiments led to the identification of multipotential stem cells within human colorectal adenomas, responsible for the development and maintenance of these tumors. The study of methylation patterns of non-expressed genes, as well as the analysis of genetic lesions in micro dissected individual crypts from colonic adenomas were used to characterize clonal evolution of these tumors [93]. The analysis of individual crypts within each adenoma showed that adenomatous crypts are clonal populations maintained by multipotential stem cells; individual crypts from each adenoma display different methylation patterns; intratumor clones present in some colonic adenomas are epigenetically homogeneous [93]. The results of this study were compatible with a model of colorectal adenoma evolution not based on continual steady growth but on an initial burst of tumor growth, followed by relative quiescence; the tumor clones form at the initial stages of tumor development but not sweep through the tumor and are present as localized with divergent intraclone methylation patterns. Rare subclones are generated later during tumor development, exhibit homogeneous methylation patterns, and are localized at the level of focal regions of the tumor [93].

Studies of the spatial distribution of genetic alterations within a tumor by phylogeography, an approach that combines tumor phylogeny or the ancestral relationships of tumor subclones with their spatial physical locations in the tumor, allows to visualize how tumors spread [94]. The spatial analysis of private mutations in early CRCs, combining multiregional sequencing with mathematical multiscale models showed the existence of spatial mutation patterns in these tumors, supporting the existence of early colorectal tumor cell mobility, a tumor cell property required for generating ITH [95].

The analysis of epigenetic ITH into CRCs analyzing opposite tumor sides showed evidence of little ITH or stepwise selection during tumor development, suggesting that the epigenome observed in various tumor regions reflects that of its founder cells; despite epigenomic conservation, RNA expression displayed significant variation between individual tumor regions, seemingly due to mechanisms of continue adaptation related to phenotypic plasticity [96].

Saturation microdissection and targeted deep resequencing have shown that CRCs are jigsaw arrayed in millimeter-wide columns sharing common phenotypes rather than being arranged horizontally by phenotype [97]. Most of the large subclones thus identified shared both invasive and superficial phenotype; subclones with invasive phenotypes arose from both early and late phylogenetic branches [97]. This pattern of phylogeography is consistent with single tumor expansions by founder cells possessing all the driver mutations required to sustain tumor growth rather than a stepwise mechanism involving progressive invasions by a minority of subclones at various levels of progression [97]. Particularly, on 11 CRCs analyzed in this study, two out of 11 displayed private driver mutations, while nine in 11 did not have private driver mutations, showing evidence of multiclonal invasion, and invasive and metastatic subclones originate early during tumor development [97].

In conclusion, the analysis of the genetic heterogeneity observed at the level of CRCs is compatible with a "Big Bang" expansion model, characterized by an early phase of tumor growth consisting in a single cell expansion; this initial tumor expansion generates a large number of early-arising clones, coexisting within the tumor for long periods of time for the absence of a selective pressure [98]. This weak selection was insufficient to determine large clonal expansions in short times. This finding supports the view that the large part of tumor heterogeneity is generated early during tumor development, at a stage where the tumor is still undetectable at clinical level [98].

9. Conclusions

About half of CRCs develop metastases and metastatic spreading is the main cause of CRC-related death. The dynamics and the molecular processes remain largely unknown. Several recent studies have shown that systemic spread can occur early in CRC development. Recent studies have reported a detailed analysis of the genomic landscape of metastatic CRC patients underlying the molecular heterogeneity of these patients and the possibility to identify some therapeutic targets in these patients. The study of molecular evolution of CRCs suggest that these tumors may evolve either through a process of subclonal selection or neutral evolution.

A better understanding of the cellular and molecular processes governing CRC metastasis spreading will be necessary to improve the outcome of metastatic CRC patients.

Although the survival rate of patients with metastatic CRC patients improved in the last years, the response to current treatments and prognosis of patients bearing *KRAS*, *NRAS*, and *BRAF* mutations remain still poor. Therefore, there is an absolute need to identify these patients and to discover new improvements for therapeutic vulnerabilities and to formulate rational prospective personalized therapies aiming to improve their survival chances.

Funding: This research received no external funding.

Conflicts of Interest: The authors declare no conflict of interest.

References

1. Dekker, E.; Tanis, P.J.; Valengels, J.; Kass, P.M.; Wallace, M.B. Colorectal cancer. *Lancet* **2019**, *394*, 1467–1480. [CrossRef]
2. Mullert, M.F.; Ibrahim, A.; Arends, M.J. Molecular pathological classification of colorectal cancer. *Wirchows Arch.* **2016**, *469*, 125–134. [CrossRef] [PubMed]
3. Walther, A.; Houlston, R.; Toulinson, I. Association between chromosomal instability and prognosis in colorectal cancer: A meta-analysis. *Gut* **2008**, *57*, 941–950. [CrossRef] [PubMed]
4. The Cancer Genome Atlas Network. Comprehensive molecular characterization of human colon and rectal cancer. *Nature* **2012**, *487*, 330–337. [CrossRef] [PubMed]
5. Zhang, B.; Wang, J.; Wang, X.; Zhu, J.; Liu, Q.; Shi, Z.; Chambers, M.C.; Zimmerman, L.J.; Shaddox, K.F. Proteogenomic characterization of human colon and rectal cancer. *Nature* **2014**, *513*, 382–387. [CrossRef]
6. Ried, T.; Meijer, G.A.; Harrison, D.J.; Grech, G.; Franch-Esposito, S.; Briffa, R.; Carvalho, B.; Campos, J. The landscape of genomic copy number alterations in colorectal cancer and their consequences on gene expression levels and disease outcome. *Mol. Asp. Med.* **2019**, *69*, 48–61. [CrossRef]
7. Guinney, J.; Dienstmann, R.; Wang, X.; De Reynies, A.; Schilker, A.; Soneson, C.; Marisa, L.; Roepman, P.; Nyamundanda, G.; Angelino, P.; et al. The consensus molecular subtypes of colorectal cancer. *Nat. Med.* **2015**, *21*, 1350–1356. [CrossRef]
8. Okita, A.; Takahashi, S.; Ouchi, K.; Inuoe, M.; Watanabe, M.; Endo, M.; Honda, H.; Yamada, Y.; Ishioka, C. Consensus molecular subtypes classification of colorectal cancer as a predictive factor for chemotherapeutic efficacy again st metastatic colorectal cancer. *Oncotarget* **2018**, *9*, 18698–18711. [CrossRef]

9. Mooi, J.K.; Wirapati, P.; Asher, R.; Lee, C.K.; Savas, P.; Price, T.J.; Towsend, A.; Hardingham, J.; Buchanan, D.; Williams, D.; et al. The prognostic impact of consensus molecular subtypes (CMS) and its predictive effects for bevacizumab benefit in metastatic colorectal cancer: Molecular analysis of the AGITG MAX clinical trial. *Ann. Oncol.* **2018**, *29*, 2240–2246. [CrossRef]
10. Stintzing, S.; Wirapati, P.; Lenz, H.J.; Neureiter, D.; Fisher von Weikersthal, L.; Decker, T.; Kiani, A.; Kaiser, F.; Al-Batran, S.; Heingtes, T.; et al. Consensus molecular subgroups (CMS) of colorectal cancer (CRC) and first-line efficacy of FOLFIRI plus cetuximab or bevacizumab in the FIRE3 (AIO KRK-0306) trial. *Ann. Oncol.* **2019**, *30*, 1796–1803. [CrossRef]
11. Becht, E.; de Reyniès, A.; Giraldo, N.A.; Pilati, C.; Buttard, B.; Lacroix, L.; Selves, J.; Sautès-Fridman, C.; Laurent-Puig, P.; Fridman, W.H. Immune and stromal classification of colorectal cancer is associated with molecular subtypes and relevant for precision immunotherapy. *Clin. Cancer Res.* **2016**, *22*, 4057–4066. [CrossRef] [PubMed]
12. Isella, C.; Brundu, F.; Bellomo, S.E.; Galimi, F.; Zanella, E.; Porporato, R.; Petti, C.; Fiori, A.; Orzan, F.; Senetta, R.; et al. Selective analysis of cancer-cell intrinsic transcriptional traits defines novel clinically relevant subtypes of colorectal cancer. *Nat. Commun.* **2017**, *8*, 15107. [CrossRef] [PubMed]
13. Tieng, F.; Baharudin, R.; Abu, N.; Yunos, R.I.; Lee, L.H.; Mutalib, N.S. Single cell transcriptomic in colorectal cancer-current updates on its application in metastasis, chemoresistance and the roles of circulating tumor cells. *Fron. Pharmacol.* **2020**, *11*, 135. [CrossRef] [PubMed]
14. Li, H.; Courtois, E.; Sengupta, D.; Tan, Y.; Chen, K.H.; Goh, J.; Kong, S.L.; Chua, C.; Hon, L.K.; Tan, W.S.; et al. Reference component analysis of single-cell transcriptomes elucidates cellular heterogeneity in human colorectal tumors. *Nat. Genet.* **2017**, *49*, 708–718. [CrossRef] [PubMed]
15. Uhlitz, F.; Bischoff, P.; Sieber, A.; Obermayer, B.; Blanc, E.; Luthen, M.; Sawitzki, B.; Kamphues, C.; Beule, D.; Sers, C.; et al. A census of cell types and paracrine interactions in colorectal cancer. *bioRxiv* **2020**. [CrossRef]
16. Zhang, Y.; Zheng, L.; Zhang, L.; Hu, X.; Ren, X.; Zhang, Z. Deep single-cell RNA sequencing data of individual T cells from treatment-naïve colorectal cancer patients. *Sci. Data* **2019**, *6*, 131. [CrossRef]
17. Zhang, L.; Li, Z.; Skrzypczynska, K.M.; Fang, Q.; Zhang, W.; O'Brien, S.; He, Y.; Wang, L.; Zhang, Q.; Kim, A.; et al. Single-cell analyses inform mechanisms of myeloid-targeted therapies in colon cancer. *Cell* **2020**, *181*, 442–459. [CrossRef]
18. Kamal, Y.; Schmit, S.L.; Hoehn, H.J.; Amos, C.I.; Frost, H.R. Transcriptomic differences between primary colorectal adenocarcinomas and distant metastases reveal metastatic colorectal cancer subtypes. *Cancer Res.* **2019**, *79*, 4227–4241. [CrossRef]
19. Lieu, C.H.; Golemis, E.A.; Serebriiskii, I.G.; Newberg, J.; Hemmerich, A.; Connelly, C.; Messersmith, W.A.; Eng, C.; Eckardt, S.G.; Frampton, G.; et al. Comprehensive genomic landscapes in early and later onset colorectal cancer. *Clin. Cancer Res.* **2019**, *25*, 5852–5858. [CrossRef]
20. Dienstmann, R.; Salazar, R.; Tabernero, J. Molecular subtypes and the evolution of treatment decisions in metastatic colorectal cancer. *ASCO Educ. Book* **2018**, *38*, 231–238. [CrossRef]
21. Xie, Y.H.; Chen, Y.X.; Fang, J.Y. Comprehensive review of targeted therapy for colorectal cancer. *Signal Transduct. Target. Ther.* **2020**, *5*, 22. [CrossRef] [PubMed]
22. Zehir, A.; Benayed, R.; Shahm, R.K.; Syed, A.; Middha, S.; Kiom, H.R.; Srinivasan, P.; Gao, J.; Chakravarty, D.; Sevlin, S.M.; et al. Mutational landscape of metastatic cancer revealed from prospective clinical sequencing of 10,000 patients. *Nat. Med.* **2017**, *23*, 703–713. [CrossRef] [PubMed]
23. Priestley, P.; Baber, J.; Lolkema, M.P.; Steeghs, N.; de Brujn, E.; Shale, C.; Duyvesteyn, K.; Haidari, S.; van Hoeck, A.; Onstenk, W.; et al. Pan-cancer whole-genome analyses of metastatic solid tumours. *Nature* **2019**, *575*, 210–216. [CrossRef] [PubMed]
24. Yaeger, R.; Chatila, W.; Lipsyc, M.; Hechtman, J.; Cercek, A.; Sanchez-Vega, F.; Jayakumaran, G.; Middha, S.; Zehir, A.; Donoghue, M.; et al. Clinical sequencing defines the genomic landscape of metastatic colorectal cancer. *Cancer Cell* **2018**, *33*, 125–136. [CrossRef]
25. Belardinilli, F.; Capalbo, C.; Malapelle, U.; Pisapia, P.; Raimondo, D.; Milanetti, E.; Yasaman, M.; Liccardi, C.; Paci, P.; Sibilio, P.; et al. Clinical multigene panel sequencing identifies mutational association patterns in metastatic colorectal cancer. *Front. Oncol.* **2020**, *10*, 560. [CrossRef]
26. Barras, D.; Missiagnia, E.; Wirapati, P.; Sieber, O.M.; Jorissen, R.N.; Love, C.; Molloy, P.L.; Jones, I.T.; McLaughlin, S.; Gibbs, P.; et al. BRAF V600E mutant colorectal cancer subtypes based on gene expression. *Clin. Cancer Res.* **2017**, *23*, 104–115. [CrossRef]

27. Jones, J.C.; Renfro, L.A.; Al-Shamsi, O.; Achrock, A.B.; Rankin, A.; Zhang, B.Y.; Kasi, P.M.; Voss, J.S.; Leal, A.D.; Sun, J.; et al. Non-V600BRAF mutations define a clinically distinct molecular subtype of metastatic colorectal cancer. *J. Clin. Oncol.* **2017**, *35*, 2624–2630. [CrossRef]
28. Yao, Z.; Yaeger, R.; Rodrik-Outmezguine, V.S.; Tao, A.; Torres, N.M.; Chang, M.T.; Drosten, M.; Zhao, H.; Cecchi, F.; Hembrough, T.; et al. Tumours with class 3 BRAF mutants are sensitive to the inhibition of activated RAS. *Nature* **2017**, *548*, 234–238. [CrossRef]
29. Cremolini, C.; Di Bartolomeo, M.; Amatu, A.; Antoniotti, C.; Moretto, R.; Berenato, R.; Perrone, F.; Tamborini, E.; Aprile, G.; Lonerdi, S.; et al. BRAF codons 594 and 596 mutations identify a new molecular subtype of metastatic colorecxtal cancer at favorable prognosis. *Ann. Oncol.* **2015**, *26*, 2092–2097. [CrossRef]
30. Schrippa, M.; Biason, P.; Lonardi, S.; Pella, N.; Pina, M.S.; Urbano, F.; Antoniotti, C.; Cremolini, C.; Corallo, S.; Pietrantonio, F.; et al. Class 1, 2, and 3 BRAF-mutated metastatic colorectal cancer: A detailed clinical, pathologic, and molecular characterization. *Clin. Cancer Res.* **2019**, *27*, 3954–3961. [CrossRef]
31. Riihimaki, M.; Hemminki, A.; Sundquist, J.; Hemminki, K. Patterns of metastasis in colon and rectal cancer. *Sci. Rep.* **2016**, *6*, 29765. [CrossRef] [PubMed]
32. Jones, B.; Chen, W.; Parmigiani, G.; Diehl, F.; Beerenwinkel, N.; Antal, T.; Traulsen, A.; Nowak, M.A.; Siegel, C.; Velculescu, A.; et al. Comparative lesion sequencing provides insights into tumor evolution. *Proc. Natl. Acad. Sci. USA* **2008**, *105*, 4283–4288. [CrossRef]
33. Vakiani, E.; Janakiraman, M.; Shen, R.; Sinha, R.; Zeng, Z.; Shia, J.; Cercek, A.; Kemeny, N.; D'Angelica, M.; Viale, A. Comparative genomic analysis of primary versus metastatic colorectal carcinomas. *J. Clin. Oncol.* **2012**, *30*, 2956–2962. [CrossRef] [PubMed]
34. Brannon, A.R.; Vakiani, E.; Sylvester, B.E.; Scott, S.N.; McDermott, G.; Shah, R.H.; Kania, K.; Viale, A.; Oschwald, D.M.; Vacic, V.; et al. Comparative sequencing analysis reveals high genomic concordance between matched primary and metastatic colorectal cancer lesions. *Genome Biol.* **2014**, *13*, 454. [CrossRef] [PubMed]
35. Vermaat, J.S.; Nijman, I.J.; Koudjis, M.J.; Gerritse, F.L.; Scherer, F.J.; Mokry, M.; Roessingh, W.M.; Lansu, N.; de Brujin, E.; van Hillegersberg, R.; et al. Primary colorectal cancers and their subsequent hepatic metastases are genetically different: Implications for selection of patients for targeted treatment. *Clin. Cancer Res.* **2012**, *18*, 688–699. [CrossRef] [PubMed]
36. Lim, B.; Mun, J.; Kim, J.H.; Kim, C.W.; Roh, S.A.; Cho, D.H.; Kim, Y.S.; Kim, S.Y.; Kim, J.C. Genome-wide mutation profiles of colorectal tumors and associated liver metastases at the exome and transcriptome levels. *Oncotarget* **2015**, *26*, 22179–22190. [CrossRef] [PubMed]
37. Vignot, S.; Lefebvre, C.; Frampton, G.M.; Stephens, P.J.; Soria, J.C.; Spano, J.P. Comparative analysis of primary tumour and matched metastases in colorectal cancer patients: Evaluation of concordance between genomic and transcriptomic profiles. *Eur. J. Cancer* **2015**, *51*, 791–799. [CrossRef] [PubMed]
38. Tan, I.B.; Malik, S.; Ramnarayanan, K.; McPherson, J.R.; Ho, D.L.; Suzuki, Y.; Ng, S.B.; Yan, S.; Lim, K.H.; Koh, D.; et al. High-depth sequencing of over 750 genes supports linear progression of primary tumors and metastases in most patients with liver-limited metastatic colorectal cancer. *Genome Biol.* **2019**, *16*, 32. [CrossRef]
39. Kim, K.P.; Kim, J.E.; Hong, Y.S.; Ahn, S.M.; Chun, S.M.; Hong, S.M.; Jang, S.J.; Yu, C.S.; Kim, J.C.; Kim, T.W. Paired primary and metastatic tumor analysis of somatic mutations in synchronous and metachronous colorectal cancer. *Cancer Res. Treat.* **2017**, *49*, 161–167. [CrossRef]
40. Fujiyoshi, K.; Yamamoto, G.; Takahashi, A.; Arai, Y.; Yamada, M.; Kakuta, M.; Yamaguchi, K.; Akagi, Y.; Nishimura, Y.; Sakamoto, H.; et al. High concordance rate of KRAS/BRAF mutations and MSI-H between primary and corresponding metastases. *Oncol. Rep.* **2017**, *37*, 785–792. [CrossRef]
41. Jesinghaus, M.; Wolf, T.; Pfarr, N.; Muckenhuber, A.; Ahadova, A.; Warth, A.; Goeppert, B.; Sers, C.; Kloor, M.; Endris, V.; et al. Distinctive spatiotemporal stability of somatic mutations in metastasized microsatellite-stable colorectal cancer. *Am. J. Surg. Pathol.* **2015**, *39*, 1140–1147. [CrossRef] [PubMed]
42. Isaque, N.; Abba, M.L.; Huaser, C.; Patil, N.; Paramasivan, N.; Huebschmann, D.; Leupold, J.H.; Balusabramanian, G.P.; Kleinheinz, K.; Poprak, U.H.; et al. Whole genome sequencing put forward hypotheses on metastasis evaluation and therapy in colorectal cancer. *Nat. Commun.* **2018**, *9*, 4782. [CrossRef] [PubMed]

43. Kawamata, F.; Patch, A.M.; Nones, K.; Bond, C.; McKeone, K.; Pearson, S.A.; Homma, S.; Liu, C.; Fennell, L.; Dumenil, T.; et al. Copy number profiles of paired primary and metastatic colorectal cancers. *Oncotarget* **2018**, *9*, 3394–3405. [CrossRef]
44. Smeets, D.; Miller, I.S.; O'Connor, D.P.; Das, S.; Moran, B.; Boeckx, B.; Gaiser, T.; Betge, J.; Barat, A.; Klinger, R.; et al. Copy number load predicts outcome of metastatic colorectal cancer patients receiving bevacizumab combination therapy. *Nat. Commun.* **2008**, *9*, 4112. [CrossRef] [PubMed]
45. Bhullar, D.S.; Barriuso, J.; Mullamitha, S.; Saunders, M.P.; O'Dwyer, S.T.; Aziz, O. Biomarker concordance between primary colorectal cancer and its metastases. *EBioMedicine* **2019**, *40*, 363–374. [CrossRef]
46. Molinari, C.; Marisi, G.; Passardi, A.; Matteucci, L.; De Maio, G.; Ulivi, P. Heterogeneity in colorectal cancer: A challenge for personalized medicine? *Int. J. Med. Sci.* **2018**, *19*, 3733. [CrossRef]
47. Baisse, B.; Bouzorene, H.; Saraga, E.P.; Bosman, F.T.; Benhattar, J. Intratumor genetic heterogeneity in advanced human colorectal adenocarcinoma. *Int. J. Cancer* **2001**, *93*, 346–352. [CrossRef]
48. Jeantet, M.; Tougeron, D.; Tachon, G.; Cortes, U.; Archambaut, C.; Fromont, G.; Karayan-Tapon, L. High intra- and inter-tumoral heterogeneity of RAS mutations in colorectal cancer. *Int. J. Mol.* **2016**, *17*, 2015. [CrossRef]
49. Kim, T.M.; Jung, S.H.; An, C.H.; Lee, S.H.; Baek, I.P.; Kim, M.S.; Park, S.W.; Rhee, J.K.; Lee, S.H.; Chung, Y.J. Subclonal genomic architectures of primary and metastatic colorectal cancer based on intratumoral genetic heterogeneity. *Clin. Cancer Res.* **2015**, *21*, 4461–4472. [CrossRef]
50. Sveen, A.; Loes, I.M.; Alagaratnam, S.; Nilsen, G.; Høland, M.; Lingjærde, O.C.; Sorbye, H.; Berg, K.C.; Horn, A.; Angelsen, J.H.; et al. Intra-patient inter-metastatic genetic heterogeneity in colorectal cancer as a key determinant of survival after curative liver resection. *PLoS Genet.* **2016**, *12*, e1006225. [CrossRef]
51. Uchi, R.; Takahashi, Y.; Niida, A.; Shimamura, T.; Hirata, H.; Sugimachi, K.; Sawada, G.; Iwaya, T.; Kurashige, J.; Shinden, Y.; et al. Integrated multiregional analysis proposing a new model of colorectal cancer evolution. *PLoS Genet.* **2016**, *12*, e1005778. [CrossRef] [PubMed]
52. Saito, T.; Niida, A.; Uchi, R.; Hirata, H.; Komatsu, H.; Sakimura, S.; Hayashi, S.; Nambara, S.; Kurada, Y. A temporal shift of the evolutionary principle shaping intratumor heterogeneity in colorectal cancer. *Nat. Commun.* **2018**, *9*, 2884. [CrossRef] [PubMed]
53. Wei, Q.; Ye, Z.; Zhong, X.; Li, L.; Wang, C.; Myers, R.E.; Palazzo, J.P.; Fortuna, D.; Yan, A.; Waldman, S.A.; et al. Multiregion whole-exome sequencing of matched primary and metastatic tumors revealed genomic heterogeneity and suggested polyclonal seeding in colorectal cancer metastasis. *Ann. Oncol.* **2017**, *28*, 2135–2141. [CrossRef] [PubMed]
54. Suzuki, Y.; Ng, S.B.; Chua, C.; Leow, W.Q.; Chng, J.; Liu, S.Y.; Ramnarayanan, K.; Gan, A.; Ho, D.L. Multiregion ultra-deep sequencing reveals early intermixing and variable levels of intratumoral heterogeneity in colorectal cancer. *Mol. Oncol.* **2017**, *11*, 124–139. [CrossRef] [PubMed]
55. Oh, B.; Shin, H.T.; Yun, J.W.; Kim, K.T.; Kim, J.; Bae, J.S.; Cho, Y.B.; Lee, W.Y.; Park, Y.A.; Im, Y.H.; et al. Intratumor heterogeneity inferred from targeted deep sequencing as a prognostic indicator. *Scient. Rep.* **2019**, *9*, 4542. [CrossRef] [PubMed]
56. Kreso, A.; O'Brien, C.A.; van Galen, P.; Gan, O.I.; Notta, F.; Brown, A.; Ng, K.; Ma, J.; Wienholds, E.; Dumont, C.; et al. Variable clonal repopulation dynamics influence chemotherapy response in colorectal cancer. *Science* **2013**, *339*, 543–548. [CrossRef]
57. Chun, Y.S.; Passot, G.; Yamashita, S.; Nusrat, M.; Katsonis, P.; Loree, J.M.; Conrad, C.; Tzeng, C.W.; Xiao, L.; Aloia, T.A.; et al. Deleterious effect of RAS and evolutionary high-risk TP53 double mutation in colorectal liver metastases. *Ann. Surg.* **2019**, *269*, 917–923. [CrossRef]
58. Margonis, G.; Buettner, S.; Andreatos, N.; Kim, Y.; Wagner, D.; Sasaki, K.; Beer, A.; Schwartz, C.; Loes, I.M.; Smolle, M.; et al. Association of BRAF mutations with survival and recurrence in surgically treated patients with metastatic colorectal liver cancer. *JAMA Surg.* **2018**, *153*, e180996. [CrossRef]
59. Datta, J.; Smith, J.J.; Cjhatila, W.K.; McAuliffe, J.C.; Kandoth, C.; Valdani, E.; Frankel, T.L.; Ganesh, K.; Wasserman, I.; Lipsyc-Sharf, M.; et al. Co-altered Ras/B-raf and TP53 is associated with extremes of survivorship and distinct patterns of metastasis in patients with metastatic colorectal cancer. *Clin. Cancer Res.* **2020**, *26*, 1077–1085. [CrossRef]
60. Kawaguchi, Y.; Kopetz, S.; Newhook, T.E.; De Bellis, M.; Chey, J.N.; Chun, Y.S.; Tzeng, C.W.; Aloia, T.A.; Vauthey, J.N. Mutation status of RAS, TP53, and SMAD4 is superior to mutation status of RAS alone for predicting prognosis after resection of colorectal liver metastases. *Clin. Cancer Res.* **2019**, *25*, 5843–5851. [CrossRef]

61. Smith, J.J.; Chatila, W.K.; Sanchez-Vega, F.; Datta, J.; Connell, L.C.; Szeglin, B.C.; Basunia, A.; Boucher, T.M.; Hauser, H.; Wasserman, I.; et al. Genomic stratification beyond Ras/B-Raf in colorectal liver metastasis patients treated with hepatic arterial infusion. *Cancer Med.* **2019**, *8*, 6538–6548. [CrossRef] [PubMed]
62. Leung, M.L.; Davis, A.; Gao, R.; Casasent, A.; Wang, Y.; Sei, E.; Vilar, E.; Maru, D.; Kopetz, S.; Navin, N.E.; et al. Single-cell DNA sequencing reveals a late-dissemination model in metastatic colorectal cancer. *Genome Res.* **2017**, *27*, 1287–1299. [CrossRef] [PubMed]
63. Chang, G.J.; Rodrigiuez-Bigas, M.A.; Skibber, J.M.; Mayer, V.A. Lymph nodes evaluation and survival after curative resection of colon cancer: Systematic review. *J. Natl. Cancer Inst.* **2007**, *99*, 433–441. [CrossRef]
64. Naxerova, K.; Reiter, J.G.; Bratchel, E.; Lennerz, J.; Van de Wetering, M.; Rowan, A.; Cai, T.; Clevers, H.; Swanton, C.; Nowak, M.A.; et al. Origins of lymphatic and distant metastases in human colorectal cancer. *Science* **2017**, *357*, 55–60. [CrossRef]
65. Ulintz, P.J.; Greenson, J.K.; Wu, R.; Fearon, E.R.; Hardiman, K.M. Lymph node metastases in colon cancer are polyclonal. *Clin. Cancer Res.* **2017**, *24*, 2214–2224. [CrossRef] [PubMed]
66. Hu, Z.; Ding, J.; Ma, Z.; Sun, R.; Soane, J.A.; Shaffer, J.S.; Suarez, C.J.; Berghoff, A.S.; Cremolini, C.; Falcone, A.; et al. Quantitative evidence for early metastatic seeding in colorectal cancer. *Nat. Genet.* **2019**, *51*, 1113–1122. [CrossRef] [PubMed]
67. Hu, Z.; Li, Z.; Ma, Z.; Curtis, C. Multi-cancer analysis of clonality and the timing of systemic spread in paired primary tumors and metastases. *Nat. Genet* **2020**, *52*, 701–708. [CrossRef] [PubMed]
68. Garcia-Carbonero, N.; Martinez-Useros, J.; Li, W.; Orta, A.; Perez, N.; Carames, C.; Hernandez, T.; Moreno, I.; Serrano, G.; Garcia-Foncillas, J. KRAS and BRAF mutations as prognostic and predictive biomarkers for standard chemotherapy response in metastatic colorectal cancer: A single institutional study. *Cells* **2020**, *9*, 219. [CrossRef]
69. Misala, S.; Yaeger, R.; Hober, S.; Scala, E.; Janckraman, M.; Liska, D.; Valtorta, E.; Schiavo, R.; Buscarino, M.; Siravegna, G.; et al. Emergence of KRAS mutations and acquired resistance to anti EGFR therapy in colorectal cancer. *Nature* **2012**, *486*, 532–536. [CrossRef]
70. Bertotti, A.; Papp, E.; Jones, S.; Adleff, V.; Anagnostou, V.; Lupo, B.; Sausen, M.; Phallen, J.; Hrubau, C.A.; Tokheim, C.; et al. The genomic landscape of response to EGFR blockade in colorectal cancer. *Nature* **2015**, *526*, 263–267. [CrossRef]
71. Russo, M.; Siravegna, G.; Blazkowsky, L.S.; Corti, G.; Crisafulli, G.; Ahronian, L.G.; Mussolin, B.; Kwak, E.L.; Buscorino, M.; Lazzari, L.; et al. Tumor heterogeneity and lesion-specific response to targeted therapy in colorectal cancer. *Cancer Discov.* **2016**, *6*, 147–153. [CrossRef] [PubMed]
72. Bertotti, A.; Milgiardi, G.; Galimi, F.; Sassi, F.; Torti, D.; Isella, C.; Corà, D.; Di Nicolantonio, F.; Buscarino, M.; Petti, F.; et al. A molecularly annotated platform of patient-derived xenografts ("xenopatients") identified HER2 as an effective therapeutic target in cetuximab-resistant colorectal cancer. *Cancer Discov.* **2011**, *1*, 508–523. [CrossRef]
73. Sartore-Bianchi, A.; Trusolino, L.; Martino, C.; Bencardino, K.; Lonardi, S.; Bergamo, F.; Zagonel, V.; Leone, F.; Depetris, I.; Martinelli, E. Dual-targeted therapy with trastuzumab and lapatinib in tretament-refractory, KRas codon 12/13 wild-type, HER2-positive metastatic colorectal cancer (HERACLES): A proof-of-concept, multicentre, open-label phase 2 trial. *Lancet Oncol.* **2016**, *17*, 738–746. [CrossRef]
74. Siravegna, G.; Lazzari, L.; Crisafulli, G.; Sartore-Bianchi, A.; Mussolin, B.; Cossingena, A.; Martiono, C.; Lanman, R.B.; Nagy, R.J.; Fairalough, S.; et al. Radiologic and genomic evolution of individual metastases during HER2 blockade in colorectal cancer. *Cancer* **2018**, *34*, 148–162. [CrossRef]
75. Barker, N.; Ridgway, R.A.; van Es, J.H.; van de Wetering, M.; Begthel, H.; van den Born, M.; Danenberg, E.; Clarke, A.R.; Sansom, O.J.; Clevers, H. Crypt stem cells as the cells-of-origin of intestinal cancer. *Nature* **2009**, *457*, 608–611. [CrossRef] [PubMed]
76. Lee-Six, H.; Olafasson, S.; Ellis, P.; Osborne, R.J.; Sanders, M.A.; Moore, L.; Georgakopoulos, N.; Torrente, F.; Noorani, A.; Goddard, M.; et al. The landscape of somatic mutation in normal colorectal epithelial cells. *Nature* **2019**, *574*, 532–537. [CrossRef]
77. Olafsson, S.; McIntyre, R.E.; Coorens, T.; Butler, T.; Jung, H.; Robinson, P.S.; Lee-Six, H.; Sanders, M.A.; Arestang, K.; Dawson, C.; et al. Somatic evolution in non-neoplastic IBD-affected colon. *Cell* **2020**, *182*, 1–13. [CrossRef]

78. Nicholson, A.M.; Olpe, C.; Hoyle, A.; Thorsen, A.S.; Rus, T.; Colombé, M.; Brunton-Sim, R.; Kemp, R.; Marks, K.; Quirk, P.; et al. Fixation and spread of somatic mutations in adult human colonic epithelium. *Cell Stem Cell* **2018**, *22*, 909–918. [CrossRef]
79. Nikolaev, S.I.; Sotiriou, S.K.; Pateras, J.S.; Santoni, F.; Sougioultzis, S.; Edgren, H.; Almusa, H.; Robyr, D.; Guipponi, M.; Saarela, J.; et al. A single-nucleotide substitution mutator phenotype revealed by exome sequencing of human colon adenomas. *Cancer Res.* **2012**, *72*, 6279–6289. [CrossRef]
80. Lin, S.H.; Raju, G.; Huff, C.; Ye, Y.; Gu, J.; Chen, J.S.; Hildebrandt, M.; Liang, H.; Menter, D.G.; Morris, J. The somatic mutation landscape of premalignant colorectal adenoma. *Gut* **2017**, in press. [CrossRef]
81. Lee, S.H.; Jung, S.H.; Kim, T.M.; Rhee, J.K.; Park, H.C.; Kim, M.S.; Chang, H.A.; Lee, S.H.; Chung, H.J. Whole-exome sequencing identified mutational profiles of high-grade colon adenomas. *Oncotarget* **2017**, *8*, 6579–6588. [CrossRef]
82. Druliner, B.R.; Wang, P.; Bae, T.; Baheti, S.; Slettedahl, S.; Mahoney, D.; Vasmastzis, N.; Xu, H.; Kim, M.; Bockol, M.; et al. Molecular characterization of colorectal adenomas with and without malignancy reveals distinguishing genome, transcriptome and methylome alterations. *Scient. Rep.* **2018**, *8*, 3161. [CrossRef] [PubMed]
83. Cross, W.; Kanc, M.; Mustonen, V.; Temko, D.; Davis, H.; Baker, A.M.; Biswas, S.; Arnold, R.; Chegwidden, L.; Gatenbeee, C.; et al. The evolutionary landscape of colorectal cancer tumorigenesis. *Nat. Ecol. Evol.* **2018**, *2*, 1661–1672. [CrossRef] [PubMed]
84. Fearon, E.R.; Volgstein, B. A genetic model for colorectal tumorigenesis. *Cell* **1990**, *61*, 759–767. [CrossRef]
85. Sottoriva, A.; Kang, H.; Ma, Z.; Graham, T.A.; Salomon, M.P.; Zhao, J.; Marjoram, P.; Siegmund, K.; Press, M.F.; Shibata, D.; et al. A Big Bang model of human colorectal tumor growth. *Nat. Genet.* **2015**, *47*, 209–216. [CrossRef]
86. Kang, H.; Salomon, M.P.; Sottoriva, A.; Zhao, J.; Toy, M.; Press, M.F.; Curtis, C.; Marjoram, P.; Siegmund, K.; Shibata, D. Many private mutations originate from the first few divisions of a human colorectal adenoma. *J. Pathol.* **2015**, *237*, 355–362. [CrossRef]
87. Sievers, C.K.; Zou, L.; Pickhardt, P.J.; Matkowskyj, K.A.; Albrecht, D.M.; Clipson, L.; Bacher, J.W.; Pooler, B.D.; Moawad, F.J.; Cash, B.D.; et al. Subclonal diversity arises early even in small colorectal tumours and contributes to differential growth fates. *Gut* **2017**, *66*, 2131–2140. [CrossRef]
88. Reiter, J.G.; Makahon-Moore, A.P.; Gerold, J.M.; Heyde, A.; Attieh, M.A.; Kohutek, Z.A.; Tokheim, C.J.; Brown, A.; De Blasio, R.M.; Niyazov, J.; et al. Minimal functional driver gene heterogeneity among untreated metastases. *Science* **2018**, *361*, 1033–1037. [CrossRef]
89. Williams, M.J.; Werner, B.; Heide, T.; Curtis, C.; Barnes, C.; Sottoriva, A.; Graham, T.A. Quantification of subclonal selection in cancer from bulk sequencing data. *Nat. Genet.* **2018**, *50*, 895–903. [CrossRef]
90. Williams, M.J.; Werner, B.; Barnes, C.; Graham, T.A.; Sottoriva, A. Identification of neutral evolution across cancer types. *Nat. Genet.* **2016**, *48*, 238–244. [CrossRef]
91. McFarland, C.D.; Korolev, K.; Kryukov, G.; Sunyaev, S.R.; Mirny, L.A. Impact of deleterious passenger mutations on cancer progression. *Proc. Natl. Acad. Sci. USA* **2013**, *110*, 2910–2913. [CrossRef] [PubMed]
92. Mc Farland, C.D.; Mirny, L.A.; Korolev, K.S. Tug-of-war between driver and passenger mutations in cancer and other adaptive processes. *Proc. Natl. Acad. Sci. USA* **2014**, *111*, 15138–15143. [CrossRef]
93. Humphries, A.; Cereser, B.; Gay, L.J.; Miller, D.S.; Das, B.; Gutteridge, A.; Elia, G.; Nye, E.; Jeffery, R.; Poulsom, R.; et al. Lineage tracing reveals multipotent stem cells maintain human adenomas and the pattern of clonal expansion in tumor evolution. *Proc. Natl. Acad. Sci. USA* **2013**, *110*, E2490–E2499. [CrossRef] [PubMed]
94. Shibata, D. Visualizing human colorectal cancer intratumor heterogeneity with phylogeography. *iScience* **2020**, *23*, 101304. [CrossRef]
95. Ryser, M.D.; Min, B.H.; Siegmund, K.D.; Shibata, D. Spatial mutation patterns as markers of early colorectal tumor cell mobility. *Proc. Natl. Acad. Sci. USA* **2018**, *115*, 5774–5779. [CrossRef] [PubMed]
96. Ryser, M.D.; Yu, M.; Grady, W.; Siegmund, K.; Shibata, D. Epigenetic heterogeneity in human colorectal tumors reveals preferential conservation and evidence of immune surveillance. *Sci. Rep.* **2018**, *8*, 17292. [CrossRef]

97. Ryser, M.D.; Mallo, D.; Hall, A.; Hardman, T.; King, L.M.; Tatischev, S.; Sorribes, K.; Maley, C.C.; Marks, J.R.; Hwang, E.S.; et al. Normal barriers to invasion driving human colorectal tumor growth. *Nat. Commun.* **2020**, *11*, 1280. [CrossRef] [PubMed]
98. Sottoriva, A.; Barnes, C.P.; Graham, T.A. Catch my drift? Making sense of genomic intra-tumor heterogeneity. *Biochim. Biophys. Acta* **2017**, *1867*, 95–100.

Publisher's Note: MDPI stays neutral with regard to jurisdictional claims in published maps and institutional affiliations.

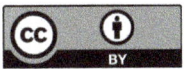 © 2020 by the authors. Licensee MDPI, Basel, Switzerland. This article is an open access article distributed under the terms and conditions of the Creative Commons Attribution (CC BY) license (http://creativecommons.org/licenses/by/4.0/).

Article

Identification and Validation of New Cancer Stem Cell-Related Genes and Their Regulatory microRNAs in Colorectal Cancerogenesis

Kristian Urh, Margareta Žlajpah, Nina Zidar and Emanuela Boštjančič *

Faculty of Medicine, Institute of Pathology, University of Ljubljana, 1000 Ljubljana, Slovenia; kristian.urh@mf.uni-lj.si (K.U.); margareta.zlajpah@mf.uni-lj.si (M.Ž.); nina.zidar@mf.uni-lj.si (N.Z.)
* Correspondence: emanuela.bostjancic@mf.uni-lj.si; Tel.: +386-15437195

Abstract: Significant progress has been made in the last decade in our understanding of the pathogenetic mechanisms of colorectal cancer (CRC). Cancer stem cells (CSC) have gained much attention and are now believed to play a crucial role in the pathogenesis of various cancers, including CRC. In the current study, we validated gene expression of four genes related to CSC, *L1TD1*, *SLITRK6*, *ST6GALNAC1* and *TCEA3*, identified in a previous bioinformatics analysis. Using bioinformatics, potential miRNA-target gene correlations were prioritized. In total, 70 formalin-fixed paraffin-embedded biopsy samples from 47 patients with adenoma, adenoma with early carcinoma and CRC without and with lymph node metastases were included. The expression of selected genes and microRNAs (miRNAs) was evaluated using quantitative PCR. Differential expression of all investigated genes and four of six prioritized miRNAs (*hsa-miR-199a-3p*, *hsa-miR-335-5p*, *hsa-miR-425-5p*, *hsa-miR-1225-3p*, *hsa-miR-1233-3p* and *hsa-miR-1303*) was found in at least one group of CRC cancerogenesis. *L1TD1*, *SLITRK6*, *miR-1233-3p* and *miR-1225-3p* were correlated to the level of malignancy. A negative correlation between *miR-199a-3p* and its predicted target *SLITRK6* was observed, showing potential for further experimental validation in CRC. Our results provide further evidence that CSC-related genes and their regulatory miRNAs are involved in CRC development and progression and suggest that some them, particularly *miR-199a-3p* and its *SLITRK6* target gene, are promising for further validation in CRC.

Keywords: colorectal cancer; differentially expressed genes; cancer stem cells; qPCR

1. Introduction

Colorectal cancer (CRC) is ranked as the third most common cause of morbidity due to cancer worldwide [1]. The five-year survival of patients with CRC can vary, with five-year survival rates of approximately 90% in patients with adenoma with early carcinoma and approximately 8–12% in patients with advanced CRC [2]. Despite the introduction of new treatment modalities, 40–50% of CRC patients develop metastases [1–4]. The prognosis can be improved significantly with the detection of early lesions through population screening programs [5,6].

CRC development is divided into discrete stages, ranging from normal mucosa to invasive carcinoma. The majority of CRC cases develop from precursor lesions, adenomas and serrated polyps [4]. Molecular pathways involved in CRC development include stepwise accumulation of mutations, epigenetic changes, and changes in gene expression, leading to uncontrolled cell division and an invasive phenotype [4,7]. Most genetic events that are associated with tumour development occur early, before the formation of the adenoma, leading to an urgent need to define mechanisms responsible for the switch from adenoma to carcinoma.

It is believed that the bulk of any given neoplasm consists of cells incapable of metastatic seeding or tumour progression. A minority of cancer cells, referred to as cancer stem cells (CSC) or CSC-like cells [8], are capable of self-renewal, differentiation and mobility. They are mostly found as a subpopulation on the invasive tumour front, and are believed to be responsible for invasiveness, metastatic spread and relapse [9,10]. Additionally, turnover of CSCs is slow, which in turn allows greater resistance to therapies that target rapidly replicating cells [9,10].

Two separate mechanisms have been suggested for the development of CSC in CRC. According to the first, oncogenic mutations accumulate within the colonic crypt stem cells, located in the bottom area of a normal crypt. These CSCs are able to differentiate into mature cancer cells and exhibit uncontrolled proliferation. According to the second mechanism, cancer cells undergoing an accumulation of genetic changes and/or epithelial-mesenchymal transition dedifferentiate from normal mature epithelial cells into a state similar to stem cells [11].

In a previous study, we used a bioinformatics analysis of publicly available gene expression microarray projects [12] and identified potential markers for differentiation between normal colon mucosa, adenoma and CRC. Some of the differentially expressed genes were associated with CSC-like cells, namely *L1TD1*, *SLITRK6*, *ST6GALNAC1* and *TCEA3*. *L1TD1*, a gene-encoding RNA-binding protein, has been identified as a marker for human embryonic stem cells, their renewal and cancer cell proliferation. It has been associated with RNA transcription, splicing, processing, localization, stability and translation [13–16]. *SLITRK6*, an integral membrane protein, has been found to be highly expressed in human adult neural stem-like cells and in several cancers. It has been associated with cell adhesion and actin cytoskeleton [17–19], cell features that are closely related to cell differentiation, stemness, cancer cell migration and invasion [20–22]. *ST6GALNAC1*, encoding an enzyme, has been associated with cell migration, contact and maintenance of isolated CRC stem cells. It is involved in the activation of akt pathway and it is a potential candidate for CSC targeting therapy [23]. *TCEA3*, a transcription elongation factor, has been shown to regulate differentiation of mouse embryonal stem cells through the Lefty1-Nodal-Smad2 pathway [24].

However, there is very limited information about their role in CRC. We therefore analysed the expression of these four genes during CRC cancerogenesis, from normal mucosa, adenoma and adenoma with early carcinoma to advanced CRC, predicted miRNAs that could regulate these genes and analysed their expression as well.

2. Materials and Methods

2.1. Patient and Tissue Selection

Patients who underwent excision or resection of adenoma, adenoma with early carcinoma and CRC from 2015 to 2019 were included in the study. For routine histopathologic examination, tissue samples were fixed in 10% buffered formalin and embedded in paraffin (FFPE). During routine examination, all specimens were evaluated by a pathologist according to standard procedures and, after histopathologic examination, pTNM (pathologic Tumour Node Metastasis) classification was assessed on the basis of the depth of invasion and extent of the primary tumour, the number of lymph nodes with metastases and the presence of distant metastases (AJCC 8th edition [25]). For the purpose of this study, biopsy samples were collected retrospectively from the archives of the Institute of Pathology, Faculty of Medicine, University of Ljubljana. After re-evaluation of consecutive cases for each group by a pathologist and initial quality check, representative samples were selected for further study. Samples of normal mucosa obtained from resected CRC specimens were used as control samples. Patients treated by radiotherapy, chemotherapy or biologic drugs prior to surgery were not included in this study. Patients with mucinous carcinomas or signet cell carcinomas were also excluded. Only sporadic CRC cases were included. Tissue samples were grouped as normal mucosa, adenoma, adenoma with early carcinoma, CRC without lymph node metastases (CRC N0) or CRC with lymph node metastases (CRC N+).

The study was conducted according to the guidelines of the Declaration of Helsinki, and approved by the National Medical Ethics Committee (Republic of Slovenia, Ministry of Health), approval number 0120-54/2020/4.

2.2. Target miRNAs Identification and Prioritization

For the identified differentially expressed genes (DEGs), we searched for miRNA targets that might be involved in the regulation of their expression. The databases MiRTar [26], miRDB [27], Mirna-coadread [28], TarBase [29], TargetScan [30], miRBase [31] and a literature based search on Pubmed, as well as the settings used in the miRNA mining, are given in Table S1.

miRNAs that could target selected DEGs were checked in the miRBase [31] for annotation, method of identification and validation. Cases in which the miRNAs were identified as not true miRNAs were discarded. Only miRNAs either with a known functional association with cancer or that appeared in at least two databases as related to the target gene were considered as potential regulators of DEGs. The identified miRNAs from Table S1 were further prioritized as explained below.

Alignment between the miRNA and gene sequence was inspected manually and mismatches in the seed region were noted. In cases in which there was a maximum of one mismatch in the miRNA seed binding region in the binding relevant 2–7 bp, the matching was considered sufficient for further analysis [32]. Additionally, in cases in which a relevant reference for cancer associations was identified, the miRNA was also considered for further analysis. We identified the sequence 70 bp and 30 bp upstream and downstream of the mature miRNA binding site, the former for minimum free energy (ΔG) determination in regard to the folding of the sequence and 30 bp for secondary structure analysis [33,34]. Higher ΔG upstream or downstream of the binding site may imply binding issues, whereas a lower ΔG suggests a locally linear RNA structure around the target mRNA-binding site [34]. We also identified ΔG of the potential binding site and identified cases in which the difference between the potential binding site and the 70 bp flanking 3′ and 5′ was at least 10 kcal/mol [35]. ΔG and secondary structure analysis was performed using mFold [36] and Vienna RNAfold [37]. Identification of secondary structures and destabilising elements (DSE) or stabilising elements (SE) was performed for each miRNA-binding site and the 30 bp flanking sequence on each side. Potential DSEs with the following cut-off lengths include a hairpin loop, $\geq$11 bp; interior loop, $\geq$9 bp; bulge loop, $\geq$7 bp; multiple branching loop $\geq$ 11 bp; and joint sequence or free end, $\geq$11 bp. DSE could aid in miRNA binding while stabilising elements (SE) including stems, as explained by Zhao, Samal and Srivastava [34]. Structures were considered significant for inhibition of miRNA binding if the ΔG of the structure was lower than -6 kcal/mol [38]. Identification of potential conservation of miRNA-target gene binding site sequences between human, mouse, rat and chicken was performed using TargetScan 7.2 [30].

RNA22 [39] was used for identification of statistically significant ($p \leq 0.05$) alignments between DEG target 3′-UTR sites and miRNAs. The settings used in the analysis were: 8-mer or 7-mer seed binding, 1 unpaired sequence in seed region, 1 G:U wobble, maximum folding energy for heteroduplex -12.0 and 20.0 kcal/mol. The heteroduplex energies with cut-off -12.0 and -20.0 kcal/mol used in RNA22 were the energies suggested by the software and the typical setting described in the study by Miranda, Huynh, Tay, Ang, Tam, Thomson, Lim and Rigoutsos [39]. Results of individual analyses were compared for possible overlaps. The full workflow of the prioritization is shown in Figure 1.

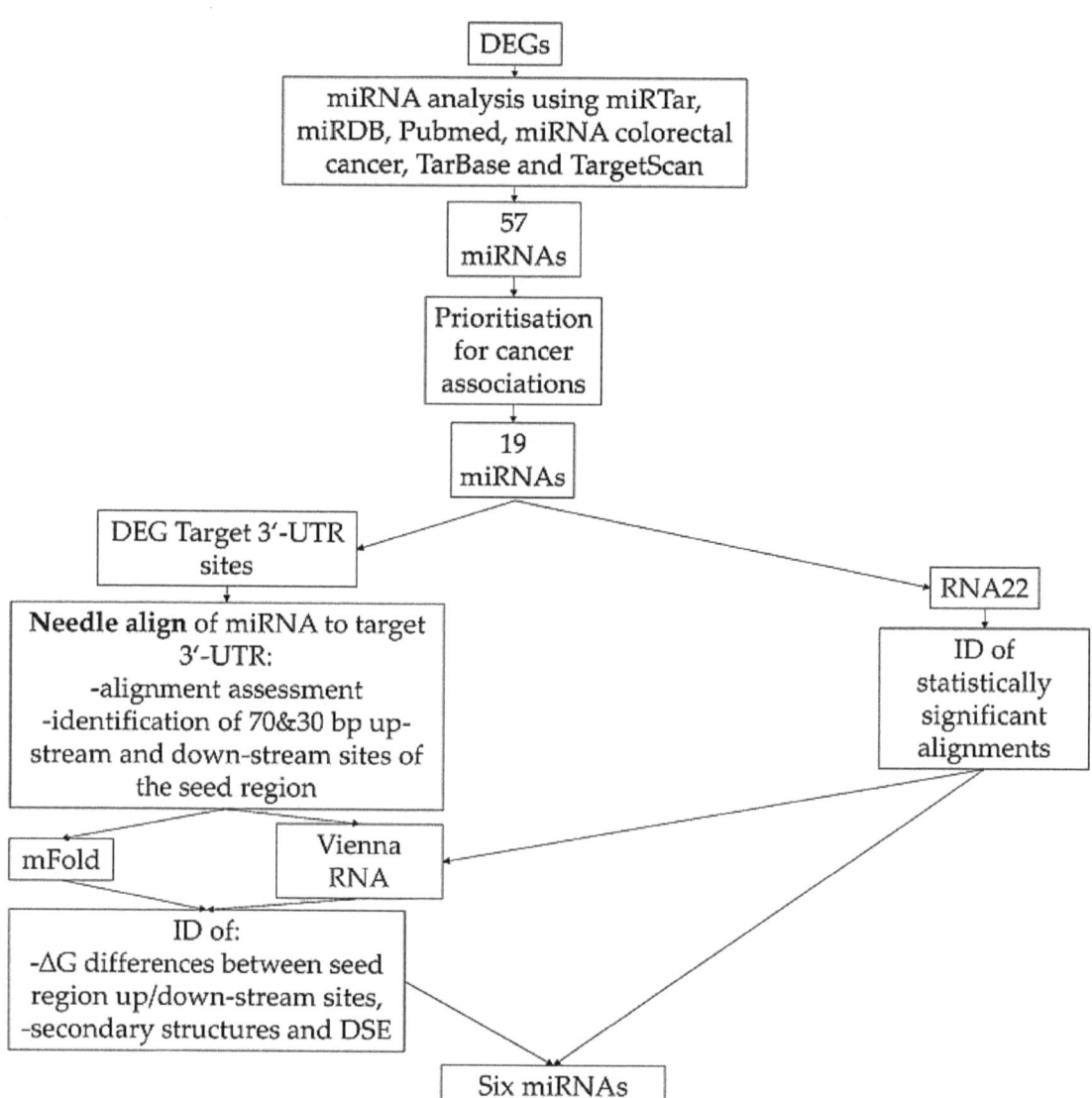

Figure 1. Identification and prioritization of miRNAs. Legend: DEG, differentially expressed genes; DSE, destabilising elements; ΔG, minimum free energy; ID, identification.

2.3. RNA Isolation and Quality Assessment

RNA was obtained from FFPE tissue slides using a microtome (4 × 10 μm-thick slides). RNA, including miRNAs, was isolated using an AllPrep DNA/RNA FFPE kit (Qiagen, Hilden, Germany) kit according to the manufacturer's protocol. Concentration and quality assessment of the isolated RNA was performed using a spectrophotometer ND-1000 or ND-One (Nanodrop, Thermo Fisher Scientific, Waltham, MA, USA) at wavelengths 260 nm and 280 nm. Prior to further analysis, RNA quality was tested using reverse transcription and amplification of *GAPDH* (Hs_GAPDH_vb.1_SG, 100 bp) by SybrGreen technology. Samples that did not amplify during this initial control step were excluded from further analysis.

2.4. Reverse Transcription (RT) and Pre-Amplification

Reverse transcription (RT) of the isolated mRNA was performed using OneTaq®® RT-PCR Kit (New England Biolabs, Ipswich, MA, USA) using a mix of random hexamers and oligo-dT primers according to the manufacturer's protocol. We used 60 ng of RNA in the total 10 µL RT reaction and 1 µL of random hexamers, and incubated for 5 min at 70 °C. Afterward, we added 5 µL of the Reaction mix and 1 µL of Enzyme mix to the reaction and incubated at 25 °C for 5 min, 42 °C for 1 h and 80 °C for 5 min.

Preamplification of the obtained cDNA was performed using the TaqMan®® Preamp Master Mix (Thermo Fisher Scientific, Waltham, MA, USA) according to the manufacturer's instructions. For a 10 µL reaction, we added 5 µL of PreAmp Master Mix (2×), 2.5 µL of Pooled TaqMan®® Gene Expression probes (Thermo Fisher Scientific, Waltham, MA, USA) (0.2×, diluted in TE buffer) and 2.5 µL of cDNA. Incubation was performed at 95 °C for 10 min, 95 °C for 15 s and 60 °C for 4 min.

RT of the isolated miRNAs was performed using the TaqMan™ MicroRNA Reverse Transcription Kit (Applied Biosystems, Foster City, CA, USA) according to the manufacturer's protocol. The reaction volume was a total of 10 µL, including 10 ng of RNA, 2 µL of RT primer, 0.1 µL of 100 mM dNTPs, 1 µL of MultiScribe™ Reverse Transcriptase 50 U/µL, 1 µL of 10× Reverse Transcription Buffer, 0.19 µL of the RNase Inhibitor 20 U/µL and 0.71 µL nuclease-free water. The conditions for the reverse transcription were 30 min at 16 °C, 30 min at 42 °C and 5 min at 85 °C.

2.5. Selection of Primers and Probes

The TaqMan-based approach (Thermo Fisher Scientific, Waltham, MA, USA) was used for the quantitative real-time PCR (qPCR) methodology. A predesigned mixture of primers and probes was used for expression analysis of mRNAs of DEGs and their potential regulatory miRNAs relative to reference genes (RGs). The candidate genes were selected after a bioinformatics analysis performed in a previous study [12]. The potential regulatory miRNAs were selected as described above. Selected probes are shown in Table 1, with reference genes (RGs) presented in bold.

Table 1. Selected probes.

Gene/miRNA	Assay ID	Sequence (Probe Sequence or Mature miRNA Sequence)
B2M	Hs99999907_m1	GTTAAGTGGGATCGAGACATGTAAG
IPO8	Hs00183533_m1	GGGGAATTGATCAGTGCATTCCACT
L1TD1	Hs00219458_m1	TTTTTCGCCAGGCACCAAGGCACAG
SLITRK6	Hs00536106_s1	TTTCCATGGACTGGAAAACCTGGAA
ST6GALNAC1	Hs01027885_m1	AGGAGGCCTTCAGACGACTTGCCCT
TCEA3	Hs00957468_m1	GAAATCGAAGATCATATCTACCAAG
hsa-miR-199a-3p	002304	ACAGUAGUCUGCACAUUGGUUA
hsa-miR-335-5p	000546	UCAAGAGCAAUAACGAAAAAUGU
hsa-miR-425-5p	001516	AAUGACACGAUCACUCCCGUUGA
hsa-miR-1225-3p	002766	UGAGCCCCUGUGCCGCCCCAG
hsa-miR-1233-3p	002768	UGAGCCCUGUCCUCCCGCAG
hsa-miR-1274b	**002884**	UCCCUGUUCGGGCGCCA
hsa-miR-1303	002792	UUUAGAGACGGGGUCUUGCUCU
RNU6B	**001093**	CGCAAGGATGACACGCAAATTCGTGAAGCGTTCCATATTTT

2.6. Quantitative Real-Time PCR (qPCR)

Prior to qPCR amplification, efficiencies were determined in triplicate reactions for each probe and for each group of samples. The dilution series included 4-point dilutions ranging from 5-fold to 625-fold for mRNAs/miRNAs. A Rotor Gene Q (Qiagen, Hilden, Germany) machine was used for all qPCR analyses, and all 10 µL testing reactions were performed in duplicate. For mRNAs, the cycling protocol was 50 °C for 2 min, 95 °C for 10 min, 40 cycles of 95 °C for 15 s and 62 °C for 1 min. For miRNAs, the cycling protocol was 95 °C for 10 min, 40 cycles of 95 °C for 15 s and 60 °C for 60 s. The reactions included 5.0 µL of the FastStart™ PCR Master mix (Roche Diagnostics, Basel, Switzerland), 0.5 µL of the TaqMan probe and 4.5 µL of cDNA (pre-amplified cDNA diluted 5-fold for mRNAs and for miRNAs cDNA diluted 100–fold).

After efficiency correction, the obtained ΔCq (normalized Cq of analysed mRNAs/miRNAs relative to geometric mean of RGs) were used for analysis of target gene/miRNA expression. The fold difference in the expression was calculated against the normal mucosa samples group using the ΔΔCq method [40].

2.7. Statistics

Differences in expression were compared between tumour and corresponding normal mucosa using ΔCq and the Willcoxon Rank test (nonparametric test for dependent samples). For comparison of relative quantification of mRNAs/miRNAs between independent groups of samples (e.g., adenoma vs. normal mucosa), ΔCq and the Mann–Whitney U test were used (nonparametric test for independent group of samples). ΔΔCq and the Mann–Whitney U test were used for comparison between CRC N0 and CRC N+ sample groups. Using the Spearman coefficient, we analysed whether miRNAs and the target mRNA were in reverse correlation and whether miRNAs and mRNAs were associated with cancerogenesis. All statistical analyses of experimental data were performed using SPSS version 24 (SPSS Inc., Chicago, IL, USA). Differences in expression between groups were considered significant at $p \leq 0.05$.

3. Results

3.1. Patient Characteristics

Approximately 30% of retrospectively selected cases successfully passed initial quality control. Our study therefore included 70 biopsy samples from 47 patients with adenoma (n = 11), adenoma with early carcinoma (n = 13), CRC without lymph node metastases (n = 10) and CRC with lymph node metastases (n = 13). There were 15 women and 32 men, aged 73.7 ± 8.4 and 65.7 ± 11.4 years, respectively. As a control group, microscopically normal mucosa from CRC resected specimens was used (n = 23). Demographic characteristics of the included patients are shown in Table 2.

Table 2. Demographic characteristics of the included patients.

Patients	Adenoma	Adenoma with Early Carcinoma	CRC without Lymph Node Metastases	CRC with Lymph Node Metastases
M:F	10:1	9:4	4:6	9:4
Age	62.3 ± 10.7	64.9 ± 5.7	72.7 ± 11.6	73.2 ± 11.8

Legend: CRC, colorectal cancer; F, female; M, male.

Among adenomas, there were six cases of tubular adenoma with high-grade dysplasia, three tubulovillous adenomas with high-grade dysplasia and two tubulovillous adenomas with low-grade dysplasia. Among adenomas with early carcinoma, there were six tubulovillous adenomas, six tubular adenomas and one villous adenoma, all with high grade dysplasia and with malignant transformation, evidenced by invasion of the dysplastic glands in the submucosa (pT1). Among CRC cases, there were two stage I carcinomas, five stage IIA, two stage IIB, eight stage IIIB, one stage IIIC, four stage IVA and one stage IVB carcinomas. Of the CRC cases, 7 cases were poorly differentiated and 16 were moderately differentiated.

3.2. Differential Gene Expression

3.2.1. Differential Gene Expression in Adenoma and Adenoma with Early Carcinoma

ΔCq for the investigated genes in adenoma and adenoma with early carcinoma were statistically evaluated independently against normal mucosa samples. Statistically significant results include 6.20-fold downregulation of *SLITRK6* (p = 0.010) in adenomas, and

3.22-fold upregulation of *TCEA3* in adenomas with early carcinoma ($p = 0.006$). The results are shown in Figure 2.

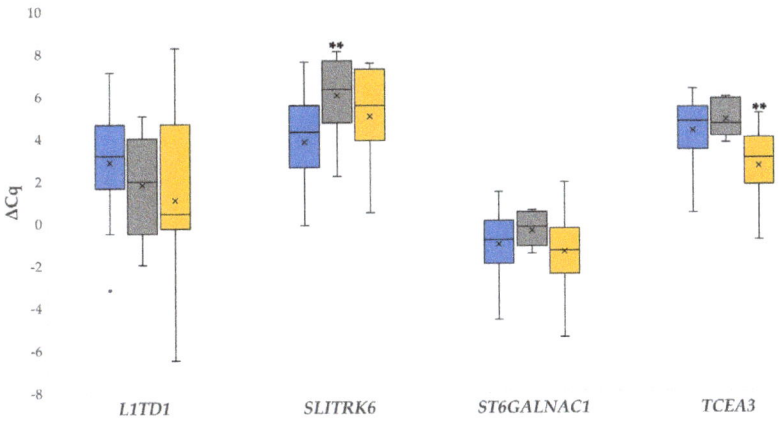

Figure 2. Expression (ΔCq) of four genes (*L1TD1*, *SLITRK6*, *ST6GALNAC1*, *TCEA3*) in normal mucosa, adenoma and adenoma with early carcinoma. Legend: x, mean; ○, outlier; ** $p \leq 0.01$.

We also observed statistically significant 4.58-fold upregulation in adenoma with early carcinoma compared to adenoma for the gene *TCEA3* ($p \leq 0.001$).

3.2.2. Differential Gene Expression in Carcinoma Compared to Normal Mucosa

Differences in expression of the investigated genes between CRC N0 or CRC N+ and corresponding normal mucosa were calculated using ΔCq. Statistically significant results include the 7.16-fold upregulation of *L1TD1* in CRC N+ ($p = 0.008$) and 6.16-fold downregulation of *SLITRK6* ($p = 0.039$) and 3.10-fold for *ST6GALNAC1* ($p = 0.02$) in CRC N+. Additionally, 7.97-fold upregulation of *TCEA3* in the CRC N0 ($p = 0.004$) was also observed. The results are shown in Figure 3.

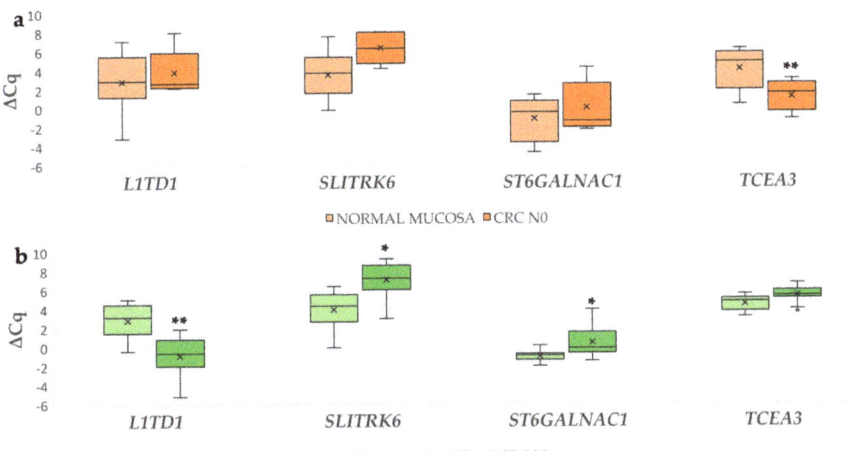

Figure 3. Expression (ΔCq) of the investigated genes in carcinoma without (**a**) and with lymph node metastases (**b**) and corresponding normal mucosa. Legend: CRC N0, colorectal carcinoma without lymph node metastases; CRC N+, colorectal carcinoma with lymph node metastases; x, mean; ○, outlier; * $p \leq 0.05$; ** $p \leq 0.01$.

3.2.3. Gene Expression in Carcinoma with Lymph Node Metastases Compared to Carcinoma without Lymph Node Metastases

ΔCq values for each carcinoma case were first calculated against the corresponding normal mucosa. Then, the independent $\Delta\Delta Cq$ comparisons for the investigated genes between the CRC N0 and CRC N+ were performed. Statistical significance was identified for *TCEA3*, which was upregulated in the CRC N0 group compared to CRC N+ ($p \leq 0.000$). The results are shown in Figure 4. The complete statistical comparisons are available in Table S2.

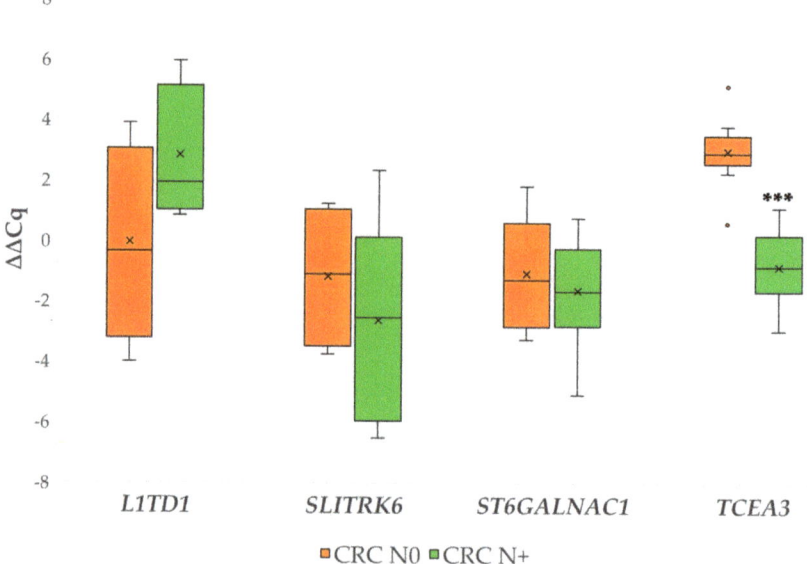

Figure 4. Expression ($\Delta\Delta Cq$) of the investigated genes (*L1TD1*, *SLITRK6*, *ST6GALNAC1*, *TCEA3*) in carcinoma without and carcinoma with lymph node metastases. Legend: CRC N0, colorectal carcinoma without lymph node metastases; CRC N+, colorectal carcinoma with lymph node metastases; x, mean; o, outlier; *** $p \leq 0.001$.

3.3. Prioritization of Potential miRNA-Target Gene Associations

Only miRNAs with a known functional association with cancer or which appeared in at least two databases in correlation with the target gene were considered for further prioritization. The complete results of the miRNA prioritization for target genes correlations with relevant information and manual alignment with free energy comparisons and secondary structure identification are available in Tables S3 and S4. The complete results of the RNA22 analysis are presented in Table S5.

After comparison of the results of analyses presented in Tables S3–S5, we identified several miRNAs for further validation. A condensed view of choosing a specific miRNA for further validation in association with a potential target gene is presented in Table 3. The minimum requirements are in bold. Only cases with DSEs present in the sequence, a known previous association with the target gene and a previous association with CRC, are included.

Table 3. Condensed view of prioritization results for the miRNAs identified for further validation.

Gene	miRNA	Association with at Least Two Databases	Folding Free Energy Constraints	RNA22	Direct Validation
L1TD1	hsa-miR-1303	+	+	−	−
SLITRK6	hsa-miR-199a-3p	+	−	+	−
	hsa-miR-425-5p	−	+	−	+
ST6GALNAC1	hsa-miR-335-5p	+	+	−	−
	hsa-miR-335-5p	+	+	−	−
TCEA3	hsa-miR-1225-3p	+	+	−	−
	hsa-miR-1233-3p	+	+	+ *	−

Legend: CRC, colorectal carcinoma; *, did not appear as a significant binding pair, but had a folding energy higher than the software cut-off.

3.4. Differential miRNA Expression

3.4.1. Differential Expression of miRNAs in Adenoma and Adenoma with Early Carcinoma

We compared ΔCq values of the investigated miRNAs in adenomas and adenoma with early carcinoma to normal mucosa samples. Among the investigated miRNAs, *miR-335-5p* was not expressed in normal mucosa, adenoma and adenoma with early carcinoma.

Statistically significant changes in expression included upregulation for the majority of miRNAs in both adenoma and adenoma, with early carcinoma in comparison to normal mucosa: 13.43-fold and 6.07-fold for *miR-425-5p* ($p < 0.001$, $p < 0.001$), respectively; 16.97-fold and 6.78-fold for *miR-1225-3p* ($p < 0.001$, $p < 0.001$), respectively; and 11.86-fold and 4.40-fold for *miR-1233-3p* ($p < 0.001$, $p = 0.003$), respectively. *miR-1303* was significantly 4.29-fold upregulated only in the adenoma group ($p = 0.025$). The results are shown in Figure 5.

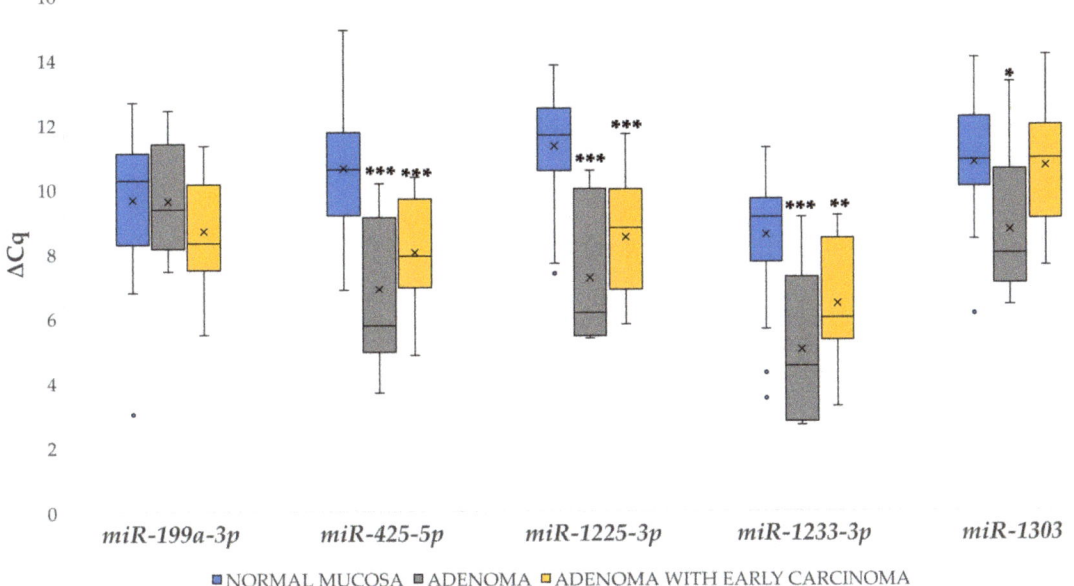

Figure 5. Expression (ΔCq) of the investigated miRNAs in normal mucosa, adenoma and adenoma with early carcinoma. Legend: x, mean; ○, outlier; * $p \leq 0.05$; ** $p \leq 0.01$; *** $p \leq 0.001$.

3.4.2. Differential miRNA Expression in Carcinoma with and without Lymph Node Metastases Compared to Corresponding Normal Mucosa

ΔCq values for the investigated miRNAs were compared between CRC N0 and CRC N+ and their corresponding normal mucosa, as shown in Figure 6. Statistically significant results include the 7.38-fold upregulation of *miR-425-5p* ($p = 0.002$), 6.60-fold for *miR-1225-3p* ($p = 0.001$) and 6.95-fold for *miR-1233-3p* ($p = 0.001$) in CRC N0 and 3.28-fold for *miR-1225-3p* ($p = 0.019$) in CRC N+. Among the investigated miRNAs, *miR-335-5p* was expressed neither in normal mucosa nor in CRC.

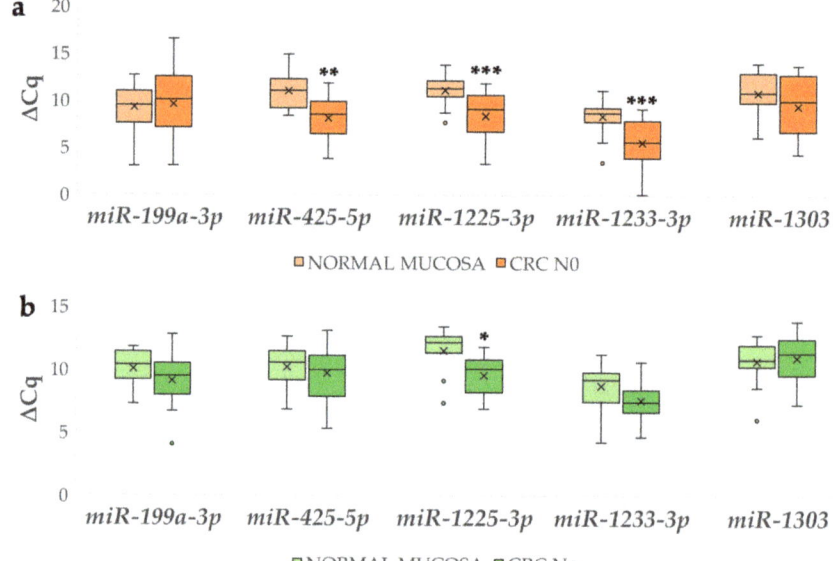

Figure 6. Expression (ΔCq) of the investigated miRNAs in carcinoma without (**a**) and with lymph node metastases (**b**) in comparison to corresponding normal mucosa. Legend: CRC N0, colorectal carcinoma without lymph node metastases; CRC N+, colorectal carcinoma with lymph node metastases; x, mean; ○, outlier; * $p \leq 0.05$, ** $p \leq 0.01$; *** $p \leq 0.001$.

3.4.3. Differential Expression of miRNAs Between Carcinoma with and without Lymph Node Metastases

Figure 7 shows independent ΔΔCq comparisons for the investigated miRNAs between the CRC N0 and CRC N+, which revealed a statistically significant difference in the expression of *miR-425-5p* ($p = 0.003$). Additional statistical comparisons are available in Table S6.

3.5. Correlation between Expression of Investigated Genes and Their Potentially Regulatory miRNAs

The expression of *L1TD1* to *miR-1303*, as shown in Figure 8, showed an inverse trend in all analysed groups except the adenoma group. However, we were not able to confirm a negative correlation between *L1TD1* and *miR-1303* (Table 4).

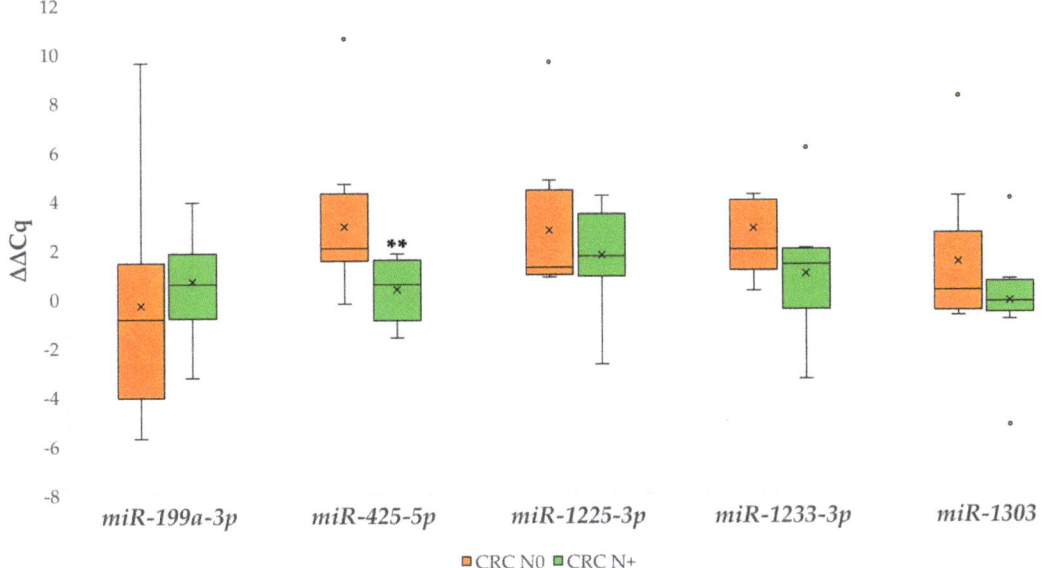

Figure 7. Expression (ΔΔCq) of the investigated miRNAs in carcinoma without and with lymph node metastases. Legend: CRC N0, colorectal carcinoma without lymph node metastases; CRC N+, colorectal carcinoma with lymph node metastases; x, mean; ○, outlier; ** $p \leq 0.01$.

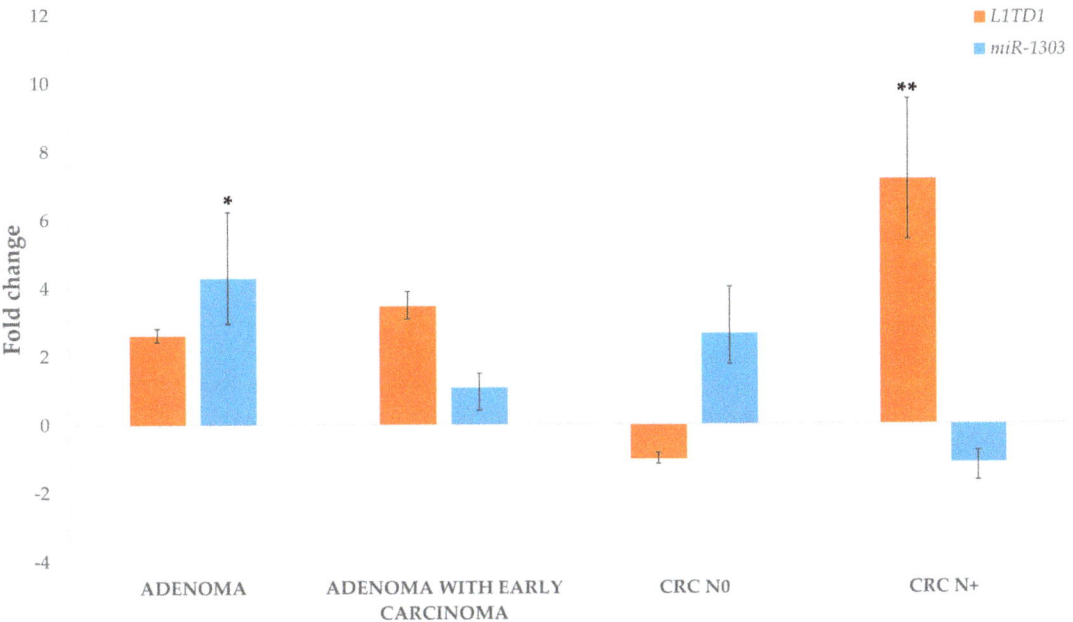

Figure 8. Expression of *L1TD1* and *miR*-1303 in adenoma, adenoma with early carcinoma and carcinoma without and with lymph node metastases. Legend: CRC N0, colorectal carcinoma without lymph node metastases; CRC N+, colorectal carcinoma with lymph node metastases; * $p \leq 0.05$; ** $p \leq 0.01$.

Table 4. Spearman's correlation coefficients between expression of genes and their potentially regulatory miRNAs.

Gene and miRNA		Correlation Coefficient	Significance (2-Tailed)
L1TD1	miR-1303	−0.024	0.862
SLITRK6	miR-425-5p	−0.187	0.176
	miR-199a-3p	−0.323	0.017 *
TCEA3	miR-1233-3p	0.116	0.360
	miR-1225-3p	0.056	0.660

Legend: * $p \leq 0.05$.

Comparing the fold change expression data for *SLITRK6* with the predicted miRNAs *miR-425-5p* and *miR-199a-3p*, we observed an inverse trend of expression between *miR-425-5p* and *SLITRK6* in all tested groups. Expression of *miR-199a-3p* remained at similar levels throughout the adenoma-carcinoma progression. The results are shown in Figure 9a. However, we were able to confirm a negative correlation between *SLITRK6* and *miR-199a-3p*, as shown in Figure 9b. The correlation testing results are given in Table 4.

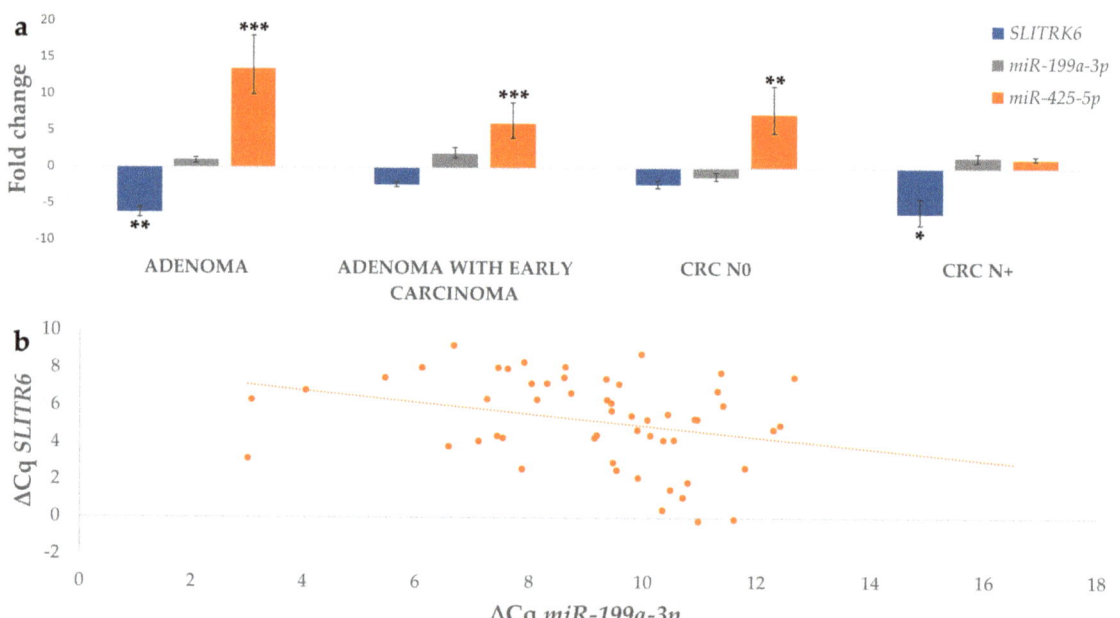

Figure 9. (**a**) Expression of *SLITRK6*, *miR-199a-3p* and *miR-425*-5p in adenoma, adenoma with early carcinoma and carcinoma without and with lymph node metastases; (**b**) Correlation between expression (ΔCq) of *miR-199a-3p* and target gene *SLITRK6*. Legend: CRC N0, colorectal carcinoma without lymph node metastases; CRC N+, colorectal carcinoma with lymph node metastases; * $p \leq 0.05$; ** $p \leq 0.01$; *** $p \leq 0.001$.

Expression of the *TCEA3* gene showed a similar trend in adenoma with early carcinoma and CRC N0 to both miRNAs, *miR-1225-3p* and *miR-1233-3p*. In adenoma and CRC N+, both miRNAs showed opposite trends in expression to its potential target gene *TCEA3*. The results are shown in Figure 10. We were not able to confirm any correlation between *TCEA3* and *miR-1225-3p* or *miR-1233-3p* (Table 4).

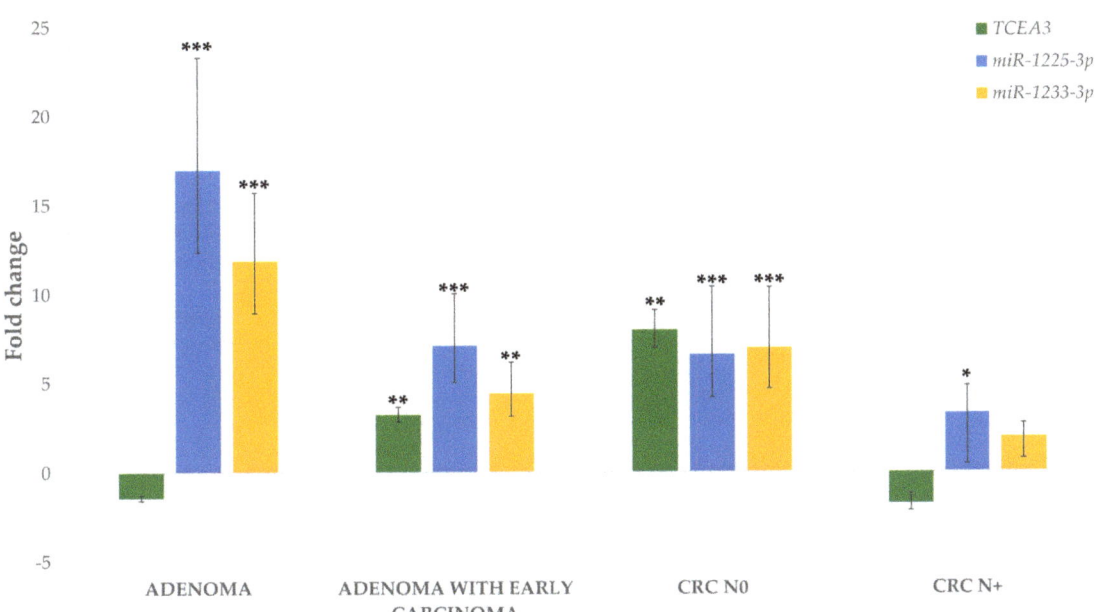

Figure 10. Expression of *TCEA3*, *miR-1225-3p* and *miR-1233-3p* in adenoma, adenoma with early carcinoma and carcinoma without and with lymph node metastases. Legend: CRC, colorectal carcinoma; N0, without lymph node metastases; N+, with lymph node metastases; * $p \leq 0.05$; ** $p \leq 0.01$; *** $p \leq 0.001$.

3.6. Gene and miRNA Correlation to the Level of Malignancy

The Spearman correlation coefficient showed that *L1TD1* and *SLITRK6* were significantly correlated to level of malignancy. *L1TD1* was weakly positively correlated, *SLITRK6* was moderately negatively correlated and *miR-1225-3p* and *miR-1233-3p* were significantly positively correlated to the level of malignancy (Table 5).

Table 5. Spearman correlation coefficients of the association between ΔCq of analysed genes and miRNAs and level of malignancy (from normal mucosa to adenoma, adenoma with early carcinoma, carcinoma without and carcinoma with lymph node metastases).

Gene and miRNA	Correlation Coefficient	Significance (2-Tailed)
L1TD1	0.336	0.011
SLITRK6	−0.433	<0.001
ST6GALNAC1	−0.186	0.141
TCEA3	0.102	0.419
miR-199a-3p	0.128	0.291
miR-425-5p	0.209	0.083
miR-1225-3p	0.345	0.003
miR-1233-3p	0.276	0.021
miR-1303	0.014	0.912

4. Discussion

We validated four genes related to CSC and CSC-like properties which were previously identified using bioinformatics analysis as differentially expressed between normal mucosa, adenoma and CRC [12]. We also validated miRNAs postulated by a bioinformatics approach as regulating these genes. We found that in CRC, expression of *ST6GALNAC1* decreased and expression of *L1TD1* increased with level of malignancy, whereas *SLITRK6* and *TCEA3* showed variable expression. *TCEA3* was also related to the malignant transformation of adenoma to adenoma with early carcinoma and the development of lymph node metastases in CRC. Furthermore, we found differential expression of miRNAs that potentially regulate these genes (*miR-199a-3p, miR-425-5p, miR-1225-3p, miR-1233-3p* and *miR-1303*) and a negative correlation between *miR-199a-3p* and its potential target gene *SLITRK6*.

Expression of the *L1TD1* gene in our study progressively increased from adenoma to CRC, with the highest expression in CRC with lymph node metastases. L1TD1 has been shown to be associated with RNA binding, renewal of undifferentiated embryonal stem cells [13] and embryonal carcinoma cell lines [14]. In human embryonal stem cells, L1TD1 has also been associated with canonical markers of pluripotency that are also involved in cancerogenesis, such as *OCT4*, *NANOG*, *LIN28* and *SOX2* [15]. With the use of bioinformatics analysis, a higher expression of *L1TD1* in CRC was shown to be associated with longer disease-free survival [16]. Our results showed a positive trend of expression of *L1TD1* to CRC cancerogenesis. However, its role remains speculative due to limited information on *L1TD1* in cancerogenesis.

Our study showed variable expression of gene *SLITRK6* during CRC cancerogenesis. It was downregulated in all stages of CRC development, except in adenoma with early carcinoma, in which it was upregulated. SLITRK6 has been shown to be highly expressed in neural stem and progenitor cells [17], and it has been associated with cytoskeletal dynamics, axon guidance and cell adhesion [18]. In other cancer types, it was expressed at high levels in bladder cancer and, to a lesser extent, in lung cancer, breast cancer and glioblastomas. Moreover, in bladder cancer, it was suggested as a promising target for conjugate therapy [19]. A bioinformatics study on CRC showed differentially expressed *SLITRK6* together with *L1TD1* and *ST6GALNAC1* [16], and it was downregulated in CRC compared to adenomas using microarray expression analysis [41]. However, our results showed no significant differences in expression between adenomas and CRC. This difference may be explained by the use of different methodologies for expression analysis of *SLITRK6* (microarrays versus qPCR).

Gene expression of *ST6GALNAC1* in our study progressively decreased from adenoma to CRC, with the lowest expression in CRC with lymph node metastases. This gene, and its product STn antigen, has been demonstrated to be associated with cell contact, cell migration and prognosis of patients with carcinoma of the colon, stomach, pancreas, breast, prostate and ovaries [23]. STn antigen has been used as a target in immunotherapy trials for breast, colon and ovarian cancer [23]. Data regarding its expression and function in normal human tissues are limited [16,23]. It has also been associated with stem cell maintenance in ovarian cancer [42], as well as with the maintenance of isolated stem cells of CRC [23]. Its upregulation has been associated with good prognosis in breast cancer [43] and enhanced tumorigenicity in a breast cancer cell line [44]. siRNA silencing of *ST6GALNAC1* led to reduced growth, migration and invasion of gastric cancer cells in vitro [45], whereas its overexpression enhanced their metastatic ability [46]. Due to limited data on its role in CRC and different patterns of expression in several cancers, further investigation is needed for better understanding the involvement of this gene in CRC cancerogenesis and metastatic spread.

Gene *TCEA3* showed variable expression in our study, with significant upregulation in adenoma with early carcinoma and CRC without lymph node metastases. Interestingly, its expression was also significantly different between adenoma and CRC and between CRC without and with lymph node metastases, suggesting its role in metastases development. *TCEA3* was shown to have a higher expression level in mouse embryonal cells and was involved in regulation of stem cell differentiation [24]. Expression of *TCEA3* was lower in cell lines of ovarian carcinoma in which its interaction with receptor TGFβ I induced cell death [47]. *TCEA3* has also been associated with stomach cancer, in which high expression has been associated with better prognosis, lower proliferation of carcinoma cells and induction of apoptosis [48]. In a bioinformatics study of microarray expression data of normal colon tissue and CRC, *TCEA3* downregulation was identified among differentially expressed genes [49]. Our results are therefore consistent with previous findings on stomach cancer and CRC, thus contributing to understanding the involvement of *TCEA3* in CRC cancerogenesis.

When investigating correlations of genes/miRNAs with the level of malignancy, it is important to note that *SLITRK6* showed a moderate negative correlation and *L1TD1* was positively correlated with the level of malignancy. Among miRNAs, the expression of *miR-1225-3p* and *miR-1233-3p*, targeting *TCEA3*, were in weak positive correlation with the level of malignancy.

Interestingly, when investigating the miRNA-predicted target gene correlations, only *miR-199a-3p* and its target *SLITRK6* were in significant correlation. The pair was negatively correlated, which suggests inhibition of the target gene by the miRNA [50]. This correlation has not yet been previously observed in CRC.

miR-199a-3p was downregulated in our study in all investigated groups. However, no significant differences among the groups were found. In previous studies, *miR-199a-3p* was found to be highly expressed in the late stage of differentiation of human embryonal stem cells, as well as foetal pancreas and adult islet samples [51]. Additionally, *miR-199a-3p* was shown to target stemness and mitogenic-related pathways to suppress the expansion and tumorigenic capabilities of prostate cancer stem cells in vitro [52]. In CRC, *miR-199a-3p* was described as being significantly downregulated in the microarray expression data [53]. Upregulation of *miR-199a/b* contributed to cisplatin resistance in ALDHA1+ CRC stem cells [54]. Our data are consistent with previous microarray results on CRC. Further investigation of the exact involvement of *miR-199a-3p* in cancerogenesis of CRC is needed.

miR-425-5p was significantly upregulated in all investigated groups except CRC with lymph node metastases. Additionally, significant differences in expression were observed between adenoma and CRC and between CRC without and with lymph node metastases, suggesting its role in malignant transformation and the development of metastases. *miR-425-5p* has been previously associated with CRC, showing that *miR-425-5p* regulates chemoresistance in CRC cells [55] both in vitro and in vivo. A microarray analysis comparing isogenic chemo-sensitive and chemo-resistant HCT116 cell lines identified differentially expressed *miR-425-5p*. Xenograft mouse models showed that *miR-425-5p* inhibitor sensitized HCT116-R xenografts to chemotherapeutic drugs in vivo. *miR-425-5p* was also upregulated in a microarray expression experiment on CRC [56], and it was found that *miR-425-5p* downregulation impacted stemness and cisplatin resistance in laryngeal carcinoma cells [57]. Our results are consistent with previous microarray results on CRC.

miR-1225-3p is another miRNA in our study that was significantly upregulated in all investigated groups compared to normal mucosa. Additionally, it was also significantly differentially expressed between adenoma and CRC, suggesting a role in malignant transformation. Published data have shown that it was associated with the *TCEA3* gene in project GSE42095 performed on differentiated embryonic stem cells [51] and with CRC in project GSE35602 on CRC stromal tissue, in which it was upregulated [56]. Using microarray analysis, it was identified as one of the 173 differentially expressed miRNAs between spheroid body-forming cells (which possess gastric cancer stem cell properties) and parental cells on MKN-45 gastric cancer cell line cells [58]. Our results are consistent with microarray results on CRC stromal tissue.

miR-1233-3p was significantly upregulated in all investigated groups when compared to normal mucosa except CRC with lymph node metastases. Additionally, it was also significantly differentially expressed between adenoma and CRC, suggesting a role in malignant transformation. *miR-1233-3p* was associated with the *TCEA3* gene in project GSE28260, which was performed on renal cortex and medulla [59]. It was associated with CRC in a study performed on serum miRNA profiling in patients with colon adenomas or cancer, in which it was downregulated when comparing CRC to normal samples [60]. Before comparing our results to those performed on serum samples, it is important to note that, in addition to the fact that there are numerous differences in tissue types, there are also numerous differences in the methodologies used for profiling different tissue types.

miR-1303 showed variable expression with significant upregulation in adenoma in comparison to normal mucosa. Additionally, it was also significantly differentially expressed between adenoma and CRC, suggesting a role in malignant transformation. *miR-1303* has been previously investigated in association with CRC, in which it was found to be part of a group with frequent and sometimes biallelic mutations in microsatellite instable (MSI) tumours. No direct link was found between the presence or absence of mono- or biallelic alterations and the levels of mature *miR-1303* expression in MSI cell lines. A significant increase in *miR-1303* was observed in microsatellite stable (MSS) CRC cell lines in comparison to normal colonic mucosa [61]. A correlation between *miR-1303* and *L1TD1* was also previously identified in the integrative knowledge base for miRNA-mRNA expression in colorectal cancer [28]. However, expression of this miRNA is variable, and there are limited data regarding its role in CRC cancerogenesis.

Genes associated with CSC features could be promising prognostic and therapeutic markers. It has been previously shown that CSC-associated molecular profiles can predict tumour regeneration and disease relapse after conventional therapy in CRC patients [9,62–66]. Direct targeting can be achieved by inhibiting self-renewal pathways, by interfering with antiapoptotic or metabolic pathways, by activating differentiation pathways or by acting on the protective microenvironment through the involved genes. Several potential anti-CSC targeted drugs have emerged in previous studies, with some of them making their way to the clinic [67]. As previously mentioned, *SLITRK6* is a promising candidate for conjugate therapy in bladder cancer [19] and the product of *ST6GALNAC1* has been a target in immunotherapy trials for several cancers [23]. Studying miRNAs regulating selected genes is also a promising therapeutic approach by silencing these genes using miRNAs mimic or by depleting miRNAs using antagomirs to re-express investigated genes [68].

One of the limitations of our study is related to normal samples, which were taken at least 20 cm away from the tumour and showed no microscopic abnormalities. However, genetic and protein aberrations may already be present in morphologically normal mucosa [69,70]. Despite certain limitations, these samples may be used as corresponding control samples to overcome differences in the genetic background. Additionally, the newly identified associations of these genes and miRNAs with CSCs, CRC development and progression in this study are of a preliminary nature. Further validation through a functional study may be needed for additional confirmation of the results. Another limitation is the relatively small sample size. The latter is due to the use of formalin-fixed paraffin-embedded (FFPE) tissue samples, in which nucleic acids are fragmented and therefore difficult to analyse. However, all FFPE cases were evaluated by pathologists, enabling appropriate diagnosis. Furthermore, only samples that successfully passed the initial quality control and samples with stable expression of the reference genes were selected for further analysis, thus limiting the number of included samples.

5. Conclusions

Using a bioinformatics approach, we identified and validated new CSC-related genes with a previously unknown or poorly defined role in CRC development and progression. Expression of three investigated genes progressively increased (*L1TD1*) or decreased (*ST6GALNAC1*, *SLITRK6*) with the level of malignancy. The *TCEA3* gene was also related to the malignant transformation of adenoma to adenoma with early carcinoma and development of lymph node metastases in CRC.

The expression of some of the potential regulatory miRNAs confirmed the alterations in gene expression in CRC development. Our results provide further evidence that CSC-related genes and their regulatory miRNAs are involved in CRC cancerogenesis and progression, and suggest that some of them, particularly *miR-199a-3p* and its *SLITRK6* target gene, are promising for further validation in CRC.

Supplementary Materials: The following are available online at https://www.mdpi.com/2227-9059/9/2/179/s1.

Author Contributions: Conceptualization, K.U., E.B., N.Z.; methodology, K.U., M.Ž., E.B., validation, K.U. and M.Ž.; formal analysis, K.U.; data curation, K.U.; writing—original draft preparation, K.U. and E.B., writing—review and editing, E.B., M.Ž., N.Z.; visualization, K.U.; supervision, E.B., N.Z. All authors have read and agreed to the published version of the manuscript.

Funding: This research was funded by the Slovenian Research Agency (research core funding no. P3-0054; project funding J3-1754; PhD research funding).

Institutional Review Board Statement: The study was conducted according to the guidelines of the Declaration of Helsinki, and approved by the National Medical Ethics Committee (Republic of Slovenia, Ministry of Health), approval number 0120-54/2020/4.

Informed Consent Statement: Patient consent was waived due to the following reason. As stated in the approval document, the study is retrospective, observational, performed on tissue samples that were obtained during routine diagnostic/therapeutic procedures, consisted of either excision or resection. Therefore, enough tissue was available for routine analysis and research. Moreover, tissue is still available for any additional analysis in the future. Our State Ethical Committee does not require informed consent from patients in such studies. However, the informed consent was obtained before the routine procedure.

Conflicts of Interest: The authors declare no conflict of interest.

References

1. Kudryavtseva, A.V.; Lipatova, A.V.; Zaretsky, A.R.; Moskalev, A.A.; Fedorova, M.S.; Rasskazova, A.S.; Shibukhova, G.A.; Snezhkina, A.V.; Kaprin, A.D.; Alekseev, B.Y.; et al. Important molecular genetic markers of colorectal cancer. *Oncotarget* **2016**, *7*, 53959–53983. [CrossRef] [PubMed]
2. Cao, H.; Xu, E.; Liu, H.; Wan, L.; Lai, M.-D. Epithelial–mesenchymal transition in colorectal cancer metastasis: A system review. *Pathol. Res. Pr.* **2015**, *211*, 557–569. [CrossRef]
3. Balch, C.; Ramapuram, J.B.; Tiwari, A.K. The epigenomics of embryonic pathway signaling in colorectal cancer. *Front. Pharmacol.* **2017**, *8*, 267. [CrossRef]
4. Sepulveda, A.R.; Portillo, A.J.D. Molecular basis of diseases of the gastrointestinal tract. In *Molecular Pathology*, 2nd ed.; Coleman, W.B., Tsongalis, G.J., Eds.; Elsevier BV: Amsterdam, The Netherlands, 2018; pp. 387–415. [CrossRef]
5. Järvinen, H.J.; Mecklin, J.-P.; Sistonen, P. Screening reduces colorectal cancer rate in families with hereditary nonpolyposis colorectal cancer. *Gastroenterology* **1995**, *108*, 1405–1411. [CrossRef]
6. Brenner, H.; Jansen, L.; Ulrich, A.; Chang-Claude, J.; Hoffmeister, M. Survival of patients with symptom- and screening-detected colorectal cancer. *Oncotarget* **2016**, *7*, 44695–44704. [CrossRef]
7. Fischer, J.; Walker, L.C.; Robinson, B.A.; Frizelle, F.A.; Church, J.M.; Eglinton, T.W. Clinical implications of the genetics of sporadic colorectal cancer. *ANZ J. Surg.* **2019**, *89*, 1224–1229. [CrossRef] [PubMed]
8. Blank, A.; Roberts, D.E.I.; Dawson, H.; Zlobec, I.; Lugli, A. Tumor heterogeneity in primary colorectal cancer and corresponding metastases. Does the apple fall far from the tree? *Front. Med.* **2018**, *5*, 234. [CrossRef]
9. Dylla, S.J.; Beviglia, L.; Clarke, M.F.; Hoey, T.; Lewicki, J.; Gurney, A.L.; Park, I.-K.; Chartier, C.; Raval, J.; Ngan, L.; et al. Colorectal cancer stem cells are enriched in xenogeneic tumors following chemotherapy. *PLoS ONE* **2008**, *3*, e2428. [CrossRef]
10. Saiki, Y.; Ishimaru, S.; Mimori, K.; Takatsuno, Y.; Nagahara, M.; Ishii, H.; Yamada, K.; Mori, M. Comprehensive analysis of the clinical significance of inducing pluripotent stemness-related gene expression in colorectal cancer cells. *Ann. Surg. Oncol.* **2009**, *16*, 2638–2644. [CrossRef]
11. Munro, M.J.; Wickremesekera, S.K.; Peng, L.; Tan, S.T.; Itinteang, T. Cancer stem cells in colorectal cancer: A review. *J. Clin. Pathol.* **2018**, *71*, 110–116. [CrossRef]
12. Hauptman, N.; Boštjančič, E.; Žlajpah, M.; Ranković, B.; Zidar, N. Bioinformatics analysis reveals most prominent gene candidates to distinguish colorectal adenoma from adenocarcinoma. *BioMed Res. Int.* **2018**, *2018*, 1–10. [CrossRef] [PubMed]
13. Wong, R.C.-B.; Ibrahim, A.; Fong, H.; Thompson, N.; Lock, L.F.; Donovan, P.J. L1TD1 is a marker for undifferentiated human embryonic stem cells. *PLoS ONE* **2011**, *6*, e19355. [CrossRef] [PubMed]
14. Närvä, E.; Rahkonen, N.; Rao, A.; Lahesmaa, R.; Emani, M.R.; Lund, R.; Pursiheimo, J.-P.; Nästi, J.; Autio, R.; Rasool, O.; et al. RNA-binding protein L1TD1 interacts with LIN28 via RNA and is required for human embryonic stem cell self-renewal and cancer cell proliferation. *Stem Cells* **2011**, *30*, 452–460. [CrossRef] [PubMed]
15. Emani, M.R.; Närvä, E.; Stubb, A.; Chakroborty, D.; Viitala, M.; Rokka, A.; Rahkonen, N.; Moulder, R.; Denessiouk, K.; Trokovic, R.; et al. The L1TD1 protein interactome reveals the importance of post-transcriptional regulation in human pluripotency. *Stem Cell Rep.* **2015**, *4*, 519–528. [CrossRef] [PubMed]
16. Chakroborty, D.; Emani, M.; Klén, R.; Böckelman, C.; Hagström, J.; Haglund, C.; Ristimäki, A.; Lahesmaa, R.; Elo, L.L. L1TD1-a prognostic marker for colon cancer. *BMC Cancer* **2019**, *19*, 727. [CrossRef] [PubMed]
17. Sandberg, C.J.; Vik-Mo, E.O.; Behnan, J.; Helseth, E.; Langmoen, I.A. Transcriptional profiling of adult neural stem-like cells from the human brain. *PLoS ONE* **2014**, *9*, e114739. [CrossRef] [PubMed]

18. Proenca, C.C.; Gao, P.; Shmelkov, S.V.; Rafii, S.; Lee, F.S. Slitrks as emerging candidate genes involved in neuropsychiatric disorders. *Trends Neurosci.* **2011**, *34*, 143–153. [CrossRef]
19. Morrison, K.; Challita-Eid, P.M.; Verlinsky, A.; Aviña, H.; Doñate, F.; Joseph, I.B.; Pereira, D.S.; Morrison, K.; Stover, D.R.; Raitano, A.; et al. Development of ASG-15ME, a novel antibody-drug conjugate targeting *SLITRK6*, a new urothelial cancer biomarker. *Mol. Cancer Ther.* **2016**, *15*, 1301–1310. [CrossRef] [PubMed]
20. Farahani, E.; Patra, H.K.; Jangamreddy, J.R.; Rashedi, I.; Kawalec, M.; Pariti, R.K.R.; Batakis, P.; Wiechec, E. Cell adhesion molecules and their relation to (cancer) cell stemness. *Carcinogenesis* **2014**, *35*, 747–759. [CrossRef]
21. Ambriz, X.; De Lanerolle, P.; Ambrosio, J.R. The mechanobiology of the actin cytoskeleton in stem cells during differentiation and interaction with biomaterials. *Stem Cells Int.* **2018**, *2018*, 1–11. [CrossRef]
22. Yamaguchi, H.; Condeelis, J. Regulation of the actin cytoskeleton in cancer cell migration and invasion. *Biochim. Biophys. Acta (BBA) Mol. Cell Res.* **2007**, *1773*, 642–652. [CrossRef]
23. Ogawa, T.; Hirohashi, Y.; Murai, A.; Nishidate, T.; Okita, K.; Wang, L.; Ikehara, Y.; Satoyoshi, T.; Usui, A.; Kubo, T.; et al. *ST6GALNAC1* plays important roles in enhancing cancer stem phenotypes of colorectal cancer via the Akt pathway. *Oncotarget* **2017**, *8*, 112550–112564. [CrossRef]
24. Park, K.-S.; Cha, Y.; Han, Y.-M.; Kim, J.; Song, J.; Kim, J.Y.; Tesar, P.J.; Lanza, R.; Lee, K.-A.; Kim, K.-S.; et al. Transcription elongation factor Tcea3 regulates the pluripotent differentiation potential of mouse embryonic stem cells, via the Lefty1-Nodal-Smad2 pathway. *Stem Cells* **2012**, *31*, 282–292. [CrossRef] [PubMed]
25. Brierley, J.D.; Gospodarowicz, M.K.; Wittekind, C. (Eds.) *TNM Classification of Malignant Tumours*, 8th ed.; Wiley Blackwell: Oxford, UK, 2017.
26. Chou, C.H.; Shrestha, S.; Yang, C.D.; Chang, N.W.; Lin, Y.L.; Liao, K.W.; Huang, W.C.; Sun, T.H.; Tu, S.J.; Lee, W.H.; et al. miRTarBase update 2018: A resource for experimentally validated microRNA-target interactions. *Nucleic Acids Res.* **2018**, *46*, D296–D302. [CrossRef] [PubMed]
27. Liu, W.; Wang, X. Prediction of functional microRNA targets by integrative modeling of microRNA binding and target expression data. *Genome Biol.* **2019**, *20*, 1–10. [CrossRef] [PubMed]
28. Skok, D.J.; Hauptman, N.; Boštjančič, E.; Zidar, N. The integrative knowledge base for miRNA-mRNA expression in colorectal cancer. *Sci. Rep.* **2019**, *9*, 1–9. [CrossRef]
29. Karagkouni, D.; Paraskevopoulou, M.D.; Chatzopoulos, S.; Vlachos, I.S.; Tastsoglou, S.; Kanellos, I.; Papadimitriou, D.; Kavakiotis, I.; Maniou, S.; Skoufos, G.; et al. DIANA-TarBase v8: A decade-long collection of experimentally supported miRNA–gene interactions. *Nucleic Acids Res.* **2018**, *46*, D239–D245. [CrossRef] [PubMed]
30. Agarwal, V.; Bell, G.W.; Nam, J.-W.; Bartel, D.P. Predicting effective microRNA target sites in mammalian mRNAs. *eLife* **2015**, *4*, e05005. [CrossRef]
31. Kozomara, A.; Birgaoanu, M.; Griffiths-Jones, S. miRBase: From microRNA sequences to function. *Nucleic Acids Res.* **2019**, *47*, D155–D162. [CrossRef]
32. Brennecke, J.; Stark, A.; Russell, R.B.; Cohen, S.M. Principles of microRNA–target recognition. *PLoS Biol.* **2005**, *3*, e85. [CrossRef]
33. Kertesz, M.; Iovino, N.; Unnerstall, U.; Gaul, U.; Segal, E. The role of site accessibility in microRNA target recognition. *Nat. Genet.* **2007**, *39*, 1278–1284. [CrossRef]
34. Zhao, Y.; Samal, E.; Srivastava, D. Serum response factor regulates a muscle-specific microRNA that targets Hand2 during cardiogenesis. *Nat. Cell Biol.* **2005**, *436*, 214–220. [CrossRef]
35. Boštjančič, E.; Zidar, N.; Glavač, D. MicroRNAs and cardiac sarcoplasmic reticulum calcium ATPase-2 in human myocardial infarction: Expression and bioinformatic analysis. *BMC Genom.* **2012**, *13*, 552. [CrossRef]
36. Benias, P.C.; Wells, R.G.; Theise, N.D.; Sackey-Aboagye, B.; Klavan, H.; Reidy, J.; Buonocore, D.; Miranda, M.; Kornacki, S.; Wayne, M.; et al. Structure and distribution of an unrecognized interstitium in human tissues. *Sci. Rep.* **2018**, *8*, 1–8. [CrossRef]
37. Lorenz, R.; Bernhart, S.H.F.; Zu Siederdissen, C.H.; Tafer, H.; Flamm, C.; Stadler, P.F.; Hofacker, I.L. ViennaRNA package 2.0. *Algorithms Mol. Biol.* **2011**, *6*, 26. [CrossRef] [PubMed]
38. Doench, J.G. Specificity of microRNA target selection in translational repression. *Genes Dev.* **2004**, *18*, 504–511. [CrossRef] [PubMed]
39. Miranda, K.C.; Huynh, T.; Tay, Y.; Ang, Y.-S.; Tam, W.-L.; Thomson, A.M.; Lim, B.; Rigoutsos, I. A pattern-based method for the identification of microrna binding sites and their corresponding heteroduplexes. *Cell* **2006**, *126*, 1203–1217. [CrossRef]
40. Latham, G.J. Normalization of microRNA quantitative RT-PCR data in reduced scale experimental designs. *Methods Mol. Biol.* **2010**, *667*, 19–31. [CrossRef] [PubMed]
41. Carvalho, B.; Sillars-Hardebol, A.H.; Postma, C.; Mongera, S.; Droste, J.T.S.; Obulkasim, A.; Van De Wiel, M.; Van Criekinge, W.; Ylstra, B.; Fijneman, R.J.A.; et al. Colorectal adenoma to carcinoma progression is accompanied by changes in gene expression associated with ageing, chromosomal instability, and fatty acid metabolism. *Cell. Oncol.* **2012**, *35*, 53–63. [CrossRef] [PubMed]
42. Wang, W.-Y.; Cao, Y.-X.; Zhou, X.; Wei, B.; Zhan, L.; Sun, S.-Y. Stimulative role of *ST6GALNAC1* in proliferation, migration and invasion of ovarian cancer stem cells via the Akt signaling pathway. *Cancer Cell Int.* **2019**, *19*, 86. [CrossRef]
43. Patani, N.; Jiang, W.; Mokbel, K. Prognostic utility of glycosyltransferase expression in breast cancer. *Cancer Genom. Proteom.* **2009**, *5*, 333–340.

44. Julien, S.; Adriaenssens, E.; Ottenberg, K.; Furlan, A.J.; Courtand, G.; Vercoutter-Edouart, A.-S.; Hanisch, F.-G.; Delannoy, P.; Le Bourhis, X. ST6GalNAc I expression in MDA-MB-231 breast cancer cells greatly modifies their O-glycosylation pattern and enhances their tumourigenicity. *Glycobiology* **2005**, *16*, 54–64. [CrossRef]
45. Tamura, F.; Sato, Y.; Hirakawa, M.; Yoshida, M.; Ono, M.; Osuga, T.; Okagawa, Y.; Uemura, N.; Arihara, Y.; Murase, K.; et al. RNAi-mediated gene silencing of ST6GalNAc I suppresses the metastatic potential in gastric cancer cells. *Gastric Cancer* **2016**, *19*, 85–97. [CrossRef]
46. Ozaki, H.; Matsuzaki, H.; Ando, H.; Kaji, H.; Nakanishi, H.; Ikehara, Y.; Narimatsu, H. Enhancement of metastatic ability by ectopic expression of ST6GalNAcI on a gastric cancer cell line in a mouse model. *Clin. Exp. Metastasis* **2012**, *29*, 229–238. [CrossRef]
47. Cha, Y.; Kim, D.-K.; Hyun, J.; Kim, S.-J.; Park, K.-S. TCEA3 binds to TGF-beta receptor I and induces Smad-independent, JNK-dependent apoptosis in ovarian cancer cells. *Cell. Signal.* **2013**, *25*, 1245–1251. [CrossRef]
48. Li, J.; Jin, Y.; Pan, S.; Chen, Y.; Wang, K.; Lin, C.; Jin, S.; Wu, J. TCEA3 attenuates gastric cancer growth by apoptosis induction. *Med. Sci. Monit.* **2015**, *21*, 3241–3246. [CrossRef]
49. Guo, Y.; Bao, Y.; Ma, M.; Yang, W. Identification of key candidate genes and pathways in colorectal cancer by integrated bioinformatical analysis. *Int. J. Mol. Sci.* **2017**, *18*, 722. [CrossRef]
50. Diaz, G.; Zamboni, F.; Tice, A.; Farci, P. Integrated ordination of miRNA and mRNA expression profiles. *BMC Genom.* **2015**, *16*, 1–13. [CrossRef]
51. Liao, X.; Xue, H.; Wang, Y.-C.; Nazor, K.L.; Guo, S.; Trivedi, N.N.; Peterson, S.E.; Liu, Y.; Loring, J.F.; Laurent, L. Matched miRNA and mRNA signatures from an hESC-based in vitro model of pancreatic differentiation reveal novel regulatory interactions. *J. Cell Sci.* **2013**, *126*, 3848–3861. [CrossRef]
52. Liu, R.; Liu, C.; Zhang, D.; Liu, B.; Chen, X.; Rycaj, K.; Jeter, C.; Calhoun-Davis, T.; Li, Y.; Yang, T.; et al. miR-199a-3p targets stemness-related and mitogenic signaling pathways to suppress the expansion and tumorigenic capabilities of prostate cancer stem cells. *Oncotarget* **2016**, *7*, 56628–56642. [CrossRef]
53. Shen, Z.-L.; Wang, B.; Jiang, K.-W.; Ye, C.-X.; Cheng, C.; Yan, Y.-C.; Zhang, J.-Z.; Yang, Y.; Gao, Z.-D.; Ye, Y.-J.; et al. Downregulation of miR-199b is associated with distant metastasis in colorectal cancer via activation of SIRT1 and inhibition of CREB/KISS1 signaling. *Oncotarget* **2016**, *7*, 35092–35105. [CrossRef]
54. Chen, B.; Zhang, D.; Kuai, J.; Cheng, M.; Fang, X.; Li, G. Upregulation of miR-199a/b contributes to cisplatin resistance via Wnt/β-catenin-ABCG2 signaling pathway in ALDHA1+ colorectal cancer stem cells. *Tumor Biol.* **2017**, *39*. [CrossRef]
55. Zhang, Y.; Hu, X.; Miao, X.; Zhu, K.; Cui, S.; Meng, Q.; Sun, J.; Wang, T. Micro RNA-425-5p regulates chemoresistance in colorectal cancer cells via regulation of Programmed Cell Death 10. *J. Cell. Mol. Med.* **2016**, *20*, 360–369. [CrossRef]
56. Nishida, N.; Nagahara, M.; Mori, M.; Sato, T.; Mimori, K.; Sudo, T.; Tanaka, F.; Shibata, K.; Ishii, H.; Sugihara, K.; et al. Microarray analysis of colorectal cancer stromal tissue reveals upregulation of two oncogenic mirna clusters. *Clin. Cancer Res.* **2012**, *18*, 3054–3070. [CrossRef]
57. Yuan, Z.; Xiu, C.; Liu, D.; Zhou, G.; Yang, H.; Pei, R.; Ding, C.; Cui, X.; Sun, J.; Song, K. Long noncoding RNA LINC-PINT regulates laryngeal carcinoma cell stemness and chemoresistance through miR-425-5p/PTCH1/SHH axis. *J. Cell. Physiol.* **2019**, *234*, 23111–23122. [CrossRef]
58. Liu, J.; Ma, L.; Wang, Z.; Wang, L.; Liu, C.; Chen, R.; Zhang, J. MicroRNA expression profile of gastric cancer stem cells in the MKN-45 cancer cell line. *Acta Biochim. Biophys. Sin.* **2014**, *46*, 92–99. [CrossRef]
59. Marques, F.Z.; Campain, A.E.; Tomaszewski, M.; Zukowska-Szczechowska, E.; Yang, Y.H.J.; Charchar, F.J.; Morris, B.J. Gene expression profiling reveals renin mRNA overexpression in human hypertensive kidneys and a role for microRNAs. *Hypertension* **2011**, *58*, 1093–1098. [CrossRef]
60. Zhang, Y.; Li, M.; Ding, Y.; Fan, Z.; Zhang, J.; Zhang, H.; Jiang, B.; Zhu, Y. Serum MicroRNA profile in patients with colon adenomas or cancer. *BMC Med. Genom.* **2017**, *10*, 23. [CrossRef]
61. El-Murr, N.; Abidi, Z.; Wanherdrick, K.; Svrcek, M.; Gaub, M.-P.; Flejou, J.-F.; Hamelin, R.; Duval, A.; Lesuffleur, T. MiRNA genes constitute new targets for microsatellite instability in colorectal cancer. *PLoS ONE* **2012**, *7*, e31862. [CrossRef]
62. Giampieri, R.; Scartozzi, M.; Cecchini, L.; Guerrieri, F.; Bearzi, I.; Cascinu, S.; Loretelli, C.; Piva, F.; Mandolesi, A.; Lezoche, G.; et al. Cancer stem cell gene profile as predictor of relapse in high risk stage II and stage III, radically resected colon cancer patients. *PLoS ONE* **2013**, *8*, e72843. [CrossRef]
63. Merlos-Suárez, A.; Barriga, F.M.; Clevers, H.; Sancho, E.; Mangues, R.; Batlle, E.; Jung, P.; Iglesias, M.; Céspedes, M.V.; Rossell, D.; et al. The intestinal stem cell signature identifies colorectal cancer stem cells and predicts disease relapse. *Cell Stem Cell* **2011**, *8*, 511–524. [CrossRef]
64. Colak, S.; Zimberlin, C.D.; Fessler, E.; Hogdal, L.J.; Prasetyanti, P.R.; Grandela, C.; Letai, A.; Medema, J.P. Decreased mitochondrial priming determines chemoresistance of colon cancer stem cells. *Cell Death Differ.* **2014**, *21*, 1170–1177. [CrossRef]
65. Lombardo, Y.; Scopelliti, A.; Cammareri, P.; Todaro, M.; Iovino, F.; Ricci–Vitiani, L.; Gulotta, G.; Dieli, F.; De Maria, R.; Stassi, G. Bone morphogenetic protein 4 induces differentiation of colorectal cancer stem cells and increases their response to chemotherapy in mice. *Gastroenterology* **2011**, *140*, 297–309.e6. [CrossRef]
66. Lotti, F.; Jarrar, A.M.; Pai, R.K.; Hitomi, M.; Lathia, J.; Mace, A.; Gantt, G.A.; Sukhdeo, K.; DeVecchio, J.; Vasanji, A.; et al. Chemotherapy activates cancer-associated fibroblasts to maintain colorectal cancer-initiating cells by IL-17A. *J. Exp. Med.* **2013**, *210*, 2851–2872. [CrossRef]

67. Zeuner, A.; Todaro, M.; Stassi, G.; De Maria, R. Colorectal cancer stem cells: From the crypt to the clinic. *Cell Stem Cell* **2014**, *15*, 692–705. [CrossRef]
68. Wang, V.; Wu, W. MicroRNA-based therapeutics for cancer. *BioDrugs* **2009**, *23*, 15–23. [CrossRef]
69. Sanz-Pamplona, R.; Berenguer, A.; Cordero, D.; Molleví, D.G.; Crous-Bou, M.; Sole, X.; Paré-Brunet, L.; Guino, E.; Salazar, R.; Santos, C.; et al. Aberrant gene expression in mucosa adjacent to tumor reveals a molecular crosstalk in colon cancer. *Mol. Cancer* **2014**, *13*, 46. [CrossRef]
70. Polley, A.C.; Mulholland, F.; Pin, C.; Williams, E.A.; Bradburn, D.M.; Mills, S.J.; Mathers, J.C.; Johnson, I.T. Proteomic analysis reveals field-wide changes in protein expression in the morphologically normal mucosa of patients with colorectal neoplasia. *Cancer Res.* **2006**, *66*, 6553–6562. [CrossRef]

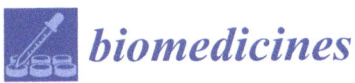

Review

TRIM Proteins in Colorectal Cancer: TRIM8 as a Promising Therapeutic Target in Chemo Resistance

Flaviana Marzano [1], Mariano Francesco Caratozzolo [1], Graziano Pesole [1,2], Elisabetta Sbisà [3] and Apollonia Tullo [1,*]

[1] Institute of Biomembranes, Bioenergetics and Molecular Biotechnologies, National Research Council, CNR, 70126 Bari, Italy; f.marzano@ibiom.cnr.it (F.M.); mf.caratozzolo@ibiom.cnr.it (M.F.C.); g.pesole@ibiom.cnr.it (G.P.)

[2] Department of Biosciences, Biotechnology and Biopharmaceutics, University of Bari, "Aldo Moro", 70125 Bari, Italy

[3] Institute for Biomedical Technologies, National Research Council, CNR, 70126 Bari, Italy; elisabetta.sbisa@ba.itb.cnr.it

* Correspondence: a.tullo@ibiom.cnr.it

Abstract: Colorectal cancer (CRC) represents one of the most widespread forms of cancer in the population and, as all malignant tumors, often develops resistance to chemotherapies with consequent tumor growth and spreading leading to the patient's premature death. For this reason, a great challenge is to identify new therapeutic targets, able to restore the drugs sensitivity of cancer cells. In this review, we discuss the role of TRIpartite Motifs (TRIM) proteins in cancers and in CRC chemoresistance, focusing on the tumor-suppressor role of TRIM8 protein in the reactivation of the CRC cells sensitivity to drugs currently used in the clinical practice. Since the restoration of TRIM8 protein levels in CRC cells recovers chemotherapy response, it may represent a new promising therapeutic target in the treatment of CRC.

Keywords: CRC; chemoresistance; TRIM8; miR-17-5p

Citation: Marzano, F.; Caratozzolo, M.F.; Pesole, G.; Sbisà, E.; Tullo, A. TRIM Proteins in Colorectal Cancer: TRIM8 as a Promising Therapeutic Target in Chemo Resistance. *Biomedicines* 2021, 9, 241. https://doi.org/10.3390/biomedicines9030241

Academic Editor: Veronique Baud

Received: 14 January 2021
Accepted: 23 February 2021
Published: 27 February 2021

Publisher's Note: MDPI stays neutral with regard to jurisdictional claims in published maps and institutional affiliations.

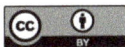

Copyright: © 2021 by the authors. Licensee MDPI, Basel, Switzerland. This article is an open access article distributed under the terms and conditions of the Creative Commons Attribution (CC BY) license (https://creativecommons.org/licenses/by/4.0/).

1. The CRC Therapy

Colorectal cancer (CRC) is one of the most prevalent malignancy tumors with high morbidity and mortality. Risk factors for the occurrence of CRC are related to both external factors such as diet, obesity, smoking, old age, chronic intestinal inflammation and genetic factors. The majority of CRC (70–80%) is sporadic, while around 20–30% of CRC has a hereditary component, such as Lynch Syndrome (LS) (3–4%) and the familial adenomatous polyposis (FAP) (~1%) [1]. A high percentage of sporadic CRC is characterized by deletions, translocations and other chromosomal rearrangements identified as chromosomal instability (CIN) [2]. A smaller percentage of sporadic CRC show a defective DNA mismatch repair (MMR), caused by hypermutated regions and microsatellite instability (MSI) [3].

Moreover, CpG island methylation phenotype (CIMP), is an epigenetic cause of CRC, as it induces silencing of a range of tumor suppressor genes, including MutL Homolog 1 (*MLH1*), and one of the *MMR* genes [4,5]. Recently, a classification of CRC into four Consensus Molecular Subtypes (CMS) has been reported in the literature: CMS1 (MSI Immune, 14%), hypermutated, microsatellite unstable, strong immune activation; CMS2 (Canonical, 37%), epithelial, chromosomally unstable, marked WNT and MYC signaling activation; CMS3 (Metabolic, 13%), epithelial, evident metabolic dysregulation; and CMS4 (Mesenchymal, 23%), prominent transforming growth factor β activation, stromal invasion, and angiogenesis [6].

All of the studies carried out so far have demonstrated that an earlier diagnosis is correlated with a better prognosis [7,8]. Current treatments used for CRC include some combination of surgery, radio-/chemotherapies and targeted therapy [8]. Unfortunately, despite some advances in pharmacological therapies, the 5-year survival rate of patients with late stage CRC is very poor because of recurrence and metastasis; moreover, one essential reason for treatment failure is the presence of innate or acquired resistance, which affects 90% of patients with metastatic cancer [7–9].

The main therapy for CRC patients has been, since the 1950s, chemotherapy based on 5-fluorouracil (5-FU) [8–10]. This drug inhibits DNA replication, replacing thymidine with fluorinated nucleotides into the DNA, hereby causing cell death. The active metabolite of 5-FU, fluorodeoxyuridine mono-phosphate (FdUMP), inhibits thymidylate synthase (TS), the enzyme essential for the conversion of deoxyuridine mono-phosphate to deoxythymidine monophosphate in the DNA synthesis pathway [11]. Different studies show that high TS levels are closely associated with the 5-FU resistance of cancer cells [12,13]. It follows that 5-FU resistance is closely related to the expression of thymidylate synthase (TS) and patients with low TS expression show a better prognosis [14,15].

Other enzymes involved in the metabolism and degradation of 5-FU, such as Thymidine phosphorylase (TP), uridine phosphorylase (UP), orotate phosphoribosyl transferase (OPRT) and dihydropyrimidine dehydrogenase (DPD), are correlated with sensitivity of CRC cells to 5-FU. It is reported that higher levels of TP, UP and OPRT displayed enhanced sensitivity to 5-FU therapy [16–18], by contrast, DPD expression level is inversely correlated with chemosensitivity [17].

Capecitabine was the first oral chemotherapy drug for CRC. Thymidylate synthase (TS), is the enzyme that converts capecitabine to 5-FU and for this reason loss of function of this enzyme confers the resistance of Capecitabine [19,20].

Moreover, the literature reports that changes in the status of *p53* affects the sensitivity to TS inhibitors, suggesting that analysis of the status of *p53* (e.g., wild type or mutant and functionally active or not) could be useful to predict the clinical outcome of the chemotherapy with TS inhibitors [21].

FOLFOX is the first combined chemotherapeutic strategy which integrates the use of 5-FU with Leucovorin and Oxaliplatin (a platinum-based chemotherapeutic drug approved for the treatment of CRC).

Oxaliplatin causes DNA breaks that are difficult to repair, hereby improving its tumor cell killing potential [22]. Oxaliplatin effectiveness is related to the expression level of nucleotide excision repair (*NER*) genes; indeed, ERCC1, XRCC1 and XDP, and WBSCR22 proteins represent novel oxaliplatin resistance biomarkers.

TGF-β1-treated CRC cells have been shown to increase epithelial mesenchymal transition, indicating the involvement of TGF-β1 in resistance to oxaliplatin [23–25].

Irinotecan (CPT-11), a semi-synthetic derivative of the plant extract camptothecin, is another chemotherapeutic drug used in CRC, that inhibits topoisomerase I (Topo I). In cells, Irinotecan becomes an active metabolite, SN-38, with a stronger anticancer activity, and forms a topoisomerase-inhibitor-DNA complex affecting the DNA function. Elevated levels of Topo I make cells more sensitive to irinotecan [26,27]. Furthermore, carboxylesterases (CES), uridine diphosphate glucuronosyltransferase (UGT), hepatic cytochrome P-450 enzymes CYP3A, β-glucuronidase and ATP-binding cassette (ABC) transporter protein, involved in the uptake and metabolism of Irinotecan, have a role in chemoresistance [28,29]. If the Irinotecan resistance is due to the epigenetic changes occurring in CRC, the use of histone deacetylase (HDAC) inhibitors could solve the resistance of the CRC cells to Irinotecan [30].

A second-line option for the combined treatment of mCRC (metastatic CRC), is represented by Capecitabine and Irinotecan therapy (XELIRI) with or without Bevacizumab [31,32]. The advent of monoclonal antibodies such as Bevacizumab and Cetuximab permitted great development in the CRC therapy.

In the last few years, studies have focused on stem cells and their prognostic value for CRC [33,34]. In fact, these cells show an enrichment of surface markers such as CD133, EphB2high, EpCAMhigh, CD44+, CD166+, ALDH+, LGR5+ and CD44v6+, which are useful for prognosis and follow the course of the pathology [35]; moreover, these cells show a higher expression of ATP binding cassette (ABC) family members, the efflux pumps that promote the transport of drugs outside the cell [36,37].

In addition to those described, other drugs in recent years have been used to treat CRC, including tyrosine kinase inhibitors (TKI) such as Sorafenib and Axitinib that block cell proliferation by inhibiting the mitogen-activated protein kinase (MAPK) pathway and prevent tumor-associated angiogenesis. Several studies have shown that the single use of TKIs is ineffective to increase patient survival and combined approaches are under investigation. Some clinical data suggested the use of Sorafenib in combination with oxaliplatin and irinotecan in metastatic CRC patients as it appears to block cell proliferation [38,39]; in other studies, sorafenib, used in combination with standard FOLFOX chemotherapy, was not effective [40–42]. Axitinib seems to have a better effect used in combination therapy with other chemotherapeutic drugs such as Erlotinib and Dasatinib [42].

Furthermore, Cisplatin is employed for the treatment of CRC, inducing the formation of platinum–DNA adducts [43], which in turn trigger the apoptotic process [44]. Cisplatin treatment often results in the development of resistance, leading to therapeutic failure. Intense research has identified several mechanisms underlying Cisplatin resistance [45,46].

Nutlin-3 is a chemotherapeutic drug that inhibits the interaction between Mouse double minute 2 homolog (MDM2) and tumor suppressor p53 causing the stabilization of p53 and its consequent activation. In this way p53 leads to the inhibition of cancer cell proliferation and the induction of cellular senescence.

The Doxorubicin is an antineoplastic antibiotic of the anthracycline family with a broad antitumor spectrum. The drug binds to cellular DNA, inhibiting nucleic acid synthesis and mitosis and causing chromosomal aberrations. The literature shows that a combination of Nutlin-3 and Doxorubicin was more effective in treatment [47].

A novel important approach in cancer therapy is represented by the application of proteasome inhibitors [48–51]. In particular E3 ligases, enzymes that perform the final step in the ubiquitination cascade, represent drug targets for its ability to regulate protein stability and functions [52,53]. For this reason researchers are exploring the role of E3 ligases in tumor chemotherapy resistance and the underlying mechanism [54–60]. Indeed, a growing number of E3 ligases and related substrate proteins, such as the RING finger protein (RNFs), MDM2, the apoptotic protein inhibitor (IAPs), and tripartite proteins (TRIMs), have emerged as crucial players in drug resistance of several cancers, including CRC [61,62]. The literature reports that both C3HC4-typezinc finger-containing 1 (RBCK1), also known as HOIL-1L (a protein with an N-terminal ubiquitin like (UBL) domain) and the 3-ubiquitin ligase FBXW7 (a protein that influences the epithelial–stromal micro environmental interactions) increase epithelial-mesenchymal transition (EMT) and contribute to chemoresistance and stemness in CRC [63]. The miR-223/FBXW7 pathway has been reported to play a crucial role in the mechanism of chemoresistance in many human cancers, such as gastric, breast, and non-small cell lung cancers. However, it is unclear whether similar mechanisms of doxorubicin resistance are involved in particular in CRC. The miR-223/FBXW7 axis regulates doxorubicin sensitivity through EMT in CRC [64]. Moreover, the overexpression of RNF126, RING finger protein 126 (RNF126), a novel E3 ubiquitin ligase, was remarkably associated with multiple advanced clinical features of CRC patients independent of *p53* status. RNF126 promotes cell proliferation, mobility, and drug resistance in CRC via enhancing p53 ubiquitination and degradation [65]. Considering the resistance mechanisms described for the CRC, more research is needed to clarify the role in this mechanism of others E3 ligases such as TRIM proteins.

2. TRIM Proteins in Cancer

The TRIpartite Motifs (TRIM) protein family is composed of more than 70 known TRIM proteins in humans and mice, which are encoded by approximately 71 genes in humans. The TRIpatite Motif is composed by three zinc-binding domains, a RING domain (R), a B-box type 1 (B1) and a B-box type 2 (B2), followed by a coiled-coil (CC) region [66,67]. Functionally, the RING finger domain is involved in the ubiquitination system, mediating the transfer of ubiquitin from E2-Ub ligase enzyme to its substrates: this domain is therefore a characteristic signature of many E3 ubiquitin ligases [68]. Genes encoding for TRIM proteins are present in all metazoans [69] and mutations in these genes are implicated in a variety of human diseases including cancer.

This is not surprising if we consider that TRIM family proteins are involved in a plethora of cellular functions, such as regulation of gene expression, signal transduction pathways, autophagy, cell growth, migration, protein stability through the ubiquitination system, regulation of development and immune response, effects on cell survival and metabolism and direct antiviral action. Alterations of TRIM expression levels represent biomarker and prognostic factors of specific cancers including osteosarcoma, gastric, liver, breast, ovarian, prostate, lung, cervical and CRC [70–72].

Depending on tumor type and on their deregulation mechanisms, TRIMs proteins can exert their action both as onco-protein and tumor-suppressor proteins in cancers. To date, many TRIMs proteins have resulted to be overexpressed in one or more cancers. TRIMs 11, 14, 22, 24, 25, 27, 28, 32, 37, 44, 47, 49, 59, 65 are upregulated in some of the high incidence cancers (breast, gastric, liver, lung, osteosarcoma, prostate, kidney) [73–114], while some others TRIM are upregulated in a cancer-specific way (e.g., TRIM22 in lung, TRIM31 and TRIM35 in liver, TRIM63 in breast, TRIM66 in osteosarcoma, TRIM68 in prostate). The altered expression of this TRIMs has been correlated with poor prognosis [115–119] (Table 1). On the contrary, there are also many TRIMs downregulated in tumors. TRIMs 3, 8, 13, 16, 21, 62 are downregulated in many of the main cancers worldwide (breast, gastric, liver, lung, osteosarcoma, prostate, kidney) [120–131], while some TRIMs are under-expressed in a cancer-specific way (e.g., TRIM15 in gastric cancer, TRIM26 in liver, TRIM58 in lung). In these cases, their downregulation is correlated with early-onset and poor overall survival among cancer patients [132–134] (Table 1).

Interestingly, there are some TRIM proteins, which result in being up- or down- regulated depending on cancer type. Among them are TRIM2 (up-regulated in osteosarcoma, down-regulated in kidney cancer), TRIM29 (up-regulated in lung cancer and osteosarcoma, down-regulated in liver and prostate cancers), TRIM33 (up-regulated in breast cancer, down-regulated in liver and kidney cancers) [135–143].

Table 1. TRIM proteins in tumors. Tripartite motif (TRIM) proteins described in the manuscript are listed based on their expression levels in the main cancer types worldwide.

Cancer Type	Upregulated TRIMs	Downregulated TRIMs
Breast	11 [112], 24 [77], 25 [73], 27 [75], 28 [74], 32 [107], 33 [138], 37 [82], 44 [97], 47 [113], 59 [104], 63 [119]	8 [131], 13 [130], 16 [127], 21 [128], 62 [120]
Gastric	14 [144], 24 [84], 28 [76], 32 [96], 37 [106], 44 [79], 59 [105]	3 [145], 15 [134]
Liver	11 [92], 14 [101], 24 [108], 28 [90], 31 [117], 32 [85], 35 [116], 37 [83], 65 [100]	3 [121], 16 [125], 21 [123], 26 [132], 29 [146], 33 [135]
Lung	11 [109], 22 [98], 24 [80], 25 [88], 27 [78], 28 [81], 29 [139], 32 [111], 37 [102], 44 [91], 47 [93], 59 [94], 65 [89]	13 [129], 16 [124], 58 [133], 62 [122]
Osteosarcoma	2 [142,143], 29 [147], 37 [99], 59 [87], 66 [118]	8 [148]
Prostate	24 [110], 25 [149], 28 [103], 47 [86], 68 [115]	16 [126], 29 [136]
Renal	44 [114], 59 [95]	2 [141], 8 [150,151], 33 [137,140]

At the basis of the correlation between TRIMs, altered expression and tumor onset, there are, generally, several mechanisms, not fully understood, such as chromosomal translocations (resulting in oncogenic gain-of-function fusion genes), that likely contribute to oncogenesis through the constitutive activation of oncogenic signaling pathways, hyper- or hypo- methylation of CpG islands present in the TRIMs promoter regions [70,152–156]. Alternatively, the low expression of the tumor-suppressive TRIMs is inversely correlated with specific micro RNAs (miRs) overexpression (e.g., TRIM8 vs. miR17-92 family). On the contrary, overexpression of some oncogenic TRIMs in various cancers is frequently due to the loss of miR dependent gene suppression (e.g., TRIM11, TRIM14, TRIM24, TRIM25, and TRIM44) [144,150,157–163].

The pivotal role of TRIMs, in the pathological as well as in the physiological cellular life, is now clear if we consider that one or more TRIM members can influence diverse key downstream effector cellular pathways, such as p53 controlled pathways, the Wnt/β-catenin signaling, Transforming Growth Factor-β (TGF-β), Phosphoinositide-3-kinase /Protein Kinase B (PI3K/Akt) pathways and the pro-inflammatory Signal transducer and activator of transcription 3- Nuclear Factor kappa-light-chain-enhancer of activated B cells (STAT3-NF-κB) pathways.

2.1. TRIM Family and the p53 Controlled Pathways

The tumor suppressor protein p53 is a key player in the regulation of cell cycle, apoptosis, and in the maintenance of genome stability. A high percentage of tumors show inactivation of p53 function due to gene mutation (with a consequent not-functional p53 protein) or to network inactivation (also in the presence of a wild-type p53 protein). In several human malignancies, it has been shown that TRIMs are able to modulate chemoresistance by exerting their role on p53 stability and/or activity [164,165].

The oncogenic TRIMs are able to negatively regulate p53 by increasing its polyubiquitination and subsequent proteasomal degradation or by impairing its transcriptional activity both directly and indirectly (e.g., TRIM11, TRIM21, TRIM23, TRIM24, TRIM25, TRIM28, TRIM29, TRIM31, TRIM32, TRIM39, TRIM59 and TRIM66) [149,166–179]. On the contrary, a group of tumor suppressive TRIMs are showed to have positive stabilizing effects on p53 protein. They mainly work by enhancing p53 stability by interfering with MDM2 ubiquitin ligase activity and/or inhibiting the p53–MDM2 interaction. These TRIMs are downregulated in tumors (e.g., TRIM3, TRIM8, TRIM13, TRIM19 and TRIM67) [145,150,151,180–184] (Table 1).

2.2. TRIM Family and the Wnt/β -Catenin Signaling Pathway

The Wnt signaling pathway is involved in controlling several main cellular processes (e.g., proliferation, migration, cell adhesion). Moreover, it is important for normal embryonic development and adult tissue homeostasis [185,186].

TRIM29 and TRIM58 are the only two TRIM family members which have been identified to act by modulating the Wnt/β-catenin signaling pathway, and they act in an opposite way. TRIM29 (pro-proliferative) is upregulated in several human tumors. It induces the Wnt/β-catenin signaling pathway through upregulation of CD44 expression, linking this network to the progression of other human tumors. On the contrary, TRIM58 (anti-proliferative) is downregulated in human lung tumor. It exerts its tumor-suppressive activity by suppressing the expression of EMT and matrix metalloproteinase (MMP) genes and, consequently, by inhibiting cell invasion. Moreover, its overexpression significantly increases β-catenin ubiquitination and proteasomal degradation in gastrointestinal (GI) tumors [147,187–192].

2.3. TRIM Family and the TGF-β Pathway

Several members of TRIM proteins are implicated in the regulation of TGF-β signaling. The members of the TGF-β family are cytokines crucially involved in the regulation of cellular processes (e.g., cell growth, differentiation, migration, autophagy, and apoptosis). The TRIM family proteins work by specifically degrading signaling modules involved in this pathway (TGF-β-receptors, R-Smads, and Co-Smads) [193–197].

Different TRIM proteins have been demonstrated to modulate the canonical TGF-β-Smad signaling pathway both positively and negatively, depending on the TRIM protein involved. In particular, TRIM14, TRIM25, TRIM27, TRIM44, TRIM47, TRIM59 are significantly linked to the TGF-β signaling pathway [198–200].

2.4. TRIM Family and the PI3K/Akt Signaling Pathway

The PI3K/Akt pathway has also been correlated with tumor onset and progression. Its deregulation is frequently observed in most human malignancies due to the altered transmission of extracellular growth factor-derived signals [201–204]. The activation of the PI3K/Akt pathway has been frequently observed in various cancers, but only for a few years has this activation been also linked to an increased expression of some TRIM proteins.

For example, TRIM14, TRIM27, TRIM44 and TRIM59 are linked to the activation of the PI3K/Akt pathway in different tumors. These TRIM members are upregulated in cancer tissues and this correlates with a poor prognosis and an increase in some characteristic tumor features including invasion, metastasis, and apoptosis resistance [205–209]. They act by degrading its antagonist Phosphatase and tensin homolog (PTEN), with the increase in Akt phosphorylation and PI3K/Akt signaling activity, or by directly inducing the Akt signaling pathway, through the regulation of phosphorylated PI3K and Akt levels. Both these mechanisms lead to an increase in cell proliferation and EMT, with the consequent poor patients' prognosis [144,210,211].

2.5. TRIM Family and the Pro-Inflammatory STAT3-NF-κB Pathway

Many tumors show a constitutive activation of transcription factors involved in the pro-inflammatory response. These include transcription factors like STAT3 and members of the NF-κB protein family, that seem to be crucial in linking chronic inflammation to cancer development. In particular, the aberrant STAT3 signaling is mainly due to persisting signaling events caused by the deregulation of specific signaling modules [212–218]. The aberrant TRIMs expression seems to be clinically relevant for constitutive STAT signaling in several tumors, particularly those of the gastrointestinal (GI) tract. Indeed, excessive TRIM-mediated *STAT3* activation has been reported for several TRIMs (e.g., TRIM14, TRIM27, TRIM29 and TRIM52) and this is associated with an overall poor survival of patients [219–222]. Oncogenic TRIMs, in particular, exert their effects mainly through the activation of the Janus kinase/signal transducers and activators of transcription 3 (JAK/STAT3) signaling pathway by inducing the formation of the constitutively active JAK1-2/STAT3 complex or by promoting the poly-ubiquitination and consequent degradation of a protein tyrosine phosphatase involved in the negative regulation of *STAT3* (named Shp2), thus activating a STAT3 signal. By promoting the activation of *STAT3*, TRIMs indirectly induce STAT3-target genes, such as *MMP-2*, *MMP-9* and the vascular endothelial derived growth factor (VEGF), thus promoting cancer cell migration and invasion [220].

Moreover, the aberrant NF-κB activation is linked with several tumors' onset. The NF-kB canonical pathway can be mainly activated by proteasomal degrading the NF-κB inhibitor IκBα, leading to a release and subsequent activation of dimeric complexes of the NF-κB/Rel transcription family members p50, p65 (RelA) and c-Rel. Alternatively, the NF–κB activation relies on the inducible phosphorylation–dependent ubiquitination and processing of the NF–κB precursor protein p100 by the action of the NF–κB-inducing kinase (NIK) (non-canonical pathway). Once activated, NF-κB promotes tumorigenesis by inducing proinflammatory genes such as cyclooxygenase-2 (*COX-2*).

Several oncogenic TRIMs are able to activate both the NF–κB dependent routes: the canonical NF-κB pathway, triggered by different pro-inflammatory cytokines, or the non-canonical NF-κB pathway, also by interfering with autophagy [223–227].

Contrary to oncogenic TRIMs, there are also some tumor suppressors, TRIMs protein that are able to antagonize NF-kB activity by promoting inhibitor of nuclear factor kappaB kinase subunit gamma (IKKγ) neddylation with the consequent stabilization of the IκBα protein and the impairing of the NF–κB activation, even in the presence of NF-κB activating cytokines [228].

3. TRIMs Involved in CRC

Different TRIM proteins are involved in development and progression of CRC. They can regulate various aspects of tumorigenesis, including proliferation, apoptosis, autophagy, transcriptional regulation, chromatin remodeling, invasion, metastasis and chemoresistance [229]. Cancer cells, through different mechanisms such as inactivation of the tumor suppressor gene *p53*, may acquire resistance to chemotherapy. For this reason, the reactivation of wild type *p53*, through the TRIM proteins, could be a promising strategy to restore sensitivity to the treatment of chemotherapy in all tumors including CRC [164,165]. Below we describe the role and the levels of the different TRIMs in the CRC.

TRIM23 is upregulated in CRC, it binds p53, inducing its ubiquitination and promoting colorectal cell proliferation [149]; TRIM24 (transcription intermediary factor 1α-TIF1α), mRNA and protein levels were higher in CRC tissues compared to controls, indicating this TRIM is a potential negative prognostic marker. In particular, TRIM24 promotes the degradation of p53 via ubiquitination [230].

The literature reports that TRIM25 negatively regulates the expression of Caspase-2, and consequently the reduction of TRIM25 levels in the colorectal cell increases their sensibility to drugs [230]; moreover, TRIM25 reduction induces p53 acetylation and p53-dependent cell death in HCT116 cells [173,231,232]. This TRIM regulates p53 levels and activity in the HCT116 cell line in two opposite ways. From one side, TRIM25 prevents the formation of the ternary complex constituted by p53, MDM2, and p300, which is essential for p53-polyubiquitination and degradation, leading to the increase in p53 stability. Despite this, from another side, p53 transcriptional activity is inhibited in the presence of TRIM25, since the same p53-MDM2-p300 complex is required for p53 acetylation and, consequently, it is able to block the p53-dependent activation of p53-controlled apoptotic genes, following DNA damage [173].

TRIM59 is upregulated in CRC patients and correlates with a poor prognosis. Therefore, the reduction of TRIM59 levels reversed the expression of epithelial-mesenchymal transformation-related proteins vimentin, in *p53* wild-type and *p53* mutated cells, demonstrating that the TRIM59 oncogenic action is *p53* independent [209,233]. In CRC, it has not been studied whether the oncogenic role of TRIM59 is through direct degradation of p53; only in stomach cancer does the literature report a direct TRIM59-p53 interaction and subsequent p53 degradation [170].

TRIM28 and TRIM29 are markers for patient survival in CRC. TRIM28 binds MDM2 and promotes the degradation of p53 [234]. In addition, TRIM28, in concert with MDM2, promotes the formation of a p53 complex with histone deacetylase 1 (HDAC1), thus preventing acetylation of p53 [166]. To date, it is unclear by which molecular mechanism TRIM29 regulates the development of CRC; in fact, this TRIM could prevent p53-mediated transcription of its target genes in the nucleus by sequestering p53 outside the nucleus and thus preventing its p300-dependent acetylation [168]. Alternatively, it could promote p53 degradation by degrading and/or changing the localization of TIP60, a transcriptional coactivator of p53, consequently reducing TIP60-dependent p53 acetylation [146]. In contrast, histone deacetylase9 (HDAC9) can inhibit the action of TRIM29, resulting in increased p53 activity and reduced cell survival [168].

Some TRIM proteins behave like oncogenes because they are involved in the activation of pro-proliferative pathways such as Akt/mTOR and NF-κB signaling pathways. In particular, TRIM2 and TRIM47 are potential targets for therapy in CRC, since they promote cell proliferation, epithelial-mesenchymal transition (EMT) and metastasis in vitro and in vivo [143,199]. TRIM6 is upregulated in CRC and its reduction increases the anti-proliferative effects of 5-fluorouracil and oxaliplatin [235]. TRIM27 and TRIM44 are involved in activation of the Akt/mTOR signaling pathway inducing cell proliferation, migration, invasion and metastasis in CRC [206,207]. Additionally, TRIM66, TRIM52 and

TRIM14 also play an oncogenic role in CRC, since they are involved in cancer proliferation and metastasis through the regulation of STAT3 pathway expression [118,144,220,222]. Instead, TRIM27 is involved in proliferation, invasion and metastasis of CRC in vitro and in vivo regulating AKT [206]. TRIM14, together with TRIM1, have a role in autophagy. Indeed, TRIM14 negatively interferes with the autophagic degradation of the NF-κB family member p100/p52, inducing a non-canonical NF-κB signaling pathway [227]. By contrast, TRIM11 mediates the degradation of the receptor-interacting protein kinase 3 (RIPK3). RIPK3 activation is linked to necrotic cell death and represents a causative role for both pediatric and adult IBDs (inflammatory bowel diseases). TRIM11 counteracts mTOR-induced activation of RIPK3, inducing RIPK3 degradation through autophagy and thus representing a novel regulatory mechanism important for antagonizing necroptosis [236]. In this way, TRIM11 shows a protective role in the gut, mainly through antagonizing intestinal inflammation and cancer.

Finally, TRIM31 and TRIM40 interfere with the canonical NF–κB pathway, promoting invasion and metastasis in CRC [226,227]. In particular, TRIM40 is downregulated in gastrointestinal cancers. It is able to inhibit the NF–κB activity by promoting the neddylation of the IKKγ, also called NEMO (NF–κB essential modulator), a key regulator for NF-κB activation, thus preventing inflammation-associated carcinogenesis in the GI tract [202]. In contrast to the oncogenic action of the TRIMs described so far, TRIM67, TRIM58 and TRIM8 are downregulated in CRC, playing a tumor suppressor role. The reduction of TRIM67 levels in CRC is caused by methylation of two loci (cg21178978 and cg27504802). Mechanistically, TRIM67 binds p53, thus inhibiting MDM2 binding to p53 and following ubiquitination [184]. TRIM58 plays a critical role of tumor suppressor by limiting Wnt/β-catenin dependent EMT; indeed, the recovery of TRIM58 reduces tumor invasion [191]. TRIM8 seems to be down-regulated in CRC and in restoring TRIM8 levels, p53 is stabilized, and cells become sensitive again to chemotherapeutics (The Human protein Atlas, available from http://www.proteinatlas.org, accessed on 25 February 2021) [151,182,229,237] (Table 2).

Table 2. TRIM proteins involved in CRC. Tripartite motif (TRIM) proteins described in the manuscript are listed based on their expression levels in different types of cancer, also below is indicated where the TRIM gene expression levels or mechanisms of action were obtained. The arrows indicate if that TRIM protein was found up- (↑) or down- (↓) regulated; nd indicates not detected levels.

TRIMs	Levels	Action		References
TRIM11	nd	Has a protective role in the gut mainly through antagonizing intestinal inflammation and cancer	HEK293 and HT29 cell line	[236]
TRIM14	↑	promotes migration and invasion of CRC regulating the SPHK1/STAT3 pathway	CRC tissue and HT-29, SW620, and LoVo cell lines	[220]
TRIM2	↑	promotes Epithelial-mesenchymal transition in CRC	CRC tissue and SW620, RKO cell lines	[143]
TRIM23	↑	induces p53 ubiquitination promoting cell proliferation	CRC tissue, SW480, HT29, SW1116, HCT116, SW620 and FHC cell lines, xenograft	[179]
TRIM24	↑	mRNA and protein levels are elevated in CRC tissue	CRC tissue	[230]
TRIM25	↑	its reduction increases the CRC chemo sensibility	DLD-1RKO and HEK293 cell lines	[231]
TRIM27	↑	involved in proliferation, invasion and metastasis of CRC	CRC tissue, LoVo, HCT116, SW480, DLD-1, HT29 and normal epithelial colon cells (NCM460), xenograft	[206]
TRIM28	↑	promotes MDM2-mediated p53 degradation reducing the CRC patient survival	CRC tissue	[234]
TRIM29	↑	prevents p53-mediated transcription of its target genes	CRC tissue, CT116, SW620, SW480, SW1116, LOVO, HT29 and RKO cell lines	[219]

Table 2. *Cont.*

TRIMs	Levels	Action		References
TRIM31	↑	involves in canonical NF–κB pathway, promotes invasion and metastasis in CRC	CRC tissue, HT-29, SW 116, SW 620, SW 480 cell lines	[226]
TRIM40	↑	involves in activation of the Akt/mTOR signaling pathway, inducing cell proliferation, migration, and invasion in CRC	CRC tissue, HEK293T, HeLa and SW480 cell lines	[228]
TRIM44	↑	involves in activation of the Akt/mTOR signaling pathway, induces cell proliferation, migration, and invasion in CRC	CRC tissue, Intestinal mucosal epithelial cells (NCM460) and SW620, LOVO, and HCT116 cell lines	[207]
TRIM47	↑	promotes proliferation and metastasis in CRC	CRC tissue, HCT116, HT29, SW480, RKO, SW620, Caco2, LoVo and SW1116 cell lines, nude mice	[200]
TRIM52	↑	with an oncogenic role in CRC via regulating the STAT3 signaling pathway	CRC tissue, SW480, LoVo, SW620, HT29 and RKO) and normal human intestinal crypt cells (HIEC), xenografts	[222]
TRIM59	↑	the reduction of TRIM59 levels reduce the expression of EMT related proteins	CRC tissue, Caco-2, SW480, HT-29, LoVo, DLD-1, HCT116 cell lines and normal human colorectal epithelial cells (NCM460)	[208]
TRIM6	↑	its reduction increases the anti-proliferative effects of 5-fluorouracil and oxaliplatin	CRC tissue, FHC, and CRC cell lines, LOVO, Sw620, HCT-8 and HCT116 cell lines and nude mice	[235]
TRIM66	↑	regulates migration and invasion in CRC through JAK2/STAT3 pathway	CRC tissue, Human normal colorectal cell lines NCM460 and human CRC cell lines including HCT116, HT29, CaCo2 and SW620	[118]
TRIM58	↓	inhibits CRC invasion through EMT and MMP activation.	CRC tissue, HCT8, KM12, Caco-2, DLD-1, HCT116, LoVo, HT-29, SW480, SW620, RKO and HCT15 cell lines	[191]
TRIM67	↓	inhibits metastasis by mediating mitogen-activated protein kinase 11 (MAPK11) in CRC	CRC tissue and xenografts	[184]
TRIM8	↓	restoring levels of TRIM8 the CRC becomes sensitive to chemotherapeutic drugs	HCT116 cell line and xenografts	[151,182]

4. *TRIM8* Tumor Suppressor Gene

The *TRIM8* gene is located on the 10q24.3 chromosome and transcribes an mRNA of about 3.0 kbp that is translated into a protein of 551 aa with a molecular weight of 61.5 kDa. TRIM8 is expressed in many human tissues such as lungs, intestine, breast, brain, placenta, muscles, kidneys. TRIM8 performs activities involved in embryonic development and cell differentiation, in response to the innate immune system and in different human tumors [238,239]. Although a role of *TRIM8* as an oncogene is reported by affecting the NF-κB and JAK-STAT pathways, much experimental evidence support a role for *TRIM8* as a tumor suppressor [240–243]. Over the years it has been demonstrated how these two pathways are involved in several processes, including inflammatory ones that are associated with the onset and development of CRC [244–246].

The first role of TRIM8 in cancer was demonstrated by Vincent et al., in 2000. The authors showed frequent deletion or loss of heterozygosity in the *TRIM8* gene in glioblastomas [238]. Then, Carinci et al. performed the transcriptome analysis of larynx squamous cell carcinoma (LSCC) tissue and they observed a large reduction of TRIM8 expression which correlated with metastatic progression, suggesting a tumor suppressor role of TRIM8 [148]. Over the years, the suppression role of TRIM8 has been observed in different tumors. Zelin et al. demonstrated that TRIM8 is downregulated in breast cancer and the protein level of TRIM8 is negatively correlated with estrogen receptor α. Moreover, knockdown of TRIM8 can significantly enhance breast cancer cell proliferation and migration both in vitro and in vivo [131]. As in breast cancer, and also in other cancers, low expression levels of TRIM8 are associated with a poor prognosis for the patients; in fact, TRIM8 is downregulated in Glioma, Chronic lymphocytic leukemia (CLL), Renal Clear Cell Carcinoma (ccRCC), CRC and in melanoma [148,150,247–249].

In particular, the literature reports that the downregulation of TRIM8 in tumors is often caused by the action of specific miRNAs. In fact, in patients affected by ccRCC, CRC (The Human protein Atlas, available from http://www.proteinatlas.org, accessed on 25 February 2021) [237], Glioma, and CLL, the overexpression of miR-17-5p causes TRIM8 downregulation that affects cell proliferation and is associated with patient's survival [150,229,247,248]. One of the reasons why TRIM8 plays a tumor suppressor role is its capacity to regulate the stability and activity of *p53* tumor suppressor gene. Indeed, *TRIM8* is a direct p53 target gene, and by a feedback mechanism, displaces p53-MDM2 binding, thus stabilizing p53 and promoting MDM2 degradation. As final outcome, TRIM8 promotes the p53-dependent suppression of cell proliferation and DNA repair [182].

Generally, the most aggressive chemo-resistant tumors have mutations in the *p53* gene or inactivation in its pathway through alterations of its regulators. This is the case with tumors like the clear cell renal cell carcinoma (ccRCC) and the CRC in which the reactivation of the p53 pathway could be one of the best treatment strategies [250–252]. Strikingly, it has been demonstrated that in HCT116 colon, carcinoma and in ccRCC cell lines, TRIM8 silencing induced p53 inactivation and MDM2 stabilization impairing Cisplatin and Nutlin-3 effect. This suggests that TRIM8 levels are relevant to the p53-mediated cellular responses to chemotherapeutic drugs. Conversely, the overexpression of TRIM8 in HCT116 cells induced a great reduction in proliferation rate, which became more pronounced when the cells were treated with Nutlin-3 and Cisplatin [150].

Another case of resistance to chemotherapy is represented by Anaplastic Thyroid Cancer (ATC), where it has been demonstrated that TRIM8 is a direct target of miR-182, which is upregulated in ATC tissue and cell lines. Suppressing the action of TRIM8, miR-182 promotes cellular growth and enhances the cisplatin resistance of ATC cells [253].

5. TRIM8 and miR-17-92 Cluster in CRC Progression and Chemo Resistance

The downregulation of TRIM8 expression in tumors, including CRC, is explained by the upregulation of the miR-17-5p belonging to the miR-17-92 cluster. MiR-17-5p directly targets the 3' UTR of TRIM8 repressing its expression [150,247,248]. The human genome contains two paralogues of the miR-17-92 cluster, the miR-106b/25 cluster and the miR-106a/363 cluster. The miR-17-92 and miR-106b/25 clusters are emerging as key actors in a wide range of biological processes including tumorigenesis [254,255]. An increasing number of recent papers has reported that miR-106b-5p and miR-17-5p are overexpressed in many different chemo/radio-resistant cancers, including CRC, ccRCC and glioma, playing a role in early metastatic progression [256] and contributing to oncogenesis and chemo-resistance [150]. MiR-17-5p and miR-106b-5p are transactivated by N-MYC, and this oncogene is negatively regulated by miR-34a, which is transactivated by p53. Interestingly, miR-17-5p and miR-106b-5p silencing increases TRIM8 expression levels, which in turn stabilizes and activates p53 towards a cell proliferation arrest program. Moreover, p53 promotes the transcription of miR-34a, which turns off the oncogenic effect of N-MYC, linking p53 to N-MYC. By restoring normal TRIM8 levels, CRC cells recover sensitivity to chemotherapy treatments such as Sorafenib, Axitinib, which are among the Tyrosine Kinase inhibitors currently in use for treatment of both renal and colorectal carcinoma [257–260], and also to Nutlin-3 and Cisplatin [150]. In conclusion, TRIM8, among all miR-17-5p targets, is pivotal in controlling cell sensitivity to chemotherapy and its role in tumor growth has been demonstrated also in human tumor xenografts generated in nude mice. Indeed, in TRIM8-treated tumors, cell proliferation stops completely compared to tumors treated with a control vector. This evidence confirmed in vivo the pathway identified in vitro, underlying TRIM8 as a key factor in the p53/N-MYC/miR-17 axis [150].

Another important role of TRIM8 in counteracting the proliferation of cancer cells is highlighted by its effects on the stability and activity of the oncogenic transcription factor

ΔNp63α, belonging to the *p53* gene family. ΔNp63α is upregulated in different tumors, in fact the expression level of this transcription factor is correlated with a poor prognosis of patients [261–263]. It has been demonstrated that TRIM8 promotes the degradation of ΔNp63α in both a proteasomal and caspase-1-dependent way. It is important to point out that ΔNp63α is able to downregulate TRIM8 expression, thus preventing the stabilization of p53. This dual role of TRIM8 demonstrates an enhanced activity in the inhibition of tumor development and therefore in the role played in chemoresistance and offers more possible therapeutic benefits [264].

6. Conclusions

Studies are increasingly focusing on the molecular basis of chemoresistance in CRC. The identification of new molecular targets and the development of drugs able to regulate their activity opens a positive landscape for CRC patients. Specifically, in this review we reported the tumor suppressor role of TRIM8 in the resistance to drugs administered for the treatment of CRC. TRIM8 is downregulated in colon carcinoma cells due to the inhibitory action of miR-17-5p and miR-106b. Suppressing the activity of these miRNAs, the level of TRIM8 proteins increase, and the activity of p53 tumor suppressor protein is restored and cells respond again to chemotherapy treatment. TRIM8 is therefore a promising therapeutic target for CRC treatment.

Author Contributions: Conceptualization, F.M. and A.T.; methodology F.M., M.F.C., A.T.; software, F.M. and M.F.C.; formal analysis, F.M. and A.T.; investigation, F.M., M.F.C., E.S., A.T.; resources, G.P.; writing—original draft preparation, F.M. and A.T.; writing—review and editing, M.F.C., E.S. and G.P. visualization, A.T.; supervision, A.T.; project administration, F.M.; funding acquisition, G.P. All authors have read and agreed to the published version of the manuscript.

Funding: This research received no external funding.

Institutional Review Board Statement: Not applicable.

Informed Consent Statement: Not applicable.

Acknowledgments: We thank the native English-speaking Catriona Isobel Macleod for English revision, Laura Marra for technical assistance, and the project "Cluster in Bioimaging" (QZYCUM0) by the Apulian Region.

Conflicts of Interest: The authors declare no conflict of interest. The funders had no role in the design of the study; in the collection, analyses, or interpretation of data; in the writing of the manuscript, or in the decision to publish the results.

References

1. Medina Pabón, M.A.; Babiker, H.M. *A Review of Hereditary Colorectal Cancers*; StatPearls Publishing: Treasure Island, FL, USA, 2020.
2. Poulogiannis, G.; Ichimura, K.; Hamoudi, R.A.; Luo, F.; Leung, S.Y.; Yuen, S.T.; Harrison, D.J.; Wyllie, A.H.; Arends, M.J. Prognostic relevance of DNA copy number changes in colorectal cancer. *J. Pathol.* **2010**, *220*, 338–347. [CrossRef]
3. Arends, M.J. Pathways of colorectal carcinogenesis. *Appl. Immunohistochem. Mol. Morphol.* **2013**, *21*, 97–102. [CrossRef] [PubMed]
4. Ibrahim, A.E.; Arends, M.J.; Silva, A.L.; Wyllie, A.H.; Greger, L.; Ito, Y.; Vowler, S.L.; Huang, T.H.; Tavaré, S.; Murrell, A.; et al. Sequential DNA methylation changes are associated with DNMT3B overexpression in colorectal neoplastic progression. *Gut* **2011**, *60*, 499–508. [CrossRef]
5. Müller, M.F.; Ibrahim, A.E.K.; Arends, M.J. Molecular pathological classification of colorectal cancer. *Virchows Arch.* **2016**, *469*, 125–134. [CrossRef] [PubMed]
6. Guinney, J.; Dienstmann, R.; Wang, X.; de Reyniès, A.; Schlicker, A.; Soneson, C.; Marisa, L.; Roepman, P.; Nyamundanda, G.; Angelino, P.; et al. The consensus molecular subtypes of colorectal cancer. *Nat. Med.* **2015**, *21*, 1350–1356. [CrossRef]
7. Brenner, H.; Kloor, M.; Pox, C.P. Colorectal cancer. *Lancet* **2014**, *383*, 1490–1502. [CrossRef]
8. Salonga, D.; Danenberg, K.D.; Johnson, M.; Metzger, R.; Groshen, S.; Tsao-Wei, D.D.; Lenz, H.J.; Leichman, C.G.; Leichman, L.; Diasio, R.B.; et al. Colorectal tumors responding to 5-fluorouracil have low gene expression levels of dihydropyrimidine dehydrogenase, thymidylate synthase, and thymidine phosphorylase. *Clin. Cancer Res.* **2000**, *6*, 1322–1327. [PubMed]
9. Showalter, S.L.; Showalter, T.N.; Witkiewicz, A.; Havens, R.; Kennedy, E.P.; Hucl, T.; Kern, S.E.; Yeo, C.J.; Brody, J.R. Evaluating the drug-target relationship between thymidylate synthase expression and tumor response to 5-fluorouracil. Is it time to move forward? *Cancer Biol. Ther.* **2008**, *7*, 986–994. [CrossRef] [PubMed]

10. Blondy, S.; David, V.; Verdier, M.; Mathonnet, M.; Perraud, A.; Christou, N. 5-Fluorouracil resistance mechanisms in colorectal cancer: From classical pathways to promising processes. *Cancer Sci.* **2020**, *111*, 3142–3154. [CrossRef]
11. Pinedo, H.M.; Peters, G.F. Fluorouracil: Biochemistry and pharmacology. *J. Clin. Oncol.* **1988**, *6*, 1653–1664. [CrossRef] [PubMed]
12. Beck, A.; Etienne, M.C.; Cheradame, S.; Fischel, J.L.; Formento, P.; Renee, N.; Milano, G. A role for dihy-dropyrimidine dehydrogenase and thymidylate synthase intumour sensitivity to fluorouracil. *Eur. J. Cancer* **1994**, *30A*, 1517–1522. [CrossRef]
13. Peters, G.J.; van der Wilt, C.L.; van Groeningen, C.J. Predictive value of thymidylate synthase and dihydropyrimidine dehydrogenase. *Eur. J. Cancer* **1994**, *30A*, 1408–1411. [CrossRef]
14. Qiu, L.X.; Tang, Q.Y.; Bai, J.L.; Qian, X.P.; Li, R.T.; Liu, B.R.; Zheng, M.H. Predictive value of thymidylate synthase expression in advanced colorectal cancer patients receiving fluoropyrimidine-based chemotherapy: Evidence from 24 studies. *Int. J. Cancer* **2008**, *123*, 384–2389. [CrossRef]
15. Abdallah, E.A.; Fanelli, M.F.; Buim, M.E.; Machado Netto, M.C.; Gasparini Junior, J.L.; Souza, E.; Silva, V.; Dettino, A.L.; Mingues, N.B.; Romero, J.V.; et al. Thymidylate synthase expression in circulating tumor cells: A new tool to predict 5-fluorouracil resistance in metastatic colorectal cancer patients. *Int. J. Cancer* **2015**, *137*, 1397–1405. [CrossRef]
16. Yanagisawa, Y.; Maruta, F.; Iinuma, N.; Ishizone, S.; Koide, N.; Nakayama, J.; Miyagawa, S. Modified Irinotecan/5FU/Leucovorin therapy in advanced colorectal cancer and predicting therapeutic efficacy by expression of tumor-related enzymes. *Scand. J. Gastroenterol.* **2007**, *42*, 477–484. [CrossRef] [PubMed]
17. Sakowicz-Burkiewicz, M.; Przybyla, T.; Wesserling, M.; Bielarczyk, H.; Maciejewska, I.; Pawelczyk, T. Suppression of TWIST1 enhances the sensitivity of colon cancer cells to 5-fluorouracil. *Int. J. Biochem. Cell Biol.* **2016**, *78*, 268–278. [CrossRef] [PubMed]
18. Che, J.; Pan, L.; Yang, X.; Liu, Z.; Huang, L.; Wen, C.; Lin, A.; Liu, H. Thymidine phosphorylase expression and prognosis in colorectal cancer treated with 5-fluorouracil-based chemotherapy: A metaanalysis. *Mol. Clin. Oncol.* **2017**, *7*, 943–952. [CrossRef]
19. Stark, M.; Bram, E.E.; Akerman, M.; Mandel-Gutfreund, Y.; Assaraf, Y.G. Heterogeneous nuclear ribonucleoprotein H1/H2-dependent unsplicing of thymidine phosphorylase results in anticancer drug resistance. *J. Biol. Chem.* **2011**, *286*, 3741–3754. [CrossRef] [PubMed]
20. Lin, S.; Lai, H.; Qin, Y.; Chen, J.; Lin, Y. Thymidine phosphorylase and hypoxia-inducible factor 1-α expression in clinical stage II/III rectal cancer: Association with response to neoadjuvant chemoradiation therapy and prognosis. *Int. J. Clin. Exp. Pathol.* **2015**, *8*, 10680–10688.
21. Giovannetti, E.; Backus, H.H.; Wouters, D.; Ferreira, C.G.; van Houten, V.M.; Brakenhoff, R.H.; Poupon, M.F.; Azzarello, A.; Pinedo, H.M.; Peters, G.J. Changes in the status of *p53* affect drug sensitivity to thymidylate synthase (TS) inhibitors by altering TS levels. *Br. J. Cancer* **2007**, *96*, 769–775. [CrossRef] [PubMed]
22. Chaney, S.G.; Campbell, S.L.; Bassett, E.; Wu, Y. Recognition and processing of cisplatin- and oxaliplatin-DNA adducts. *Crit. Rev. Oncol. Hematol.* **2005**, *53*, 3–11. [CrossRef]
23. Gnoni, A.; Russo, A.; Silvestris, N.; Maiello, E.; Vacca, A.; Marech, I.; Numico, G.; Paradiso, A.; Lorusso, V.; Azzariti, A. Pharmacokinetic and metabolism determinants of fluoropyrimidines and oxaliplatin activity in treatment of colorectal patients. *Curr. Drug Metab.* **2011**, *12*, 918–931. [CrossRef]
24. Yan, D.; Tu, L.; Yuan, H.; Fang, J.; Cheng, L.; Zheng, X.; Wang, X. WBSCR22 confers oxaliplatin resistance in human colorectal cancer. *Sci. Rep.* **2017**, *7*, 15443. [CrossRef]
25. Mao, L.; Li, Y.; Zhao, J.; Li, Q.; Yang, B.; Wang, Y.; Zhu, Z.; Sun, H.; Zhai, Z. Transforming growth factor-β1 contributes to oxaliplatin resistance in colorectal cancer via epithelial to mesenchymal transition. *Oncol. Lett.* **2017**, *14*, 647–654. [CrossRef] [PubMed]
26. Meisenberg, C.; Gilbert, D.C.; Chalmers, A.; Haley, V.; Gollins, S.; Ward, S.E.; El-Khamisy, S.F. Clinical and cellular roles for TDP1and TOP1 in modulating colorectal cancer response to irinotecan. *Mol. Cancer Ther.* **2015**, *14*, 575–585. [CrossRef] [PubMed]
27. Palshof, J.A.; Høgdall, E.V.; Poulsen, T.S.; Linnemann, D.; Jensen, B.V.; Pfeiffer, P.; Tarpgaard, L.S.; Brünner, N.; Stenvang, J.; Yilmaz, M.; et al. Topoisomerase 1 copy number alterations as biomarker for irinotecan efficacy in metastatic colorectal cancer. *BMC Cancer* **2017**, *17*, 48. [CrossRef] [PubMed]
28. Nielsen, D.L.; Palshof, J.A.; Brünner, N.; Stenvang, J.; Viuff, B.M. Implications of ABCG2 Expression on Irinotecan Treatment of Colorectal Cancer Patients: A Review. *Int. J. Mol. Sci.* **2017**, *18*, 1926. [CrossRef] [PubMed]
29. De Man, F.M.; Goey, A.K.L.; van Schaik, R.H.N.; Mathijssen, R.H.J.; Bins, S. Individualization of Irinotecan Treatment: A Review of Pharmacokinetics, Pharmacodynamics and Pharmacogenetics. *Clin. Pharmacokinet.* **2018**, *57*, 1229–1254. [CrossRef] [PubMed]
30. Meisenberg, C.; Ashour, M.E.; El-Shafie, L.; Liao, C.; Hodgson, A.; Pilborough, A.; Khurram, S.A.; Downs, J.A.; Ward, S.E.; El-Khamisy, S.F. Epigenetic changes in histone acetylation underpin resistance to the topoisomerase I inhibitor irinotecan. *Nucleic Acids Res.* **2017**, *45*, 1159–1176. [CrossRef]
31. Kotaka, M.; Xu, R.; Muro, K.; Park, Y.S.; Morita, S.; Iwasa, S.; Uetake, H.; Nishina, T.; Nozawa, H.; Matsumoto, H.; et al. Study protocol of the Asian XELIRI ProjecT (AXEPT): A multinational, randomized, non-inferiority, phase III trial of second-line chemotherapy for metastatic colorectal cancer, comparing the efficacy and safety of XELIRI with or without bevacizumab versus FOLFIRI with or without bevacizumab. *Chin. J. Cancer* **2016**, *35*, 102. [PubMed]
32. Garcia-Alfonso, P.; Chaves, M.; Muñoz, A.; Salud, A.; GarcíaGonzalez, M.; Grávalos, C.; Massuti, B.; González-Flores, E.; Queralt, B.; López-Ladrón, A.; et al. Spanish Cooperative Group for the Treatment of Digestive Tumors (TTD). Capecitabine and irinotecan with bevacizumab 2-weekly for metastatic colorectal cancer: The phase II AVAXIRI study. *BMC Cancer* **2015**, *15*, 327. [CrossRef]

33. Hu, J.; Li, J.; Yue, X.; Wang, J.; Liu, J.; Sun, L.; Kong, D. Expression of the cancer stem cell markers ABCG2 and OCT-4 in right-sided colon cancer predicts recurrence and poor outcomes. *Oncotarget* **2017**, *8*, 28463–28470. [CrossRef]
34. De Sousa, E.; Melo, F.; Colak, S.; Buikhuisen, J.; Koster, J.; Cameron, K.; de Jong, J.H.; Tuynman, J.B.; Prasetyanti, P.R.; Fessler, E.; et al. Methylation of cancer-stem-cell-associated Wnt target genes predicts poor prognosis in colorectal cancer patients. *Cell Stem Cell* **2011**, *9*, 476–485.
35. Zeuner, A.; Todaro, M.; Stassi, G.; De Maria, R. Colorectal cancer stem cells: From the crypt to the clinic. *Cell Stem Cell* **2014**, *15*, 692–705. [CrossRef] [PubMed]
36. Vermeulen, L.; De Sousa, E.M.F.; van der Heijden, M.; Cameron, K.; de Jong, J.H.; Borovski, T.; Tuynman, J.B.; Todaro, M.; Merz, C.; Rodermond, H.; et al. Wnt activity defines colon cancer stem cells and is regulated by the microenvironment. *Nat. Cell Biol.* **2010**, *12*, 468–476. [CrossRef]
37. Paquet-Fifield, S.; Koh, S.L.; Cheng, L.; Beyit, L.M.; Shembrey, C.; Mølck, C.; Behrenbruch, C.; Papin, M.; Gironella, M.; Guelfi, S.; et al. Tight Junction Protein Claudin-2 Promotes Self Renewal of Human Colorectal Cancer Stem-like Cells. *Cancer Res.* **2018**, *78*, 2925–2938. [CrossRef]
38. Kupsch, P.; Henning, B.F.; Passarge, K.; Richly, H.; Wiesemann, K.; Hilger, R.A.; Scheulen, M.E.; Christensen, O.; Brendel, E.; Schwartz, B.; et al. Results of a phase I trial of sorafenib (bay 43–9006) in combination with oxaliplatin in patients with refractory solid tumors, including colorectal cancer. *Clin. Colorectal Cancer* **2005**, *5*, 188–196. [CrossRef] [PubMed]
39. Mross, K.; Steinbild, S.; Baas, F.; Gmehling, D.; Radtke, M.; Voliotis, D.; Brendel, E.; Christensen, O.; Unger, C. Results from an in vitro and a clinical/pharmacological phase I study with the combination irinotecan and sorafenib. *Eur. J. Cancer* **2007**, *43*, 55–63. [CrossRef] [PubMed]
40. Tabernero, J.; Garcia-Carbonero, R.; Cassidy, J.; Sobrero, A.; van Cutsem, E.; Kohne, C.H.; Tejpar, S.; Gladkov, O.; Davidenko, I.; Salazar, R.; et al. Sorafenib in combination with oxaliplatin, leucovorin, and fluorouracil (modified folfox6) as first-line treatment of metastatic colorectal cancer: The respect trial. *Clin. Cancer Res.* **2013**, *19*, 2541–2550. [CrossRef]
41. Pehserl, A.M.; Ress, A.L.; Stanzer, S.; Resel, M.; Karbiener, M.; Stadelmeyer, E.; Stiegelbauer, V.; Gerger, A.; Mayr, C.; Scheideler, M.; et al. Comprehensive Analysis of miRNome Alterations in Response to Sorafenib Treatment in Colorectal Cancer Cell. *Int. J. Mol. Sci.* **2016**, *17*, 2011. [CrossRef] [PubMed]
42. Berndsen, R.H.; Swier, N.; van Beijnum, J.R.; Nowak-Sliwinska, P. Colorectal Cancer Growth Retardation through Induction of Apoptosis, Using an Optimized Synergistic Cocktail of Axitinib, Erlotinib, and Dasatinib. *Cancers* **2019**, *11*, 1878. [CrossRef] [PubMed]
43. Huang, H.; Zhu, L.; Reid, B.R.; Drobny, G.P.; Hopkins, P.B. Solution structure of a cisplatin-induced DNA interstrand cross-link. *Science* **1995**, *270*, 1842–1845. [CrossRef]
44. Wang, D.; Lippard, S.J. Cellular processing of platinum anticancer drugs. *Nat. Rev. Drug Discov.* **2005**, *4*, 307–320. [CrossRef]
45. Galluzzi, L.; Vitale, I.; Michels, J.; Brenner, C.; Szabadkai, G.; Harel-Bellan, A.; Castedo, M.; Kroemer, G. Systems biology of Cisplatin resistance: Past, present and future. *Cell Death Dis.* **2014**, *5*, e1257. [CrossRef] [PubMed]
46. Pillozzi, S.; D'Amico, M.; Bartoli, G.; Gasparoli, L.; Petroni, G.; Crociani, O.; Marzo, T.; Guerriero, A.; Messori, L.; Severi, M.; et al. The combined activation of K Ca 3.1 and inhibition of K v 11.1/hERG1 currents contribute to overcome Cisplatin resistance in colorectal cancer cells. *Br. J. Cancer* **2018**, *118*, 200–212. [CrossRef] [PubMed]
47. Nadler-Milbauer, M.; Apter, L.; Haupt, Y.; Haupt, S.; Barenholz, Y.; Minko, T.; Rubinstein, A. Synchronized release of Doxil and Nutlin-3 by remote degradation of polysaccharide matrices and its possible use in the local treatment of colorectal cancer. *J. Drug Target.* **2011**, *19*, 859–873. [CrossRef] [PubMed]
48. Di Napoli, M.; Papa, F. The proteasome system and proteasome inhibitors in stroke: Controlling the inflammatory response. *Curr. Opin. Investig. Drugs* **2003**, *4*, 1333–1342. [PubMed]
49. Landis-Piwowar, K.R.; Milacic, V.; Chen, D.; Yang, H.; Zhao, Y.; Chan, T.H.; Yan, B.; Dou, Q.P. The proteasome as a potential target for novel anticancer drugs and chemosensitizers. *Drug Resist. Updat.* **2006**, *9*, 263–273. [CrossRef]
50. Zhao, Z.; Zhu, J.; Quan, H.; Wang, G.; Li, B.; Zhu, W.; Xie, C.; Lou, L. X66, a novel N-terminal heat shock protein 90 inhibitor, exerts antitumor effects without induction of heat shock response. *Oncotarget* **2016**, *7*, 29648–29663. [CrossRef]
51. Lub, S.; Maes, K.; Menu, E.; De Bruyne, E.; Vanderkerken, K.; Van Valckenborgh, E. Novel strategies to target the ubiquitin proteasome system in multiple myeloma. *Oncotarget* **2016**, *7*, 6521–6537. [CrossRef]
52. Liu, J.; Shaik, S.; Dai, X.; Wu, Q.; Zhou, X.; Wang, Z.; Wei, W. Targeting the ubiquitin pathway for cancer treatment. *Biochim. Biophys. Acta* **2015**, *1855*, 50–60. [CrossRef]
53. Yang, L.; Chen, J.; Huang, X.; Zhang, E.; He, J.; Cai, Z. Novel Insights into E3 Ubiquitin Ligase in Cancer Chemoresistance. *Am. J. Med. Sci.* **2018**, *355*, 368–376. [CrossRef]
54. Petzold, G.; Fischer, E.S.; Thoma, N.H. Structural basis of lenalidomide-induced CK1alpha degradation by the CRL4 ubiquitin ligase. *Nature* **2016**, *532*, 127–130. [CrossRef] [PubMed]
55. Nelson, J.K.; Cook, E.C.; Loregger, A.; Hoeksema, M.A.; Scheij, S.; Kovacevic, I.; Hordijk, P.L.; Ovaa, H.; Zelcer, N. Deubiquitylase Inhibition Reveals Liver X Receptor-independent Transcriptional Regulation of the E3 Ubiquitin Ligase IDOL and Lipoprotein Uptake. *J. Biol. Chem.* **2016**, *291*, 4813–4825. [CrossRef]
56. Zhang, X.; Li, C.F.; Zhang, L.; Wu, C.Y.; Han, L.; Jin, G.; Rezaeian, A.H.; Han, F.; Liu, C.; Xu, C.; et al. TRAF6 Restricts p53 Mitochondrial Translocation, Apoptosis and Tumor Suppression. *Mol. Cell* **2016**, *64*, 803–814. [CrossRef]

57. Yoshino, S.; Hara, T.; Nakaoka, H.J.; Kanamori, A.; Murakami, Y.; Seiki, M.; Sakamoto, T. The ERK signaling target RNF126 regulates anoikis resistance in cancer cells by changing the mitochondrial metabolic flux. *Cell Discov.* **2016**, *2*, 16019. [CrossRef] [PubMed]
58. Xu, Q.; Hou, Y.X.; Langlais, P.; Erickson, P.; Zhu, J.; Shi, C.X.; Luo, M.; Zhu, Y.; Xu, Y.; Mandarino, L.J.; et al. Expression of the cereblon binding protein argonaute 2 plays an important role for multiple myeloma cell growth and survival. *BMC Cancer* **2016**, *16*, 297. [CrossRef] [PubMed]
59. Tanaka, N.; Kosaka, T.; Miyazaki, Y.; Mikami, S.; Niwa, N.; Otsuka, Y.; Minamishima, Y.A.; Mizuno, R.; Kikuchi, E.; Miyajima, A.; et al. Acquired platinum resistance involves epithelial to mesenchymal transition through ubiquitin ligase FBXO32 dysregulation. *JCI Insight* **2016**, *1*, e83654. [CrossRef] [PubMed]
60. Jeon, Y.K.; Kim, C.K.; Koh, J.; Chung, D.H.; Ha, G.H. Pellino-1 confers chemoresistance in lung cancer cells by upregulating cIAP2 through Lys63-mediated polyubiquitination. *Oncotarget* **2016**, *7*, 41811–41824. [CrossRef]
61. Liu, L.; Wong, C.C.; Gong, B.; Yu, J. Functional significance and therapeutic implication of ring-type E3ligases in colorectal cancer. *Oncogene* **2018**, *37*, 148–159. [CrossRef]
62. Liu, M.L.; Zang, F.; Zhang, S.J. RBCK1 contributes to chemoresistance and stemness in colorectal cancer (CRC). *Biomed. Pharmacother.* **2019**, *118*, 109250. [CrossRef]
63. Li, N.; Babaei-Jadidi, R.; Lorenzi, F.; Spencer-Dene, B.; Clarke, P.; Domingo, E.; Tulchinsky, E.; Vries, R.G.J.; Kerr, D.; Pan, Y.; et al. An FBXW7-ZEB2 axis links EMT and tumour microenvironment to promote colorectal cancer stem cells and chemoresistance. *Oncogenesis* **2019**, *8*, 13. [CrossRef] [PubMed]
64. Ding, J.; Zhao, Z.; Song, J.; Luo, B.; Huang, L. MiR-223 promotes the doxorubicin resistance of colorectal cancer cells via regulating epithelial-mesenchymal transition by targeting FBXW7. *Acta Biochim. Biophys. Sin.* **2018**, *50*, 597–604. [CrossRef] [PubMed]
65. Wang, S.; Wang, T.; Wang, L.; Zhong, L.; Li, K. Overexpression of RNF126 Promotes the Development of Colorectal Cancer via Enhancing p53 Ubiquitination and Degradation. *OncoTargets Ther.* **2020**, *13*, 10917–10929. [CrossRef] [PubMed]
66. Reddy, B.A.; Etkin, L.D.; Freemont, P.S. A novel zinc finger coiled-coil domain in a family of nuclear proteins. *Trends Biochem. Sci.* **1992**, *17*, 344–345. [CrossRef]
67. Borden, K.L.; Boddy, M.N.; Lally, J.; O'Reilly, N.J.; Martin, S.; Howe, K.; Solomon, E.; Freemont, P.S. The solution structure of the RING finger domain from the acute promyelocytic leukaemia proto-oncoprotein PML. *EMBO J.* **1995**, *14*, 1532–1541. [CrossRef] [PubMed]
68. Joazeiro, C.A.; Weissman, A.M. RING finger proteins: Mediators of ubiquitin ligase activity. *Cell* **2000**, *102*, 549–552. [CrossRef]
69. Meroni, G.; Diez-Roux, G. TRIM/RBCC, a novel class of 'single protein RING finger' E3 ubiquitin ligases. *Bioessays* **2005**, *27*, 1147–1157. [CrossRef]
70. Watanabe, M.; Hatakeyama, S. TRIM proteins and diseases. *J. Biochem.* **2017**, *161*, 135–144. [CrossRef] [PubMed]
71. Park, J.S.; Burckhardt, C.J.; Lazcano, R.; Solis, L.M.; Isogai, T.; Li, L.; Chen, C.S.; Gao, B.; Minna, J.D.; Bachoo, R.; et al. Mechanical regulation of glycolysis via cytoskeleton architecture. *Nature* **2020**, *578*, 621–626. [CrossRef] [PubMed]
72. Mandell, M.A.; Saha, B.; Thompson, T.A. The Tripartite Nexus: Autophagy, Cancer, and Tripartite Motif-Containing Protein Family Members. *Front Pharmacol.* **2020**, *11*, 308. [CrossRef] [PubMed]
73. Suzuki, T. Estrogen-responsive finger protein as a new potential biomarker for breast cancer. *Clin. Cancer Res.* **2005**, *11*, 6148–6154. [CrossRef]
74. Ho, J.; Kong, J.W.F.; Choong, L.Y.; Loh, M.C.S.; Toy, W.; Chong, P.K.; Wong, C.H.; Wong, C.Y.; Shah, N.; Lim, Y.P. Novel Breast Cancer Metastasis-Associated Proteins. *J. Proteome Res.* **2009**, *8*, 583–594. [CrossRef] [PubMed]
75. Tezel, G.G.; Uner, A.; Yildiz, I.; Guler, G.; Takahashi, M. RET finger protein expression in invasive breast carcinoma: Relationship between RFP and ErbB2 expression. *Pathol. Res. Pract.* **2009**, *205*, 403–408. [CrossRef] [PubMed]
76. Yokoe, T.; Toiyama, Y.; Okugawa, Y.; Tanaka, K.; Ohi, M.; Inoue, Y.; Mohri, Y.; Miki, C.; Kusunoki, M. KAP1 is associated with peritoneal carcinomatosis in gastric cancer. *Ann. Surg. Oncol.* **2010**, *17*, 821–828. [CrossRef]
77. Tsai, W.W.; Wang, Z.; Yiu, T.T.; Akdemir, K.C.; Xia, W.; Winter, S.; Tsai, C.Y.; Shi, X.; Schwarzer, D.; Plunkett, W.; et al. TRIM24 links a non-canonical histone signature to breast cancer. *Nature* **2010**, *468*, 927–932. [CrossRef]
78. Iwakoshi, A.; Murakumo, Y.; Kato, T.; Kitamura, A.; Mii, S.; Saito, S.; Yatabe, Y.; Takahashi, M. RET finger protein expression is associated with prognosis in lung cancer with epidermal growth factor receptor mutations. *Pathol. Int.* **2012**, *62*, 324–330. [CrossRef] [PubMed]
79. Kashimoto, K.; Komatsu, S.; Ichikawa, D.; Arita, T.; Konishi, H.; Nagata, H.; Takeshita, H.; Nishimura, Y.; Hirajima, S.; Kawaguchi, T.; et al. Overexpression of TRIM44 contributes to malignant outcome in gastric carcinoma. *Cancer Sci.* **2012**, *103*, 2021–2026. [CrossRef]
80. Li, H.; Tang, Z.; Fu, L.; Xu, Y.; Li, Z.; Luo, W.; Qiu, X.; Wang, E. Overexpression of TRIM24 Correlates with Tumor Progression in Non-Small Cell Lung Cancer. *PLoS ONE* **2012**, *7*, e37657. [CrossRef]
81. Liu, L.; Zhao, E.; Li, C.; Huang, L.; Xiao, L.; Cheng, L.; Huang, X.; Song, Y.; Xu, D. TRIM28, a new molecular marker predicting metastasis and survival in early-stage non-small cell lung cancer. *Cancer Epidemiol.* **2013**, *37*, 71–78. [CrossRef]
82. Bhatnagar, S.; Gazin, C.; Chamberlain, L.; Ou, J.; Zhu, X.; Tushir, J.S.; Virbasius, C.M.; Lin, L.; Zhu, L.J.; Wajapeyee, N.; et al. TRIM37 is a new histone H2A ubiquitin ligase and breast cancer oncoprotein. *Nature* **2014**, *516*, 116–120. [CrossRef] [PubMed]
83. Jiang, J.; Yu, C.; Chen, M.; Tian, S.; Sun, C. Over-expression of TRIM37 promotes cell migration and metastasis in hepatocellular carcinoma by activating Wnt/b-catenin signaling. *Biochem. Biophys. Res. Commun.* **2015**, *464*, 1120–1127. [CrossRef] [PubMed]

84. Miao, Z.F.; Wang, Z.N.; Zhao, T.T.; Xu, Y.Y.; Wu, J.H.; Liu, X.Y.; Xu, H.; You, Y.; Xu, H.M. TRIM24 is upregulated in human gastric cancer and promotes gastric cancer cell growth and chemoresistance. *Virchows Arch.* **2015**, *466*, 525–532. [CrossRef] [PubMed]
85. Cui, X.; Lin, Z.; Chen, Y.; Mao, X.; Ni, W.; Liu, J.; Zhou, H.; Shan, X.; Chen, L.; Lv, J.; et al. Upregulated TRIM32 correlates with enhanced cell proliferation and poor prognosis in hepatocellular carcinoma. *Mol. Cell Biochem.* **2016**, *421*, 127–137. [CrossRef] [PubMed]
86. Fujimura, T.; Inoue, S.; Urano, T.; Takayama, K.; Yamada, Y.; Ikeda, K.; Obinata, D.; Ashikari, D.; Takahashi, S.; Homma, Y. Increased expression of tripartite motif (TRIM) 47 is a negative prognostic predictor in human prostate cancer. *Clin. Genitourin. Cancer* **2016**, *14*, 298–303. [CrossRef]
87. Liang, J.; Xing, D.; Li, Z.; Shen, J.; Zhao, H.; Li, S. TRIM59 is upregulated and promotes cell proliferation and migration in human osteosarcoma. *Mol. Med. Rep.* **2016**, *13*, 5200–5206. [CrossRef]
88. Qi, Y.; Cui, C.; Zhang, H. Overexpression of TRIM25 in Lung Cancer Regulates Tumor Cell Progression. *Technol. Cancer Res. Treat.* **2016**, *15*, 707–715.
89. Wang, X.L.; Shi, W.P.; Shi, H.C.; Lu, S.C.; Wang, K.; Sun, C.; He, J.S.; Jin, W.G.; Lv, X.X.; Zou, H.; et al. Knockdown of TRIM65 inhibits lung cancer cell proliferation, migration and invasion: A therapeutic target in human lung cancer. *Oncotarget* **2016**, *7*, 81527–81540. [CrossRef]
90. Wang, Y.; Jiang, J.; Li, Q.; Ma, H.; Xu, Z.; Gao, Y. KAP1 is overexpressed in hepatocellular carcinoma and its clinical significance. *Int. J. Clin. Oncol.* **2016**, *21*, 927–933. [CrossRef] [PubMed]
91. Xing, Y.; Meng, Q.; Chen, X.; Zhao, Y.; Liu, W.; Hu, J.; Xue, F.; Wang, X.; Cai, L. TRIM44 promotes proliferation and metastasis in nonsmall cell lung cancer via mTOR signaling pathway. *Oncotarget* **2016**, *7*, 30479–30491. [CrossRef] [PubMed]
92. Chen, Y.; Li, L.; Qian, X.; Ge, Y.; Xu, G. High expression of TRIM11 correlates with poor prognosis in patients with hepatocellular carcinoma. *Clin. Res. Hepatol. Gastroenterol.* **2017**, *41*, 190–196. [CrossRef]
93. Han, Y.; Tian, H.; Chen, P.; Lin, Q. TRIM47 overexpression is a poor prognostic factor and contributes to carcinogenesis in non-small cell lung carcinoma. *Oncotarget* **2017**, *8*, 22730–22740. [CrossRef]
94. Hao, L.; Du, B.; Xi, X. TRIM59 is a novel potential prognostic biomarker in patients with non-small cell lung cancer: A research based on bioinformatics analysis. *Oncol. Lett.* **2017**, *14*, 2153–2164. [CrossRef] [PubMed]
95. Hu, S.H.; Zhao, M.J.; Wang, W.X.; Xu, C.W.; Wang, G.D. TRIM59 is a key regulator of growth and migration in renal cell carcinoma. *Cell Mol. Biol.* **2017**, *63*, 68–74. [CrossRef] [PubMed]
96. Ito, M.; Migita, K.; Matsumoto, S.; Wakatsuki, K.; Tanaka, T.; Kunishige, T.; Nakade, H.; Nakatani, M.; Nakajima, Y. Overexpression of E3 ubiquitin ligase tripartite motif 32 correlates with a poor prognosis in patients with gastric cancer. *Oncol. Lett.* **2017**, *13*, 3131–3138. [CrossRef]
97. Kawabata, H.; Azuma, K.; Ikeda, K.; Sugitani, I.; Kinowaki, K.; Fujii, T.; Osaki, A.; Saeki, T.; Horie-Inoue, K.; Inoue, S. TRIM44 Is a Poor Prognostic Factor for Breast Cancer Patients as a Modulator of NF-kappaB Signaling. *Int. J. Mol. Sci.* **2017**, *18*, 1931. [CrossRef] [PubMed]
98. Liu, L.; Zhou, X.M.; Yang, F.F.; Miao, Y.; Yin, Y.; Hu, X.J.; Hou, G.; Wang, Q.Y.; Kang, J. TRIM22 confers poor prognosis and promotes epithelial-mesenchymal transition through regulation of AKT/GSK3beta/beta-catenin signaling in non-small cell lung cancer. *Oncotarget* **2017**, *8*, 62069–62080. [CrossRef]
99. Tao, Y.; Xin, M.; Cheng, H.; Huang, Z.; Hu, T.; Zhang, T.; Wang, J. TRIM37 promotes tumor cell proliferation and drug resistance in pediatric osteosarcoma. *Oncol. Lett.* **2017**, *14*, 6365–6372. [CrossRef]
100. Yang, Y.F.; Zhang, M.F.; Tian, Q.H.; Zhang, C.Z. TRIM65 triggers b-catenin signaling via ubiquitylation of Axin1 to promote hepatocellular carcinoma. *J. Cell Sci.* **2017**, *130*, 3108–3115. [CrossRef] [PubMed]
101. Dong, B.; Zhang, W. High Levels of TRIM14 Are Associated with poor prognosis in hepatocellular carcinoma. *Oncol. Res. Treat.* **2018**, *41*, 129–134. [CrossRef]
102. Dong, S.; Pang, X.; Sun, H.; Yuan, C.; Mu, C.; Zheng, S. TRIM37 targets AKT in the growth of lung cancer cells. *OncoTargets Ther.* **2018**, *11*, 7935–7945. [CrossRef]
103. Fong, K.W.; Zhao, J.C.; Song, B.; Zheng, B.; Yu, J. TRIM28 protects TRIM24 from SPOP-mediated degradation and promotes prostate cancer progression. *Nat. Commun.* **2018**, *9*, 5007. [CrossRef]
104. Liu, Y.; Dong, Y.; Zhao, L.; Su, L.; Diao, K.; Mi, X. TRIM59 overexpression correlates with poor prognosis and contributes to breast cancer progression through AKT signaling pathway. *Mol. Carcinog.* **2018**, *57*, 1792–1802. [CrossRef] [PubMed]
105. Wang, Y.; Zhou, Z.; Wang, X.; Zhang, X.; Chen, Y.; Bai, J.; Di, W. TRIM59 is a novel marker of poor prognosis and promotes malignant progression of ovarian cancer by inducing annexin A2 expression. *Int. J. Biol. Sci.* **2018**, *14*, 2073–2082. [CrossRef]
106. Wu, G.; Song, L.; Zhu, J.; Hu, Y.; Cao, L.; Tan, Z.; Zhang, S.; Li, Z.; Li, J. An ATM/TRIM37/NEMO axis counteracts genotoxicity by activating nuclear-to-cytoplasmic NFkB signaling. *Cancer Res.* **2018**, *78*, 6399–6412. [CrossRef]
107. Zhao, T.T.; Jin, F.; Li, J.G.; Xu, Y.Y.; Dong, H.T.; Liu, Q.; Xing, P.; Zhu, G.L.; Xu, H.; Yin, S.C.; et al. TRIM32 promotes proliferation and confers chemoresistance to breast cancer cells through activation of the NF-kappaB pathway. *J. Cancer* **2018**, *9*, 1349–1356. [CrossRef] [PubMed]
108. Zhu, Y.; Zhao, L.; Shi, K.; Huang, Z.; Chen, B. TRIM24 promotes hepatocellular carcinoma progression via AMPK signaling. *Exp. Cell Res.* **2018**, *367*, 274–281. [CrossRef] [PubMed]
109. Huang, J.; Tang, L.; Zhao, Y.; Ding, W. TRIM11 promotes tumor angiogenesis via activation of STAT3/VEGFA signaling in lung adenocarcinoma. *Am. J. Cancer Res.* **2019**, *9*, 2019–2027. [PubMed]

110. Offermann, A.; Roth, D.; Hupe, M.C.; Hohensteiner, S.; Becker, F.; Joerg, V.; Carlsson, J.; Kuempers, C.; Ribbat-Idel, J.; Tharun, L.; et al. TRIM24 as an independent prognostic biomarker for prostate cancer. *Urol. Oncol. Semin. Orig. Investig.* **2019**, *37*, 576.e1–576.e10. [CrossRef]
111. Yin, H.; Li, Z.; Chen, J.; Hu, X. Expression and the potential functions of TRIM32 in lung cancer tumorigenesis. *J. Cell. Biochem.* **2019**, *120*, 5232–5243. [CrossRef] [PubMed]
112. Song, W.; Wang, Z.; Gu, X.; Wang, A.; Chen, X.; Miao, H.; Chu, J.F.; Tian, Y. TRIM11 promotes proliferation and glycolysis of breast cancer cells via targeting AKT/GLUT1 pathway. *OncoTargets Ther.* **2019**, *12*, 4975–4984. [CrossRef]
113. Wang, Y.; Liu, C.; Xie, Z.; Lu, H. Knockdown of TRIM47 inhibits breast cancer tumorigenesis and progression through the inactivation of PI3K/ Akt pathway. *Chem. Biol. Interact.* **2020**, *317*, 108960. [CrossRef] [PubMed]
114. Yamada, Y.; Kimura, N.; Takayama, K.I.; Sato, Y.; Suzuki, T.; Azuma, K.; Fujimura, T.; Ikeda, K.; Kume, H.; Inoue, S. TRIM44 promotes cell proliferation and migration by inhibiting FRK in renal cell carcinoma. *Cancer Sci.* **2020**, *111*, 881–890. [CrossRef] [PubMed]
115. Miyajima, N.; Maruyama, S.; Bohgaki, M.; Kano, S.; Shigemura, M.; Shinohara, N.; Nonomura, K.; Hatakeyama, S. TRIM68 regulates ligand-dependent transcription of androgen receptor in prostate cancer cells. *Cancer Res.* **2008**, *68*, 3486–3494. [CrossRef]
116. Jia, D.; Wei, L.; Guo, W.; Zha, R.; Bao, M.; Chen, Z.; Zhao, Y.; Ge, C.; Zhao, F.; Chen, T.; et al. Genome-wide copy number analyses identified novel cancer genes in hepatocellular carcinoma. *Hepatology* **2011**, *54*, 1227–1236. [CrossRef]
117. Guo, P.; Ma, X.; Zhao, W.; Huai, W.; Li, T.; Qiu, Y.; Zhang, Y.; Han, L. TRIM31 is upregulated in hepatocellular carcinoma and promotes disease progression by inducing ubiquitination of TSC1–TSC2 complex. *Oncogene* **2018**, *37*, 478–488. [CrossRef] [PubMed]
118. He, T.; Cui, J.; Wu, Y.; Sun, X.; Chen, N. Knockdown of TRIM66 inhibits cell proliferation, migration and invasion in colorectal cancer through JAK2/STAT3 pathway. *Life Sci.* **2019**, *235*, 116799. [CrossRef]
119. Li, K.; Pan, W.; Ma, Y.; Xu, X.; Gao, Y.; He, Y.; Wei, L.; Zhang, J. A novel oncogene TRIM63 promotes cell proliferation and migration via activating Wnt/b-catenin signaling pathway in breast cancer. *Pathol. Res. Pract.* **2019**, *215*, 152573. [CrossRef]
120. Lott, S.T.; Chen, N.; Chandler, D.S.; Yang, Q.; Wang, L.; Rodriguez, M.; Xie, H.; Balasenthil, S.; Buchholz, T.A.; Sahin, A.A.; et al. DEAR1 is a dominant regulator of acinar morphogenesis and an independent predictor of local recurrence-free survival in early-onset breast cancer. *PLoS Med.* **2009**, *6*, e1000068. [CrossRef]
121. Chao, J.; Zhang, X.-F.; Pan, Q.-Z.; Zhao, J.-J.; Jiang, S.-S.; Wang, Y.; Zhang, J.H.; Xia, J.C. Decreased expression of TRIM3 is associated with poor prognosis in patients with primary hepatocellular carcinoma. *Med. Oncol.* **2014**, *31*, 102. [CrossRef]
122. Quintás-Cardama, A.; Post, S.M.; Solis, L.M.; Xiong, S.; Yang, P.; Chen, N.; Wistuba, I.I.; Killary, A.M.; Lozano, G. Loss of the novel tumour suppressor and polarity gene *Trim62* (Dear1) synergizes with oncogenic Ras in invasive lung cancer. *J. Pathol.* **2014**, *234*, 108–119. [CrossRef]
123. Ding, Q.; He, D.; He, K.; Zhang, Q.; Tang, M.; Dai, J.; Lv, H.; Wang, X.; Xiang, G.; Yu, H. Downregulation of TRIM21 contributes to hepatocellular carcinoma carcinogenesis and indicates poor prognosis of cancers. *Tumour Biol.* **2015**, *36*, 8761–8772. [CrossRef] [PubMed]
124. Huo, X.; Li, S.; Shi, T.; Suo, A.; Ruan, Z.; Yao, Y. Tripartite motif 16 inhibits epithelial-mesenchymal transition and metastasis by down-regulating sonic hedgehog pathway in non-small cell lung cancer cells. *Biochem. Biophys. Res. Commun.* **2015**, *460*, 1021–1028. [CrossRef]
125. Li, L.; Dong, L.; Qu, X.; Jin, S.; Lv, X.; Tan, G. Tripartite motif 16 inhibits hepatocellular carcinoma cell migration and invasion. *Int. J. Oncol.* **2016**, *48*, 1639–1649. [CrossRef]
126. Qi, L.; Lu, Z.; Sun, Y.H.; Song, H.T.; Xu, W.K. TRIM16 suppresses the progression of prostate tumors by inhibiting the Snail signaling pathway. *Int. J. Mol. Med.* **2016**, *38*, 1734–1742. [CrossRef] [PubMed]
127. Yao, J.; Xu, T.; Tian, T.; Fu, X.; Wang, W.; Li, S.; Shi, T.; Suo, A.; Ruan, Z.; Guo, H.; et al. Tripartite motif 16 suppresses breast cancer stem cell properties through regulation of Gli-1 degradation via the ubiquitin-proteasome pathway. *Oncol. Rep.* **2016**, *35*, 1204–1212. [CrossRef]
128. Zhou, W.; Zhang, Y.; Zhong, C.; Hu, J.; Hu, H.; Zhou, D.; Cao, M.Q. Decreased expression of TRIM21 indicates unfavorable outcome and promotes cell growth in breast cancer. *Cancer Manag. Res.* **2018**, *10*, 3687–3696. [CrossRef] [PubMed]
129. Xu, L.; Wu, Q.; Zhou, X.; Wu, Q.; Fang, M. TRIM13 inhibited cell proliferation and induced cell apoptosis by regulating NF-kappaB pathway in nonsmall-cell lung carcinoma cells. *Gene* **2019**, *715*, 144015. [CrossRef]
130. Chen, W.X.; Cheng, L.; Xu, L.Y.; Qian, Q.; Zhu, Y.L. Bioinformatics analysis of prognostic value of *TRIM13* gene in breast cancer. *Biosci. Rep.* **2019**, *39*, BSR20190285–BSR20190294. [CrossRef] [PubMed]
131. Tian, Z.; Tang, J.; Liao, X.; Gong, Y.; Yang, Q.; Wu, Y.; Wu, G. TRIM8 inhibits breast cancer proliferation by regulating estrogen signaling. *Am. J. Cancer Res.* **2020**, *10*, 3440–3457. [PubMed]
132. Wang, Y.; He, D.; Yang, L.; Wen, B.; Dai, J.; Zhang, Q.; Kang, J.; He, W.; Ding, Q.; He, D. TRIM26 functions as a novel tumor suppressor of hepatocellular carcinoma and its downregulation contributes to worse prognosis. *Biochem. Biophys. Res. Commun.* **2015**, *463*, 458–465. [CrossRef] [PubMed]
133. Diaz-Lagares, A.; Mendez-Gonzalez, J.; Hervas, D.; Saigi, M.; Pajares, M.J.; Garcia, D.; Crujerias, A.B.; Pio, R.; Montuenga, L.M.; Zulueta, J.; et al. A Novel Epigenetic Signature for Early Diagnosis in Lung Cancer. *Clin. Cancer Res. Cancer Res.* **2016**, *22*, 3361–3371. [CrossRef] [PubMed]

134. Chen, W.; Lu, C.; Hong, J. TRIM15 exerts anti-tumor effects through suppressing cancer cell invasion in gastric adenocarcinoma. *Med. Sci. Monit.* **2018**, *24*, 8033–8041. [CrossRef]
135. Ding, Z.; Jin, G.; Wang, W.; Chen, W.; Wu, Y.; Ai, X.; Chen, L.; Zhang, W.; Liang, H.F.; Laurence, A.; et al. Reduced expression of transcriptional intermediary factor 1 gamma promotes metastasis and indicates poor prognosis of hepatocellular carcinoma. *Hepatology* **2014**, *60*, 1620–1636. [CrossRef] [PubMed]
136. Kanno, Y.; Watanabe, M.; Kimura, T.; Nonomura, K.; Tanaka, S.; Hatakeyama, S. TRIM29 as a novel prostate basal cell marker for diagnosis of prostate cancer. *Acta Histochem.* **2014**, *116*, 708–712. [CrossRef]
137. Jingushi, K.; Ueda, Y.; Kitae, K.; Hase, H.; Egawa, H.; Ohshio, I.; Kawakami, R.; Kashiwagi, Y.; Tsukada, Y.; Kobayashi, T.; et al. miR629 targets TRIM33 to promote TGFβ/Smad signaling and metastatic phenotypes in ccRCC. *Mol. Cancer Res.* **2015**, *13*, 565–574. [CrossRef]
138. Kassem, L.; Deygas, M.; Fattet, L.; Lopez, J.; Goulvent, T.; Lavergne, E.; Chabaud, S.; Carrabin, N.; Chopin, N.; Bachelot, T.; et al. TIF1γ interferes with TGFβ1/SMAD4 signaling to promote poor outcome in operable breast cancer patients. *BMC Cancer* **2015**, *15*, 453. [CrossRef]
139. Song, X.; Fu, C.; Yang, X.; Sun, D.; Zhang, X.; Zhang, J. Tripartite motif-containing 29 as a novel biomarker in non-small cell lung cancer. *Oncol. Lett.* **2015**, *10*, 2283–2288. [CrossRef]
140. Xue, J.; Chen, Y.; Wu, Y.; Wang, Z.; Zhou, A.; Zhang, S.; Lin, K.; Aldape, K.; Majumder, S.; Lu, Z.; et al. Tumour suppressor TRIM33 targets nuclear β-catenin degradation. *Nat. Commun.* **2015**, *6*, 6156. [CrossRef]
141. Xiao, W.; Wang, X.; Wang, T.; Xing, J. TRIM2 downregulation in clear cell renal cell carcinoma affects cell proliferation, migration, and invasion and predicts poor patients' survival. *Cancer Manag. Res.* **2018**, *10*, 5951–5964. [CrossRef] [PubMed]
142. Qin, Y.; Ye, J.; Zhao, F.; Hu, S.; Wang, S. TRIM2 regulates the development and metastasis of tumorous cells of osteosarcoma. *Int. J. Oncol.* **2018**, *53*, 1643–1656. [CrossRef] [PubMed]
143. Cao, H.; Fang, Y.; Liang, Q.; Wang, J.; Luo, B.; Zeng, G.; Zhang, T.; Jing, X.; Wang, X. TRIM2 is a novel promoter of human colorectal cancer. *Scand. J. Gastroenterol.* **2019**, *54*, 210–218. [CrossRef]
144. Wang, F.; Ruan, L.; Yang, J.; Zhao, Q.; Wei, W. TRIM14 promotes the migration and invasion of gastric cancer by regulating epithelial-to-mesenchymal transition via activation of AKT signaling regulated by miR-195-5p. *Oncol. Rep.* **2018**, *40*, 3273–3284. [CrossRef]
145. Piao, M.Y.; Cao, H.L.; He, N.N.; Xu, M.Q.; Dong, W.X.; Wang, W.Q.; Wang, B.M.; Zhou, B. Potential role of TRIM3 as a novel tumour suppressor in colorectal cancer (CRC) development. *Scand. J. Gastroenterol.* **2016**, *51*, 572–582. [CrossRef] [PubMed]
146. Sho, T.; Tsukiyama, T.; Sato, T.; Kondo, T.; Cheng, J.; Saku, T.; Asaka, M.; Hatakeyama, S. TRIM29 negatively regulates p53 via inhibition of Tip60. *Biochim. Biophys. Acta* **2011**, *1813*, 1245–1253. [CrossRef]
147. Sun, J.; Zhang, T.; Cheng, M.; Hong, L.; Zhang, C.; Xie, M.; Sun, P.; Fan, R.; Wang, Z.; Wang, L.; et al. TRIM29 facilitates the epithelial-to-mesenchymal transition and the progression of colorectal cancer via the activation of the Wnt/β-catenin signaling pathway. *J. Exp. Clin. Cancer Res.* **2019**, *38*, 104. [CrossRef] [PubMed]
148. Carinci, F.; Arcelli, D.; Lo Muzio, L.; Francioso, F.; Valentini, D.; Evangelisti, R.; Volinia, S.; D'Angelo, A.; Meroni, G.; Zollo, M.; et al. Molecular classification of nodal metastasis in primary larynx squamous cell carcinoma. *Transl. Res.* **2007**, *150*, 233–245. [CrossRef]
149. Takayama, K.I.; Suzuki, T.; Tanaka, T.; Fujimura, T.; Takahashi, S.; Urano, T.; Ikeda, K.; Inoue, S. TRIM25 enhances cell growth and cell survival by modulating p53 signals via interaction with G3BP2 in prostate cancer. *Oncogene* **2018**, *37*, 2165–2180. [CrossRef] [PubMed]
150. Mastropasqua, F.; Marzano, F.; Valletti, A.; Aiello, I.; Di Tullio, G.; Morgano, A.; Liuni, S.; Ranieri, E.; Guerrini, L.; Gasparre, G.; et al. TRIM8 restores p53 tumour suppressor function by blunting N-MYC activity in chemo-resistant tumours. *Mol. Cancer* **2017**, *16*, 67. [CrossRef]
151. Caratozzolo, M.F.; Valletti, A.; Gigante, M.; Aiello, I.; Mastropasqua, F.; Marzano, F.; Ditonno, P.; Carrieri, G.; Simonnet, H.; D'Erchia, A.M.; et al. TRIM8 anti-proliferative action against chemo-resistant renal cell carcinoma. *Oncotarget* **2014**, *5*, 7446–7457. [CrossRef]
152. Cambiaghi, V.; Giuliani, V.; Lombardi, S.; Marinelli, C.; Toffalorio, F.; Pelicci, P.G. TRIM proteins in cancer. *Adv. Exp. Med. Biol.* **2012**, *770*, 77–91.
153. Hutchinson, K.E.; Lipson, D.; Stephens, P.J.; Otto, G.; Lehmann, B.D.; Lyle, P.L.; Vnencak-Jones, C.L.; Ross, J.S.; Pietenpol, J.A.; Sosman, J.A.; et al. BRAF fusions define a distinct molecular subset of melanomas with potential sensitivity to MEK inhibition. *Clin. Cancer Res.* **2013**, *19*, 6696–6702. [CrossRef] [PubMed]
154. Nakaoku, T.; Tsuta, K.; Ichikawa, H.; Shiraishi, K.; Sakamoto, H.; Enari, M.; Furuta, K.; Shimada, Y.; Ogiwara, H.; Watanabe, S.; et al. Druggable oncogene fusions in invasive mucinous lung adenocarcinoma. *Clin. Cancer Res.* **2014**, *20*, 3087–3093. [CrossRef] [PubMed]
155. Shim, H.S.; Kenudson, M.; Zheng, Z.; Liebers, M.; Cha, Y.J.; Hoang Ho, Q.; Onozato, M.; Phi Le, L.; Heist, R.S.; Iafrate, A.J. Unique Genetic and Survival Characteristics of Invasive Mucinous Adenocarcinoma of the Lung. *J. Thorac. Oncol.* **2015**, *10*, 1156–1162. [CrossRef]
156. Alfonso, A.; Montalban-Bravo, G.; Takahashi, K.; Jabbour, E.J.; Kadia, T.; Ravandi, F.; Cortes, J.; Estrov, Z.; Borthakur, G.; Pemmaraju, N.; et al. Natural history of chronic myelomonocytic leukemia treated with hypomethylating agents. *Am. J. Hematol.* **2017**, *92*, 599–606. [CrossRef]

157. Yin, Y.; Zhong, J.; Li, S.W.; Li, J.Z.; Zhou, M.; Chen, Y.; Sang, Y.; Liu, L. TRIM11, a direct target of miR-24-3p, promotes cell proliferation and inhibits apoptosis in colon cancer. *Oncotarget* **2016**, *7*, 86755–86765. [CrossRef]
158. Fang, Z.; Zhang, L.; Liao, Q.; Wang, Y.; Yu, F.; Feng, M.; Xiang, X.; Xiong, J. Regulation of TRIM24 by miR-511 modulates cell proliferation in gastric cancer. *J. Exp. Clin. Cancer Res.* **2017**, *36*, 17. [CrossRef] [PubMed]
159. Li, Y.H.; Zhong, M.; Zang, H.L.; Tian, X.F. The E3 ligase for metastasis associated 1 protein, TRIM25, is targeted by microRNA-873 in hepatocellular carcinoma. *Exp. Cell Res.* **2018**, *368*, 37–41. [CrossRef] [PubMed]
160. Han, Q.; Cheng, P.; Yang, H.; Liang, H.; Lin, F. Altered expression of microRNA-365 is related to the occurrence and development of non-small-cell lung cancer by inhibiting TRIM25 expression. *J. Cell. Physiol.* **2019**, *234*, 22321–22330. [CrossRef] [PubMed]
161. Zhang, W.; Zhu, L.; Yang, G.; Zhou, B.; Wang, J.; Qu, X.; Yan, Z.; Qian, S.; Liu, R. Hsa_circ_0026134 expression promoted TRIM25- and IGF2BP3-mediated hepatocellular carcinoma cell proliferation and invasion via sponging miR-127-5p. *Biosci. Rep.* **2020**, *40*. [CrossRef]
162. Sun, S.; Li, W.; Ma, X.; Luan, H. Long Noncoding RNA LINC00265 Promotes Glycolysis and Lactate Production of Colorectal Cancer through Regulating of miR-216b-5p/TRIM44 Axis. *Digestion* **2020**, *101*, 391–400. [CrossRef]
163. Lei, R.; Feng, L.; Hong, D. ELFN1-AS1 accelerates the proliferation and migration of colorectal cancer via regulation of miR-4644/TRIM44 axis. *Cancer Biomark. Sect. Dis. Markers.* **2020**, *27*, 433–443. [CrossRef] [PubMed]
164. Elabd, S.; Meroni, G.; Blattner, C. TRIMming p53's anticancer activity. *Oncogene* **2016**, *35*, 5577–5584. [CrossRef] [PubMed]
165. Valletti, A.; Marzano, F.; Pesole, G.; Sbisà, E.; Tullo, A. Targeting Chemoresistant Tumors: Could TRIM Proteins-p53 Axis Be a Possible Answer? *Int. J. Mol. Sci.* **2019**, *20*, 20. [CrossRef]
166. Wang, C.; Ivanov, A.; Chen, L.; Fredericks, W.J.; Seto, E.; Rauscher, F.J.; Chen, J. MDM2 interaction with nuclear corepressor KAP1 contributes to p53 inactivation. *EMBO J.* **2005**, *24*, 3279–3290. [CrossRef] [PubMed]
167. Jain, A.K.; Barton, M.C. Regulation of p53: TRIM24 enters the RING. *Cell Cycle* **2009**, *8*, 3668–3674. [CrossRef]
168. Yuan, Z.; Villagra, A.; Peng, L.; Coppola, D.; Glozak, M.; Sotomayor, E.M.; Chen, J.; Lane, W.S.; Seto, E. The ATDC (TRIM29) protein binds p53 and antagonizes p53-mediated functions. *Mol. Cell. Biol.* **2010**, *30*, 3004–3015. [CrossRef]
169. Zhang, L.; Huang, N.J.; Chen, C.; Tang, W.; Kornbluth, S. Ubiquitylation of p53 by the APC/C inhibitor Trim39. *Proc. Natl. Acad. Sci. USA* **2012**, *109*, 20931–20936. [CrossRef] [PubMed]
170. Zhou, Z.; Ji, Z.; Wang, Y.; Li, J.; Cao, H.; Zhu, H.H.; Gao, W.Q. TRIM59 is up-regulated in gastric tumors, promoting ubiquitination and degradation of p53. *Gastroenterology* **2014**, *147*, 1043–1054. [CrossRef] [PubMed]
171. Liu, J.; Zhu, Y.; Hu, W.; Feng, Z. TRIM32 is a novel negative regulator of p53. *Mol. Cell Oncol.* **2014**, *2*, e970951. [CrossRef]
172. Jain, A.K.; Allton, K.; Duncan, A.D.; Barton, M.C. TRIM24 is a p53-induced E3-ubiquitin ligase that undergoes ATM-mediated phosphorylation and autodegradation during DNA damage. *Mol. Cell Biol.* **2014**, *34*, 2695–2709. [CrossRef]
173. Zhang, P.; Elabd, S.; Hammer, S.; Solozobova, V.; Yan, H.; Bartel, F.; Inoue, S.; Henrich, T.; Wittbrodt, J.; Loosli, F.; et al. TRIM25 has a dual function in the p53/MDM2 circuit. *Oncogene* **2015**, *34*, 5729–5738. [CrossRef]
174. Chen, Y.; Guo, Y.; Yang, H.; Shi, G.; Xu, G.; Shi, J.; Yin, N.; Chen, D. TRIM66 overexpresssion contributes to osteosarcoma carcinogenesis and indicates poor survival outcome. *Oncotarget* **2015**, *6*, 23708–23719. [CrossRef]
175. Liu, J.; Rao, J.; Lou, X.; Zhai, J.; Ni, Z.; Wang, X. Upregulated TRIM11 exerts its oncogenic effects in hepatocellular carcinoma through inhibition of P53. *Cell Physiol. Biochem.* **2017**, *44*, 255–266. [CrossRef]
176. Nguyen, J.Q.; Irby, R.B. TRIM21 is a novel regulator of Par-4 in colon and pancreatic cancer cells. *Cancer Biol. Ther.* **2017**, *18*, 16–25. [CrossRef] [PubMed]
177. Czerwinska, P.; Mazurek, S.; Wiznerowicz, M. The complexity of TRIM28 contribution to cancer. *J. Biomed. Sci.* **2017**, *24*, 63. [CrossRef]
178. Guo, P.; Qiu, Y.; Ma, X.; Li, T.; Ma, X.; Zhu, L.; Lin, Y.; Han, L. Tripartite motif 31 promotes resistance to anoikis of hepatocarcinoma cells through regulation of p53-AMPK axis. *Exp. Cell Res.* **2018**, *368*, 59–66. [CrossRef]
179. Han, Y.; Tan, Y.; Zhao, Y.; Zhang, Y.; He, X.; Yu, L.; Jiang, H.; Lu, H.; Tian, H. TRIM23 overexpression is a poor prognostic factor and contributes to carcinogenesis in colorectal cancer. *J. Cell. Mol. Med.* **2020**, *24*, 5491–5500. [CrossRef] [PubMed]
180. Joo, H.M.; Kim, J.Y.; Jeong, J.B.; Seong, K.M.; Nam, S.Y.; Yang, K.H.; Kim, C.S.; Kim, H.S.; Jeong, M.; An, S.; et al. Ret finger protein 2 enhances ionizing radiation-induced apoptosis via degradation of AKT and MDM2. *Eur. J. Cell Biol.* **2011**, *90*, 420–431. [CrossRef] [PubMed]
181. Hatakeyama, S. TRIM proteins and cancer. *Nat. Rev. Cancer* **2011**, *11*, 792–804. [CrossRef]
182. Caratozzolo, M.F.; Micale, L.; Turturo, M.G.; Cornacchia, S.; Fusco, C.; Marzano, F.; Augello, B.; D'Erchia, A.M.; Guerrini, L.; Pesole, G.; et al. TRIM8 modulates p53 activity to dictate cell cycle arrest. *Cell Cycle* **2012**, *11*, 511–523. [CrossRef]
183. Stramucci, L.; Pranteda, A.; Bossi, G. Insights of crosstalk between p53 protein and the MKK3/MKK6/p38 MAPK signaling pathway in cancer. *Cancers* **2018**, *10*, 131. [CrossRef]
184. Wang, S.; Zhang, Y.; Huang, J.; Wong, C.C.; Zhai, J.; Li, C.; Wei, G.; Zhao, L.; Wang, G.; Wei, H.; et al. TRIM67 Activates p53 to Suppress Colorectal Cancer Initiation and Progression. *Cancer Res.* **2019**, *79*, 4086–4098. [CrossRef] [PubMed]
185. Clevers, H. Wnt/beta-catenin signaling in development and disease. *Cell* **2006**, *127*, 469–480. [CrossRef]
186. White, B.D.; Chien, A.J.; Dawson, D.W. Dysregulation of Wnt/β-catenin signaling in gastrointestinal cancers. *Gastroenterology* **2012**, *142*, 219–232. [CrossRef] [PubMed]
187. Clevers, H.; Nusse, R. Wnt/β-catenin signaling and disease. *Cell* **2012**, *149*, 1192–1205. [CrossRef] [PubMed]

188. Chang, G.; Zhang, H.; Wang, J.; Zhang, Y.; Xu, H.; Wang, C.; Zhang, H.; Ma, L.; Li, Q.; Pang, T. CD44 targets Wnt/β-catenin pathway to mediate the proliferation of K562 cells. *Cancer Cell Int.* **2013**, *13*, 117. [CrossRef]
189. Novellasdemunt, L.; Antas, P.; Li, V.S.W. Targeting Wnt signaling in colorectal cancer. A Review in the Theme: Cell Signaling: Proteins, Pathways and Mechanisms. *Am. J. Physiol. Cell Physiol.* **2015**, *309*, C511–C521.
190. Xu, R.; Hu, J.; Zhang, T.; Jiang, C.; Wang, H.Y. TRIM29 overexpression is associated with poor prognosis and promotes tumor progression by activating Wnt/b-catenin. *Oncotarget* **2016**, *7*, 28579–28591. [CrossRef] [PubMed]
191. Liu, M.; Zhang, X.; Cai, J.; Li, Y.; Luo, Q.; Wu, H.; Yang, Z.; Wang, L.; Chen, D. Downregulation of TRIM58 expression is associated with a poor patient outcome and enhances colorectal cancer cell invasion. *Oncol. Rep.* **2018**, *40*, 1251–1260. [CrossRef] [PubMed]
192. Liu, X.; Long, Z.; Cai, H.; Yu, S.; Wu, J. TRIM58 suppresses the tumor growth in gastric cancer by inactivation of β-catenin signaling via ubiquitination. *Cancer Biol. Ther.* **2020**, *21*, 203–212. [CrossRef] [PubMed]
193. Derynck, R.; Zhang, Y.E. Smad-dependent and Smad-independent pathways in TGF-beta family signalling. *Nature* **2003**, *425*, 577–584. [CrossRef]
194. Moustakas, A.; Heldin, C.H. Non-Smad TGF-beta signals. *J. Cell Sci.* **2005**, *118*, 3573–3584. [CrossRef] [PubMed]
195. Zhang, Y.E. Non-Smad pathways in TGF-beta signaling. *Cell Res.* **2009**, *19*, 128–139. [CrossRef]
196. Massagué, J. TGFβ signalling in context. *Nat. Rev. Mol. Cell Biol.* **2012**, *13*, 616–630. [CrossRef] [PubMed]
197. De Boeck, M.; ten Dijke, P. Key role for ubiquitin protein modification in TGFβ signal transduction. *Upsala J. Med. Sci.* **2012**, *117*, 153–165. [CrossRef]
198. Sun, N.; Xue, Y.; Dai, T.; Li, X.; Zheng, N. Tripartite motif containing 25 promotes proliferation and invasion of colorectal cancer cells through TGF-β signaling. *Biosci. Rep.* **2017**, *37*. [CrossRef] [PubMed]
199. Lee, H.-J. The Role of Tripartite Motif Family Proteins in TGF-β Signaling Pathway and Cancer. *J. Cancer Prev.* **2018**, *23*, 162–169. [CrossRef]
200. Liang, Q.; Tang, C.; Tang, M.; Zhang, Q.; Gao, Y.; Ge, Z. TRIM47 is up-regulated in colorectal cancer, promoting ubiquitination and degradation of SMAD4. *J. Exp. Clin. Cancer Res.* **2019**, *38*, 159. [CrossRef] [PubMed]
201. Cantley, L.C. The phosphoinositide 3-kinase pathway. *Science* **2002**, *296*, 1655–1657. [CrossRef] [PubMed]
202. Papadatos-Pastos, D.; Rabbie, R.; Ross, P.; Sarker, D. The role of the PI3K pathway in colorectal cancer. *Crit. Rev. Oncol. Hematol.* **2015**, *94*, 18–30. [CrossRef]
203. Tiwari, A.; Saraf, S.; Verma, A.; Panda, P.K.; Jain, S.K. Novel targeting approaches and signaling pathways of colorectal cancer: An insight. *World J. Gastroenterol.* **2018**, *24*, 4428–4435. [CrossRef] [PubMed]
204. Fruman, D.A.; Chiu, H.; Hopkins, B.D.; Bagrodia, S.; Cantley, L.C.; Abraham, R.T. The PI3K Pathway in Human Disease. *Cell* **2017**, *170*, 605–635. [CrossRef] [PubMed]
205. Shen, W.; Jin, Z.; Tong, X.; Wang, H.; Zhuang, L.; Lu, X.; Wu, S. TRIM14 promotes cell proliferation and inhibits apoptosis by suppressing PTEN in colorectal cancer. *Cancer Manag. Res.* **2019**, *11*, 5725–5735. [CrossRef]
206. Zhang, Y.; Feng, Y.; Ji, D.; Wang, Q.; Qian, W.; Wang, S.; Zhang, Z.; Ji, B.; Zhang, C.; Sun, Y.; et al. TRIM27 functions as an oncogene by activating epithelial-mesenchymal transition and p-AKT in colorectal cancer. *Int. J. Oncol.* **2018**, *53*, 620–632. [CrossRef] [PubMed]
207. Li, C.G.; Hu, H.; Yang, X.J.; Huang, C.Q.; Yu, X.Q. TRIM44 Promotes Colorectal Cancer Proliferation, Migration, and Invasion through the Akt/mTOR Signaling Pathway. *OncoTargets Ther.* **2019**, *12*, 10693–10701. [CrossRef]
208. Sun, Y.; Ji, B.; Feng, Y.; Zhang, Y.; Ji, D.; Zhu, C.; Wang, S.; Zhang, C.; Zhang, D.; Sun, Y. TRIM59 facilitates the proliferation of colorectal cancer and promotes metastasis via the PI3K/AKT pathway. *Oncol. Rep.* **2017**, *38*, 43–52. [CrossRef]
209. Wang, M.; Chao, C.; Luo, G.; Wang, B.; Zhan, X.; Di, D.; Qian, Y.; Zhang, X. Prognostic significance of TRIM59 for cancer patient survival: A systematic review and meta-analysis. *Medicine* **2019**, *98*, e18024. [CrossRef]
210. Saxton, R.A.; Sabatini, D.M. mTOR Signaling in Growth, Metabolism, and Disease. *Cell* **2017**, *168*, 960–976. [CrossRef]
211. Ma, L.; Yao, N.; Chen, P.; Zhuang, Z. TRIM27 promotes the development of esophagus cancer via regulating PTEN/AKT signaling pathway. *Cancer Cell Int.* **2019**, *19*, 283. [CrossRef]
212. Bromberg, J.; Wang, T.C. Inflammation and cancer: IL-6 and STAT3 complete the link. *Cancer Cell.* **2009**, *15*, 79–80. [CrossRef]
213. Bollrath, J.; Greten, F.R. IKK/NF-kappaB and STAT3 pathways: Central signalling hubs in inflammation-mediated tumour promotion and metastasis. *EMBO Rep.* **2009**, *10*, 1314–1319. [CrossRef]
214. Yu, H.; Pardoll, D.; Jove, R. STATs in cancer inflammation and immunity: A leading role for STAT3. *Nat. Rev. Cancer* **2009**, *9*, 798–809. [CrossRef]
215. Sakamoto, K.; Maeda, S.; Hikiba, Y.; Nakagawa, H.; Hayakawa, Y.; Shibata, W.; Yanai, A.; Ogura, K.; Omata, M. Constitutive NF-kappaB activation in colorectal carcinoma plays a key role in angiogenesis, promoting tumor growth. *Clin. Cancer Res.* **2009**, *15*, 2248–2258. [CrossRef]
216. Terzic, J.; Grivennikov, S.; Karin, E.; Karin, M. Inflammation and colon cancer. *Gastroenterology* **2010**, *138*, 2101–2114. [CrossRef] [PubMed]
217. Fan, Y.; Mao, R.; Yang, J. NF-κB and STAT3 signaling pathways collaboratively link inflammation to cancer. *Protein Cell* **2013**, *4*, 176–185. [CrossRef] [PubMed]
218. Yu, H.; Lee, H.; Herrmann, A.; Buettner, R.; Jove, R. Revisiting STAT3 signalling in cancer: New and unexpected biological functions. *Nat. Rev. Cancer* **2014**, *14*, 736–746. [CrossRef] [PubMed]

219. Xu, W.; Xu, B.; Yao, Y.; Yu, X.; Cao, H.; Zhang, J.; Liu, J.; Sheng, H. RNA interference against TRIM29 inhibits migration and invasion of colorectal cancer cells. *Oncol. Rep.* **2016**, *36*, 1411–1418. [CrossRef]
220. Jin, Z.; Li, H.; Hong, X.; Ying, G.; Lu, X.; Zhuang, L.; Wu, S. TRIM14 promotes colorectal cancer cell migration and invasion through the SPHK1/STAT3 pathway. *Cancer Cell Int.* **2018**, *18*, 202. [CrossRef] [PubMed]
221. Zhang, H.X.; Xu, Z.S.; Lin, H.; Li, M.; Xia, T.; Cui, K.; Wang, S.Y.; Li, Y.; Shu, H.B.; Wang, Y.Y. TRIM27 mediates STAT3 activation at retromer-positive structures to promote colitis and colitis-associated carcinogenesis. *Nat. Commun.* **2018**, *9*, 3441. [CrossRef] [PubMed]
222. Pan, S.; Deng, Y.; Fu, J.; Zhang, Y.; Zhang, Z.; Ru, X.; Qin, X. TRIM52 promotes colorectal cancer cell proliferation through the STAT3 signaling. *Cancer Cell Int.* **2019**, *19*, 57. [CrossRef] [PubMed]
223. Hayden, M.S.; Ghosh, S. Shared principles in NF-kappaB signaling. *Cell* **2008**, *132*, 344–362. [CrossRef] [PubMed]
224. Sun, S.C. The non-canonical NF-κB pathway in immunity and inflammation. *Nat. Rev. Immunol.* **2017**, *17*, 545–558. [CrossRef]
225. Choudhury, N.R.; Heikel, G.; Trubitsyna, M.; Kubik, P.; Nowak, J.S.; Webb, S.; Granneman, S.; Spanos, C.; Rappsilber, J.; Castello, A.; et al. RNA-binding activity of TRIM25 is mediated by its PRY/SPRY domain and is required for ubiquitination. *BMC Biol.* **2017**, *15*, 105. [CrossRef]
226. Wang, H.; Yao, L.; Gong, Y.; Zhang, B. TRIM31 regulates chronic inflammation via NF-κB signal pathway to promote invasion and metastasis in colorectal cancer. *Am. J. Transl. Res.* **2018**, *10*, 1247–1259. [PubMed]
227. Chen, M.; Zhao, Z.; Meng, Q.; Liang, P.; Su, Z.; Wu, Y.; Huang, J.; Cui, J. TRIM14 Promotes Noncanonical NF-κB Activation by Modulating p100/p52 Stability via Selective Autophagy. *Adv. Sci. Weinh. Baden Wurtt. Ger.* **2020**, *7*, 1901261. [CrossRef] [PubMed]
228. Noguchi, K.; Okumura, F.; Takahashi, N.; Kataoka, A.; Kamiyama, T.; Todo, S.; Hatakeyama, S. TRIM40 promotes neddylation of IKKγ and is downregulated in gastrointestinal cancers. *Carcinogenesis* **2011**, *32*, 995–1004. [CrossRef] [PubMed]
229. Eberhardt, W.; Haeussler, K.; Nasrullah, U.; Pfeilschifter, J. Multifaceted Roles of TRIM Proteins in Colorectal Carcinoma. *Int. J. Mol. Sci.* **2020**, *21*, 7532. [CrossRef]
230. Wang, F.Q.; Han, Y.; Yao, W.; Yu, J. Prognostic relevance of tripartite motif containing 24 expression in colorectal cancer. *Pathol. Res. Pract.* **2017**, *213*, 1271–1275. [CrossRef]
231. Nasrullah, U.; Haeussler, K.; Biyanee, A.; Wittig, I.; Pfeilschifter, J.; Eberhardt, W. Identification of TRIM25 as a Negative Regulator of Caspase-2 Expression Reveals a Novel Target for Sensitizing Colon Carcinoma Cells to Intrinsic Apoptosis. *Cells* **2019**, *8*, 1622. [CrossRef]
232. Barlev, N.A.; Liu, L.; Chehab, N.H.; Mansfield, K.; Harris, K.G.; Halazonetis, T.D.; Berger, S.L. Acetylation of p53 activates transcription through recruitment of coactivators/histone acetyltransferases. *Mol. Cell* **2001**, *8*, 1243–1254.
233. Wu, W.; Chen, J.; Wu, J.; Lin, J.; Yang, S.; Yu, H. Knockdown of tripartite motif-59 inhibits the malignant processes in human colorectal cancer cells. *Oncol. Rep.* **2017**, *38*, 2480–2488. [CrossRef]
234. Fitzgerald, S.; Espina, V.; Liotta, L.; Sheehan, K.M.; O'Grady, A.; Cummins, R.; O'Kennedy, R.; Kay, E.W.; Kijanka, G.S. Stromal TRIM28-associated signaling pathway modulation within the colorectal cancer microenvironment. *J. Transl. Med.* **2018**, *16*, 89. [CrossRef] [PubMed]
235. Zheng, S.; Zhou, C.; Wang, Y.; Li, H.; Sun, Y.; Shen, Z. TRIM6 promotes colorectal cancer cells proliferation and response to thiostrepton by TIS21/FoxM1. *J. Exp. Clin. Cancer Res.* **2020**, *39*, 23. [CrossRef]
236. Xie, Y.; Zhao, Y.; Shi, L.; Li, W.; Chen, K.; Li, M.; Chen, X.; Zhang, H.; Li, T.; Matsuzawa-Ishimoto, Y.; et al. Gut epithelial TSC1/mTOR controls RIPK3-dependent necroptosis in intestinal inflammation and cancer. *J. Clin. Investig.* **2020**, *130*, 2111–2128. [CrossRef] [PubMed]
237. Uhlén, M.; Fagerberg, L.; Hallström, B.M.; Lindskog, C.; Oksvold, P.; Mardinoglu, A.; Sivertsson, Å.; Kampf, C.; Sjöstedt, E.; Asplund, A.; et al. Tissue-based map of the human proteome. *Science* **2015**, *347*, 1260419, The Human protein Atlas.
238. Vincent, S.R.; Kwasnicka, D.A.; Fretier, P. A novel RING finger-B box-coiled-coil protein, GERP. *Biochem. Biophys. Res. Commun.* **2000**, *279*, 482–486. [CrossRef]
239. Maarifi, G.; Smith, N.; Maillet, S.; Moncorgé, O.; Chamontin, C.; Edouard, J.; Sohm, F.; Blanchet, F.P.; Herbeuval, J.P.; Lutfalla, G.; et al. TRIM8 is required for virus-induced IFN response in human plasmacytoid dendritic cells. *Sci. Adv.* **2019**, *5*, eaax3511. [CrossRef] [PubMed]
240. Caratozzolo, M.F.; Marzano, F.; Mastropasqua, F.; Sbisà, E.; Tullo, A. TRIM8: Making the Right Decision between the Oncogene and Tumour Suppressor Role. *Genes* **2017**, *8*, 354. [CrossRef]
241. Bhaduri, U.; Merla, G. Rise of TRIM8: A Molecule of Duality. *Mol. Ther. Nucleic Acids* **2020**, *22*, 434–444. [CrossRef] [PubMed]
242. Tomar, D.; Sripada, L.; Prajapati, P.; Singh, R.; Singh, A.K.; Singh, R. Nucleo-cytoplasmic trafficking of TRIM8, a novel oncogene, is involved in positive regulation of TNF induced NF-κB pathway. *PLoS ONE* **2012**, *7*, e48662. [CrossRef]
243. Venuto, S.; Castellana, S.; Monti, M.; Appolloni, I.; Fusilli, C.; Fusco, C.; Pucci, P.; Malatesta, P.; Mazza, T.; Merla, G.; et al. TRIM8-driven transcriptomic profile of neural stem cells identified glioma-related nodal genes and pathways. *Biochim. Biophys. Acta Gen. Subj.* **2019**, *1863*, 491–501. [CrossRef]
244. Xiong, H.; Zhang, Z.G.; Tian, X.Q.; Sun, D.F.; Liang, Q.C.; Zhang, Y.J.; Lu, R.; Chen, Y.X.; Fang, J.Y. Inhibition of JAK1, 2/STAT3 signaling induces apoptosis, cell cycle arrest, and reduces tumor cell invasion in colorectal cancer cells. *Neoplasia* **2008**, *10*, 287–297. [CrossRef]

245. Zhuang, Q.; Hong, F.; Shen, A.; Zheng, L.; Zeng, J.; Lin, W.; Chen, Y.; Sferra, T.J.; Hong, Z.; Peng, J. Pien Tze Huang inhibits tumor cell proliferation and promotes apoptosis via suppressing the STAT3 pathway in a colorectal cancer mouse model. *Int. J. Oncol.* **2012**, *40*, 1569–1574. [PubMed]
246. Patel, M.; Horgan, P.G.; McMillan, D.C.; Edwards, J. NF-kappaB pathways in the development and progression of colorectal cancer. *Transl. Res.* **2018**, *197*, 43–56. [CrossRef] [PubMed]
247. Bomben, R.; Gobessi, S.; Dal Bo, M.; Volinia, S.; Marconi, D.; Tissino, E.; Benedetti, D.; Zucchetto, A.; Rossi, D.; Gaidano, G.; et al. The miR-17~92 family regulates the response to Toll-like receptor 9 triggering of CLL cells with unmutated IGHV genes. *Leukemia* **2012**, *26*, 1584–1593. [CrossRef] [PubMed]
248. Micale, L.; Fusco, C.; Fontana, A.; Barbano, R.; Augello, B.; De Nittis, P.; Copetti, M.; Pellico, M.T.; Mandriani, B.; Cocciadiferro, D.; et al. TRIM8 downregulation in glioma affects cell proliferation and it is associated with patients survival. *BMC Cancer* **2015**, *15*, 470. [CrossRef] [PubMed]
249. Xia, Y.J.; Zhao, J.; Yang, C. Identification of key genes and pathways for melanoma in the TRIM family. *Cancer Med.* **2020**, *9*, 8989–9005. [CrossRef] [PubMed]
250. Toledo, F.; Wahl, G.M. Regulating the p53 pathway: In vitro hypotheses, in vivo veritas. *Nat. Rev. Cancer* **2006**, *6*, 909–923. [CrossRef] [PubMed]
251. Zambetti, G.P. The p53 mutation "gradient effect" and its clinical implications. *J. Cell Physiol.* **2007**, *213*, 370–373. [CrossRef]
252. Robles, A.I.; Harris, C.C. Clinical outcomes and correlates of TP53 mutations and cancer. *Cold Spring Harb. Perspect. Biol.* **2010**, *2*, a001016. [CrossRef]
253. Liu, Y.; Zhang, B.; Shi, T.; Qin, H. miR-182 promotes tumor growth and increases chemoresistance of human anaplastic thyroid cancer by targeting tripartite motif 8. *OncoTargets Ther.* **2017**, *10*, 1115–1122. [CrossRef]
254. Mogilyansky, E.; Rigoutsos, I. The miR-17/92 cluster: A comprehensive update on its genomics, genetics, functions and increasingly important and numerous roles in health and disease. *Cell Death Differ.* **2013**, *20*, 1603–1614. [CrossRef]
255. Arabi, L.; Gsponer, J.R.; Smida, J.; Nathrath, M.; Perrina, V.; Jundt, G.; Ruiz, C.; Quagliata, L.; Baumhoer, D. Upregulation of the miR-17-92 cluster and its two paraloga in osteosarcoma—Reasons and consequences. *Genes Cancer* **2014**, *5*, 56–63. [CrossRef] [PubMed]
256. Jepsen, R.K.; Novotny, G.W.; Klarskov, L.L.; Bang-Berthelsen, C.H.; Haakansson, I.T.; Hansen, A.; Christensen, I.J.; Riis, L.B.; Høgdall, E. Early metastatic colorectal cancers show increased tissue expression of miR-17/92 cluster members in the invasive tumor front. *Hum. Pathol.* **2018**, *80*, 231–238. [CrossRef] [PubMed]
257. Radulovic, S.; Bjelogrlic, S.K. Sunitinib, sorafenib and mTOR inhibitors in renal cancer. *J. BUON* **2007**, *12* (Suppl. S1), S151–S162.
258. Bielecka, Z.F.; Czarnecka, A.M.; Solarek, W.; Kornakiewicz, A.; Szczylik, C. Mechanisms of Acquired Resistance to Tyrosine Kinase Inhibitors in Clear-Cell Renal Cell Carcinoma (ccRCC). *Curr. Signal Transduct. Ther.* **2014**, *8*, 218–228. [CrossRef]
259. Martchenko, K.; Schmidtmann, I.; Thomaidis, T.; Thole, V.; Galle, P.R.; Becker, M.; Möhler, M.; Wehler, T.C.; Schimanski, C.C. Last line therapy with sorafenib in colorectal cancer: A retrospective analysis. *World J. Gastroenterol.* **2016**, *22*, 5400–5405. [CrossRef]
260. Thomas, V.A.; Balthasar, J.P. Sorafenib decreases tumor exposure to an anti-carcinoembryonic antigen monoclonal antibody in a mouse model of colorectal cancer. *AAPS J.* **2016**, *18*, 923–932. [CrossRef]
261. Moergel, M.; Abt, E.; Stockinger, M.; Kunkel, M. Overexpression of p63 is associated with radiation resistance and prognosis in oral squamous cell carcinoma. *Oral Oncol.* **2010**, *46*, 667–671. [CrossRef] [PubMed]
262. Matin, R.N.; Chikh, A.; Law Pak Chong, S.; Mesher, D.; Graf, M.; Sanza', P.; Senatore, V.; Scatolini, M.; Moretti, F.; Leigh, I.M.; et al. p63 is an alternative p53 repressor in melanoma that confers chemoresistance and a poor prognosis. *J. Exp. Med.* **2013**, *210*, 581–603. [CrossRef] [PubMed]
263. Loljung, L.; Coates, P.J.; Nekulova, M.; Laurell, G.; Wahlgren, M.; Wilms, T.; Widlöf, M.; Hansel, A.; Nylander, K. High expression of p63 is correlated to poor prognosis in squamous cell carcinoma of the tongue. *J. Oral Pathol. Med.* **2014**, *43*, 14–19. [CrossRef] [PubMed]
264. Caratozzolo, M.F.; Marzano, F.; Abbrescia, D.I.; Mastropasqua, F.; Petruzzella, V.; Calabrò, V.; Pesole, G.; Sbisà, E.; Guerrini, L.; Tullo, A. TRIM8 Blunts the Pro-proliferative Action of deltaNp63alpha in a p53 Wild-Type Background. *Front. Oncol.* **2019**, *9*, 1154. [CrossRef] [PubMed]

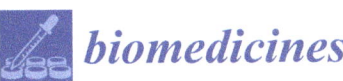

Article

Reinforcement of Colonic Anastomosis with Improved Ultrafine Nanofibrous Patch: Experiment on Pig

Jachym Rosendorf [1,2,*], Marketa Klicova [3], Lenka Cervenkova [1], Jana Horakova [3], Andrea Klapstova [3], Petr Hosek [1], Richard Palek [1,2], Jan Sevcik [1], Robert Polak [1,2], Vladislav Treska [2], Jiri Chvojka [3] and Vaclav Liska [1,2,*]

[1] Biomedical Center, Faculty of Medicine in Pilsen, Charles University, 301 00 Pilsen, Czech Republic; lenka.cervenkova@lfp.cuni.cz (L.C.); petr.hosek@lfp.cuni.cz (P.H.); palekr@fnplzen.cz (R.P.); sevcik.jan97@seznam.cz (J.S.); polakr@fnplzen.cz (R.P.)
[2] Department of Surgery, Faculty of Medicine in Pilsen, Charles University, 301 00 Pilsen, Czech Republic; treska@fnplzen.cz
[3] Department of Nonwovens and Nanofibrous Materials, Faculty of Textile Engineering, Technical University of Liberec, 460 01 Liberec, Czech Republic; marketa.klicova@seznam.cz (M.K.); horakova2222@gmail.com (J.H.); a.klapstova@centrum.cz (A.K.); jiri.chvojka@tul.cz (J.C.)
* Correspondence: jachymrosendorf@gmail.com (J.R.); vena.liska@skaut.cz (V.L.)

Abstract: Anastomotic leakage is a dreadful complication in colorectal surgery. It has a negative impact on postoperative mortality, long term life quality and oncological results. Nanofibrous polycaprolactone materials have shown pro-healing properties in various applications before. Our team developed several versions of these for healing support of colorectal anastomoses with promising results in previous years. In this study, we developed highly porous biocompatible polycaprolactone nanofibrous patches. We constructed a defective anastomosis on the large intestine of 16 pigs, covered the anastomoses with the patch in 8 animals (Experimental group) and left the rest uncovered (Control group). After 21 days of observation we evaluated postoperative changes, signs of leakage and other complications. The samples were assessed histologically according to standardized protocols. The material was easy to work with. All animals survived with no major complication. There were no differences in intestinal wall integrity between the groups and there were no signs of anastomotic leakage in any animal. The levels of collagen were significantly higher in the Experimental group, which we consider to be an indirect sign of higher mechanical strength. The material shall be further perfected in the future and possibly combined with active molecules to specifically influence the healing process.

Keywords: colorectal surgery; nanofibrous materials; anastomotic leakage; intestinal anastomosis; anastomotic patch; polycaprolactone; electrospinning; experiment; peritoneal adhesions

1. Introduction

Anastomotic leakage (AL) is a severe and feared complication in colorectal surgery. There used to be a lack of consensus over the classification of such conditions in the past, making it difficult to compare complication rates after specific types of procedures. Rahbari et al. [1] created a clear classification of the leaks depending on the type of approach to the complication, which is generally accepted by the wider medical community. However, different hospitals have different approaches and what could be treated conservatively in one department (classified as grade A or B [1]), could also end up with an anastomosis resection and a Hartmann procedure in another (classified as grade C [1]). It is therefore very difficult to assess the real incidence of AL, however it is usually reported to be as high as 5 to 19% [2–4]. The majority of colorectal procedures are performed for colorectal cancer and the number of performed procedures is enormous. Therefore, these complications form a great medical problem [5,6].

Many risk factors have been identified and one of the strongest is the position of anastomosis. Especially low anastomoses (within 5 or 6 cm from the anal verge [7,8]) show high risk of AL [9,10]. Other known factors are age, gender, smoking, steroid therapy and more [9–11]. All of the risk conditions are assumed to decrease the patient's healing abilities generally or locally. However, the specific pathophysiological mechanisms are not well described. As postoperative life quality is often terribly compromised after such complications and the complication itself is in many cases (especially grade C) fatal, AL is considered a large socioeconomic burden [12,13].

Peritoneal adhesions (PAs) are a common problem in abdominal surgery. They are formed in various extents after all surgical procedures and also other damage to the peritoneal cavity. Their purpose is protective, however they are in many cases a source of long term postoperative complications such as gastrointestinal obstruction, infertility or abdominal discomfort [14].

Some kind of patch seems to be a promising solution for local prevention of AL (and possibly PAs). Many materials have been tested for these purposes yet none of them are currently accepted in routine clinical practice [15–17]. There also has not been any material developed and tested for prevention of both PAs and AL according to our knowledge and a literature search.

Nanofibrous materials are nonwoven fabrics created by different techniques, usually from polymeric biomaterials. The variety of source materials and range of fabrication protocols offer an enormous spectrum of such fabrics, naturally resulting in novel applications in medical use. Some versions of nanofibrous planar biodegradable materials have been described to have a positive effect on wound healing by several authors [18–20]. It is assumed to be caused, among other factors, by its structural similarities to collagenous extracellular matrix [19]. There are a variety of synthetic biodegradable materials suitable for fabrication of nanofibrous scaffolds such as polycaprolactone (PCL), polylactide, polyglycolide, polydioxanone, polyhydroxybutyrate and others [21]. PCL is among the most used for implantable devices because of its good mechanical and biological properties and for the fact that it is a substance already in use in clinical medicine [22–24].

Electrospinning is one of the most commonly used approaches for scaffold production. The versatility of the process together with easily controlled parameters has led to wide use of electrospun scaffolds in the field of regenerative medicine and tissue engineering [25]. In our study, the planar nanofibrous PCL layers were fabricated via a needleless electrospinning technique called Nanospider™. The chosen method contrasts with commonly used needle electrospinning by allowing large-scale industrial production, thus supporting further introduction of the material to the market.

Our team developed and tested several versions of these materials [26,27]. A complex histological, clinical and macroscopic evaluation system has been perfected in recent works [26].

The healing process of both a skin wound or an anastomosis on the small or the large intestine is a complicated process that is yet to be fully explored and understood [28]. However, some parts of the process are known and it is certain that this process must remain well balanced for a successful outcome. A healthy peritoneum is a well-perfused metabolically active structure capable of relatively high metabolic exchange with its surroundings including both peritoneal fluid and other viscera and neighboring peritoneal surfaces [29,30]. Based on the results of our previous experiments and on the presumption that a certain level of metabolic exchange between the sutured intestine and the surrounding peritoneal surfaces is needed to maintain the healing process rather than creating a sealed barrier, we decided to create a very fine porous nanofibrous patch. Such a patch should allow this metabolic exchange while maintaining the pro-healing properties of a nanofibrous mesh we proposed in the previous studies [26,27]. The process conditions for fabricating a material with a low surface density were optimized via needleless electrospinning.

According to our knowledge, our study is the first to propose the idea of a porous anastomotic patch for healing support that should not act only as a mechanical barrier, but support the healing process of the intestinal anastomosis. We intend to develop such a patch into a product that could be routinely used in colorectal surgery for healing support in either all or high risk anastomoses.

In this study we aimed to develop an ultrafine porous polycaprolactone nanofibrous patch, use it in a perfected model of complicated anastomotic healing on the large intestine, and further develop current assessment methods for evaluation of anastomotic healing in experimental settings.

2. Materials and Methods

2.1. Material Preparation (Electrospinning Method)

A mixture of 16% w/w PCL (Mw 45,000 g/mol, Sigma Aldrich, St. Louis, MI, USA) in chloroform/ethanol/acetic acid in ratio 8/1/1 (Penta Chemicals, Prague, Czech Republic) was stirred 24 h until complete dissolution of the PCL granulate. Subsequently, the solution was electrospun using the needleless NanospiderTM 1WS500U electrospinning device (Elmarco, Liberec, Czech Republic) (scheme in Supplementary Figure S1). The environmental parameters such as the relative humidity and temperature were controlled via the climatic system NS AC150 (Elmarco). The nanofibers were collected on a polypropylene spunbond substrate. The process parameters were optimized to produce a nanofibrous layer with low surface density, namely 10 g/m^2 (listed in Appendix A, Table A1).

2.2. Material Characterization

A scanning electron microscope (SEM) VEGA 3 TESCAN (SB Easy Probe, Brno, Czech Republic) was used to obtain the surface morphology of the fabricated nanofibers. Prior to scanning, the samples were sputter coated with 10 nm of gold using QUORUM Q50ES (Quorum technologies, Lewes, UK). The fiber diameters were assessed by the software IMAGE J (NIH Image, Bethesda, MD, USA) by randomly measuring 500 fibers in the scans. The specific weight was calculated by weighing of samples in the dimension 10 × 10 cm ($n = 10$).

Sterilization and in vitro biocompatibility tests: Before in vitro testing, the materials were sterilized via low temperature ethylene oxide (Anprolene, Andersen Sterilizers, Haw River, NC, USA) according to the Czech norm CSN EN ISO 11135-1. The materials were tested one week after sterilization to eliminate the effect of ethylene oxide residues in the layers. The PCL scaffolds were seeded with 3T3 mouse fibroblasts (ATCC, Manassas, VA, USA) in a concentration 7×10^3 cells per well. Metabolic activity was evaluated after 3, 7, 14 and 21 days via colorimetric Cell Counting Kit-8 (CCK-8) (Dojindo Laboratories, Rockville, MD, USA). During the CCK-8 assay, the scaffolds were incubated with 10% (*v/v*) of CCK-8 solution in full DMEM media for 3 h at 37 °C, 5% CO_2. Absorbance was measured at 450 nm ($n = 5$). The morphology of the cells on the PCL materials was also monitored. Fluorescence imaging was performed with Nikon Eclipse-Ti-E (Nikon Imaging, Prague, Czech Republic) on fixed cells with 2.5% *v/v* glutaraldehyde (Sigma Aldrich, St. Louis, MI, USA) in PBS by adding DAPI (for cell nuclei visualization) and phalloidin-FITC (for staining actin cytoskeleton) after 3, 7, 14 and 21 days. The MATLAB software (MATLAB Student R2020b, Mathworks, Natick, MA, USA) was used to calculate the number of cells per 1 mm^2 of the scaffold from 10 random fields of view. Dehydrated samples with fixed cells were also scanned via SEM during the same time period to obtain the morphology of the cells.

2.3. Experimental Design

We used 16 Prestice black-pied pigs in two groups; this number was chosen after consultation with a statistician (Supplementary Document S1). The animals were subjected to transection of the descending colon and anastomosis with a standardized defect under general anesthesia (Figure 1).

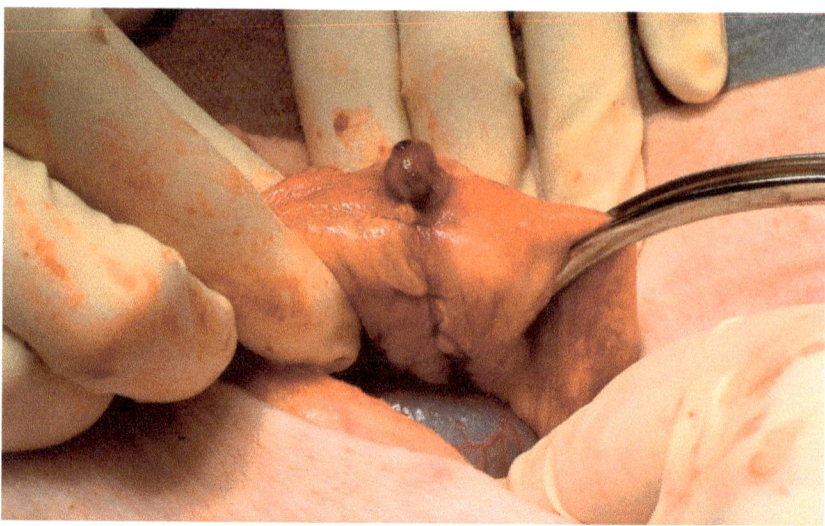

Figure 1. Construction of a defective anastomosis. Intestinal anastomosis with a defect on antimesenteric side pulled through a small incision.

The defect was covered with the nanomaterial in the Experimental group while it was left uncovered in the Control group. The animals were observed for 3 weeks. Sample collection and macroscopic evaluation were performed on the 21st postoperative day (POD). Histological evaluation followed.

2.4. Surgical Procedure

The animals were not fed on the day of the surgery, but no further intestinal preparation was applied. They were premedicated with ketamine (Narkamon 100 mg/mL, BioVeta a.s., Ivanovice na Hané, Czech Republic) and azaperone (Stresnil 40 mg/mL, Elanco AH, Prague, Czech Republic) administered intramuscularly. The animals were weighed prior to the surgical procedure. General anesthesia was maintained by continual application of propofolum MCT/LCT (Propofol 2% MCT/LCT Fresenius Medical Care a.s.). Nalbuphin (Nalbuphin, Torrex Chiesi CZ s.r.o., Prague, Czech Republic) was used for analgesia. A single dose of 0.6 g Amoksiklav (Amoksiklav 1.2 g, Sandoz s.r.o., Prague, Czech Republic) was administered intravenously 30 min before the skin incision, a second 0.6 g dose was administered 2 h later.

A Pro-Port implantable central venous catheter (Deltec, Smiths medical, Minneapolis, MN, USA) was introduced in general anesthesia through the right jugular vein and attached to the subcutaneous tissue on the right lateral side of the neck in each animal for easy and stress-less manipulation with the animal during the follow-up. After the implantation, we entered the abdominal cavity via a 10-cm-long transrectal incision performed in the left caudal abdominal quadrant. We pulled the descending colon up through the incision. We then transected the colon approximately 20 cm from the anus. We used soft intestinal clamps to prevent solid intestinal contents from contaminating the abdominal cavity. We cleaned the two ends of the transected colon using wet cotton balls. We constructed a hand-sewn end-to-end anastomosis using the standard seromuscular running suture using glyconate monofilament 4/0 suture line (Monocryl 4/0, B. Braun Medical s.r.o., Prague, Czech Republic). We intentionally left a 1-cm-large defect on the ventral side of the anastomosis, simulating a technical fault. We placed a standard 2.5-cm-wide sheet of the nanomaterial onto the sutured intestine, covering the intestinal circumference with the defect and the neighboring parts of the mesocolon in the Experimental group. We left the defect uncovered in the Control group. We placed the colon back to the abdominal cavity and sutured the peritoneum with an absorbable material (Vicryl 3/0, Ethicon Inc., Johnson & Johnson, s.r.o., Prague, Czech Republic) to prevent adhesions to the abdominal wall. Then we closed the muscle layer using single non-absorbable sutures (Mersilene 1, Ethicon Inc., Johnson & Johnson, s.r.o., Prague, Czech Republic). We rinsed the subcutaneous tissue with saline solution before finally suturing the skin.

2.5. Postoperative Observation

The animals were observed for 3 weeks and they were checked daily for stool passage, body temperature and clinical signs of complications by both a surgeon and a veterinarian. Activity of the animals was scored using a 4-point scale (normal activity, decreased activity, little to no activity, irritated animal). Intravenous infusions of 250 mL 10% glucose and 250 mL Hartmann solution were applied daily in the first 3 Postoperative days (PODs). The animals were fed according to a re-alimentation schedule created for previous experiments. When feeding intolerance occurred, intravenous infusions were administered in the same way as in the first three PODs. Blood samples were obtained in defined time points (before the surgical procedure, 2 h after construction of colonic anastomosis, on the 1st POD, 3rd POD, 7th POD, 14th POD, 21st POD) and tested for blood count, level of bilirubin, liver enzymes, hemoglobin, urea and creatinine to distinguish metabolic disorders. Animals were weighed each time the blood sample was taken. A 5% weight difference from the initial weight was considered a significant weight change.

2.6. Macroscopic Evaluation

The animals were subjected to laparotomy again on the 21st POD under general anesthesia. The abdominal cavity was inspected and checked for signs of AL (visible free intestinal contents or purulent secretion, macroscopic changes of peritoneal surfaces), visible defects in the site of anastomosis, changes in the intestinal diameter (stenosis of the anastomosis, dilation of oral segments of the intestine) or any other visible postoperative changes. At same time, the extent and location of PAs (according to qualitative Zühlke's grading and quantitative Peritoneal Adhesions Amount Score (PAAS) (Supplementary Figure S2) [26]), amount and macroscopic quality of peritoneal fluid and the position and appearance of the nanofibrous material (if present) were recorded.

The intestinal specimens including the anastomoses were collected together with surrounding adhering tissues, cut on the mesenteric side longitudinally, pinned onto a cork underlay and stored in 10% buffered formalin.

2.7. Histological Evaluation

The intestinal samples were cut into 5 pieces, 5 mm thick, crosswise to the line of the anastomosis in the area of the anastomotic defect. The tissues were processed by common paraffin technique. Each sample was cut to 5 µm slides and stained with hematoxylin and eosin for comprehensive overview; a Gomori trichrom kit was used to stain connective tissues.

The samples were investigated semi-quantitatively and quantitatively. Epithelization, inflammatory infiltration and necrosis were assessed in a single overall semi-quantitative investigation (Intestinal Wall Integrity Score (Appendix B, Table A2)). The inflammatory reaction to stitches and microabscesses were not included in the score. The score was determined for all five blocks, and the three blocks with the highest score (corresponding to the area of the anastomotic defect) were used for statistical evaluation.

The blocks with the highest total score for each pig were subsequently analyzed quantitatively; 5 µm sections were stained with picrosirius red (Direct red 80) for visualization of collagen in polarized light. Immunohistochemical methods were used for detection of the vascular endothelium using Anti-Von Willebrand Factor antibody (Abcam ab6994, dilution 1:400); Calprotectin Monoclonal Antibody MAC387 (Invitrogen MA1-81381, dilution 1:200) was used for detection of granulocytes and tissue macrophages.

The area for quantitative evaluation for samples without visible defect of the muscular layer was defined as the intestinal wall excluding mucosa located 3 mm orally and aborally from the center of the anastomosis. The evaluation area for samples with a defect of the muscular layer or pseudodiverticulum was defined as 2 mm orally and aborally from the defect margins. The volume of endothelial cells, volume of MAC387 positive cells and volume of collagen was assessed using stereological methods in a similar way as in a previous study [26].

2.8. Statistics

Common descriptive statistics and frequencies were used to characterize the sample data set. Due to their non-normal distribution, the intestinal wall integrity scores and histologically determined volume fractions were compared between the Experimental and Control group using Mann–Whitney U test in STATISTICA data analysis software (Version 12, StatSoft, Inc., Tulsa, OK, USA). The material properties, presented as mean ± standard deviation (SD), were analyzed using GraphPad Prism (Version 7, GraphPad Software, San Diego, CA, USA). Firstly, the Shapiro–Wilk test was used to prove or reject the normal distribution of the data. For the normally distributed data, a parametric ANOVA test with Tukey's multiple comparison was performed. The nonparametric Kruskal–Wallis with Dunn's multiple comparison was chosen for the data following non-normal distribution. All reported p values are two-tailed and the level of statistical significance was set at $\alpha = 0.05$.

3. Results

3.1. Material Properties

Sheets of PCL nanofibrous material were successfully prepared and sterilized. The material appeared very subtle yet the manipulation with it was still comfortable. The material was easy to apply onto the intestinal surface and it remained adhered to the spot of application without any need of further fixation. The morphology of the fibrous material was assessed by SEM (Figure 2A). The fibers had no defects and were without any dominant orientation. The fiber diameter was (385 ± 239) nm (Figure 2B). The high SD is a consequence of ultrafine fibers being present together with larger ones. The specific weight of the material was calculated as (9.67 ± 0.77) g/m^2; the data are symmetrical around the mean value (Figure 2C).

3.2. Cytocompatibility

Adhesion, proliferation and morphology of the 3T3 mouse fibroblasts on the PCL scaffolds were monitored with fluorescence microscope and the scanning electron microscope after 3, 7, 14 and 21 days (Figure 3A). The length of the experiment corresponds with the duration of the in vivo study. Cell viability was determined using a colorimetric assay CCK-8 after 3, 7, 14 and 21 days of incubation of 3T3 mouse fibroblasts with the tested fiber layers. The obtained mean absorbance values express the cell viability of the cultured cells (Figure 3B). According to the CCK-8 assay, the absorbance was low during the first testing day, which is in positive correlation with the microscopy observation. On the seventh day of cultivation, an increase in viability was measured. At the same time, spreading of the cells was observable on the microscopy images, as the cells expanded across the material and began to form isolated cell islands. After 14 days of cultivation, there was a further increase in viability and the cells formed a sub-confluent layer. On the last testing day, the SEM image revealed 100% confluence of the cells. The number of the cells (Figure 3C) correlates with the remaining results. The highest cell density was observed during the 14th day (3887 ± 539) cells/mm^2, while on the last testing day it dropped to (2735 ± 880) cells/mm^2.

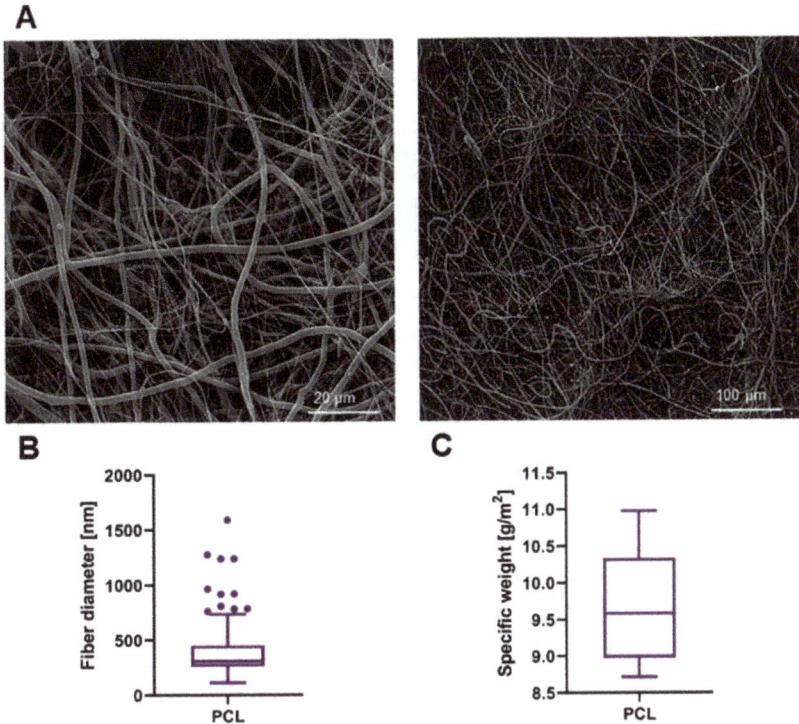

Figure 2. The SEM (scanning electron microscopy) images of the electrospun PCL (polycaprolactone) planar layer, scale bars 20 μm and 50 μm (**A**). The boxplot of fiber diameters (n = 500) (**B**). The calculated value of specific weight of the nanofibrous layer (n = 10) (**C**).

3.3. Manipulation

The material was easy to apply and no further fixation was needed. Procedure times were not prolonged by the usage of the material.

3.4. Clinical Results

All animals survived the observation period in good clinical condition. A temporary activity decrease was observed in one animal from the Control group (12.5%) and in three animals from the Experimental group (37.5%).

There were no major complications during the observation period. Laparotomy wound infection occurred in one animal from the Experimental group (12.5%) and one animal from the Control group (12.5%). Infection of the skin wound of the pro-port system occurred in the same animal from the Control group (12.5%).

No animal developed signs of gastrointestinal obstruction (vomiting, feeding intolerance). No animal developed signs of peritonitis and sepsis (abdominal wall tenderness, significant activity decrease, significant laboratory changes). Peroral intake was tolerated by all animals, all animals were fed according to the schedule with no exceptions. Only three animals from the Control group (37.5%) gained more than 5% of weight during the experiment, while six animals from the Experimental group (75%) showed such weight gain (Appendix C, Table A3).

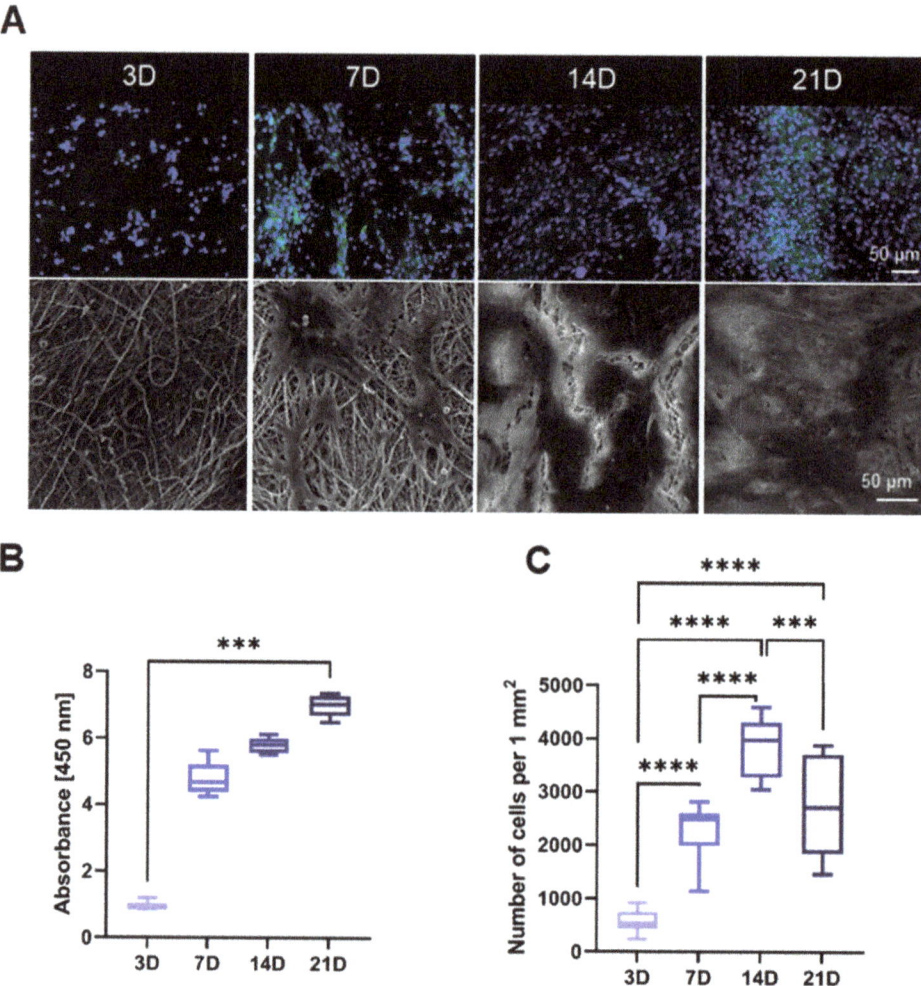

Figure 3. Fluorescence microscopy images (blue cell nuclei and green actin cytoskeleton) and SEM images of the cells on the PCL scaffold after 3, 7, 14 and 21 days of the in vitro testing, scale bars 50 µm (**A**). The result of the colorimetric CCK-8 assay after the same time period, Kruskal–Wallis *** $p = 0.0004$. (**B**). Counted number of the cells on the surface of PCL materials per 1 mm², ordinary one-way ANOVA, *** $p < 0.0006$, **** $p = 0.0001$ (**C**).

3.5. Macroscopic Results

There was no macroscopically visible pathological reactions to the material in the abdominal cavities of the animals after 3 weeks of observation. Four animals (50%) had no PAs at the site of the anastomosis in the Control group, while three animals (37.5%) from the Experimental group had no PAs there. A mean PAAS value of 1 was recorded in both the Control and the Experimental group (Tab). All PAs were scored 2 points according to the Zühlke's grading system in both groups (partially vascularized adhesions, possible to separate by combination of blunt and sharp dissection). Stenosis of the anastomosis was observed in one animal from the Control group (12.5%) with low shrinkage of the intestinal diameter (less than 1/3) (Figure 4A). No stenoses were observed in the Experimental group (Figure 4B). No signs of gastrointestinal obstruction (dilatation of oral segments) were observed in any of the animals. No macroscopic signs of AL were observed (no visible defect in the site of the colonic anastomosis, no free intestinal content in the abdominal cavity).

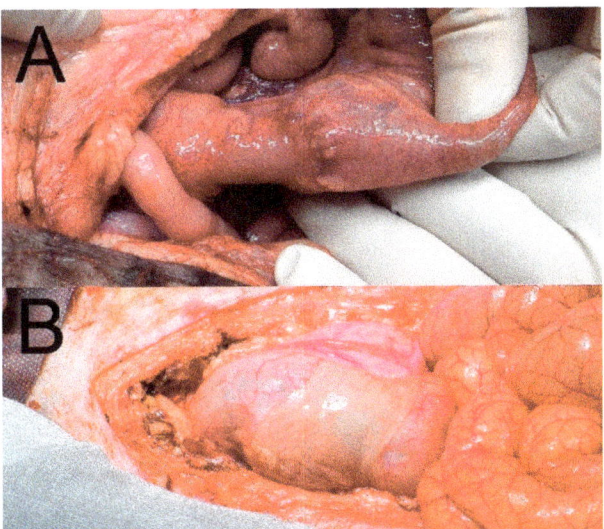

Figure 4. Macroscopic findings in situ at the end of the observation period; (**A**) stenotic anastomosis from the Control group; (**B**) anastomosis with attached material (Experimental group).

Complete dislocation of the material was not observed in any of the animals of the Experimental group. Partial dislocation was observed in three animals (37.5%), however the material always kept covering the location of the anastomotic defect (Figure 5). The defect was not visible in the Control specimens without a patch (Figure 6A). The material was well attached in the most of the specimens (Figure 6B).

Most of the adhesions in the site of the anastomosis were between the large intestine and the urinary bladder. There were no PAs observed in the rest of the abdominal cavity in any animal.

3.6. Blood Sample Results

There were no statistically significant differences in the measured parameters between the two groups and no significant deviations from normal levels of the parameters (see Supplementary Table S1).

3.7. Histological Results

The material was washed out during the histological fixation and staining. There were no microscopic signs of AL (no full-thickness defect was found in any specimen in either the Control or the Experimental group). We found normal morphology of the intestinal wall in all specimens using a comprehensive overview (Figure 7). In some cases, the muscular layer did not heal completely and pseudodiverticula were formed (three cases in the Control group (37.5%) and seven cases (87.5%) in the Experimental group; Figure 8)). There was no statistically significant difference between the groups according to our Intestinal Wall Integrity Score (Figure 9A). There were significantly higher volume fractions of collagen in the Experimental group (Figure 9B). There was no statistically significant difference between the two groups in volume fractions of MAC 387 positive cells (Figure 9D) and endothelial cells (Figure 9C).

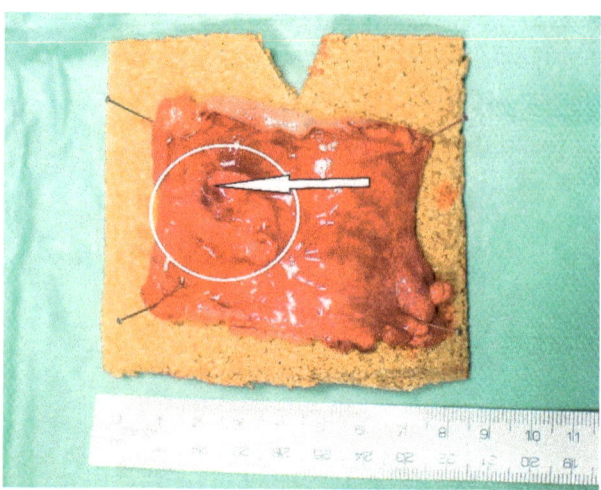

Figure 5. A specimen from the Experimental group prepared for fixation. Partial dislocation of the material (circled), residue of a PA (arrow).

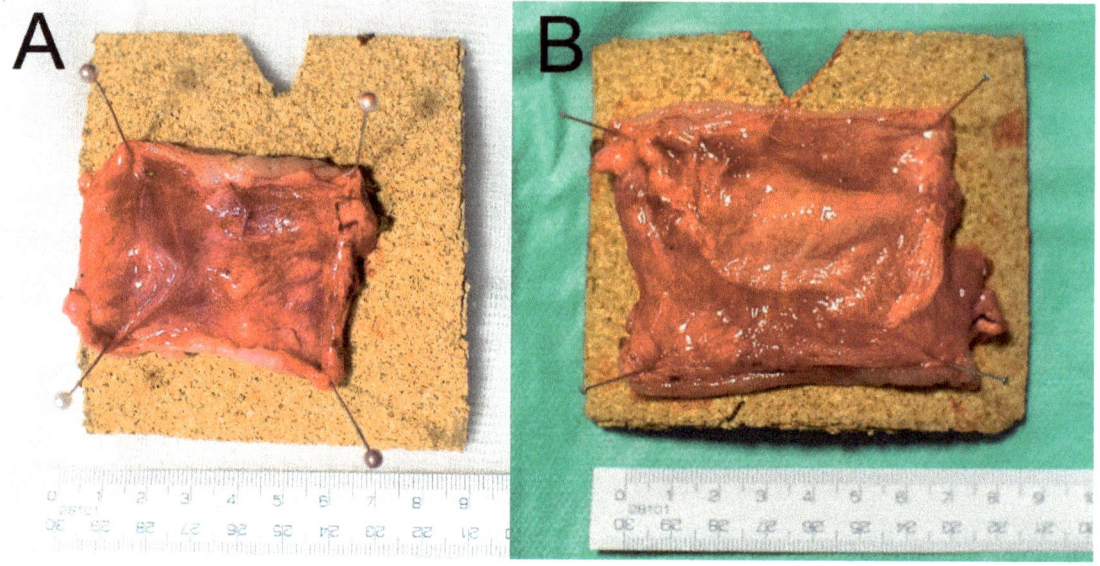

Figure 6. Specimens prepared for fixation. (**A**) A specimen from the Control group; (**B**) a specimen from the Experimental group. The material covers the line of anastomosis well.

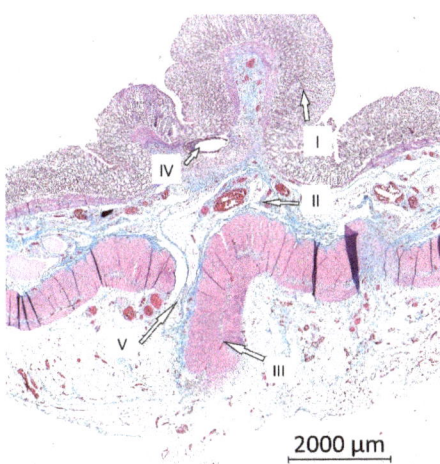

Figure 7. Example histological specimen from the Control group, Gomori trichrome staining. (I) The mucosa; (II) the submucosa; (III) the muscular layer; (IV) a defect after suture material that was washed out during histological processing; (V) location of the anastomosis with normal scar tissue.

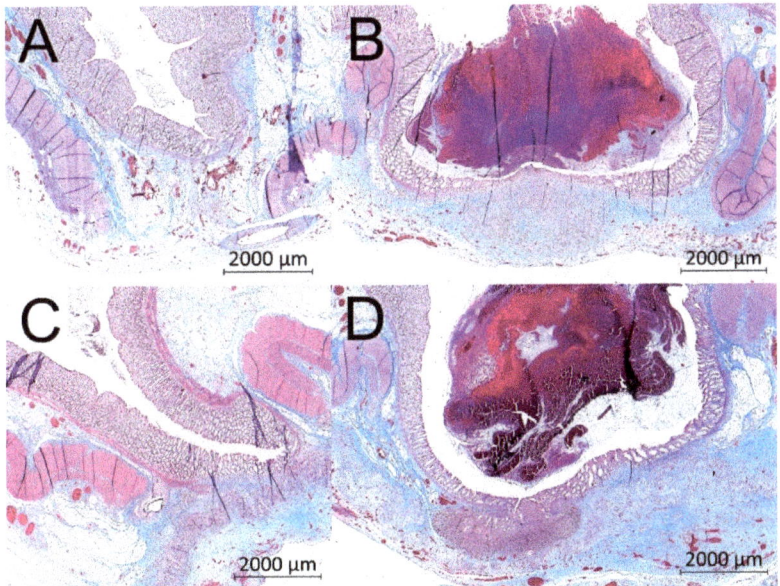

Figure 8. Example histological specimens from both groups. Gomori trichrome (**A**) Control group, optimal healing, normal morphology of the intestinal wall, muscular layer with normal scar tissue; (**B**) Control group, larger defect of the muscular layer, a pseudodiverticulus; (**C**) Experimental group, optimal healing, normal morphology of the intestinal wall, visible residues of the nanofibrous material in the bottom of the image; (**D**) Experimental group, large defect of the muscular layer, a pseudodiverticulus, visible residues of the nanofibrous material in the bottom of the image covering the incomplete defect of the intestinal wall.

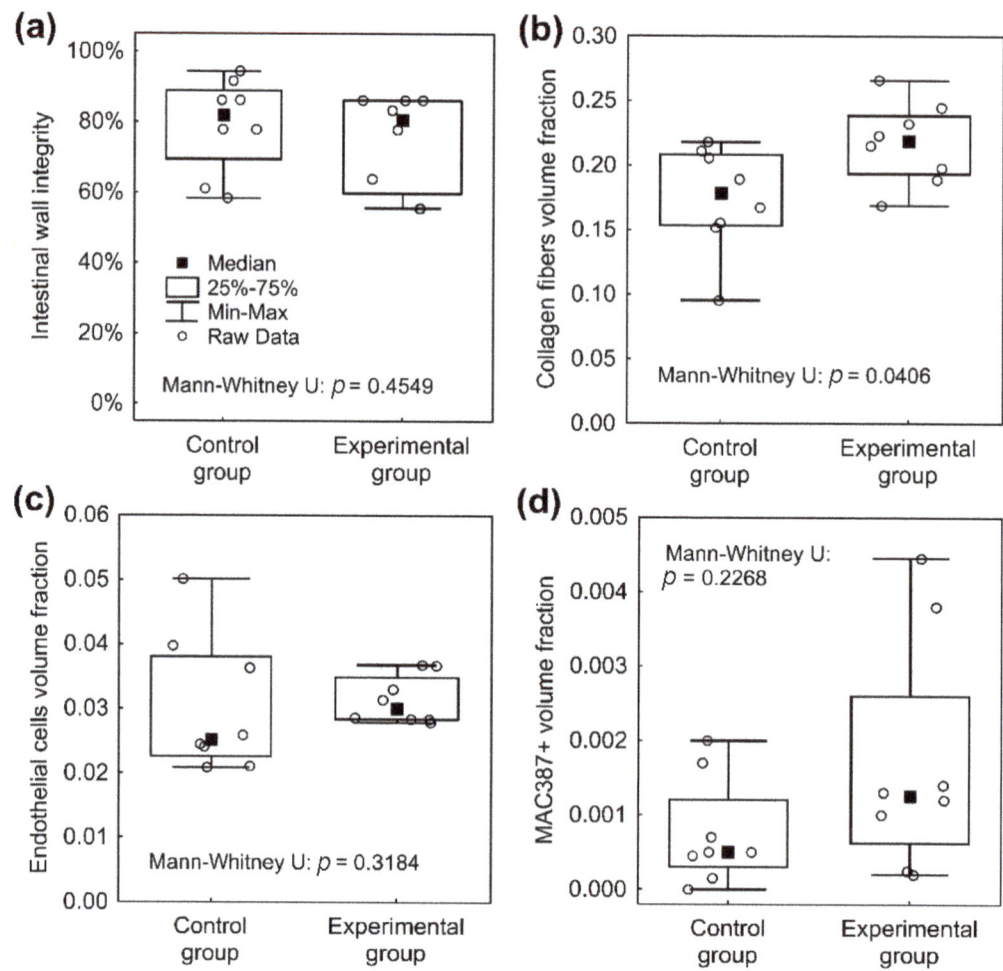

Figure 9. Graphical depiction of main histological results. (**a**) The intestinal wall integrity score in the Control group and the Experimental group with no significant differences with median value above 80%. (**b**) Significantly higher volume fractions of collagen at the site of anastomosis in the Experimental group. (**c**) No significant differences between the two groups in volume fractions of endothelial cells, lower dispersion range of values in the Experimental group. (**d**) The difference in volume fractions of inflammatory cells at the site of anastomosis between the groups is not statistically significant.

4. Discussion

We developed a nanofibrous material based on biodegradable polycaprolactone with very low specific weight. The material was uniquely designed for the reinforcement of GI anastomoses and its design was based on our previous in vitro and in vivo experiments. Polycaprolactone is often used for its biocompatibility and biodegradability [31–33]. The in vitro testing with 3T3 mouse fibroblasts proved the cytocompatibility of the material; the cells formed a fully confluent layer on the surface of the scaffold after 21 days. This observation is consistent with other literature resources, where the combination of micro- and nanofibers in PCL scaffolds supported cell growth [21,22]. Prior to the in vitro testing, the scaffolds were sterilized with low temperature ethylene oxide with respect to the low melting point of PCL. The possible effect of the ethylene oxide sterilization on PCL was already examined in our previous study by Horakova et al. [27]. The PCL patches are easy to apply and we value this as an important property. While the material is very subtle as its specific weight is only 10 g/m^2, it was still mechanically strong enough to be handled easily. The material always remained in the site of application during the surgical procedure and during reposition of the viscera without further fixation. The convenient application together with natural fixation are key properties should this approach be used in routine clinical practice.

We successfully created a model of anastomosis with a defect on the large intestine of a pig. We used the Testini's [16] modified model from previous experiments [26] in order to move the anastomosis to a location with bacterial contamination and higher risk of healing complications. The defect was chosen to be small enough to simulate a technical fault (which is also one of the contributing factors of AL [34]) and large enough to induce imperfect healing. The position of the anastomosis 20 cm from the anus was chosen for its good accessibility, no need for further preparation, possibility of small abdominal wound and therefore low non-anastomosis related complication risk. The model allowed us to focus only on imperfect anastomotic healing with no other disturbing factors. Together with the assessment methodology, the model allowed a reduction in the number of experimental animals and gave what we consider statistically reliable results. A three-week observation period was chosen based on our previous experience and the possibility of using evaluation histologic systems from previous publications. AL is typically an early complication, usually appearing within the first 10 PODs [2,35]. To verify the behavior of the material in a long term period regarding its complete absorption and impact on the risk of late complications, longer observation times would be necessary.

All of the animals in both groups survived the observation period in good clinical shape with a low complication rate. An activity decrease was observed only in the early postoperative period in both groups, which we considered as normal postoperative state. The feeding tolerance was equally good in both groups. The animals from the Experimental group gained weight in more cases than in the Control group. Weight gain is a sign of good postoperative adaption [36]. No animal developed ileus or sepsis or other serious pathological reaction to the material. This contributes to our assumption that it is safe to use in this application.

We observed slight shifting of the material in a few cases, however the material always remained covering the spot of anastomotic defect. We observed this also in the last study on the small intestine with an earlier version of the material, and therefore we assume it is not a coincidence [26]. This barrier was always present even in specimens with larger defect of muscular layer, and no macroscopic or microscopic AL was observed. It remains a question whether the material is able to prevent manifestation of AL. An anastomotic leakage is in experiments usually obtained by either large anastomotic defects or other negative influences (infection, radiation, devascularization). The model of a small defect was chosen to study the impact of the material on imperfect anastomotic healing in highly standardized conditions.

There was one partial shrinkage of the intestinal diameter at the site of the anastomosis in one animal from the Control group (12.5%), therefore we assume the material does not cause formation of anastomotic strictures. Those can however develop in longer time periods and thus a longer observation time would be needed to verify this information [37].

The level of adhesions was similarly low in both groups, suggesting the current material version to be the first in our series of polycaprolactone electrospun materials without pro-adhesive properties [26]. We consider the generally low amount of adhesions to be also a result of short procedure times with low manipulation with tissues [38]. Excessive formation of PAs is considered to be a result of a healing problem [39]. The visceral peritoneum is the superficial layer of the intestine, so wound healing of the peritoneum is a part of anastomotic wound healing. Therefore, we think, qualitative and quantitative assessment of PAs should be involved in the evaluation of anastomotic healing [26].

There were no statistically significant differences in vascularization and inflammatory cells infiltration according to the stereological measurements. This suggests a normal healing process [40]. However, the levels of collagen were found higher in the Experimental group. It was previously observed in mechanical tests of intestinal anastomoses that higher levels of collagen are associated with higher mechanical strength and higher anastomotic bursting pressure [41]. Bacterial collagenases were identified as a possible contributor to development of AL. Their activity causes collagen degradation in the site of intestinal anastomosis. Intestinal colonization with several bacterial species was identified as a strong risk factor of AL due to their production of collagenases [41–43].

We used both traditional evaluation methods [40] with those that were developed for our purposes in previous papers [26]. The intestinal wall integrity score from the previous study was adjusted for a defective model on the large intestine. Together with the rest of the involved assessment methods, it forms the most robust and complex evaluation system of anastomotic healing in similar experiments according to our knowledge and literature search.

The above-mentioned results all suggest possible contribution to AL prevention by our material only indirectly. To obtain more distinguishable results, a model with more compromised anastomotic healing with high risk of AL manifestation would be necessary. This is certainly a limitation of this study.

Because the material was washed out during the histological processing, we cannot evaluate the level of biodegradation. However, this was studied earlier for PCL in other forms [44].

The material seems to be an ideal version for use in combination with active substances like anti-inflammatory drugs, antibacterial agents or antibiotics as an anastomotic patch. Polycaprolactone was identified as a good medium for regulated drug release [33,45]; there is a broad spectrum of active molecules that could be beneficial for either AL prevention or prevention of excessive PA formation [39,46–49]. Therefore, we intend to perfect the material using these substances and to study their impact on anastomotic healing and complications further to finally offer a perfect anastomotic patch for patients with high risk of AL. Possible clinical studies will be planned afterwards.

5. Conclusions

We succeeded in creating a unique ultrafine polycaprolactone electrospun material and in applying it in a model of complicated anastomotic healing on the pig colon. The planar PCL layer was fabricated via needleless electrospinning technique, a method suitable for eventual large-scale production. The material is easy to use without any need for further fixation. The presence of the material did not cause any adverse effects in vivo. The PCL layer showed good cytocompatibility and biocompatibility and was well tolerated during the whole animal study. The material is also not pro-adhesive and did not cause anastomotic strictures or other complications. The anastomotic specimens showed significantly higher levels of collagen after the 3 weeks of observation, which is an indirect sign of higher mechanical strength. Impact on the risk of AL was not observed directly as no AL appeared in either group. We intend to develop new versions of the material with active agents and study them further in adjusted experimental settings to obtain more distinguishable results before moving to clinical studies on colorectal surgical patients.

Supplementary Materials: The following are available online at https://www.mdpi.com/2227-9059/9/2/102/s1, Figure S1: Nanospider scheme, Figure S2: Perianastomotic adhesions amount scoring system, Table S1: Leukocytosis development, Document S1: power analysis.

Author Contributions: Conceptualization, J.R., V.L., J.H.; methodology, M.K., A.K., R.P. (Richard Palek); software, P.H., M.K.; validation, P.H.; formal analysis, L.C.; investigation, L.C., R.P. (Robert Polak); resources, J.H.; data curation P.H.; writing—original draft preparation, J.R., M.K.; writing—review and editing, J.R., P.H.; visualization, J.S.; supervision, V.L., V.T., J.C.; project administration J.H., V.L.; funding acquisition, J.H., V.L. All authors have read and agreed to the published version of the manuscript.

Funding: This research was funded by the project Czech Health Research Council project AZV NU20J-08-00009 Prevention of intestinal anastomotic leakage and postoperative adhesions by using nanofibrous biodegradable materials, and by the Centrum of Clinical and Experimental Liver Surgery project UNCE/MED/006 and from European Regional Development Fund-Project Application of Modern Technologies in Medicine and Industry project CZ.02.1.01/0.0/0.0/17_048/0007280.

Institutional Review Board Statement: Work with animals: All experimental procedures with the use of piglets were certified by the Commission of Work with Experimental Animals at the Medical Faculty of Pilsen (project code: MSMT-26570/2017-2), Charles University, and were under control of the Ministry of Agriculture of the Czech Republic. All procedures were performed in compliance with the law of the Czech Republic, which is compatible with the legislation of the European Union.

Informed Consent Statement: Not applicable.

Data Availability Statement: All data included in the article or supplementary materials.

Conflicts of Interest: The authors declare no conflict of interest. The funders had no role in the design of the study; in the collection, analyses, or interpretation of data; in the writing of the manuscript, or in the decision to publish the results.

Appendix A

Table A1. Process parameters of the needless electrospinning via Nanospider^{TM}.

Distance between the electrodes [mm]	175
Voltage Electrode 1 [kV]	−10
Voltage Electrode 2 [kV]	40
Rewinding speed [mm/min]	60
Cartridge movement speed [mm/s]	450–500
Temperature [°C]	22
Relative humidity [%]	50

Appendix B

Table A2. Intestinal Wall Integrity Score.

Layer	Points	Finding
Mucosa	1/4	Completely re-epithelized
	0/4	Incompletely re-epithelized
Submucosa	1/4	Completely healed
	0/4	Purulent infiltration, necrosis
Muscularis *	3/12	No distance (≤0.09 mm)
	2/12	Distance 0.1 to 1.99 mm
	1/12	Distance 2 to 3.99 mm
	0/12	Distance over 4 mm
Serosa	3/12	No purulent infiltration and necrosis
	2/12	Purulent infiltration and/or necrosis from the muscular layer to area of nanomaterial **
	1/12	Purulent infiltration and/or necrosis from the area of nanomaterial to the peritoneum ***
	0/12	Purulent infiltration and/or necrosis passes to the peritoneum

* Distance between the two anastomosed muscle layers. ** 2/12 points for purulent infiltration and/or necrosis from muscular layer to half thickness of the serosa in the Control group. *** 1/12 points for purulent infiltration and/or necrosis from half thickness of the serosa to the peritoneum in the Control group.

Appendix C

Table A3. Weight profile of experimental animals.

Animal	POD 0 Weight (kg)	POD 3 Weight (kg)	POD 7 Weight (kg)	POD 14 Weight (kg)	POD 21 Weight (kg)
Control group					
cg 01	34	31.6	31.4	33.8	33
cg 02	31	30.1	29.4	30.7	30.7
cg 03	37	33.8	33.7	34.5	34.5
cg 04	45.5	41.3	41.1	42	42.1
cg 05	48.4	43.6	42.8	44	43.8
cg 06	30.6	30	30.7	29.5	32.5
cg 07	30	29	29.8	33.6	32.1
cg 08	27.8	25.9	27.2	30.5	30.5
Experimental group					
eg 01	28.7	28.3	29.2	29.4	29.4
eg 02	29.9	29.3	28.2	29	30.3
eg 03	35.8	35.2	35.2	39	37.9
eg 04	37.3	36.8	36	41	41
eg 05	41.7	41.5	41.3	43.4	45.2
eg 06	42.9	42.2	42.2	43.8	45.1
eg 07	27.9	27.4	26.3	29.4	30
eg 08	27.2	26.8	25.8	29.1	29

References

1. Rahbari, N.N.; Weitz, J.; Hohenberger, W.; Heald, R.J.; Moran, B.; Ulrich, A.; Holm, T.; Wong, W.D.; Tiret, E.; Moriya, Y.; et al. Definition and grading of anastomotic leakage following anterior resection of the rectum: A proposal by the International Study Group of Rectal Cancer. *Surgery* **2010**, *147*, 339–351. [CrossRef] [PubMed]
2. Gessler, B.; Eriksson, O.; Angenete, E. Diagnosis, treatment, and consequences of anastomotic leakage in colorectal surgery. *Int. J. Color. Dis.* **2017**, *32*, 549–556. [CrossRef] [PubMed]
3. Vasiliu, E.C.Z.; Zarnescu, N.O.; Costea, R.; Neagu, S. Review of Risk Factors for Anastomotic Leakage in Colorectal Surgery. *Chirurgia (Buchar. Rom. 1990)* **2015**, *110*, 26305194.
4. Iversen, H.; Ahlberg, M.; Lindqvist, M.; Buchli, C. Changes in Clinical Practice Reduce the Rate of Anastomotic Leakage after Colorectal Resections. *World J. Surg.* **2018**, *42*, 2234–2241. [CrossRef] [PubMed]
5. Kasi, P.M.; Shahjehan, F.; Cochuyt, J.J.; Li, Z.; Colibaseanu, D.T.; Merchea, A. Rising Proportion of Young Individuals with Rectal and Colon Cancer. *Clin. Color. Cancer* **2019**, *18*, e87–e95. [CrossRef] [PubMed]
6. Tsai, Y.-Y.; Chen, W.T.-L. Management of anastomotic leakage after rectal surgery: A review article. *J. Gastrointest. Oncol.* **2019**, *10*, 1229–1237. [CrossRef]
7. Fukada, M.; Matsuhashi, N.; Takahashi, T.; Imai, H.; Tanaka, Y.; Yamaguchi, K.; Yoshida, K. Risk and early predictive factors of anastomotic leakage in laparoscopic low anterior resection for rectal cancer. *World J. Surg. Oncol.* **2019**, *17*, 1–10. [CrossRef]
8. Räsänen, M.; Renkonen-Sinisalo, L.; Carpelan-Holmström, M.; Lepistö, A. Low anterior resection combined with a covering stoma in the treatment of rectal cancer reduces the risk of permanent anastomotic failure. *Int. J. Color. Dis.* **2015**, *30*, 1323–1328. [CrossRef]
9. Van Rooijen, S.; Huisman, D.; Stuijvenberg, M.; Stens, J.; Roumen, R.; Daams, F.; Slooter, G. Intraoperative modifiable risk factors of colorectal anastomotic leakage: Why surgeons and anesthesiologists should act together. *Int. J. Surg.* **2016**, *36*, 183–200. [CrossRef]
10. Sciuto, A.; Merola, G.; De Palma, G.D.; Sodo, M.; Pirozzi, F.; Bracale, U. Predictive factors for anastomotic leakage after laparoscopic colorectal surgery. *World J. Gastroenterol.* **2018**, *24*, 2247–2260. [CrossRef]
11. Kawada, K.; Sakai, Y. Preoperative, intraoperative and postoperative risk factors for anastomotic leakage after laparoscopic low anterior resection with double stapling technique anastomosis. *World J. Gastroenterol.* **2016**, *22*, 5718–5727. [CrossRef] [PubMed]

12. La Regina, D.; Di Giuseppe, M.; Lucchelli, M.; Saporito, A.; Boni, L.; Efthymiou, C.; Cafarotti, S.; Marengo, M.; Mongelli, F. Financial Impact of Anastomotic Leakage in Colorectal Surgery. *J. Gastrointest. Surg.* **2018**, *23*, 580–586. [CrossRef] [PubMed]
13. Lee, S.W.; Gregory, D.; Cool, C.L. Clinical and economic burden of colorectal and bariatric anastomotic leaks. *Surg. Endosc.* **2020**, *34*, 1–8. [CrossRef] [PubMed]
14. Ha, G.W.; Lee, M.R.; Kim, J.H. Adhesive small bowel obstruction after laparoscopic and open colorectal surgery: A systematic review and meta-analysis. *Am. J. Surg.* **2016**, *212*, 527–536. [CrossRef]
15. Trotter, J.; Onos, L.; McNaught, C.; Peter, M.; Gatt, M.; Maude, K.; MacFie, J. The use of a novel adhesive tissue patch as an aid to anastomotic healing. *Ann. R. Coll. Surg. Engl.* **2018**, *100*, 230–234. [CrossRef]
16. Testini, M.; Gurrado, A.; Portincasa, P.; Scacco, S.; Marzullo, A.; Piccinni, G.; Lissidini, G.; Greco, L.; De Salvia, M.A.; Bonfrate, L.; et al. Bovine Pericardium Patch Wrapping Intestinal Anastomosis Improves Healing Process and Prevents Leakage in a Pig Model. *PLoS ONE* **2014**, *9*, e86627. [CrossRef]
17. Yaita, A.; Nakamura, T.; Sugimachi, K.; Inokuchi, K. Use of free peritoneal patch in reenforcing alimentary tract anastomosis. *Surg. Today* **1975**, *5*, 56–63. [CrossRef]
18. Zhong, W.; Xing, M.M.; Maibach, H.I. Nanofibrous materials for wound care. *Cutan. Ocul. Toxicol.* **2010**, *29*, 143–152. [CrossRef]
19. Fu, X.; Gao, W.; Fu, X.; Shi, M.; Xie, W.; Zhang, W.; Zhao, F.; Chen, X. Enhanced wound healing in diabetic rats by nanofibrous scaffolds mimicking the basketweave pattern of collagen fibrils in native skin. *Biomater. Sci.* **2018**, *6*, 340–349. [CrossRef]
20. Adeli, H.; Khorasani, M.T.; Parvazinia, M. Wound dressing based on electrospun PVA/chitosan/starch nanofibrous mats: Fabrication, antibacterial and cytocompatibility evaluation and in vitro healing assay. *Int. J. Biol. Macromol.* **2019**, *122*, 238–254. [CrossRef]
21. Gunatillake, P.A. Biodegradable synthetic polymers for tissue engineering. *Eur. Cells Mater.* **2003**, *5*, 1–16. [CrossRef] [PubMed]
22. Luo, L.; He, Y.; Chang, Q.; Xie, G.; Zhan, W.; Wang, X.; Zhou, T.; Xing, M.; Lu, F. Polycaprolactone nanofibrous mesh reduces foreign body reaction and induces adipose flap expansion in tissue engineering chamber. *Int. J. Nanomed.* **2016**, *11*, 6471–6483. [CrossRef] [PubMed]
23. Townsend, J.M.; Ott, L.M.; Salash, J.R.; Fung, K.-M.; Easley, J.T.; Seim, H.B.; Johnson, J.K.; Weatherly, R.A.; Detamore, M.S. Reinforced Electrospun Polycaprolactone Nanofibers for Tracheal Repair in an In Vivo Ovine Model. *Tissue Eng. Part A* **2018**, *24*, 1301–1308. [CrossRef] [PubMed]
24. Fuchs, J.; Mueller, M.; Daxböck, C.; Stückler, M.; Lang, I.; Leitinger, G.; Bock, E.; El-Heliebi, A.; Moser, G.; Glasmacher, B.; et al. Histological processing of un-/cellularized thermosensitive electrospun scaffolds. *Histochem. Cell Biol.* **2018**, *151*, 343–356. [CrossRef] [PubMed]
25. Vasita, R.; Katti, D.S. Nanofibers and their applications in tissue engineering. *Int. J. Nanomed.* **2006**, *1*, 15–30. [CrossRef] [PubMed]
26. Rosendorf, J.; Horakova, J.; Klicova, M.; Palek, R.; Cervenkova, L.; Kural, T.; Hošek, P.; Kriz, T.; Tegl, V.; Moulisova, V.; et al. Experimental fortification of intestinal anastomoses with nanofibrous materials in a large animal model. *Sci. Rep.* **2020**, *10*, 1–12. [CrossRef] [PubMed]
27. Horakova, J.; Klicova, M.; Erben, J.; Klapstova, A.; Novotny, V.; Behalek, L.; Chvojka, J. Impact of Various Sterilization and Disinfection Techniques on Electrospun Poly-ε-caprolactone. *ACS Omega* **2020**, *5*, 8885–8892. [CrossRef]
28. Childs, D.R.; Murthy, A.S. Overview of Wound Healing and Management. *Surg. Clin. N. Am.* **2017**, *97*, 189–207. [CrossRef]
29. Mehrotra, R.; Devuyst, O.; Davies, S.J.; Johnson, D.W. The Current State of Peritoneal Dialysis. *J. Am. Soc. Nephrol.* **2016**, *27*, 3238–3252. [CrossRef]
30. Giffin, D.M.; Gow, K.W.; Warriner, C.B.; Walley, K.R.; Phang, P.T. Oxygen uptake during peritoneal ventilation in a porcine model of hypoxemia. *Crit. Care Med.* **1998**, *26*, 1564–1568. [CrossRef]
31. Cai, E.Z.; Teo, E.Y.; Jing, L.; Koh, Y.P.; Qian, T.S.; Wen, F.; Lee, J.W.K.; Hing, E.C.H.; Yap, Y.L.; Lee, H.; et al. Bio-Conjugated Polycaprolactone Membranes: A Novel Wound Dressing. *Arch. Plast. Surg.* **2014**, *41*, 638–646. [CrossRef] [PubMed]
32. Hashemi, H.; Asgari, S.; Shahhoseini, S.; Mahbod, M.; Atyabi, F.; Bakhshandeh, H.; Beheshtnejad, A.H. Application of polycaprolactone nanofibers as patch graft in ophthalmology. *Indian J. Ophthalmol.* **2018**, *66*, 225–228.
33. García-Salinas, S.; Evangelopoulos, M.; Gámez-Herrera, E.; Arruebo, M.; Irusta, S.; Taraballi, F.; Mendoza, G.; Tasciotti, E. Electrospun anti-inflammatory patch loaded with essential oils for wound healing. *Int. J. Pharm.* **2020**, *577*, 119067. [CrossRef] [PubMed]
34. Ricciardi, R.; Roberts, P.L.; Marcello, P.W.; Hall, J.F.; Read, T.E.; Schoetz, D.J. Anastomotic Leak Testing After Colorectal Resection. *Arch. Surg.* **2009**, *144*, 407–411. [CrossRef] [PubMed]
35. Bsc, C.L.S.; Van Groningen, J.T.; Lingsma, H.; Wouters, M.W.; Menon, A.G.; Kleinrensink, G.-J.; Jeekel, J.; Lange, J.F. Different Risk Factors for Early and Late Colorectal Anastomotic Leakage in a Nationwide Audit. *Dis. Colon Rectum* **2018**, *61*, 1258–1266. [CrossRef]
36. Marchant-Forde, J.N.; Herskin, M.S. Pigs as laboratory animals. In *Advances in Pig Welfare*; Elsevier: Amsterdam, The Netherlands, 2018; pp. 445–475.
37. Bertocchi, E.; Barugola, G.; Benini, M.; Bocus, P.; Rossini, R.; Ceccaroni, M.; Ruffo, G. Colorectal Anastomotic Stenosis: Lessons Learned after 1643 Colorectal Resections for Deep Infiltrating Endometriosis. *J. Minim. Invasive Gynecol.* **2019**, *26*, 100–104. [CrossRef]
38. Ergul, E.; Korukluoglu, B. Peritoneal adhesions: Facing the enemy. *Int. J. Surg.* **2008**, *6*, 253–260. [CrossRef]

39. Braun, K.M.; Diamond, M.P. The biology of adhesion formation in the peritoneal cavity. *Semin. Pediatr. Surg.* **2014**, *23*, 336–343. [CrossRef]
40. Williams, D.L.; Browder, I.W. Murine Models of Intestinal Anastomoses. In *Wound Healing: Methods and Protocols*, 1st ed.; Di Pietro, L.A., Burns, A.L., Eds.; Humana Press Inc.: Totowa, NJ, USA, 2010; pp. 133–140.
41. Shogan, B.D.; Belogortseva, N.; Luong, P.M.; Zaborin, A.; Lax, S.; Bethel, C.; Ward, M.; Muldoon, J.P.; Singer, M.; Alexander, Z.; et al. Collagen degradation and MMP9 activation byEnterococcus faecaliscontribute to intestinal anastomotic leak. *Sci. Transl. Med.* **2015**, *7*, 286ra68. [CrossRef]
42. Krarup, P.; Eld, M.; Jorgensen, L.; Hansen, M.B.; Ågren, M.S. Selective matrix metalloproteinase inhibition increases breaking strength and reduces anastomotic leakage in experimentally obstructed colon. *Int. J. Color. Dis.* **2017**, *32*, 1277–1284. [CrossRef] [PubMed]
43. Guyton, K.L.; Levine, Z.C.; Lowry, A.C.; Lambert, L.; Gribovskaja-Rupp, I.; Hyman, N.; Zaborina, O.; Alverdy, J.C. Identification of Collagenolytic Bacteria in Human Samples. *Dis. Colon Rectum* **2019**, *62*, 972–979. [CrossRef]
44. Li, Y.; Xia, X.; Zou, Q.; Ma, J.; Jin, S.; Li, J.; Zuo, Y.; Li, Y. The long-term behaviors and differences in bone reconstruction of three polymer-based scaffolds with different degradability. *J. Mater. Chem. B* **2019**, *7*, 7690–7703. [CrossRef]
45. Ranjbar-Mohammadi, M.; Bahrami, S.H. Electrospun curcumin loaded poly(ε-caprolactone)/gum tragacanth nanofibers for biomedical application. *Int. J. Biol. Macromol.* **2016**, *84*, 448–456. [CrossRef]
46. Wirth, U.; Rogers, S.; Haubensak, K.; Schopf, S.; Von Ahnen, T.; Schardey, H.M. Local antibiotic decontamination to prevent anastomotic leakage short-term outcome in rectal cancer surgery. *Int. J. Color. Dis.* **2017**, *33*, 53–60. [CrossRef]
47. Oh, J.; Kuan, K.G.; Tiong, L.U.; Trochsler, M.; Jay, G.; Schmidt, T.A.; Barnett, H.; Maddern, G.J. Recombinant human lubricin for prevention of postoperative intra-abdominal adhesions in a rat model. *J. Surg. Res.* **2017**, *208*, 20–25. [CrossRef]
48. Hirai, K.; Tabata, Y.; Hasegawa, S.; Sakai, Y. Enhanced intestinal anastomotic healing with gelatin hydrogel incorporating basic fibroblast growth factor. *J. Tissue Eng. Regen. Med.* **2016**, *10*, E433–E442. [CrossRef]
49. Landes, L.C.; Drescher, D.; Tagkalos, E.; Grimminger, P.; Thieme, R.; Jansen-Winkeln, B.; Lang, H.; Gockel, I. Upregulation of VEGFR1 in a rat model of esophagogastric anastomotic healing. *Acta Chir. Belg.* **2017**, *118*, 161–166. [CrossRef]

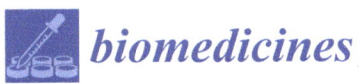

Article

MSH2 Overexpression Due to an Unclassified Variant in 3′-Untranslated Region in a Patient with Colon Cancer

Raffaella Liccardo [1,2], Antonio Nolano [1], Matilde Lambiase [1], Carlo Della Ragione [3], Marina De Rosa [1,2], Paola Izzo [1,2] and Francesca Duraturo [1,2,*]

1. Department of Molecular Medicine and Medical Biotechnology, University Federico II, via Pansini 5, 80131 Naples, Italy; raffaella.liccardo@unina.it (R.L.); nolano@ceinge.unina.it (A.N.); lambiase@ceinge.unina.it (M.L.); marina.derosa@unina.it (M.D.R.); paola.izzo@unina.it (P.I.)
2. CEINGE-BiotecnologieAvanzate, via G. Salvatore 486, 80145 Naples, Italy
3. UOC Pathological Anatomy, Azienda Ospedaliera di Rilievo Nazionale (AORN) "A. Cardarelli", via A. Cardarelli 9, 80131 Naples, Italy; c.dellaragione@hotmail.it
* Correspondence: francesca.duraturo@unina.it; Tel.: +39-0817463136; Fax: +39-0817464359

Received: 13 May 2020; Accepted: 16 June 2020; Published: 19 June 2020

Abstract: Background: The loss or low expression of DNA mismatch repair (MMR) genes can result in genomic instability and tumorigenesis. One such gene, MSH2, is mutated or rearranged in Lynch syndrome (LS), which is characterized by a high risk of tumor development, including colorectal cancer. However, many variants identified in this gene are often defined as variants of uncertain significance (VUS). In this study, we selected a variant in the 3′ untranslated region (UTR) of MSH2 (c*226A > G), identified in three affected members of a LS family and already reported in the literature as a VUS. Methods: The effect of this variant on the activity of the MMR complex was examined using a set of functional assays to evaluate MSH2 expression. Results: We found MSH2 was overexpressed compared to healthy controls, as determined by RTqPCR and Western blot analyses of total RNA and proteins, respectively, extracted from peripheral blood samples. These results were confirmed by luciferase reporter gene assays. Conclusions: We therefore speculated that, in addition to canonical inactivation via a gene mutation, MMR activity may also be modulated by changes in MMR gene expression.

Keywords: MSH2 3′UTR variant; hereditary colon cancer; Lynch syndrome; MSH2 protein; over expression MSH2; MMR gene; MMR complex deficiency; MSH2 unclassified variants

---

1. Introduction

The loss or low expression of MSH2 in particular, but also that of other DNA mismatch repair (MMR) genes, results in genomic instability and a predisposition to cancer [1,2]. It has also been described that the overexpression of *MLH1* and/or *MSH2* induces apoptosis and/or a mutator phenotype with genetic instability [3–5]. At the somatic level, genomic instability is evident, especially in repeated DNA sequences, known as microsatellite sequences. Indeed, microsatellite instability (MSI) is an important molecular marker for the characterization of a mutator phenotype linked to *MMR* genes [6]. A defective MMR system mainly results from mutations in the same *MMR* genes and is the basis of Lynch syndrome (LS). LS is an autosomal dominant condition caused by a defect in one of the *MMR* genes and is characterized by a high lifetime risk of tumor development, especially colorectal cancer (20–70%), endometrial cancer (15–70%), and other extracolonic tumors (15%) [7]. The molecular characterization of LS patients relies on the identification of point mutations and large rearrangements in the coding regions of the *MMR* genes, *MLH1*, *MSH2*, *PMS2*, and *MSH6* [8–13].

The defects are often caused by mutations in the coding regions of *MMR* genes or by the promoter methylation of these genes. However, in many cases, despite the presence of a hypermutable phenotype in a patient, no mutations/hypermethylation of *MMR* genes can be detected [14,15].

It is noteworthy that, in addition to canonical inactivation via gene mutation, MMR activity can also be modulated by changes in *MMR* gene expression [16]. To date, many hypotheses on other causes that determine loss of function in the MMR system have been postulated. Variants in some genetic regions, such as in the 3′ untranslated region (UTR), may impair the binding of putative transcriptional factors or micro (mi)RNA involved in the regulation of gene expression. In this regard, it very interesting to note a study that demonstrated a regulatory mechanism existing between miR-422a and the *MLH1* gene, following the identification of a variant of uncertain significance (VUS) in the 3′ UTR of the *MLH1* gene in a LS patient [17]. Therefore, the functional study of VUS in the 3′UTR of *MMR* genes may allow us to understand the pathogenetic significance of these variants. Here, we report a functional study of a variant identified in the 3′ UTR of *MSH2* (c*226A > G), already described as a variant of uncertain significance in an international database of *MMR* variants (www.insight-database/varints.org). This variant was found in three patients of the same family with a LS-related cancer.

2. Materials and Methods

The Clinical Department of Laboratory Medicine of the hospital affiliated to Federico II University (Naples, Italy) recruited the subjects after receiving authorization from the local ethics committee "Comitato etico per le attività Biomediche Carlo Romano" of the University of Naples, Federico II (protocol no. 120/10, approval November 2010). Once the authorization was obtained, the study received ethical approval, the participants were informed, and written consent was obtained.

The experiments were performed on DNA and on cDNA extracted from peripheral blood lymphocytes.

2.1. DNA Extraction from Patient Samples

Total genomic DNA was extracted from 4 mL peripheral blood lymphocytes collected in EDTA using a BACC2 Nucleon Kit (Amersham Life Science, Buckinghamshire, UK), according to the manufacturer's recommendations, and from formalin-fixed and paraffin-embedded (FFPE) tumor tissues using standard methods. The DNA was precipitated with two volumes of absolute ethanol and the pellet was washed with ethanol at 70% and resuspended in sterilized TE buffer (Tris 10 mM pH7.5-EDTA 1 mM pH8) [9].

2.2. DNA Amplification and Microsatellite Analysis

MSI was tested on paired samples of lymphocyte DNA and in paraffin-embedded tumor tissues of the colon. The MSI status was evaluated with a fluorescent multiplex system comprising five mononucleotide repeats (BAT-25, BAT-26, NR-21, NR-24, Bat40, and TGFβRII), four dinucleotide repeats (D2S123, D18S58, D5S346, and D17S250) and two tetranucleotide repeats (TPOX and TH01) using the CC-MSI kit (AB ANALITICA, Padova, Italy), and subsequent capillary electrophoresis analysis using an ABI 3130 Prism (Applied Biosystems, Fisher Thermo Scientific, Waltham, MA, USA). Tumors were classified as "highly unstable" (MSI-H), if at least 30% of the markers showed instabilities and "with low levels of instability" (MSI-L), if at least 10% of the markers showed instabilities. If no allele difference between the DNA extracted from normal and tumorous tissues was observed, tumors were classified as microsatellite stable (MSS) [9].

2.3. Immunohistochemistry

IHC analysis was performed on a Benchmark XT automatized immunostainer (Ventana Medical Biosystems, Tucson, USA). The primary antibody used was anti-MSH2 mouse monoclonal clone G219–1129. This antibody is supplied by the manufacturer optimally pre-diluted (3.04 µg/mL) to be compatible with VENTANA detection kits (Sigma-Aldrich). The detection system used was an iVIEW DAB Detection Kit (Ventana) based on the streptavidin–biotin-conjugated system. The antigen–positive complexes were detected by the addition of the DAB chromogen (diaminobenzidine) and its substrate (H_2O_2). The samples were finally counterstained with hematoxylin. Nuclear staining was observed using an optical microscope with positivity represented by the presence of brown staining [9]. This positivity was compared with blue nuclear epitopes in which the specific antigen was not present. The internal positive control was represented by lymphocytes, stroma, and functional mucosal crypts, while the negative control was obtained by slides without primary antibody. Strong, moderate, weak, or negative staining is revealed by this method.

2.4. RNA and Protein Analysis

Total RNA was extracted from 4 mL peripheral blood lymphocytes of the patients and from three normal controls using QIAzol reagent, according to the manufacturer's instructions (Qiagen, Hilden, Germany). cDNA was synthesized using 1 µg total RNA, 500 ng random hexamers, and 1 µL SuperScript III reverse transcriptase (Invitrogen Life Technologies, Carlsbad, CA, USA), in the presence of 4 µL 5× RT buffer, 1 µL dithiothreitol (0.1 M), and 1 mM deoxynucleotide triphosphates (Invitrogen Life Technologies, Inc.). The reaction was run on a PCR thermocycler for 50 min at 42 °C in a 20 µL reaction volume, heated to 70 °C for 15 min, and subsequently chilled on ice. Quantitative RNA analysis was performed by RT-PCR on a CFX96 Real-Time System (Bio-Rad-Laboratories, Inc., Hercules, CA, USA). Two forward and reverse primers for *MSH2* cDNA quantification were carried out by amplifying fragments spanning exons 4–5 and 13–14 (primer pair 4F-ACCGGTTGTTGAAAGGCAAA and 5R-TTGATTACCGCAGACAGTGATG; 13F-TGGTGACAGTCAATTGAAAGGA and 14R-CCCATGCTAACCCAAATCCA). A calibration curve to assess the efficiency of the PCR reaction was performed on at least three serial dilutions (1:10) of the reverse-transcriptase products. All primer sets had efficiencies of 100% ± 10%. Each RT-PCR was performed in triplicate in a 20 µL reaction mix containing 12.5 µL of 2× SYBR Green I PCR Master mix (Bio-Rad Laboratories, Inc.), 0.38 µL of a 20 µM primer mix, 2 µL of cDNA (5 ng/µL), and 7.12 µL of nuclease-free water. The cycling conditions consisted of an initial denaturation step at 95 °C for 3 min, followed by 40 cycles (95 °C for 15 s, 62 °C for 30 s, and 82 °C for 20 s) and 80 cycles performed according to the standard protocols for melting curve analysis. The CT values were determined by automated threshold analysis and the data were analyzed with the CFX Manager software version 2.1 (Bio-Rad Laboratories, Inc.). The relative expression of the target transcript was calculated with the comparative Ct method using a cDNA fragment from the glucuronidase (*GUS*) housekeeping gene as a control. The specificity of qPCR products was evaluated by melting curve analysis [9].

Total protein extracts (nuclear and cytosolic proteins) were obtained from the same blood sample used for the RNA isolation of affected patients, using QIAzol reagent (Qiagen) according to the manufacturer's instructions. The evaluation of protein concentration was performed by spectrophotometer analysis at 595 nm according to the Bradford method using the Bio-Rad Protein Assay Reagent (Bio-Rad Laboratories, Inc.). A total of 50 µg of proteins were separated by SDS-polyacrylamide gel electrophoresis and blots were prepared on an Amersham Hybond-ECL nitrocellulose membrane (Amersham Pharmacia Biotech, Inc./GE Healthcare Bio-Sciences Corp., Piscataway, NJ, USA) [18]. Membranes were incubated overnight at 4 °C with primary antibody against MSH2 (1:100, mouse monoclonal anti-human, clone GB12; Calbiochem, EMD Chemicals, Inc., Merck KGaA, Darmstadt, Germany) and subsequently normalized with anti-actin antibody (1:1000, rabbit polyclonal anti-human; clone sc-1615; Santa Cruz Biotechnology, Inc., USA). The antigen–antibody complexes were visualized with the ECL-Immobilon chemiluminescence reagents (Millipore, Life Science of Merck KGaA, Darmstadt, Germany) and subsequent autoradiography. Western blotting bands were quantified by ImageJ software.

2.5. Luciferase Constructs and Reporter Assay

The *MSH2* 3′ UTR of one of the three heterozygous carriers of the mutation, c.*226 A > G, was amplified by PCR with a primer pair containing *XhoI* and *NotI* restriction sites. Oligonucleotide sequences were as follows: *XhoI*-3′ UTR *MSH2* forward: ATACTCGAGAAAATCCCAGTAATGGAATG and *NotI*-3′ UTR *MSH2* reverse: ATAGCGGCCGCTTCAAATTCCACAAACTACA. The PCR product was cloned into the PSICHECK2 vector (Promega, Madison, WI, USA) downstream of the *Renilla* luciferase coding region (hRluc). The orientation of the wild type (WT) and mutated (MUT) inserted products was established by digestion and confirmed by sequencing. The PSICHECK2 constructs with additional mutations in the *MSH2* 3′ UTR region were generated using the QuiKChange Mutagenesis kit (Agilent Technologies, Santa Clara, CA, USA). Oligonucleotide sequences for site-directed mutagenesis were as follows: 3′UTR *MSH2* MUT1 forward, GGACTGTTTGCAATTGACATAGGTACTgATAAGTGATGTGCTG and reverse, CAGCACATCACTTATcAGTACCTATGTCAATTGCAAACAGTCC; 3′UTR *MSH2* MUT2 forward, GGACTGTTTGCAATTGACATAGGTCCGgATAAGTGATGTGCTG, and reverse, CAGCACATCACTTATcCGGACCTATGTCAATTGCAAACAGTCC (patient mutated base is in lowercase, and additional mutated bases are in bold). Luciferase activity was measured at 48 h after transfection using a dual luciferase reporter assay (Promega) according to the manufacturer's instructions and performed on a 20n/20n luminometer (Turner BioSystems, Sunnyvale, CA, USA). Relative luciferase activity was calculated by normalizing the *Renilla* luminescence to the firefly luminescence [19].

2.6. Statistical Analysis

Data from real-time quantitative PCR, Western blot analysis, and luciferase assays were analyzed using GraphPad Prism 6.0 software (GraphPad Software, Inc.). The mean values (± S.D.) were calculated. Statistical significance was determined using Student's t test or one-way analysis of variance (ANOVA). Data were considered statistically significant when p-values were ≤ 0.05

3. Results

3.1. Selected Patients

Three patients of a LS family were selected for this study. These patients were carriers of the variant c*226A > G in the 3′ UTR of *MSH2*. All patients were negative for pathogenic point mutations in the *MMR* genes (*MSH2*, *MSH6*, *MLH1* and *PMS2*) and no large rearrangements in these genes were identified.

The index case of the family was a man who had developed a sigma degenerated polyp with severe dysplasia and in situ adenocarcinoma at the age of 38 years. The mother developed a nose basal cell carcinoma at the age of 50 years, two colon mildly dysplastic tubular adenomas at the age of 69 years, and endometrial atrophy at the age of 72 years. The sister developed Hodgkin lymphoma at the age of 21 years, as shown in Figure 1. The three control subjects were used in this experimental study. The patients and the controls were of Caucasian origin and were from the Campania geographic region (Southern Italy).

In our laboratory, this variant has also been identified in another patient who developed a grade 3 (G3) endometrial cancer at 49 years of age, and who also had a familial cancer history.

3.2. Microsatellite and Immunohistochemistry Analysis

The Microsatellite analysis (MSI) was performed on two patients, the index case and his mother, respectively. The MSI-Low status was found, two dinucleotide repeats (D5S346 and D18S58) were unstable in both patients, on the sigma tissue of the index case and on the endometrial tissue of his mother. Moreover, the immunohistochemistry analysis (IHC) of the paraffin-embedded tissue stions of the two above patients revealed a strong intensity of MSH2 staining, as shown in Figure 2.

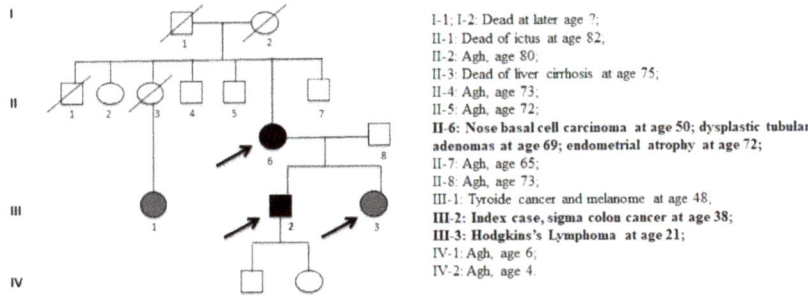

Figure 1. Pedigree with the segregation of the c.*226A > G variant. Symbols and abbreviations used are denoted as fellow: arrows, analysed members of family; black symbol, colorectal cancer or cancer associated with HNPCC; gray symbols, adenomas or cancer not associated with HNPCC. Numbers next to symbols denote age at onset; the phenotype patients are reported next to pedigree. Agh, apparent good health.

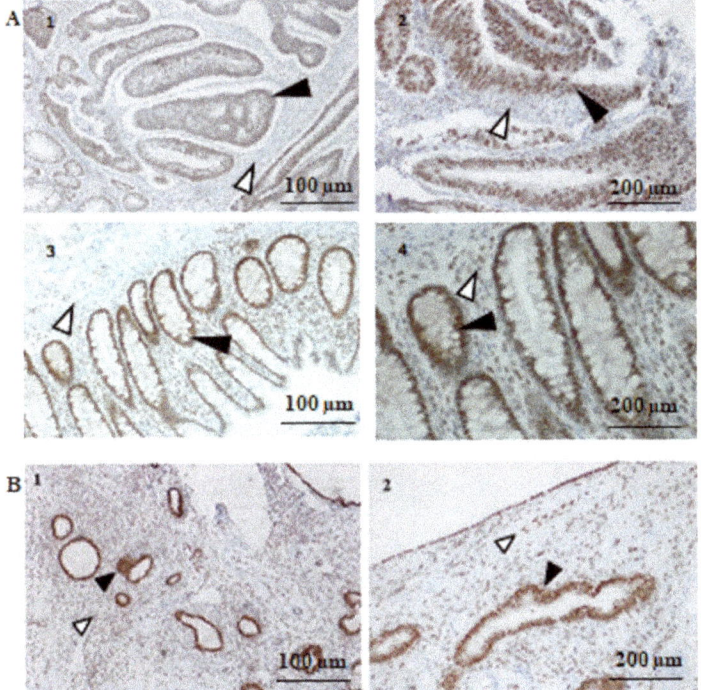

Figure 2. MSH2 immunohistochemistry (IHC) analysis. (**A**) MSH2 IHC results in index patient III-2. (1) Moderate positive IHC in the colon tumor cells (filled arrow heads point) 100 µm and (2) 200 µm; (3) strong positive IHC in the normal mucosa cells (filled arrow head point) of the patient 100 µm and (4) 200 µm, compared with IHC+ internal stromal cells (open arrow head point). (**B**) MSH2 IHC results in patient II-6. (1) Strong positive staining in the endometrial atrophic polyp cells (filled arrow head point) 100 µm and (2) 200 µm, compared with IHC+ internal stromal cells (open arrow head point).

3.3. Overexpression of MSH2 Gene and Overexpression of MSH2 Protein

To explore the possibility of *MSH2* overexpression, we performed an expression assay by RT-qPCR analysis on mRNA extracted from the peripheral blood lymphocytes of these three patients. This analysis showed an increased level of *MSH2* mRNA expression in all three patients with the variant c.*226A > G, as shown in Figure 3. Then, subsequently we performed the Western blot analysis of proteins isolated from the lymphocytes of one (III-2 index-case) of these three patients. This analysis showed an increased level of MSH2 in our patient compared with the negative control, in accordance with the real-time data, as shown in Figure 4.

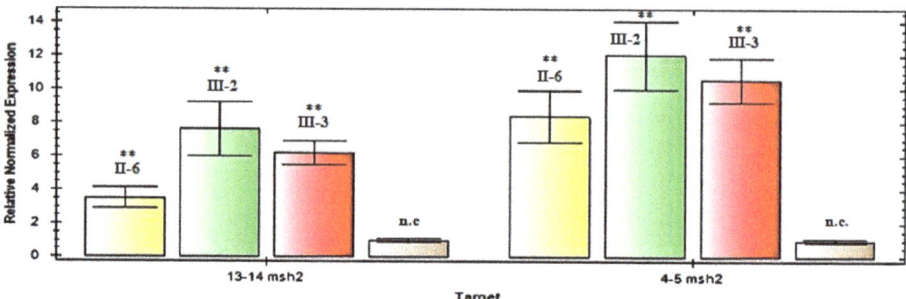

Figure 3. q-Real-Time PCR analysis of the *MSH2* mRNA in the patients with the c.*226A > G variant. Relative expression, calculated using the comparative Ct method, of *MSH2* cDNA, including fragments 13–14 and 4–5, normalized to β-glucuronidase levels, in patients II-6, II-2, III-3 and in an average of three normal controls (n.c.). The results represent the average of three independent experiments ± standard deviation. Patient numbering corresponds to that adopted in the pedigree, as shown in Figure 1. ** Statistical significance was determined by one-way ANOVA (p-values were < 0.05).

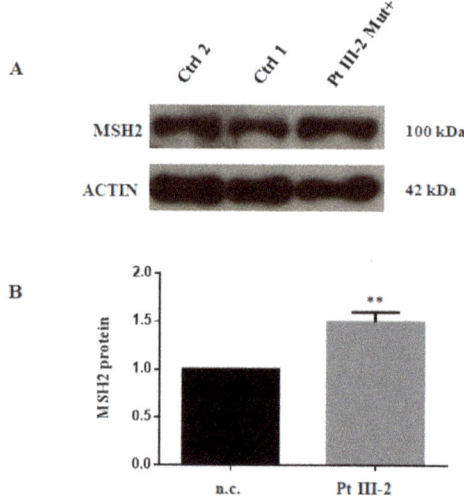

Figure 4. Patient protein analysis. (**A**) Western blot assay of MSH2 performed on protein extracts from peripheral blood cells of index-patient III-2 compared to two normal controls. Actin was used as internal positive reference. (**B**) Histogram showing density of MSH2 protein normalized versus actin protein and compared to the mean of two negative controls, controls 1 and 2 (n.c.). Density of the electrophoretic bands was obtained with ImageJ software. Data represent three independent experiments (mean ± SD). ** Statistical significance was determined by one-way ANOVA (p-values were < 0.05).

3.4. Functional Effect of the MSH2 3' UTR Variant on Reporter Luciferase Expression

To confirm whether the variant c.*226A > G altered the expression of upstream coding sequences, the wild type (WT) and 3' UTR variant were cloned downstream of the *Renilla* luciferase reporter gene, as shown in Figure 5A,B. To further investigate the correlation between *MSH2* expression and the variant region, additional substitutions in this target site were generated as reported in materials and methods and shown in Figure 5A. The reporter gene constructs were transfected into SW480 cells, and the cells were collected for luciferase assay and quantitative mRNA analysis 48 h later. The results showed that the construct bearing the 3' UTR variant consistently induced higher luciferase activity than the construct with the WT 3' UTR, as shown in Figure 5C, according to the patient data of *MSH2* expression. Moreover, greater luciferase expression was observed in proportion to the number of additional mutations, as shown in Figure 5C.

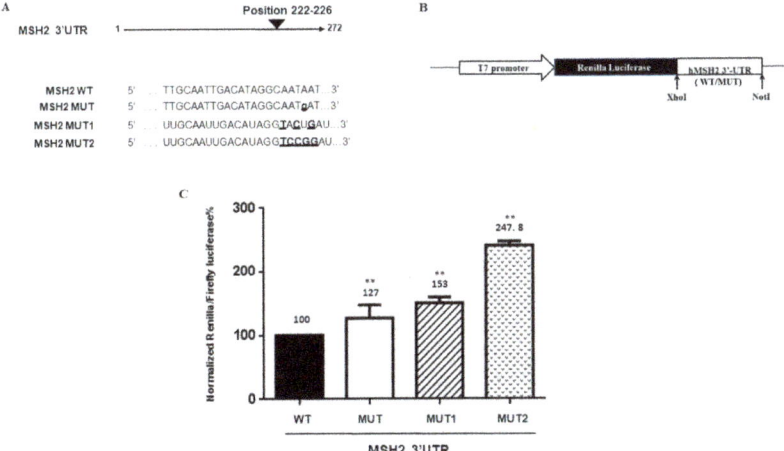

Figure 5. Luciferase *MSH2* 3'UTR constructs and reporter assay. (**A**) Sequences of wild type and mutant in the 3'UTR of *MSH2* of reporter constructs are shown. The mutated bases are underlined. (**B**) Schematic diagram of the luciferase reporter gene constructs. The constructs were cloned into the PSICHECK2 vector as indicated in Materials and Methods. (**C**) Luciferase activities of reporters carrying the wild type (WT) and mutated (MUT, MUT1, MUT2) MSH2 3'UTR were measured in SW480 cells. The data were normalized to the Firefly luciferase activity. Values are expressed in percentage as the mean ±SD of five determinations for samples assayed in three independent experiments. ** Statistical significance was determined by one-way ANOVA (p-value < 0.005).

4. Discussion

The study of a heterozygous single base substitution in the *MSH2* 3' UTR, namely c*226A > G identified in a LS family, allowed us to reach some interesting conclusions. This variant was identified in three affected patients with LS-related cancer. Point variants in other *MMR* genes (*MLH1*, *MSH6*, *PMS2*, *MLH3*, and *MSH3*) [8–10,20], and large rearrangements in these genes (*MLH1*, *MSH2*, *MSH6*, and *PMS2*) [11,12,21] were not identified in these patients. MSI analysis revealed instability in two dinucleotide repeats, D5S346 and D18S58 (of which only one repeat is of the Bethesda panel), and then a MSI-Low status. This apparent low instability may be attributed to selected tissue stions in which the tumor component was rather low. Therefore, the revealed instability may have been underestimated by the limits of the technique, even more if we consider that endometrial tissue is not a tumoral tissue. In addition, the MSI result is also compatible with the results of immunohistochemical analysis. In fact, IHC analysis on these same tissues revealed a normal expression of the MSH2 protein or even a likely MSH2 overexpression.

Therefore, we speculated that this likely MSH2 overexpression may be present at the germline level. To investigate this, we performed gene expression analysis on mRNA from peripheral blood by RTqPCR and by Western blotting for proteins. Both experimental procedures showed increased *MSH2* gene and protein levels. Finally, we confirmed these results by functional luciferase assays in vitro.

For a long time, it was known that the overexpression of *MLH1* and *MSH2* leads to potentially adverse consequences: apoptosis was induced in a human cell line when these two genes were upregulated in vitro under the control of the cytomegalovirus promoter. One possible explanation is the capture, by MLH1 and MSH2, of proteins crucial for cell-cycle progression, such as proliferating the cell nuclear antigen protein, which is involved in DNA synthesis [3]. Several reports suggest that cellular levels of MMR proteins are likely to be subject to tight regulation to prevent these proteins from sequestering other factors involved in controlling the mutation rate [3,5]. Moreover, a dangerous excess of MMR proteins can also affect the homodimerization complex, as found in a study of yeast cells by Shcherbakova et al. [5], who demonstrated that a MLH1–MLH1 homodimer replaced a MLH1/PMS1/PMS2/MLH3 heterodimer, inactivating MutSα and MutSβ functions and thus resulting in a non-functional MMR complex. This concept can also be partially extended to other minor MMR genes. The overexpression of MSH3 in cultured mammalian cells selectively inactivates MutSα because MSH2 is sequestered in the MSH2–MSH3 (MutSβ) complex, resulting in the reduced MutSα-dependent repair of base–base mismatches and a strong base substitution mutator phenotype [22]. For this reason, we plan to test the effect of this variant to alter the formation of the MutSα or MutSβ heterodimers, in the near future. Finally, elevated levels of MSH2 and MSH6 have been detected in primary melanomas with poor prognosis [23–25].

Therefore, *MSH2* overexpression may determine a MMR system deficiency, with a functional loss of the MSH2 protein.

Interestingly, this variant has also been identified in another our patients, as reported in the results stion. MSI analysis for this patient showed a MSI-high status on endometrial cancer tissue (G3). This reveals a MMR complex deficiency in this patient that could be due to this c.*226A > G variant in the 3'-UTR of the *MSH2* gene. Unfortunately, we could not confirm this result by IHC analysis.

Many hypotheses about other causes that determine loss of function in the MMR system have been postulated, such as miRNAs that can strongly influence the repair function of the MMR complex, with consequent effects on disease progression [26–31]. Thus, this overexpression effect may be related to a loss of *MSH2* downregulation, caused by a loss of base pairing with this *MSH2* 3'-untranslated region by transcription factors or miRNA. For example, the presence of single nucleotide substitutions in miRNA target sites can create or abolish miRNA interactions with their molecular targets and, therefore, determine variations in the expression of a gene [17,32]. In silico analysis of the 3' UTR of MSH2 reveals a putative binding site for hsa-miR-137 right in the region in which the variant c.*226A > G falls.

In this regard, the greater luciferase expression observed in our study, even in proportion to the number of additional mutations created in this region, allows us to speculate that this region, in which the variant c.226A > G* falls, may prevent binding with regulatory factors, as well as with the miRNA-137. A loss of regulation of the *MSH2* transcript would explain the observed overexpression, which does not enhance genomic stability but promotes hypermutability [33–35].

Author Contributions: Conceptualization, P.I. and F.D.; Data curation, F.D.; Formal analysis, R.L. and F.D.; Funding acquisition, P.I. and F.D.; Investigation, F.D.; Methodology, R.L., A.N., M.L., C.D.R., and F.D.; Project administration, P.I. and F.D.; Resources, F.D.; Software, R.L. and F.D.; Supervision, P.I. and F.D.; Validation, C.D.R. and F.D.; Visualization, F.D.; Writing—original draft, F.D.; Writing— Review and editing, R.L., M.D.R., P. I., and F.D. All authors have read and agreed to the published version of the manuscript.

Funding: This study was supported by "Fondo Ateneo-Duraturo Federico II, 2018".

Acknowledgments: CEINGE-Biotecnologie Avanzate SCarl, Naples, Italy.

Conflicts of Interest: The authors declare no conflict of interest.

References

1. Jiricny, J. The multifaceted mismatch-repair system. *Nat. Rev. Mol. Cell Biol.* **2006**, *5*, 335–346. [CrossRef] [PubMed]
2. Schmidt, M.H.; Pearson, C.E. Disease-associated repeat instability and mismatch repair. *DNA Repair* **2016**, *38*, 117–126. [CrossRef] [PubMed]
3. Zhang, H.; Richards, B. Apoptosis induced by overexpression of hMSH2 or hMLH1. *Cancer Res.* **1999**, *59*, 3021–3027. [PubMed]
4. Frosina, G. Overexpression of enzymes that repair endogenous damage to DNA. *Eur. J. Biochem.* **2000**, *267*, 2135–2149. [CrossRef] [PubMed]
5. Shcherbakova, P.V.; Hall, M.C. Inactivation of DNA mismatch repair by increased expression of yeast MLH1. *Mol. Cell Biol.* **2001**, *21*, 940–951. [CrossRef]
6. Boland, C.R.; Thibodeau, S.N. A National Cancer Institute Workshop on Microsatellite Instability for cancer detection and familial predisposition: Development of international criteria for the determination of microsatellite instability in colorectal cancer. *Cancer Res.* **1998**, *58*, 5248–5257.
7. Duraturo, F.; Liccardo, R. Genetics, diagnosis and treatment of Lynch syndrome: Old lessons and current challenges. *Oncol. Lett.* **2019**, *17*, 3048–3054. [CrossRef]
8. Liccardo, R.; Ragione, D.C. Novel variants of unknown significance in the PMS2 gene identified in patients with hereditary colon cancer. *Cancer Manag. Res.* **2019**, *11*, 6719–6725. [CrossRef]
9. Duraturo, F.; Liccardo, R. Multivariate analysis as a method for evaluating the pathogenicity of novel genetic MLH1 variants in patients with colorectal cancer and microsatellite instability. *Int. J. Mol. Med.* **2015**, *36*, 511–517. [CrossRef]
10. Liccardo, R.; De Rosa, M. Incomplete Segregation of MSH6 Frameshift Variants with Phenotype of Lynch Syndrome. *Int. J. Mol. Sci.* **2017**, *18*, 999. [CrossRef]
11. Duraturo, F.; Cavallo, A. Contribution of large genomic rearrangements in Italian Lynch syndrome patients: Characterization of a novel alu-mediated deletion. *Biomed. Res. Int.* **2013**, *2013*, 219897. [CrossRef] [PubMed]
12. Liccardo, R.; De Rosa, M. Characterization of novel, large duplications in the MSH2 gene of three unrelated Lynch syndrome patients. *Cancer Genet.* **2018**, *221*, 19–24. [CrossRef]
13. Kašubová, I.; Holubeková, V. Next Generation Sequencing in Molecular Diagnosis of Lynch Syndrome—A Pilot Study Using New Stratification Criteria. *Acta Medica (Hradec Kralove)* **2018**, *61*, 98–102. [CrossRef] [PubMed]
14. Xicola, R.M.; Clark, J.R. Implication of DNA repair genes in Lynch-like syndrome. *Fam. Cancer.* **2019**, *18*, 331–342. [CrossRef] [PubMed]
15. Liccardo, R.; De Rosa, M. Novel Implications in Molecular Diagnosis of Lynch Syndrome. Gastroenterol. *Res. Pract.* **2017**, *2017*, 2595098.
16. Wong, S.; Hui, P. Frequent loss of mutation-specific mismatch repair protein expression in nonneoplastic endometrium of Lynch syndrome patients. *Mod. Pathol.* **2020**, *33*, 1172–1181. [CrossRef]
17. Mao, G.; Pan, X. Evidence that a mutation in the MLH1 3′-untranslated region confers a mutator phenotype and mismatch repair deficiency in patients with relapsed leukemia. *J. Biol. Chem.* **2008**, *283*, 3211–3216. [CrossRef]
18. Caggiano, R.; Cattaneo, F. miR-128 Is Implicated in Stress Responses by Targeting MAFG in Skeletal Muscle Cells. *Oxidative Med. Cell. Longev.* **2017**. [CrossRef]
19. Turano, M.; Costabile, V. Characterisation of mesenchymal colon tumour-derived cells in tumourspheres as a model for colorectal cancer progression. *Int. J. Oncol.* **2018**, *53*, 2379–2396. [CrossRef]
20. Duraturo, F.; Liccardo, R. Coexistence of MLH3 germline variants in colon cancer patients belonging to families with Lynch syndrome-associated brain tumors. *J. Neuro-Oncol.* **2016**, *129*, 577–578. [CrossRef]
21. Lo Monte, A.I.; Cudia, B.; Liccardo, R.; Izzo, P.; Duraturo, F. Involvement of large rearrangements in MSH6 and PMS2 genes in southern Italian patients with Lynch syndrome. *Eur. J. Oncol.* **2018**, *23*, 47–51.
22. Marra, G.; Iaccarino, I. Mismatch repair deficiency associated with overexpression of the MSH3 gene. *Proc. Natl. Acad. Sci. USA* **1998**, *95*, 8568–8573. [CrossRef] [PubMed]
23. Winnepenninckx, V.; Lazar, V. Melanoma Group of the European Organization for Research and Treatment of Cancer. Gene expression profiling of primary cutaneous melanoma and clinical outcome. *J. Natl. Cancer Inst.* **2006**, *98*, 472–482. [CrossRef] [PubMed]

24. Kauffmann, A.; Rosselli, F. High expression of DNA repair pathways is associated with metastasis in melanoma patients. *Oncogene* **2008**, *27*, 565–573. [CrossRef]
25. Alvino, E.; Passarelli, F. High expression of the mismatch repair protein MSH6 is associated with poor patient survival in melanoma. *Am. J. Clin. Pathol.* **2014**, *142*, 121–132. [CrossRef]
26. Cummins, J.M.; He, Y. The colorectal microRNAome. *Proc. Natl. Acad. Sci. USA* **2006**, *103*, 3687–3692. [CrossRef]
27. Landau, D.A.; Frank, J.S. MicroRNAs in Mutagenesis, Genomic Instability and DNA Repair. *Semin. Oncol.* **2011**, *38*, 743–751. [CrossRef]
28. Bartel, D.P. MicroRNAs: Target recognition and regulatory functions. *Cell* **2009**, *136*, 215–233. [CrossRef]
29. Fabian, M.R.; Sonenberg, N. Regulation of mRNA translation and stability by microRNAs. *Annu. Rev. Biochem.* **2010**, *79*, 351–379. [CrossRef]
30. Valeri, N.; Gasparini, P. MicroRNA-21 induces resistance to 5-fluorouracil by down-regulating human DNA MutS homolog 2 (hMSH2). *Proc. Natl. Acad. Sci. USA* **2010**, *107*, 21098–21103. [CrossRef]
31. Svrcek, M.; El-Murr, N. Overexpression of microRNAs-155 and 21 targeting mismatch repair proteins in inflammatory bowel diseases. *Carcinogenesis* **2013**, *34*, 828–834. [CrossRef] [PubMed]
32. Mao, G.; Lee, S. Modulation of microRNA processing by mismatch repair protein MutLα. *Cell Res.* **2012**, *22*, 973–985. [CrossRef] [PubMed]
33. Sarasin, A.; Kauffmann, A. Overexpression of DNA repair genes is associated with metastasis: A new hypothesis. *Mutat. Res.* **2008**, *659*, 49–55. [CrossRef] [PubMed]
34. Wilczak, W.; Rashed, S. Up-regulation of mismatch repair genes MSH6, PMS2 and MLH1 parallels development of genetic instability and is linked to tumor aggressiveness and early PSA recurrence in prostate cancer. *Carcinogenesis* **2017**, *38*, 19–27. [CrossRef]
35. Chakraborty, U.; Dinh, T.A. Genomic Instability Promoted by Overexpression of Mismatch Repair Factors in Yeast: A Model for Understanding Cancer Progression. *Genetics* **2018**, *209*, 439–456. [CrossRef] [PubMed]

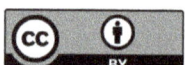 © 2020 by the authors. Licensee MDPI, Basel, Switzerland. This article is an open access article distributed under the terms and conditions of the Creative Commons Attribution (CC BY) license (http://creativecommons.org/licenses/by/4.0/).

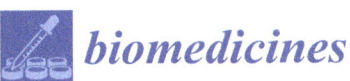

Article

Establishment of a Patient-Derived Xenograft Model of Colorectal Cancer in CIEA NOG Mice and Exploring Smartfish Liquid Diet as a Source of Omega-3 Fatty Acids

Helle Samdal [1,2], Lene C Olsen [2,3], Knut S Grøn [2], Elin S Røyset [2,4], Therese S Høiem [2], Ingunn Nervik [2], Pål Sætrom [1,2,3,5], Arne Wibe [2,6], Svanhild A Schønberg [2] and Caroline H H Pettersen [2,6,*]

1. Department of Computer Science, Faculty of Information Technology and Electrical Engineering, Norwegian University of Science and Technology (NTNU), 7491 Trondheim, Norway; helle.samdal@ntnu.no (H.S.); pal.satrom@ntnu.no (P.S.)
2. Department of Clinical and Molecular Medicine, Faculty of Medicine and Health Sciences, Norwegian University of Science and Technology (NTNU), 7491 Trondheim, Norway; lene.c.olsen@ntnu.no (L.C.O.); knut.s.gron@ntnu.no (K.S.G.); elin.s.royset@ntnu.no (E.S.R.); therese.s.hoiem@ntnu.no (T.S.H.); ingunn.nervik@ntnu.no (I.N.); arne.wibe@ntnu.no (A.W.); svanhild.schonberg@ntnu.no (S.A.S.)
3. Bioinformatics Core Facility—BioCore, Norwegian University of Science and Technology (NTNU), 7491 Trondheim, Norway
4. Department of Pathology, St. Olav's University Hospital, 7006 Trondheim, Norway
5. K.G. Jebsen Center for Genetic Epidemiology, Norwegian University of Science and Technology (NTNU), 7491 Trondheim, Norway
6. Department of Surgery, St. Olav's University Hospital, 7006 Trondheim, Norway
* Correspondence: caroline.h.pettersen@ntnu.no

Abstract: Cancer patient-derived xenografts (PDXs) better preserve tumor characteristics and microenvironment than traditional cancer cell line derived xenografts and are becoming a valuable model in translational cancer research and personalized medicine. We have established a PDX model for colorectal cancer (CRC) in CIEA NOG mice with a 50% engraftment rate. Tumor fragments from patients with CRC ($n = 5$) were engrafted in four mice per tumor ($n = 20$). Mice with established PDXs received a liquid diet enriched with fish oil or placebo, and fatty acid profiling was performed to measure fatty acid content in whole blood. Moreover, a biobank consisting of tissue and blood samples from patients was established. Histology, immunohistochemistry and in situ hybridization procedures were used for staining of tumor and xenograft tissue slides. Results demonstrate that key histological characteristics of the patients' tumors were retained in the established PDXs, and the liquid diets were consumed as intended by the mice. Some of the older mice developed lymphomas that originated from human Ki67[+], CD45[+], and EBV[+] lymphoid cells. We present a detailed description of the process and methodology, as well as possible issues that may arise, to refine the method and improve PDX engraftment rate for future studies. The established PDX model for CRC can be used for exploring different cancer treatment regimes, and liquid diets enriched with fish oil may be successfully delivered to the mice through the drinking flasks.

Keywords: PDX; patient-derived xenograft; CRC; colorectal cancer; omega-3 fatty acids

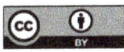

1. Introduction

In preclinical studies there has been a tradition for establishing cancer xenografts in immunosuppressed mice using cancer-derived cell lines (CDX). However, the results from CDX studies often do not correlate with the results from clinical studies, partly because cancer cell lines fail to represent the true complexity and heterogeneity of tumors (reviewed in [1–3]). This has led to a need for preclinical experimental models that better reflect the clinical situation. Patient-derived xenograft (PDX) models were first described in the 1970s [4,5], and the models have been refined over the last few decades. PDX models reflect more of the heterogeneity and individual differences of tumors compared to traditional preclinical CDX models (reviewed in [1–3,6]). However, the logistics related to the establishment of a PDX study are challenging, and there is a need for more literature guiding the initiation of PDX models.

The successful establishment of PDXs depends on several factors. The choice of animal model is important, and immunodeficient mice are found to have a higher engraftment rate for xenografts from foreign tissue as their lack of functional immune system would refrain from interfering with the foreign engrafted substance. Immunodeficient NOD/SCID/IL2Rg null (NOG) mice lack functional natural killer cells as well as B and T lymphocytes, and have defective macrophages, complement activity and dendritic cells [7]. This makes the NOG mouse an appropriate host model for establishment of PDXs, with improved tumor take rates compared to previous NOD, SCID and nude mice ([7], reviewed in [6,8]). The disruption of the interleukin 2 receptor subunit gamma (*IL2Rg*) gene reduces the chance of spontaneous lymphoma development in these animals, which was a known problem in previous NOD/SCID models [9,10]. Other important factors affecting the successful establishment of PDX models include the characteristics of the tumor subtypes, the site of implantation, the viability of the tumor cells, metastatic potential, preoperative patient treatment, contamination level in tumor specimens, time from tumor removal to implantation, the surgical procedure technique (reviewed in [1]), as well as tissue acquisition strategy [11].

In this study we aim at describing the procedure for the establishment of a PDX model of colorectal cancer (CRC). The outcome of CRC has improved significantly over the past few decades. However, CRC is still the second and third most common cancer type worldwide among women and men, respectively [12], and the second most common cancer type in Norway among both sexes [13]. Research related to improved treatment, and especially personalized treatment, for CRC patients is therefore highly needed. PDX models are currently the preferred model for preclinical studies in CRC, and studies have found the successful PDX engraftment rate to be between 56–87.5% (reviewed in [1]). We have performed a pilot study on the establishment of a PDX model for CRC in immunosuppressed CIEA NOG mice with the aim to perform preclinical combination studies of components with anticancer potential, such as cytostatic and designed diets with omega-3 polyunsaturated fatty acids (PUFAs). Combined with biobanking of healthy- and tumor tissue for whole exome- and RNA sequencing, as well as protein analyses, blood samples, and extensive clinical data via patient journals and cancer registers (e.g., the Norwegian Cancer Registry), the PDX model may be useful in the search for novel molecular biomarkers predicting responses to different anticancer drugs. The focus of this paper is to report the establishment of a PDX procedure and to test a delivery method for an omega-3 fatty acid enriched diet in mice.

2. Experimental Section
2.1. Study Design

Figure 1 gives an overview of the study design for establishing PDXs for CRC in immune suppressed mice. Surgically removed tumor fragments from 5 patients with CRC were engrafted into 4 mice per tumor. When the PDX growth was established, mice were provided with the intervention (omega-3 fatty acid (FA) or placebo enriched nutrition drinks). Follow up of the mice included assessment of animal health and weight, as well as tumor size. Mice were euthanized at humane endpoint defined by tumor volume, max latency time, and pathology, or after eight weeks treatment. Tumor and blood samples were collected for indicated analyses.

2.2. Patient Characteristics and Inclusion Criteria

Patients enrolled in the study were scheduled for cancer surgery at St. Olav's University Hospital in Trondheim between April and September 2019. Medical records of patients scheduled for consultation at the preoperative clinic at St. Olav's University Hospital were assessed. Patients were included based on the following criteria; clinically verified colon- or rectal cancer stage 1–4, tumor size exceeding 3 cm in diameter, and age > 40 years with no preoperative treatment. After signing an informed consent form, data regarding gender, age, diagnosis, tumor type, stage of disease, prior cancer treatment, use of lipid modifying medicaments, and intake of fish, cod liver oil, and omega-3 supplements were collected. Five patients who met the inclusion criteria following preoperative evaluation were included in this study. The study was approved by the Regional ethics committee for central Norway (REC ID 2017/2048, date: 10 October 2018). A Data Protection Impact Assessment (DPIA) for the project was performed in cooperation with the Norwegian Centre for Research Data (NSD) and was approved by both St. Olav's University Hospital and NTNU. Data were securely stored at the HEMIT net at St. Olav's University Hospital, locked by 2 step authorization by chip and password.

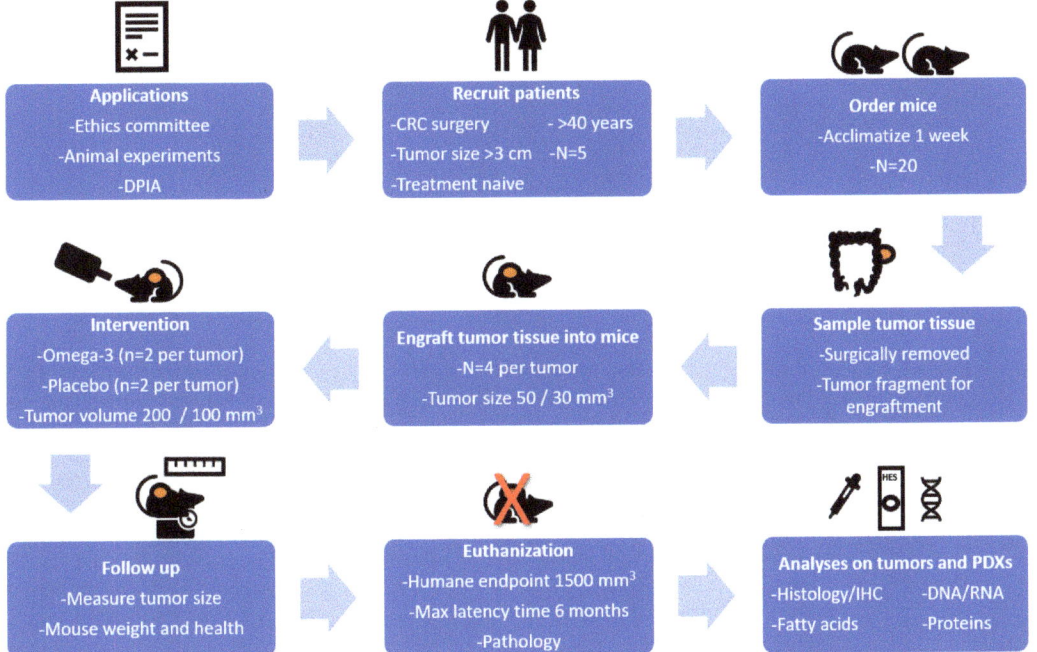

Figure 1. Study design for the establishment of patient-derived xenografts (PDXs) for colorectal cancer (CRC) in immune suppressed CIEA NOG mice.

2.3. Patient Blood Sampling

Blood samples and related information were collected, processed and stored (tubes preassigned cryptic barcode from the Biobyte® system (Biobank1®, Trondheim, Norway)) by Biobank1®. To minimize the blood sampling burden of the patients, blood samples for the study was sampled together with the standard clinical blood tests. Blood plasma and serum were frozen at −80 °C. Whole blood was stored at −80 °C for verification of germline mutations that may be found in normal colon tissue of patients and requires follow up and genetic counseling of these patients. Whole blood (2 × 50 µL) was spotted onto Whatman 903 protein saver cards (Whatman products (Cytiva), Little Chalfont, Buckinghamshire, UK), dried for 2 h at room temperature, and frozen at −80 °C for later FA profiling.

2.4. Collection of Colorectal Tumor and Healthy Tissue

Surgical personnel were informed about the request for tissue biopsies through a message in the surgery clinic's operation plan stating "Biobank Colcan". Biopsies of tumor and fresh surrounding tissue for biobanking were collected by the Biobank1® personnel. A slide of tissue was frozen in liquid nitrogen using a special clamp (Figure 2a).

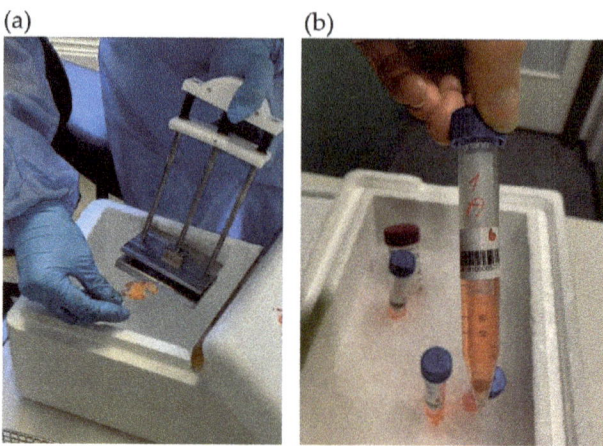

Figure 2. Tumor tissue sampling for: (**a**) biobanking and (**b**) PDX procedure.

Tissue samples of both tumor and healthy colorectal tissue were prepared for exome and RNA sequencing, protein isolation and IHC. A fresh tumor tissue sample for PDX was cut into equally sized fragments (Figure 3), placed in sterile tubes (Figure 2b) containing cold Dulbecco's modified Eagle's medium (DMEM, #D6429, Sigma Aldrich, Saint-Louis, MO, USA) supplemented with 10% fetal bovine serum (10270-098, Gibco, Thermo Fisher Scientific, Waltham, MA, USA), 1% nonessential amino acids (M7145, Sigma-Aldrich, MO, USA) and 1% gentamicin (15710049, Gibco). Location related to the tumor fragments frozen for DNA extraction was noted (Figure 3). All samples and information such as warm and cold ischemic time were registered deidentified in Biobank1®'s program Biobyte (Biobank1®, Trondheim, Norway). The CRC tissue fragments for PDX were kept on ice and transported from the clinic to the animal facility, where the mice were prepared for the surgical procedure.

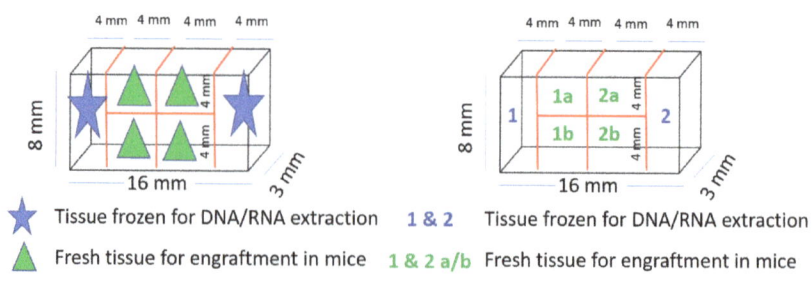

Figure 3. Tumor tissue fragmentation and naming for PDX procedure and exome sequencing.

2.5. PDX Procedure in Immunodeficient Mice

The mice were acclimatized for minimum 1 week after arrival, and four mice per cage were housed at a switched 12-h light/dark cycle at the Comparative Medicine Core Facility (CoMed), NTNU. Due to the compromised immune system of the CIEA NOG mice, all water, food, and cages were autoclaved before use. At the time of engraftment, the mice were 11 weeks or older.

CRC tissue fragments were engrafted subcutaneously into female opportunist free CIEA NOG® (NOG) mice (NOD.Cg-PrkdcscidIl2rgtm1Sug/JicTac, Taconic Biosciences, Rensselaer, NY, USA). The size of the tissue fragments from the two first patient tumors were about $4 \times 4 \times 3$ mm (~50 mm^3), and for the last three tumors about $3 \times 3 \times 3$ mm (~30 mm^3). Tissue fragments from each tumor were engrafted in four mice; in total twenty mice (see Figure 4, and Supplementary file 1).

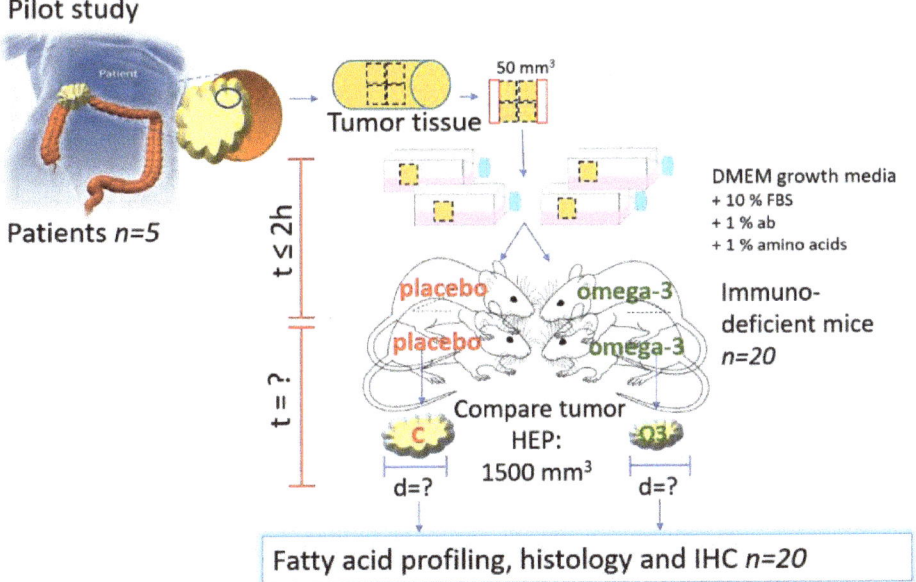

Figure 4. Experimental design of PDX of CRC in mice. C = control/placebo, ω-3 = omega-3, HEP = humane endpoint. Part of the figure is modified from [14] with approval.

The surgical table and equipment were cleaned with ethanol and the surgical equipment (scissors, forceps, cotton swabs) was autoclaved. The mice were weighed to estimate correct dosing of medications and put into an anesthesia induction chamber provided with 2% isoflurane (ESDG9623C, Baxter, Deerfield, IL, USA, 0.6% N_2 and 0.4% O_2) gas using an anesthetic vaporizer, until they were asleep. Eye gel (Viscotears, 597562, Dr. Gerhard Mann chem.-pharm. Fabrik GmbH, Wülfrath, Germany) was applied, and the mice were placed on a heating pad covered with a surgery tissue and kept anaesthetized using a nose cone with 1.5% isoflurane. The anesthetic level was checked by foot pinch using forceps and the mouse was marked by ear clip. The incision area was shaved and washed with Hibiscrub (596023, Mölnlycke, Gøteborg, Sweden) and chlorohexidine (007269, Fresenius Kabi, Bad Homburg vor der Höhe, Germany). Metacam (025388, Boehringer IngelheimVetmedica GmbH, Germany, 2–3 mg/kg) and Marcaine (169912, Aspen Pharma Traiding Limited, Ireland, 0.04 mg/kg) were given subcutaneously for systemic and local pain relief, respectively. The tumor fragments were placed in a sterile petri dish and washed briefly with sterile physiological NaCl. A small cut (3–4 mm) was made in the skin in front of the back curve, and the tissue fragment was placed in a small pocket under the skin using forceps. The wound was closed by stitching using surgical sutures (Ethicon® VicrylTM 5-0, Ethicon®, Somerville, NJ, USA), before the mice were placed on clean paper in a new cage.

A bullet point form was followed during surgery (Supplementary Figure S2-1). Details regarding surgery and anesthesia were registered in a log form (Supplementary Figure S2-2).

The animal experiments were approved by the Norwegian Food Safety Authority (Mattilsynet, FOTS ID 12823).

2.6. Postoperative Follow-Up

The mice were observed for two hours after surgery. If any stiches were opened by the mice within two hours, the mice were anesthetized and restitched. Metacam was injected subcutaneously 24 h postoperative for systemic pain relief. The mice were housed in single cages for 1–2 weeks after surgery until the wounds had healed, before placing the mice together in groups of four mice per cage. The "rat and mouse No. 1 Maintenance Autoclavable" (RMIA, Special Diets Service, Essex, UK) pellet food and water were autoclaved before use. The pellet food was available to the mice at all time. Water was available until the start of treatment regime; see details below. The mice were weighed 1–3 times per week, and observations were noted in a score sheet for each animal (Supplementary file 1). Subcutaneous tumor size was measured 1–3 times per week as soon as the xenograft was palpable using a digital caliper and registered in the score sheet. Tumor volume was calculated using the following formula V = (length × width^2)/2. In addition, tumor growth was recorded regularly by imaging.

2.7. Mouse Blood Sampling

Blood samples were taken from vena saphena before treatment was initiated (Figure 5a). The mice were restrained inside a 50 mL tube with an air opening in the tip and the sampling area was shaved and washed with 70% ethanol. A scalpel was used to punctuate the vein, and 50 µL blood was collected with a pipette and spotted on a Whatman card. The card was dried for two hours at room temperature and stored at −80 °C until FA profiling. An additional <150 µL blood was taken for blood plasma preparation and stored at −80 °C.

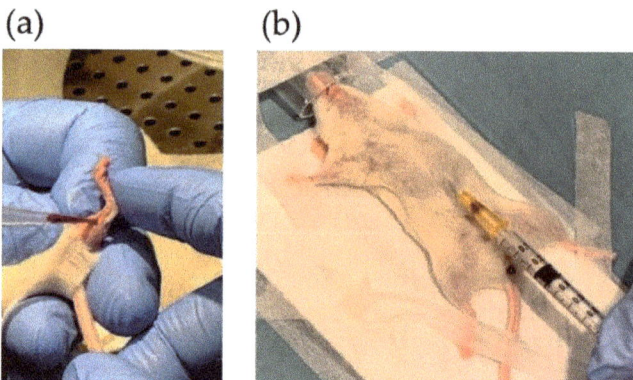

Figure 5. Blood sampling by puncturing: (**a**) vena saphena and (**b**) the heart.

At the endpoint, the mice were anesthetized, and blood was collected from the main vein/heart (Figure 5b) before euthanizing the mice by cutting the aorta. Whole blood was spotted on Whatman cards (50 µL) for FA profiling. To prepare plasma, blood was drained from the vein and transferred to Microvette CB 300 capillary tubes with EDTA (Sarstedt, Nümbrecht, Germany). Samples were mixed, centrifuged (3000 rpm, 4 °C, 10 min) and aliquoted. Whatman cards and plasma were stored at −80 °C.

2.8. Treatment with Liquid Diets

When growth of the xenograft was confirmed, mice were given either the nutrition drink Smartfish Remune with fish oil (DHA and EPA (2000 mg/200 mL), Smartfish AS, Oslo, Norway), or placebo containing an equal amount of rapeseed oil (Smartfish AS).

The diets were isocaloric and isolipidic, differing only by the type of oil. The liquid diets were aliquoted, frozen at −20 °C, thawed, and freshly provided. Mice were given nutrition drinks five days a week for seven hours a day during their active time period; otherwise fresh water was available. The drinking bottles containing the nutrition drink were weighed before and after the seven-hour feeding period to estimate daily intake. A human dose of 4 g omega-3 FAs/day is equivalent to ~1.6 mL Smartfish Remune daily. Animal equivalent dose (AED) based on body surface area was calculated by the equation: AED (mg/kg) = human dose (mg/kg) * (Human Km/Animal Km) = (4000 mg/60 kg) * (37/3) = 822.22 [15]. Oral consumption volume (OCV) was calculated by the equation: OCV (mL) = animal weight [kg] * animal dose (mg/kg)/(concentration mg/mL) = (0.020 kg * 822.22 mg/kg)/(10 mg/mL) = 1.6 mL.

2.9. Euthanasia, Necropsy and Tissue Sampling

At the humane endpoint, characterized by either a tumor volume of 1500 mm^3, reduced health/weight or a xenograft not growing after 6 months, blood sampling, and euthanization were performed as described above and in Supplementary file 3. The tumor area was shaved and washed with ethanol before a cut was made in the skin and the xenograft was collected and picture was taken. The xenograft was divided in parts for histology/IHC, RNA sequencing, and protein analysis. The remaining tumor was collected in tubes and frozen in liquid N$_2$ for protein- and RNA analysis. The samples were stored at −80 °C. Tumor tissue (both PDX and any secondary tumors) for histology/IHC was collected in neutral buffered formaldehyde (NBF, 9713.1000, BDH Chemicals, VWR, Radnor, PA, USA, equal to 10% neutral buffered formalin, >10 times tumor volume). The mice bearing xenografts from the last three patient tumors were necropsied. The abdomen was opened, and the lungs, heart, liver, kidneys, stomach, colon, spleen, and thymus were localized, inspected and collected in NBF for histology analysis. Gross findings were registered on an autopsy card (modified from [16]) for each animal (Supplementary file 1).

2.10. Fatty Acid Profiling and Omega-3 Index in Blood

The profiling of FAs in human and mouse whole blood was performed using gas chromatography with flame-ionization detection (GC-FID). Samples were analyzed by Vitas AS, Oslo, Norway. Two punches of human whole blood from the Whatman cards were diluted in sodium methylate (900 µL, 0.5 M). FA methyl esters (FAME) were formed by methylation (20 min, 600 rpm, 50 °C) and extracted with distilled water (300 µL) and hexane (500 µL) before thorough mixing (5 min) and centrifugation (5 min, 4000× g, 10 °C). The sample (3 µL) was injected into the GC-FID with an HP 7890A Gas Chromatograph System (Agilent Technologies, Palo Alto, CA, USA). FAs were separated on a Supelco 30 m × 250 µm × 0.2 µm column and the results for 11 different FAs were reported as g FAME/100 g FAME. Omega-3 index was calculated by the formula: Omega-3 index = (g DHA FAME + g EPA FAME)/total g FAME * 100.

2.11. Histology and Immunohistochemistry Analysis

To compare the histology and molecular characteristics of patient tumor tissue with the corresponding mouse xenografts, tissue samples were taken for histology and immunohistochemistry (IHC) analyses. Tumor tissue and PDX fragments were collected in tubes with 4% NBF. The Cellular and Molecular Imaging Core Facility (CMIC), Department of Clinical and Molecular Medicine (IKOM), NTNU used a histological routine procedure to process, paraffin embed (FFPE), section (4 µm) and dry (60°) the samples. The slides were stained with hematoxylin, erythrosin and saffron (HES) in the automatic slide stainer Sakura Tissue-Tek © PrismaTM. The slides were dried further in the instrument's heat chamber, before being deparaffinized through several baths of Tissue Clear and rehydrated through descending grades of ethanol to water. The slides were stained in Haematoxylin followed by bluing in water, before being stained with Erythrosine and rinsed in water for removal of excess dye. Slides were further dehydrated through ascending grades of ethanol and stained in saffron before being rinsed in several baths of absolute ethanol and cleared in Tissue Clear before cover slipping in Sakura Tissue-Tek © GlasTM automatic coverslipper. The sections were dried overnight in a well-ventilated place due to chemical evaporation. Dyes used were: Heamatoxylin (CellPath/Chemi-Tecnic, RHD-1475-100, CI No 75290), Erythrosine 239 (VWR, no 720-0179) and saffron (Chemi-Tecnic as, Chroma 5A-394, CI No 75100). Interpretation was performed by experienced pathologists using light microscopy.

For IHC analysis FFPE tissue sections (4 µm) were cut onto SuperFrost Plus slides, dried overnight at 37 °C, and then baked for 2 h at 60 °C. The sections were dewaxed in Tissue Clear and rehydrated through graded alcohols to water in an automatic slide stainer (Sakura Tissue-Tek © Prisma™). Next, the sections were pretreated in Target Retrieval Solution, High or Low pH (Dako, Agilent, Santa Clara, CA, USA, K8004/5) in PT Link (Dako) for 20 min at 97 °C to facilitate antigen retrieval. Further staining was performed on the Dako Autostainer. Following soaking in wash buffer, endogenous peroxidase activity was quenched by incubation in Peroxydase block (Dako S2023). Sections were washed in wash buffer and incubated with primary antibody for 40 min. Further, the slides were washed in wash buffer before incubating for 30 min in labelled polymer HRP anti-Mouse (Dako K4001) and DAB (Dako K3468) to develop the stain. Tris-buffered saline (TBS) (Dako K8007) was used throughout for the washing steps. In Sakura Tissue-Tek © Prisma™, the slides were lightly counterstained with Hematoxylin, dehydrated through ascending grades of ethanol, cleared in Tissue Clear, and coverslipped. For the tissue studied, appropriate negative controls were performed by omitting the primary antibody. Antibodies used were Ki67 (M7240, clone MIB-1, Dako), CD45 (M0701, clones 2B11 + PD7/26, Dako) and CD20 (M0755, clone L26, Dako). Interpretation was performed by experienced pathologists using light microscopy.

2.12. In Situ Hybridization

To detect Epstein–Barr-Virus (EBV)-encoded RNA the Inform EBER (EBV early RNA) probe (Ventana Medical Systems, Inc., Oro Valley, AZ, USA) was used for in situ hybridization (ISH) of NBF fixated paraffin embedded patient tumor and lymphoma tissue sections. The EBER ISH staining was routinely performed at the Unit of Immunohistochemistry, Department of Pathology, St. Olav's University Hospital. Paraffin embedded tissue sections were cut at 3 µm onto Superfrost slides (Thermo Scientific, Waltham, MA, USA, Superfrost plus, #J1800AMNZ). On the slides was also a known positive sample (as control). Each sample was sectioned onto two slides, one for the EBER probe and one for a Negative control probe (REF 800-2847). The section with the negative control probe was used for identification of unspecific staining. The sections were dried at 60 °C for 1 h. The analysis was performed on BenchMark Ultra instrument (Ventana, Roche, Basel, Switzerland) using the Ventana ISH IView Blue Detection Kit (Ventana, Roche, #800-092), ISH protease 3 (Ventana, Roche, #780-4149), RED II counterstain (Ventana, Roche, #780-2218) and INFORM EBER Probe (Ventana, Roche, #800-2842). After the ISH process the slides were dehydrated through ascending grades of ethanol and xylene before cover slipping in Microm CoverTech CTM6 (Thermo Scientific) automatic coverslipper. Interpretation was performed by experienced pathologists using light microscopy.

2.13. Data Analysis

All data analyses were performed in R. For the FA profiling, a hierarchical mixed linear model accounting for multiple measurements from the same mice were fitted using the lme() function from the nmle package. Overall effects of each FA was assessed using the Anova() function, and pairwise differences using the ghlt() function to perform post hoc Tukey tests. In addition to the internal adjustments of p-values for multiple testing within each model as calculated by the ghlt() function, p-values were further adjusted based on the number of FAs measured using the Bonferroni correction.

3. Results

3.1. Patient and Tumor Characteristics

All invited patients attended the preoperative information meeting and accepted enrollment of the study by signing an informed consent form. Table 1 shows the patient and tumor characteristics along with information regarding the patient's intake of fish, cod liver oil, omega-3 supplements, and lipid modifying medications recorded from the questionnaires. The included patients consisted of four males and one female (average age 67.6 years). Three tumors were surgically removed from the colon and two from the rectum. One tumor was described as ulcerating, two tumors were exophytic and ulcerating, and two stricturated the colon. All tumors were adenocarcinomas, differed in morphology (Figure 6), and the tumor sizes were between 3.7–5 cm across the largest diameter. Three tumors were staged T3 and two tumors T4. Lymph nodes close to the tumor were affected in two patients; meanwhile, no other metastases were found in any of the patients. All patients reported an intake of omega-3 supplements 0–3 times monthly, two patients had a daily intake of cod liver oil, and all patients had intake of fish 1–3 times weekly.

3.2. Establishment of Patient-Derived Xenografts of Colorectal Cancer

Fresh tissue fragments from five primary CRC tumors were engrafted in four immunodeficient CIEA NOG mice per tumor (total $n = 20$, Figure 4). Animal and engraftment details are given in Table 2. The age of the mice varied from 11 to 33 weeks. Tissue fragments were placed in DMEM on ice within ~20 min and implanted subcutaneously in the mice within 60 min after the tissue was collected (Table 2 and Figure 7).

Table 1. Patient and tumor characteristics ($n = 5$), and questionnaire answers.

	Patient 3	Patient 11	Patient 17	Patient 18	Patient 19
Gender (Male/Female)	M	F	M	M	M
Age	69	65	77	62	65
Tumor site	Colon	Colon	Colon	Rectum	Rectum
Tumor anatomy	Exophytic	Stenosing, ulcerating	Stricturating, ulcerating	Ulcerating	Exophytic, ulcerating
Tumor type	Adenocarcinoma	Signet cell carcinoma	Adenocarcinoma with mucus	Adenocarcinoma	Adenocarcinoma
Tumor stage (TMN)	T3N0M0	T3N2M0	T4N0M0	T4aN1M0	T3N0M0
Tumor differentiation grade	Medium		Medium	Medium	Medium
Tumor size (cm)	4	5	4	4	3.7
Tumor MSI status		MSI-high	MSS	MSS	MSS
Mutations		BRAF	BRAF	KRAS	
Pre-operative cancer treatment	No	No	No	No	No
Previous cancer diagnoses			Yes		No
Intake of omega-3 supplements	0–3/month	0–3/month	0–3/month	0–3/month	0–3/month
Intake of cod liver oil	0–3/month	0–3/month	Daily	0–3/month	Daily [1]
Intake of fish	1–3/week	1–3/week	1–3/week	1–3/week	1–3/week
Use of lipid reducing medication	No	No	No	Yes	No

[1] Daily intake of cod liver oil only in the wintertime (September to April). The blood sample was taken in August.

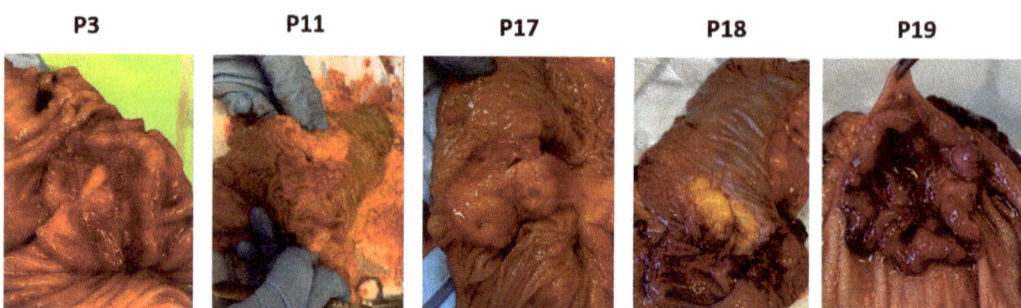

Figure 6. Pathology of CRC tumors from patients (p) 3, 11, 17, 18 and 19.

Table 2. Animal and engraftment details.

Patient ID	Patient 3				Patient 11				Patient 17				Patient 18				Patient 19			
Mouse ID	12	15	16	17	19	20	21	22	23	24	25	26	27	28	29	30	31	32	33	18
Tumor fragment ID	1a	1b	2a	2b	1a	1b	2a	2b	1a	1b	2a	2b	1a	1b	2a	2b	1a	1b	2a	2b
Ear clip	1	2	3	4	1	2	3	4	1	2	3	4	1	2	3	4	1	2	3	4
Age at engraftment (week)	11	11	11	11	17	17	17	17	31	31	31	31	31	31	31	31	33	33	33	33
Tumor fragment size (mm^3)	50	50	50	50	50	50	50	50	30	30	30	30	30	30	30	30	30	30	30	30
Days to established growth	-	64	64	99	70	34	91	34	185	-	174	52	-	-	-	-	-	-	-	-

Of the twenty mice engrafted with tumor tissue fragments, ten mice established tumor growth (Figure 8), giving a total engraftment rate of 50%. The average number of days to established xenograft growth was 87 ($\pm$51) days (Table 2). The engraftment rate and average number of days until established xenograft growth using 50 mm^3 fragments were 88% and 65 ($\pm$23) days, respectively (Table 2). When engrafting 30 mm^3 tumor fragments, only the tumor from patient 17 established growth of three xenografts after an average of 137 ($\pm$60) days. Only four PDXs exceeded humane endpoint of 1500 mm^3 before euthanization. Of these, two originated from patient tumor 3 and two from patient tumor 11 (engrafted with 50 mm^3 fragments).

Images and score sheets including animal weight and PDX size are presented in Supplementary file 1. As an example, pictures of PDX growth for mouse #26 are shown in Figure 9, which also illustrates the growth of a secondary tumor. Images of 9 of the 10 established PDXs are presented in Figure 10.

The weight for most mice was stable throughout the study (Supplementary Figure S4-1, Table 3). However, some mice were euthanized due to reduced weight and their general health condition (Table 3). Both mice #19 and #21 had a weight reduction of about 10–15% at the day of euthanization.

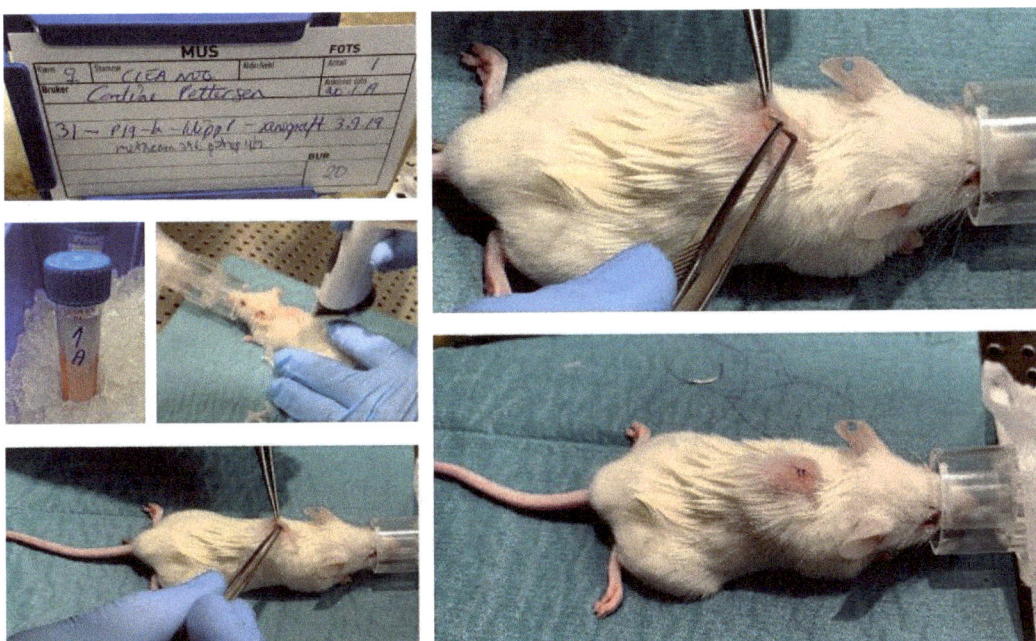

Figure 7. Implantation of a tumor fragment into immune suppressed CIEA NOG mouse #31.

3.3. Development of Secondary Tumors and Abscesses

Some mice developed growth of secondary tumors or abscesses. Mouse #23 developed a dark colored secondary tumor behind the right foreleg. At necropsy the tumor was found to contain a dark dense liquid, probably due to blood accumulation (Figure 11).

Four mice (#25, 26, 32 and 33) developed spontaneous rapidly growing secondary tumors located on the front shoulders (Figure 11). Necropsy of mouse #32 indicated red swollen legs and shoulders with bleeding areas in addition to the secondary tumor.

Three of the four mice engrafted with tumor fragments from patient 18 developed abscesses in the surgery area after tissue implantation and were euthanized. However, treatment was initialized before the "tumors" were recognized as abscesses (Figure 11 and Supplementary Figures S1-27-2, S1-28-2 and S1-29-2). For mouse #28 the abscess was intact when removed at euthanization (Figure 11).

3.4. Histological Similarity between Patient Tumors and Patient-Derived Xenografts

The histological architecture of the growing PDXs demonstrated high correlation to the primary tumors as shown by hematoxylin, erythrosine and saffron (HES) staining of tumor tissue slides (Figure 12). All five patient tumors were confirmed by pathologists to be colorectal adenocarcinomas. The histomorphology of the growing PDXs was similar to the histomorphology of the primary tumors, reflecting the heterogeneity of the primary tumors. We did not observe any direct changes in morphology between fish oil and placebo treated PDXs.

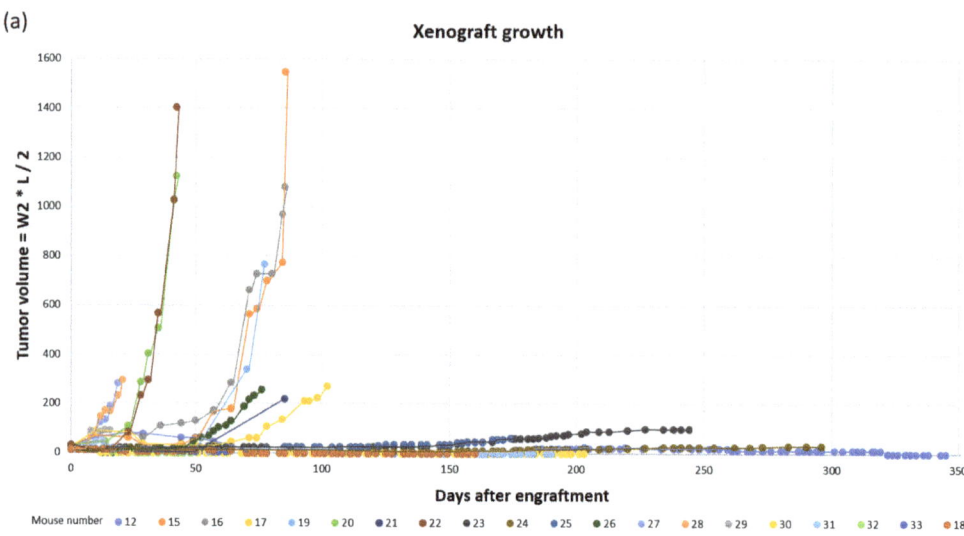
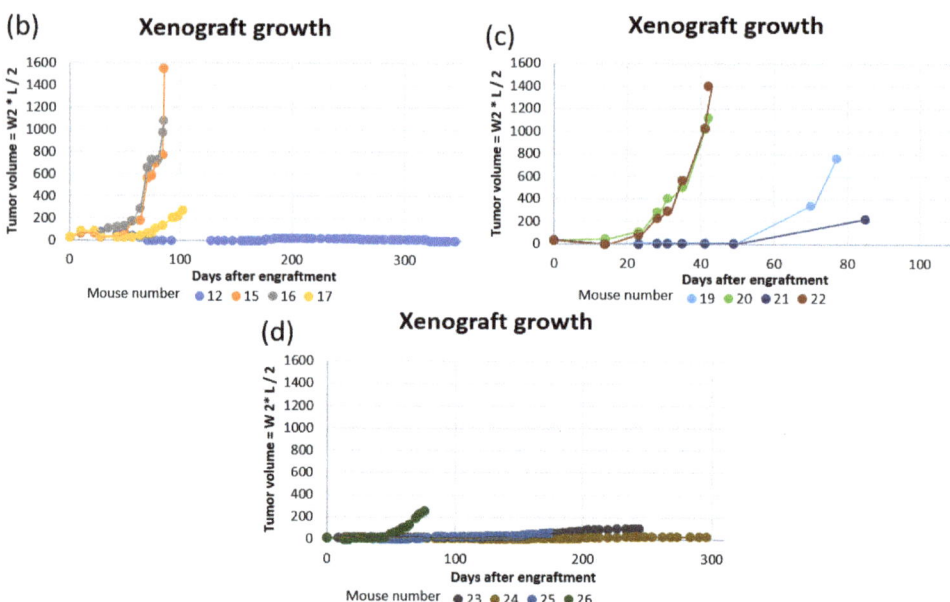

Figure 8. PDX growth curves for: (**a**) all mice; (**b**) mouse #12, 15, 16 and 17 (tumor fragments from patient 3); (**c**) mouse #19, 20, 21 and 22 (tumor fragments from patient 11) and; (**d**) mouse #23, 24, 25 and 26 (tumor fragments from patient 17).

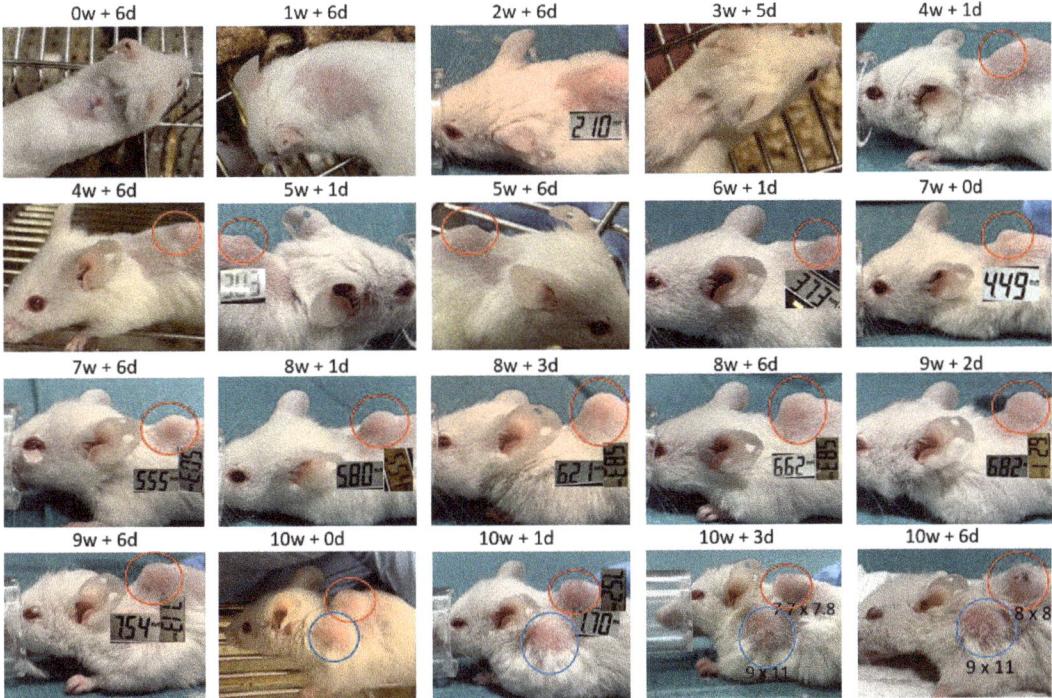

Figure 9. Images of PDX growth (red ring) for mouse #26 (patient 17). Secondary tumor from week 10 (blue ring). Numbers are millimeter (mm) length of the tumor in two dimensions. W = week, d = days.

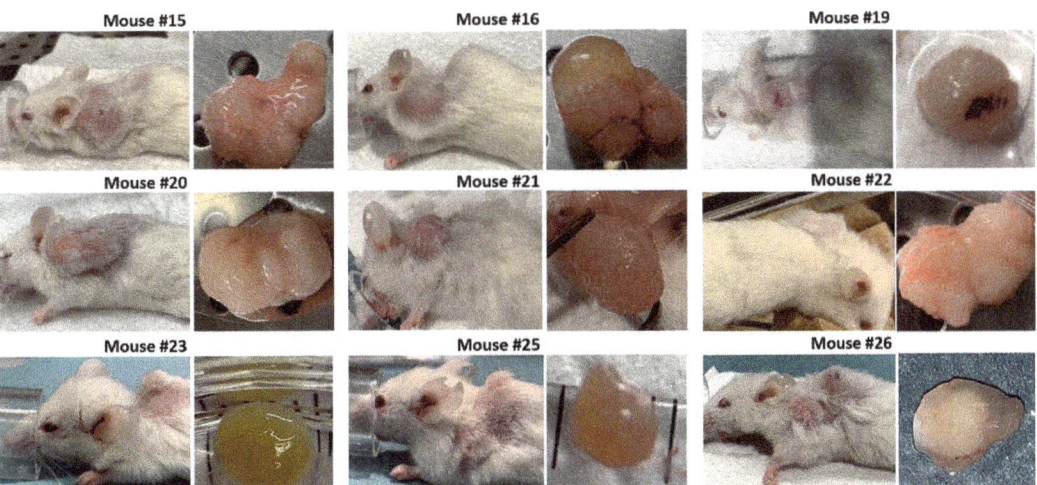

Figure 10. Images of 9 of 10 established PDXs, taken at the day of euthanization. Mouse #17 died during the anesthetic procedure (isoflurane) when assessing tumor size and the tumor was not sampled.

Table 3. Characteristics of all mice at the time of euthanization.

Mouse #	Clinical Symptoms & Comments	Necropsy Findings	Body Weight	PDX Size (mm)	Second Tumor Size (mm)
12	PDX not growing after 6 months.	Only a spot at engraftment side. Dark cystic structure close to pancreas.	Stable	-	-
15	Placebo treatment until PDX max size.	Large solid tumor.	Stable	10 × 15.5	-
16	Smartfish Remune treatment until PDX max size.	Large tumor, partly with liquid. Visible blood veins to tumor.	Stable	11.5 × 13	-
17	Smartfish Remune treatment until it died during anesthesia.	No samples taken.	Stable	7.5 × 7.5	-
19	Ulcerating xenograft. Smartfish Remune treatment.	Large solid tumor with blood traces.	Slightly reduced	11.3 × 12	-
20	Placebo treatment until PDX reached max size.	Large solid tumor.	−10–20%	11.5 × 17	-
21	Reduced general health and reduced weight. Large PDX.	Solid tumor. Low blood volume. No samples taken.	−10–15%	7 × 9	-
22	Smartfish Remune treatment until PDX max size.	Large solid tumor w/visible blood veins.	Stable	11 × 17	-
23	Reduced weight. Placebo treatment (8 weeks). Possibly rectal prolapse.	Small spleen. Second tumor with dark liquid inside. Clog of fur and food in stomach.	−10–20%	5.8 × 5.9	7 × 9
24	Did not reach "established growth" 3 months after animals without growing xenografts were euthanized.	Small slowly growing PDX. Whitish lungs. Normal organs.	Stable	3.9 × 4	-
25	Reduced general health. Large second tumor	Established growth of PDX. Whitish lungs. Large second tumor left shoulder.	Stable	5 × 5	8 × 10
26	Ulcerating xenograft. Smartfish Remune treatment. Large second tumor.	Enlarged spleen w/white fields. Whitish lungs. Two second tumors; left and right shoulder.	−10%	8 × 8	9 × 11 (left)
27	Abscess mistaken for PDX until it burst. Smartfish Remune treatment.	Wound at the abscess site. Small xenograft under the skin.	Stable	-	-
28	Abscess mistaken as PDX in the beginning. Placebo treatment	Intact abscess 9.5 × 10 mm containing green liquid. Only a spot at engraftment site	Stable	-	-

Table 3. Cont.

Mouse #	Clinical Symptoms & Comments	Necropsy Findings	Body Weight	PDX Size (mm)	Second Tumor Size (mm)
29	Abscess mistaken as PDX until it burst. Smartfish Remune treatment	Wound where abscess has burst. Small xenograft under the skin	Stable	-	-
30	Did not reach "established growth" after 6 months.	Normal organs. A small bump in the liver. Trace of PDX under the skin	Stable	-	-
31	Did not reach "established growth" after 6 months.	Small xenograft under the skin. Normal organs.	Stable	-	-
32	Reduced general health. Second tumor. Did not reach "established growth". Liquid in the eye.	Thick wounded skin at the neck. Whitish lungs. Enlarged spleen >2 cm. Red/swollen legs, shoulders and spine second tumor over the ribs.	Stable	-	-
33	Did not reach "established growth". Large second tumor.	Large second tumor. No visible xenograft. Enlarged spleen.	Stable	-	9 × 14
18	Did not reach "established growth". Rectal prolapse.	Swollen, bloody anal opening. Whitish part of one lung. Traces of xenograft under skin. Enlarged spleen ca 2.5 cm	−10%	-	-

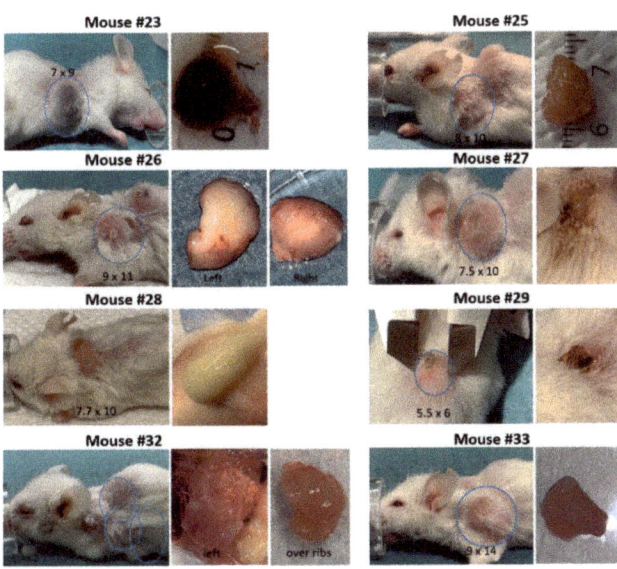

Figure 11. Pictures of mice developing secondary tumors (mouse #23, 25, 26, 32 and 33) or abscesses (mouse #27, 28 and 29). Numbers represent tumor size in mm.

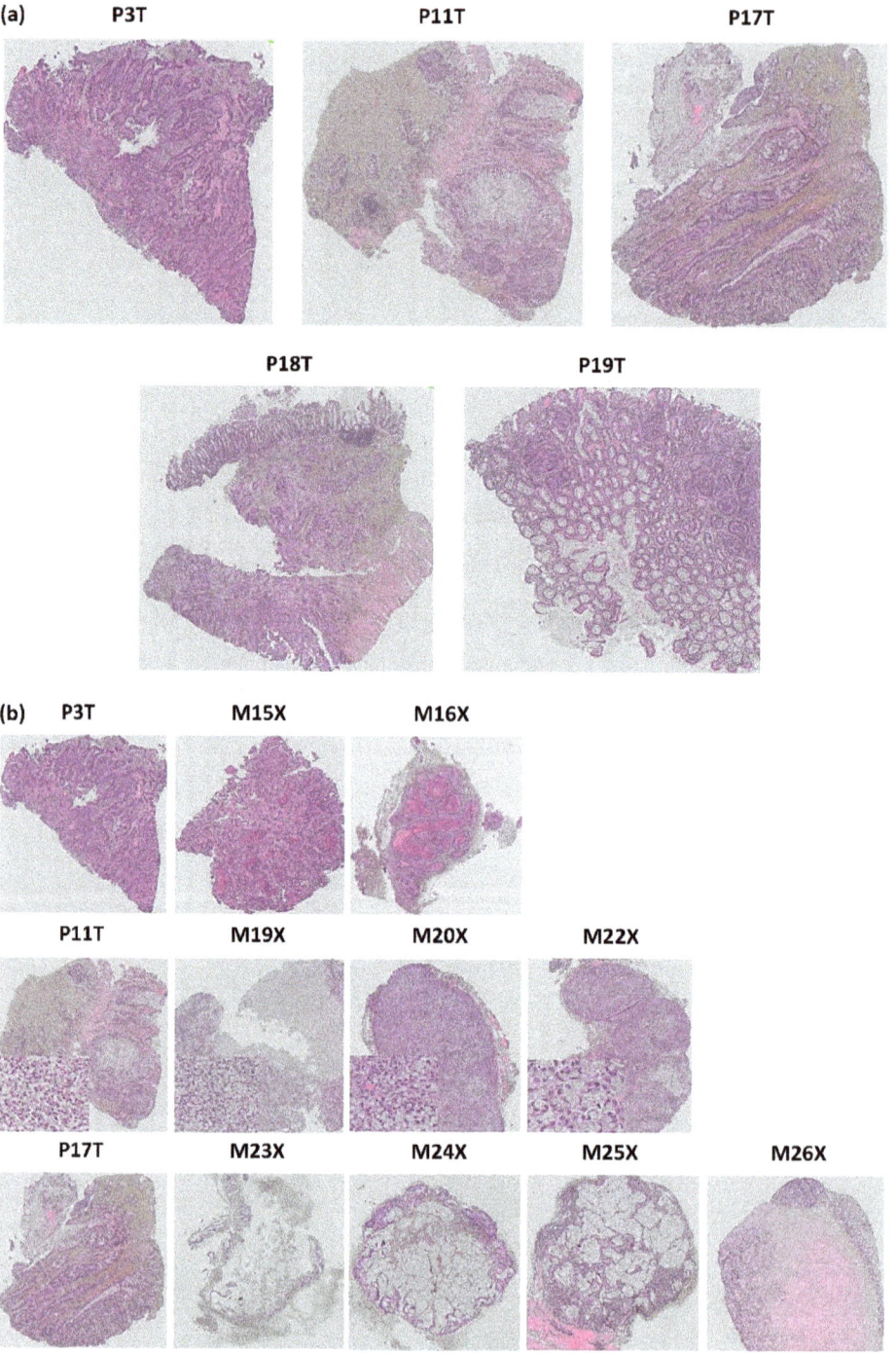

Figure 12. Histopathological comparison of: (**a**) the five patient CRC tumors and (**b**) three patient tumors and matched PDX tissue sections. The tissue sections are stained with HES. p = patient, T = tumor, M = mouse, X = xenograft.

The tumor from patient 3 was described as a typical colorectal adenocarcinoma. The glandular forms found in the HES stained section were also observed in the corresponding xenografts in mouse #15 and 16. Mouse #17 had a growing xenograft, but died due to technical problems during anesthesia and the xenograft was not sampled. Mouse #12 did not establish growth of the xenograft.

HES staining of the histology slide from patient 11 showed that the tumor was compact and mainly consisted of signet ring cells. These cells are rare CRC cells with the nucleus placed at one side and a large mucus droplet filling most of the cell. Growth was established for all four PDXs from patient tumor 11. However, mouse #21 was euthanized due to acutely reduced health and the xenograft was not sampled. HES staining confirmed that the corresponding PDXs had a high degree of histopathological similarity to the patient tumor (Figure 12).

The tumor from patient 17 had classical CRC histology with glandular forming and mucus producing cells (Figure 12). Growth was established for three out of four PDXs; mouse #23, 25 and 26. The corresponding PDXs of mice #23, 24 and 25 were adenocarcinomas with varying degree of mucus production (Figure 12). Mouse #23 was euthanized before reaching maximal tumor size due to reduced weight. Mouse #24 had a growing xenograft, but did not pass as "established PDX" due to a diameter less than 5 mm. PDXs from both mouse #23 and 24 had tumor glandules with necrotic debris in the lumen (typical for CRC tumors), as well as a necrotic core (Figure 12, Supplementary Figures S1-23-9 and S1-24-6). The PDX of mouse #25 contained glandular forming cells surrounded by a dense infiltrate of lymphoid cells (Figure 12). The outer part of the xenograft had cells with irregular nuclear membranes indicating stressed cells. The xenograft from mouse #26 had a large pale necrotic core surrounded by a dense lymphoid filtrate (Figures 12 and 13).

The tumors from patients 18 and 19 were both confirmed to be typical colorectal adenocarcinoma (Figure 12). However, none of the xenografts established growth in the host mice. The tumor from patient 18 grew in small glands and strands through the muscle layer of the bowel wall. However, as mentioned, three out of four mice engrafted with tumor fragments from patient 18 were euthanized due to rapidly developing abscesses before the xenografts were established, hence there are no histology results for these.

3.5. Histology of Secondary Tumors and Affected Organs

After euthanasia, the mice engrafted with tumor tissue from the three last patient tumors were necropsied. To study the histology by HES staining, lungs, heart, spleen, liver and any secondary tumors were sampled.

HES stained histology slides of the secondary tumors from mouse #25, 26, 32 and 33 contained malignant looking lymphoid cells (lymphoma). The secondary tumor of mouse #25 was a massive tumor consisting of lymphoid cells, while the spleen, pancreas and lungs appeared healthy (Supplementary Figure S1-25-3). Mouse #26 developed lymphoid tumors on both axes, and tumor areas with lymphoid cells were observed in the spleen, pancreas and lungs. Moreover, the lungs, spleen and pancreas had fields with pale necrotic tissue areas, and the spleen was enlarged (2.2 cm, Figure 13a,b, Supplementary Figure S1-26-4) compared to normal spleen from mouse #12 (1.3 cm, Figure 13a).

Mouse #32 developed lymphoma and was euthanized before growth of the xenograft was established. Lymphoid cancer cells were also found in the lungs and red swollen leg and shoulders of mouse #32. The spleen was enlarged (>2 cm) and contained lymphoid tumor cells (Supplementary Figures S1-32-3 and S1-32-6). Mouse #33 had lymphoid cancer cells present in the secondary tumor, lymph node from the neck and in the enlarged spleen, where we also observed pale necrotic areas (Supplementary Figure S1-33-6).

Mouse #23 developed a secondary tumor behind the right foreleg (Figure 11). At necroscopy the tumor consisted of a bladder containing dark liquid. The liquid was washed away using sterile NaCl and the rest was stored in 4% neutral buffered formaldehyde (NBF). HES staining did not indicate any lymphoid cells. The tumor appeared more like a cyst with liquid filled structures lined with benign looking epithelium (Supplementary Figure S1-23-9).

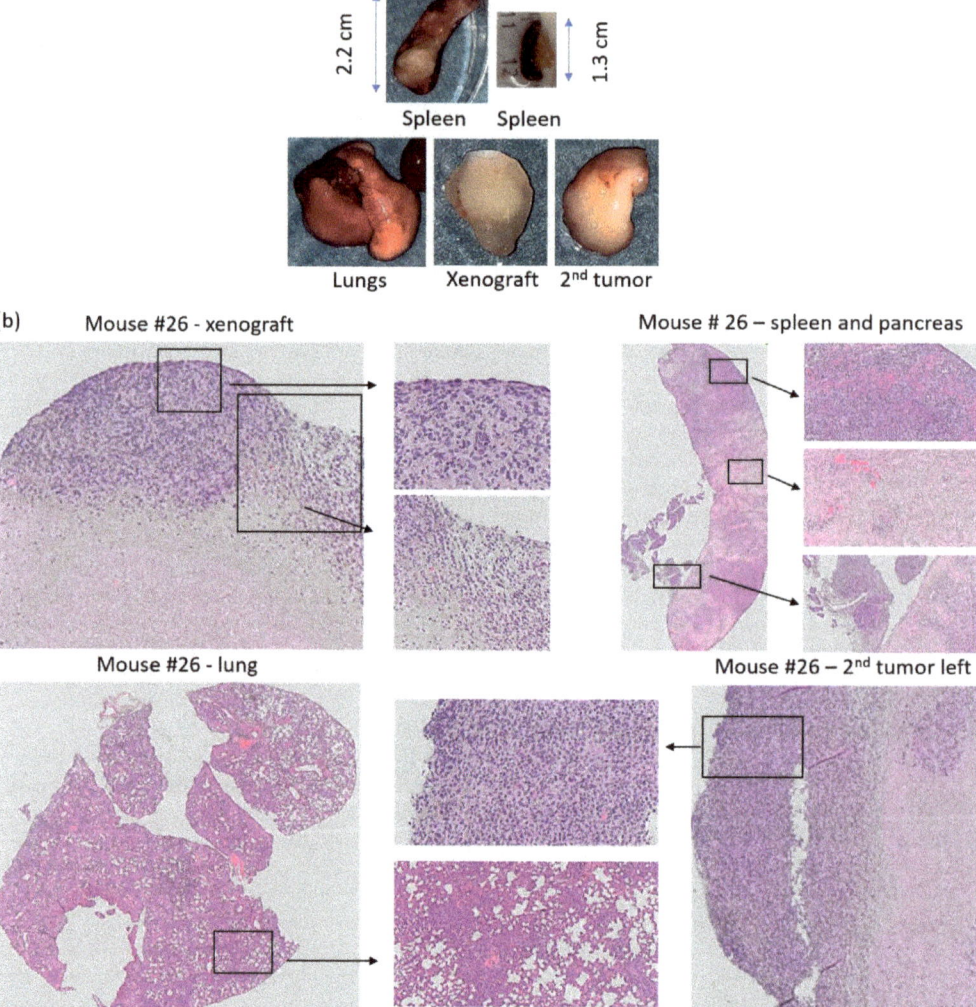

Figure 13. (**a**) Tissue collected at necroscopy from mouse #26 and spleen from mouse #12 and (**b**) HES staining of PDX, spleen, second tumor left shoulder, and lung from mouse #26. Xenograft; necrotic tissue surrounded by lymphoid cancer cells. Spleen/pancreas; lymphoid cancer cells and pale necrotic tissue areas in the spleen. Lung; dense areas with lymphoid cancer cells. Secondary tumor left shoulder; compact tumor with lymphoid cancer cells.

3.6. Origin of Cells Found in Lymphomas and Presence of Epstein–Barr Virus

All four lymphoma cases (mouse #25, 26, 32 and 33) were composed of actively proliferating neoplastic lymphoid cells including a high number of mitotic cells (Figure 14). To distinguish between human and murine cells and confirm lymphoid cell origin, lymphoma slides were IHC stained with anti Ki67 and leukocyte common antigen (LCA/CD45) specific for human cells (Figure 14). Three of the lymphomas were positive for human specific Ki67 (MIB1, Dako) indicating human cell origin, whereas the fourth was negative for the MIB1 antibody. The three MIB1 positive lymphomas were also CD45 positive (mouse #25, 26 and 33, Figure 14), while mouse #32 was negative for CD45, human specific Ki67 (Figure 11) and CD20 (Supplementary Figure S1-32-7). Hence, the lymphoma of mouse #32 is likely to have a murine origin. Other studies have reported that formation of human lymphomas in PDX models can be a result of outgrowth of Epstein–Barr-Virus (EBV) transformed lymphoid cells from the original tumor [10,17]. To address this, we tested whether the four lymphomas and the two respective patient CRC tumors were positive for EBV. The results demonstrate that three Ki67+ and CD45+ lymphomas were positive for EBV-coded RNA in the nuclei (Figure 14), indicating that EBV was latent in the tumors of patients 17 and 19 from which the lymphomas originated. However, the patient tumors (results not shown) and the lymphoma from mouse #32 (Figure 14) were negative for EBV RNA. The method controls for IHC and ISH were negative (results not shown).

3.7. Intake of Liquid Diet

When PDXs reached "established growth", mice were given liquid diets; Smartfish Remune Peach supplemented with either omega-3 FAs (fish oil) or rapeseed oil (placebo). The mice were observed to drink from the bottles (Supplementary Figure S1-23-4), and the nutrition drink was observed in the stomach of some of the animals at necroscopy. The daily intake (mL) per animal was estimated by weighing the drinking bottles before and after they were provided to the mice (density 1.047 g/mL). However, there was a considerable amount of spillage/leakage from the bottles, hence the estimated intake was inaccurate. Only mouse #23 was given the drink for the scheduled 8 weeks.

3.8. Fatty acid Profiling of Patient and Mouse Whole Blood

Whole blood from both patients and mice were spotted on Whatman filter cards to analyze FA content in blood by FA profiling. The results presented in Supplementary Table S5-1 and Figure 15 show that the FA content and Omega-3 index in whole blood varied between patients. The content of the omega-3 FAs eicosapentaenoic acid (EPA), docosapentaenoic acid (DPA) and docosahexaenoic acid (DHA), as well as the Omega-3 index, were highest in patient 17 who reported a daily intake of cod liver oil. Patient 19 had the lowest content of EPA and DHA, and Omega-3 index. This patient reported a daily intake of cod liver oil; however, only during wintertime (blood sample taken in August, Norwegian wintertime September to April).

Mouse blood samples were obtained before and after treatment to detect changes in blood FA content during treatment. In mice, the levels of EPA, DHA, and DPA significantly correlated with each other and the Omega-3 index as indicated in Supplementary Figure S5-1. An analysis of variance (ANOVA) on a hierarchical mixed model fitted to each FA and accounting for the measurements before and after treatment in the same mouse model, showed significant effects for oleic acid (OA), digamma linoleic acid (DGLA), arachidonic acid (AA), DPA, DHA, and the Omega-3 index (Figure 16). As expected, the average content of DHA as well as the Omega-3 index were higher in whole blood from the mice receiving fish oil compared to untreated mice (included blood samples from mice before treatment) as shown by a post hoc Tukey test. However, a rise in DHA content was not found in all mice within the fish oil group (mouse #22 and 27). Moreover, we also observed a trend of increased levels of DPA, DHA, and Omega-3 index for mice in the placebo group, although this was not statistically significant. The intake of long chain omega-3 FAs is known to reduce the content of long chain omega-6 FAs since they compete for the same enzymes during FA synthesis (reviewed in [18]). Mice from both treatment groups had reduced AA content in the blood compared to untreated mice; however, the level was lowest in the fish oil group.

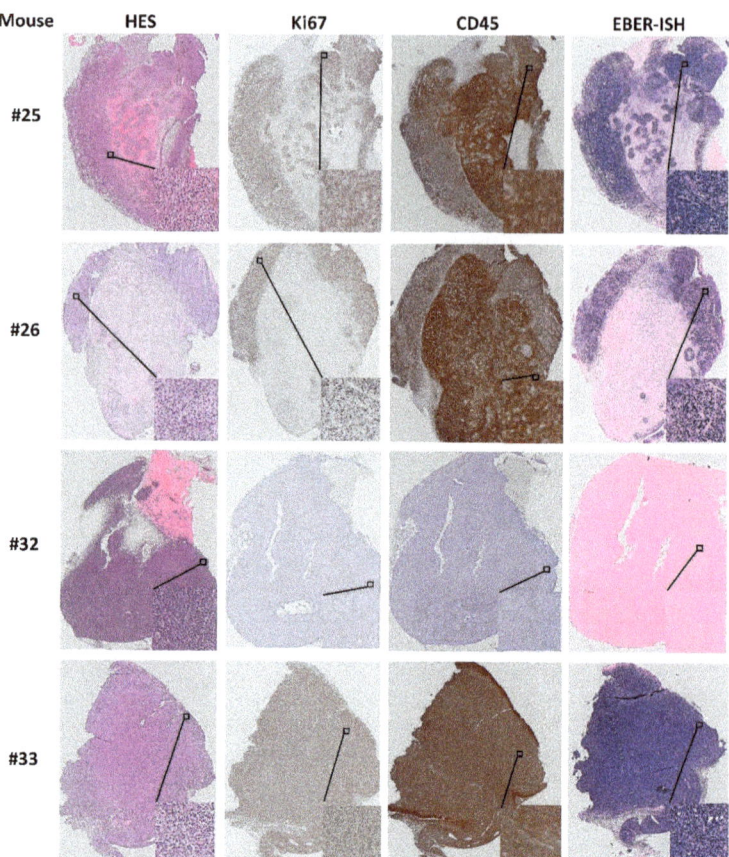

Figure 14. Characterization of lymphomas from mouse #25, 26, 32 and 33. HES, Ki67, CD45 and EBV RNA (EBER; see methods) staining.

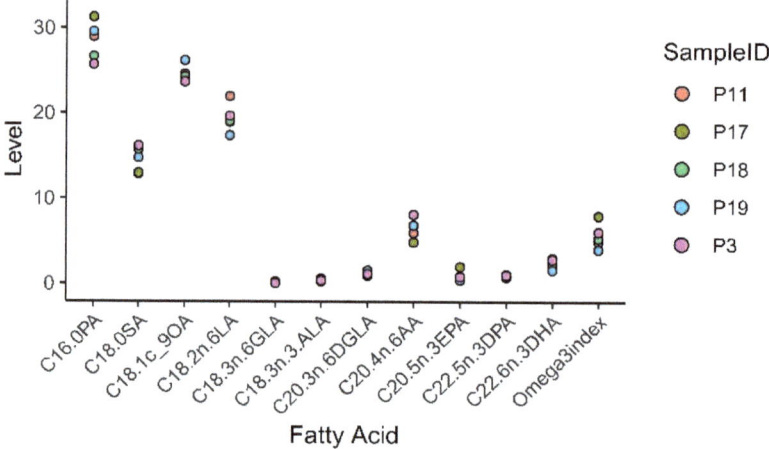

Figure 15. Patient whole blood omega-3 fatty acid (FA) profiling and Omega-3 index.

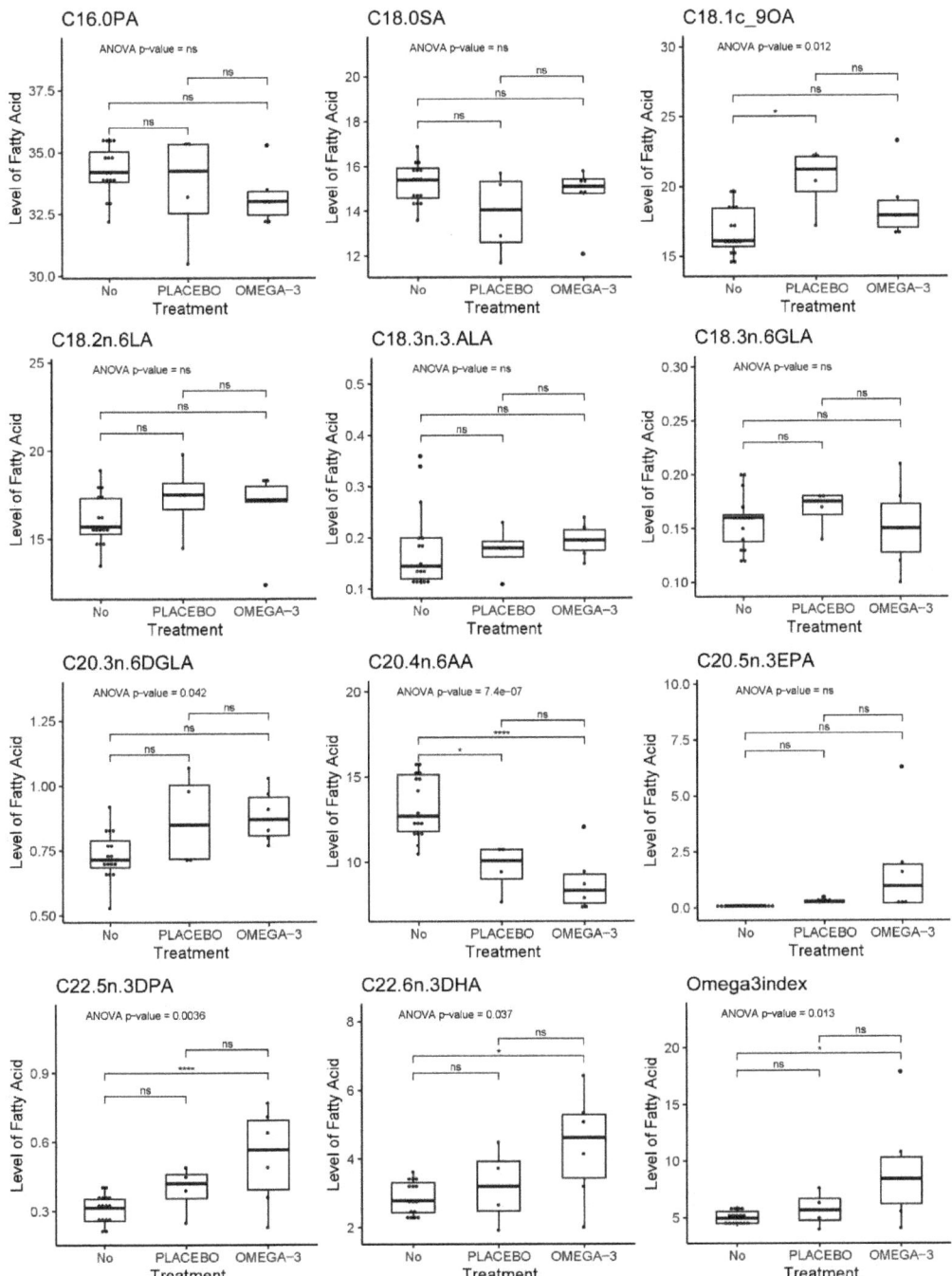

Figure 16. Mouse whole blood FA profiling and Omega-3 index. Stars indicate significant Tukey post hoc test. *p*-values indicate significance in the ANOVA model.

4. Discussion

The aim of this study was to establish a preclinical PDX model of CRC in immunodeficient mice and give a thorough presentation of the procedure. In addition, we wanted to evaluate administration of omega-3 FAs enriched in a liquid diet in this model.

PDXs preserve the biological characteristics of tumors better than CDX models, and therefore serve as a better research model for personalized cancer treatment. PDXs with established growth may be considered first generation xenografts, while several studies have made PDX lines (third generation PDX) stored in a PDX line biobank for future studies [19]. By using first generation xenografts there is a risk of failure to establish growth, while growth has already been confirmed with second or third generation PDX lines. However, in order to include more patients and use fewer mice, we decided to use first generation xenografts in this study. The study design and group sizes were based on the assumption that data obtained in animal studies typically have a standard deviation of 35%. Power calculations suggested that a sample size of $n > 10$ would allow detection of a 30% change with a significant level of 0.05 and a power of 0.08. However, we experienced that patient tumors had a high degree of heterogeneity and different tumorigenic levels. Not all tumors gave established PDXs, and if growth was established, the latency time was highly variable. Some mice developed abscesses or secondary tumors that reduced animal health and hence the PDX development time. These are important issues that we will address in future PDX studies to estimate required group sizes.

Successful PDX establishment relies on several factors, one of them being the animal host. The CIEA NOG mouse has been shown to be a good host for establishment of PDX models due to its severe immunodeficiency [7]. Tissue acquisition strategy is an important factor, and Katsiampoura et al. found that surgical tissue samples doubled the engraftment rate for PDXs compared to biopsies [11]. Based on this, we chose to use surgically removed tissue samples instead of tissue biopsies in our study. Katsiampoura et al. also found that previous cancer therapy reduced PDX engraftment rate due to the potential growth reduction effect on the tumor and reduction in viable cancer cells [11]. We therefore included treatment naïve patients that did not receive any preoperative treatment. In our study, time from tissue sampling from the tumor to engraftment in mice was up to 1 h. Others have found that implantation of tumor tissue after 12–24 h was equally effective as 2 h, which gives researchers a wider time frame to engraft the tissue samples [11]. For engraftment of tissue from the first two patient tumors, we used tumor fragments sized 50 mm^3, in line with the study by Katsiampoura et al. [11]. However, for the three last patient tumors, we reduced the size of tumor fragments to 30 mm^3 to reduce the size of the wound and possibly the distress to the mice. Other studies have used CRC tumor fragments as small as 1–2 mm^3 [20]. The engraftment site for the PDXs is also important to consider. During CDX studies, cancer cells are usually injected at the flank of the mouse. However, the CIEA NOG mice are very active and during initial tests, the mice opened the stiches and the wound within the first two hours after surgery. We therefore engrafted the tissue in front of the back curve of the mouse so that it would be less accessible. A possible drawback for studying CRC may be that this PDX model uses heterotopic subcutaneous engraftment of the CRC tissue, instead of using an orthotopic model where tissue is implanted into the original source organ in the animal. However, subcutaneous PDX models for CRC are readily used as they are easy to detect, monitor, and characterize (reviewed in [1]).

The first mice ($n = 8$) engrafted with tumor fragments were 11–13 weeks old compared to over 6 months old for the last mice ($n = 12$). The PDXs engrafted in mice at a younger age had a higher engraftment rate compared to the older mice. However, the engraftment rate may also be affected by the size of the tumor fragments, and younger mice were engrafted with larger tumor fragments compared with the older mice. In future PDX studies we will strive to use mice aged 8–12 weeks and use 3.5 × 3.5 mm tumor fragments to increase the PDX engraftment rate. When size of the tumor fragments is reduced, the amount of cancer cells implanted is also reduced, which may affect the growth of the xenografts. Larger fragments will likely represent the heterogeneity of the tumors to a larger extent.

The establishment of PDXs from gastrointestinal tumors has a higher engraftment rate compared to several other cancer types (reviewed in [6]). In this study the total successful engraftment rate was 50%, which is comparable to the engraftment rates reported in the studies by Chijiwa et al. (58% for gastrointestinal tumors) [21] and Katsiampoura et al. (56% for CRC) [11]. However, when using surgically removed CRC tumors for engraftment, Katsiampoura et al. found an engraftment rate of 72% [11], which is comparable to the study by Cho et al. and Wimsatt et al. that reported an engraftment rate of 67% and 64%, respectively [20,22]. When engrafting different types of cancer tissue in CIEA NOG mice, Fujii et al. found that CRC tissue had the highest engraftment rate at approximately 32% [23]. The engraftment rate will be affected by the latency time; that is, the time allowed for growth of the PDX to establish in the animal. In this pilot study, we chose to wait up to six months for growth to establish. However, studies have reported a latency time for CRC PDXs for up to 12 months ([11], reviewed in [24]). Hence, a longer latency time may increase the engraftment rate. In line with our findings, a recent study by Abdirahman et al. also reported an allowed six month latency period until established CRC PDX growth [19], and Chijiwa et al. stated that animals were sacrificed as "failed" if mice did not develop PDX growth over six months from engraftment [21].

The most common CRC tumor type is adenocarcinoma, representing over 90% of all colorectal carcinomas (reviewed in [25]). All five patient tumors in this study were adenocarcinomas, and most PDXs had similar differentiation as the original tumor. However, HES staining of the tumor from patient 11 showed that the tumor consisted mainly of signet ring cells. This is a rare type of CRC which is found in <1% of CRC cases (reviewed in [25]). The fact that the corresponding xenografts showed the same histology and signet ring cell type illustrates the correlation between histology of the original patient tumor and the corresponding PDXs. Signet ring cell carcinomas are often poorly differentiated (high grade) and may give a worse outcome compared to other adenocarcinomas. However, as shown in Table 1, the tumor from patient 11 was microsatellite instability high (MSI-H) and BRAF mutated, which gives an intermediate prognosis (reviewed in [25]). Whether this could affect the engraftment rate and latency time remains to be investigated.

When establishing PDX models, there is a risk of spontaneously developing mouse tumors. In our study, the secondary tumors were first detected close to the location of the xenograft. Hence, inspection and comparison of the histology and molecular markers from the primary tumors and the corresponding xenografts are necessary to be able to distinguish spontaneously growing tumors from xenografts, and to ensure that key characteristics of the original tumors are maintained in the PDXs.

The secondary tumors of mice #25, 26, 32 and 33 were recognized by pathology experts as lymphomas. However, the CIEA NOG mice are reported to have a very low incidence of developing spontaneous lymphomas [9,10]. Yasuda et al. reported spontaneously developing tumors in only 1.31% of the mice, and of these only 0.60% developed thymic lymphoma [10]. In our study, mice developing lymphoma had enlarged spleens with the presence of lymphoid cancer cells. The same was also reported by Yasuda et al. and Fujii et al. [10,17], indicating that the lymphoid cancer cells were distributed systemically. The low incidence of spontaneous lymphomas in CIEA NOG mice is due to the knockout of the *IL2Rg* gene [8]. Fujii et al. found that in 30% of the CRC PDX cases, lymphoma cells replaced the original tumor cells and that the morphology of these tumors was similar to EBV-transformed B cells in SCID mouse [23], which were reported in thirteen of fifty cases in a study by Itoh et al. [26]. Fujii et al. related the findings to the amount of B cells in the original specimen, which is known to be high in colorectal tissue, even though the tumors had nonlymphoid origin [23]. They reasoned that the severe immunodeficiency of the CIEA NOG mouse enhanced the effect of EBV [23]. Some studies have also shown the ability of EBV-transformed human B cells to form a lymphoid tumor as a result of outgrowth from the xenograft [27–31]. Both Choi et al. and Butler et al. found lymphomas with human origin only after the engraftment of the tumor tissue into NOG/NSG mice, but not nude mice [28,29]. They explained these findings by the loss of immune (NK) cells in the NOG/NSG mice compared to nude mice, which makes the NOG/NSG mice more vulnerable to the activation of EBV infected B cells compared to nude mice, which have active NK cells. Butler et al. found that the lymphoma incidence of human B cell origin could be reduced by giving the animals a single dose of the CD20 antibody rituximab at the engraftment time [28]. In our study, we found that three of four lymphomas consisted of human Ki67+ and CD45+ EBV transformed lymphoid cells. Hence the EBV was likely latent in lymphoid cells in the tumor, but at a very low level since it was not detected by EBER ISH in the patient samples. EBV is known as an oncovirus and is found latent in more than 90% of humans (reviewed in [32]). These rapidly growing lymphomas resulted in reduced time for the xenografts to establish due to increased tumor burden and/or reduced general health of the affected animals, as found in the study by Chjiwa et al. [21]. The lymphoma in mouse #32 was somewhat different from the three other lymphoma cases; the same lymphoid cancer cell type was found in the lungs, spleen, both shoulders and one hind leg, as well as in what was believed to be the remainder of the xenograft (Supplementary Figure S1-32-7). The lymphoma of mouse #32 was negative for human specific Ki67, CD20, CD45 and EBV, giving an indication that this lymphoma may be of murine origin. Despite the low rate of formation of spontaneous lymphomas in CIEA NOG mice, Yasuda et al. found thymic lymphoma to be the most common spontaneous tumors in NOG mice with a total incidence of 0.6% [10]. The NOD scid gamma (NSG) mice are also expected to have low incidence of spontaneous lymphomas. However, Moyer et al. found murine lymphomas in a PDX model in NSG mice and separated them from human-derived lymphomas using the same Ki67 MIB1 antibody as used in our study [33].

Three mice developed rapidly growing abscesses within one week after surgery. This may indicate that the tumor fragments were contaminated during the procedure or that the tumor tissue contained intracellular bacteria. For future studies we will provide the mice with antibiotics in the drinking water for 1 week after engraftment to reduce the risk of infection and the formation of abscesses.

Omega-3 PUFAs from fish oil have previously been shown to have a growth inhibitory effect on CRC cells both in vitro ([34,35], reviewed in [36]) and in vivo [37,38]. In addition, some studies have found omega-3 PUFAs to act as adjuvants to anticancer therapies [18]. Most studies that are testing treatment strategies involving omega-3 FA supplemented diets in animal studies have used omega-3 FA enriched pellet diets ([37,38], reviewed in [18]). However, Busquets et al. used oral administration of Smartfish Remune drink with omega-3 FAs as juice blocks to mice for 18 days in a CDX model, where significantly reduced primary tumor growth was observed [39]. We administered Smartfish Remune with fish oil or placebo to mice with established PDXs for 8 weeks. However, only mouse #23 completed the 8-week treatment period (placebo). The other mice were euthanized earlier (Table 3). We estimated that each mouse should drink 1.6 mL nutrition drink to achieve an adequate daily intake of DHA and EPA. Spillage was observed in cages of all mice receiving nutrition drink, meaning that the daily estimated intake was probably higher than the actual intake for all mice receiving treatment. Meanwhile, observations of mice drinking directly from the bottles, detection of nutrition drink in the stomach and results from the whole blood FA profiling, confirmed intake of the nutrition drink.

We performed FA quantification/profiling to investigate whether the patients' reported intake of fish and omega-3 supplements correlated with their FA profile. Patient 17 stated a daily intake of cod liver oil and had the highest whole blood levels of EPA, DPA and DHA, as well as the Omega-3 index. Patient 17 also had the lowest whole blood level of AA, an omega-6 PUFA known to be partially reduced in membrane phospholipids when omega-3 PUFA intake increases (reviewed in [18,40]). Patient 19 also stated to have a daily intake of cod liver oil but had the lowest Omega-3 index. However, this patient had a daily intake of cod liver oil at wintertime (Table 1), and the blood sample was taken in August. This probably influenced the EPA and DHA levels (which are included in the Omega-3 index) due to an assumed washout period for omega-3 PUFAs of about 12 weeks [41]. Although in vitro cell lines and in vivo animal studies show promising effects of omega-3 PUFAs on cancer growth, there have been few clinical trials exploring and providing evidence of a potential clinical anticancer effect of these PUFAs. However, there are studies reporting significant advantages of combining conventional cancer treatment with omega-3 PUFAs for some cancer types, and that a higher intake of marine omega-3 PUFAs after CRC diagnosis was associated with lower cancer-associated death and longer disease-free survival (reviewed in [18]).

FA profiling showed that the average content of the omega-3 PUFAs EPA, DPA, and DHA increased in both mice given fish oil and placebo compared to untreated animals, but the levels were highest and only significant in the mice provided with fish oil. Changes in the Omega-3 index and the DPA, as well as OA, DGLA, and AA content were statistically significant in the ANOVA analysis. Rapeseed oil is known to be rich in OA (over 50%) [42], and as expected, whole blood from mice given the placebo drink had the highest OA content. However, rapeseed oil does not contain EPA, DPA, or DHA, but it does contain around 8% ALA [42], which is the precursor for synthesis of EPA, DPA, and DHA in mammals. Several experimental animal studies using omega-3 enriched fish oil diets have used corn oil as control oil [18]; however, rapeseed oil was chosen due to lower concentration of omega-6 PUFAs. The reduction in the whole blood content of AA in both fish oil- and placebo treated mice may be considered positive, as AA is a precursor for omega-6 FA derived pro-inflammatory eicosanoids, while eicosanoids from the omega-3 FA EPA are considered anti-inflammatory (reviewed in [43]).

Regarding estimation of FA levels, whole blood reflects the content of both plasma and blood cells and is a more easily obtainable approach compared to using blood plasma [44]. Whole blood is readily sampled as dried blood spots (DBS) which is considered an adequate approach to analyze the content of FAs and long chain omega-3 PUFAs if FA oxidation is prevented [45,46]. Since the average levels of marine omega-3 PUFAs were highest in the mice receiving nutrition drink with fish oil, we consider the DBS analysis method for FA profiling as suitable for our study. This method also applies for analyses of cytokines and vitamin D levels.

5. Conclusions

In this study we established a method for the engraftment of CRC PDXs in CIEA NOG mice with an engraftment rate of 50%. The highest engraftment rate was obtained when engrafting larger tumor fragments in young mice. Max latency time was set to six months; however, this time frame should be extended in future PDX setups in order to increase the engraftment rate. The optimal engraftment site was in front of the back curve of the mice to prevent the mice from opening the wounds. Histological staining confirmed that the established PDXs originated from human CRC adenocarcinoma. Some of the older mice developed abscesses or secondary tumors which originated from human Ki67, CD45, and EBV positive lymphoid cells. These are important findings that researchers should be aware of when planning and performing PDX studies. We have presented a strategy to successfully provide mice with fish oil and placebo by liquid diets. The intake of omega-3 FAs was confirmed by the increased omega-3 ratio in blood. The PDX model described represents a valuable research tool for the assessment of different anticancer treatment strategies. Furthermore, the establishment of a biobank with tissue and blood samples from CRC patients will provide a unique platform for future translational research.

Supplementary Materials: The following are available online at https://www.mdpi.com/2227-9059/9/3/282/s1-s5: Supplementary file 1: Animal details; Supplementary file 2: Bullet point form for surgery and anesthesia log; Supplementary file 3: Bullet point form for euthanization, blood and tissue sampling; Supplementary file 4: Mice weight curves; Supplementary file 5: Fatty acid profiling.

Author Contributions: Conceptualization, H.S., P.S., A.W., S.A.S. and C.H.H.P.; formal analysis, L.C.O. and P.S.; funding acquisition, P.S., A.W., S.A.S. and C.H.H.P.; investigation, H.S., K.S.G., E.S.R.,

I.N. and C.H.H.P.; methodology, H.S., K.S.G., E.S.R., T.S.H., I.N. and C.H.H.P.; project administration, C.H.H.P.; resources, P.S., A.W., S.A.S. and C.H.H.P.; visualization, L.C.O., T.S.H. and C.H.H.P.; writing—original draft, H.S., L.C.O., I.N. and C.H.H.P.; writing—review and editing, H.S., L.C.O., K.S.G., E.S.R., T.S.H., I.N., P.S., A.W., S.A.S. and C.H.H.P. All authors have read and agreed to the published version of the manuscript.

Funding: This work was funded by The Joint Research Committee between the Faculty of Medicine and Health Sciences, Norwegian University of Science and Technology (NTNU), and St. Olav's University Hospital. Funding was also granted by The Cancer Fond at St. Olav's University Hospital, and the Faculty of Medicine and Health Sciences, NTNU through "strategic funding".

Institutional Review Board Statement: The study was conducted according to the guidelines of the Declaration of Helsinki, and approved by the Regional Ethics Committee for Central Norway (REC ID 2017/2048, date: 10 October 2018).

Informed Consent Statement: Informed consent was obtained from all subjects involved in the study.

Acknowledgments: The authors are especially grateful to the patients who agreed to contribute to this research project. We appreciate the effort by Line Furseth, Department of Surgery, St. Olav's University Hospital, for help during patient inclusion. We appreciate the expertise by Håkon Hov, Department of Pathology, St. Olav's University Hospital, during inspection of the HES stained lymphoma slides, and Duan Chen, IKOM, NTNU, for contribution to the project planning. The knowledge and expertise of the personnel at the Department of Surgery, Department of Pathology, and Biobank1, St. Olav's University Hospital, are highly appreciated. The animal experiments were performed at the CoMed Core Facility, NTNU. Histology and immunohistochemistry staining of tumors were performed at CMIC, NTNU. The statistical analyses were performed at BioCore, NTNU. CoMed, CMIC and BioCore are funded by the Faculty of Medicine at NTNU and Central Norway Regional Health Authority. Smartfish is acknowledged for supplementing Smartfish Remune Peach and Placebo.

Conflicts of Interest: The authors declare no conflict of interest.

References

1. Inoue, A.; Deem, A.K.; Kopetz, S.; Heffernan, T.P.; Draetta, G.F.; Carugo, A. Current and Future Horizons of Patient-Derived Xenograft Models in Colorectal Cancer Translational Research. *Cancers* **2019**, *11*, 1321. [CrossRef]
2. Yoshida, G.J. Applications of patient-derived tumor xenograft models and tumor organoids. *J. Hematol. Oncol.* **2020**, *13*, 4. [CrossRef] [PubMed]
3. Fujii, E.; Kato, A.; Suzuki, M. Patient-derived xenograft (PDX) models: Characteristics and points to consider for the process of establishment. *J. Toxicol. Pathol.* **2020**, *33*, 153–160. [CrossRef] [PubMed]
4. Cobb, L.M. The behaviour of carcinoma of the large bowel in man following transplantation into immune deprived mice. *Br. J. Cancer* **1973**, *28*, 400–411. [CrossRef] [PubMed]
5. Pickard, R.G.; Cobb, L.M.; Steel, G.G. The growth kinetics of xenografts of human colorectal tumours in immune deprived mice. *Br. J. Cancer* **1975**, *31*, 36–45. [CrossRef]
6. Brown, K.M.; Xue, A.; Mittal, A.; Samra, J.S.; Smith, R.; Hugh, T.J. Patient-derived xenograft models of colorectal cancer in pre-clinical research: A systematic review. *Oncotarget* **2016**, *7*, 66212–66225. [CrossRef] [PubMed]
7. Ito, M.; Hiramatsu, H.; Kobayashi, K.; Suzue, K.; Kawahata, M.; Hioki, K.; Ueyama, Y.; Koyanagi, Y.; Sugamura, K.; Tsuji, K.; et al. NOD/SCID/gamma(c)(null) mouse: An excellent recipient mouse model for engraftment of human cells. *Blood* **2002**, *100*, 3175–3182. [CrossRef]
8. Shultz, L.D.; Goodwin, N.; Ishikawa, F.; Hosur, V.; Lyons, B.L.; Greiner, D.L. Human cancer growth and therapy in immunodeficient mouse models. *Cold Spring Harb. Protoc.* **2014**, *2014*, 694–708. [CrossRef]
9. Kato, C.; Fujii, E.; Chen, Y.J.; Endaya, B.B.; Matsubara, K.; Suzuki, M.; Ohnishi, Y.; Tamaoki, N. Spontaneous thymic lymphomas in the non-obese diabetic/Shi-scid, IL-2R gamma (null) mouse. *Lab. Anim.* **2009**, *43*, 402–404. [CrossRef] [PubMed]
10. Yasuda, M.; Ogura, T.; Goto, T.; Yagoto, M.; Kamai, Y.; Shimomura, C.; Hayashimoto, N.; Kiyokawa, Y.; Shinohara, H.; Takahashi, R.; et al. Incidence of spontaneous lymphomas in non-experimental NOD/Shi-scid, IL-2Rgamma(null) (NOG) mice. *Exp. Anim.* **2017**, *66*, 425–435. [CrossRef]
11. Katsiampoura, A.; Raghav, K.; Jiang, Z.Q.; Menter, D.G.; Varkaris, A.; Morelli, M.P.; Manuel, S.; Wu, J.; Sorokin, A.V.; Rizi, B.S.; et al. Modeling of Patient Derived Xenografts in Colorectal Cancer. *Mol. Cancer Ther.* **2017**. [CrossRef] [PubMed]
12. Bray, F.; Ferlay, J.; Soerjomataram, I.; Siegel, R.L.; Torre, L.A.; Jemal, A. Global cancer statistics 2018: GLOBOCAN estimates of incidence and mortality worldwide for 36 cancers in 185 countries. *CA Cancer J. Clin.* **2018**, *68*, 394–424. [CrossRef] [PubMed]
13. Larsen, I.K. (Ed.) *Cancer in Norway 2016: Cancer Incidence, Mortality, Survival and Prevalence in Norway*; Cancer Registry of Norway: Oslo, Norway, 2017.

14. Constant, S.; Huang, S.; Wiszniewski, L.; Mas, C. Colon Cancer: Current Treatments and Preclinical Models for the Discovery and Development of New Therapies. In *Drug Discovery*; El-Shemy, H.A., Ed.; IntechOpen: Rijeka, Croatia, 2013. [CrossRef]
15. Nair, A.B.; Jacob, S. A simple practice guide for dose conversion between animals and human. *J. Basic Clin. Pharm.* **2016**, *7*, 27–31. [CrossRef]
16. Covelli, V. Guide to the Necroscopy of the Mouse. Available online: http://eulep.pdn.cam.ac.uk/Necropsy_of_the_Mouse/printable.php (accessed on 2 January 2020).
17. Fujii, E.; Kato, A.; Chen, Y.J.; Matsubara, K.; Ohnishi, Y.; Suzuki, M. Characterization of EBV-related lymphoproliferative lesions arising in donor lymphocytes of transplanted human tumor tissues in the NOG mouse. *Exp. Anim.* **2014**, *63*, 289–296. [CrossRef]
18. Dierge, E.; Larondelle, Y.; Feron, O. Cancer diets for cancer patients: Lessons from mouse studies and new insights from the study of fatty acid metabolism in tumors. *Biochimie* **2020**. [CrossRef] [PubMed]
19. Abdirahman, S.M.; Christie, M.; Preaudet, A.; Burstroem, M.C.U.; Mouradov, D.; Lee, B.; Sieber, O.M.; Putoczki, T.L. A Biobank of Colorectal Cancer Patient-Derived Xenografts. *Cancers* **2020**, *12*, 2340. [CrossRef]
20. Cho, Y.B.; Hong, H.K.; Choi, Y.L.; Oh, E.; Joo, K.M.; Jin, J.; Nam, D.H.; Ko, Y.H.; Lee, W.Y. Colorectal cancer patient-derived xenografted tumors maintain characteristic features of the original tumors. *J. Surg. Res.* **2014**, *187*, 502–509. [CrossRef]
21. Chijiwa, T.; Kawai, K.; Noguchi, A.; Sato, H.; Hayashi, A.; Cho, H.; Shiozawa, M.; Kishida, T.; Morinaga, S.; Yokose, T.; et al. Establishment of patient-derived cancer xenografts in immunodeficient NOG mice. *Int. J. Oncol.* **2015**, *47*, 61–70. [CrossRef] [PubMed]
22. Wimsatt, J.H.; Montgomery, C.; Thomas, L.S.; Savard, C.; Tallman, R.; Innes, K.; Jrebi, N. Assessment of a mouse xenograft model of primary colorectal cancer with special reference to perfluorooctane sulfonate. *PeerJ* **2018**, *6*, e5602. [CrossRef]
23. Fujii, E.; Suzuki, M.; Matsubara, K.; Watanabe, M.; Chen, Y.J.; Adachi, K.; Ohnishi, Y.; Tanigawa, M.; Tsuchiya, M.; Tamaoki, N. Establishment and characterization of in vivo human tumor models in the NOD/SCID/gamma(c)(null) mouse. *Pathol. Int.* **2008**, *58*, 559–567. [CrossRef]
24. Collins, A.T.; Lang, S.H. A systematic review of the validity of patient derived xenograft (PDX) models: The implications for translational research and personalised medicine. *PeerJ* **2018**, *6*, e5981. [CrossRef]
25. Fleming, M.; Ravula, S.; Tatishchev, S.F.; Wang, H.L. Colorectal carcinoma: Pathologic aspects. *J. Gastrointest. Oncol.* **2012**, *3*, 153–173. [CrossRef]
26. Itoh, T.; Shiota, M.; Takanashi, M.; Hojo, I.; Satoh, H.; Matsuzawa, A.; Moriyama, T.; Watanabe, T.; Hirai, K.; Mori, S. Engraftment of human non-Hodgkin lymphomas in mice with severe combined immunodeficiency. *Cancer* **1993**, *72*, 2686–2694. [CrossRef]
27. Bondarenko, G.; Ugolkov, A.; Rohan, S.; Kulesza, P.; Dubrovskyi, O.; Gursel, D.; Mathews, J.; O'Halloran, T.V.; Wei, J.J.; Mazar, A.P. Patient-Derived Tumor Xenografts Are Susceptible to Formation of Human Lymphocytic Tumors. *Neoplasia* **2015**, *17*, 735–741. [CrossRef]
28. Butler, K.A.; Hou, X.; Becker, M.A.; Zanfagnin, V.; Enderica-Gonzalez, S.; Visscher, D.; Kalli, K.R.; Tienchaianada, P.; Haluska, P.; Weroha, S.J. Prevention of Human Lymphoproliferative Tumor Formation in Ovarian Cancer Patient-Derived Xenografts. *Neoplasia* **2017**, *19*, 628–636. [CrossRef]
29. Choi, Y.Y.; Lee, J.E.; Kim, H.; Sim, M.H.; Kim, K.K.; Lee, G.; Kim, H.I.; An, J.Y.; Hyung, W.J.; Kim, C.B.; et al. Establishment and characterisation of patient-derived xenografts as paraclinical models for gastric cancer. *Sci. Rep.* **2016**, *6*, 22172. [CrossRef]
30. Mukohyama, J.; Iwakiri, D.; Zen, Y.; Mukohara, T.; Minami, H.; Kakeji, Y.; Shimono, Y. Evaluation of the risk of lymphomagenesis in xenografts by the PCR-based detection of EBV BamHI W region in patient cancer specimens. *Oncotarget* **2016**, *7*, 50150–50160. [CrossRef]
31. Radaelli, E.; Hermans, E.; Omodho, L.; Francis, A.; Vander Borght, S.; Marine, J.C.; van den Oord, J.; Amant, F. Spontaneous Post-Transplant Disorders in NOD.Cg- Prkdcscid Il2rgtm1Sug/JicTac (NOG) Mice Engrafted with Patient-Derived Metastatic Melanomas. *PLoS ONE* **2015**, *10*, e0124974. [CrossRef] [PubMed]
32. Fernandes, Q.; Gupta, I.; Vranic, S.; Al Moustafa, A.E. Human Papillomaviruses and Epstein-Barr Virus Interactions in Colorectal Cancer: A Brief Review. *Pathogens* **2020**, *9*, 300. [CrossRef] [PubMed]
33. Moyer, A.M.; Yu, J.; Sinnwell, J.P.; Dockter, T.J.; Suman, V.J.; Weinshilboum, R.M.; Boughey, J.C.; Goetz, M.P.; Visscher, D.W.; Wang, L. Spontaneous murine tumors in the development of patient-derived xenografts: A potential pitfall. *Oncotarget* **2019**, *10*, 3924–3930. [CrossRef] [PubMed]
34. Samdal, H.; Sandmoe, M.A.; Olsen, L.C.; Jarallah, E.A.H.; Hoiem, T.S.; Schonberg, S.A.; Pettersen, C.H.H. Basal level of autophagy and MAP1LC3B-II as potential biomarkers for DHA-induced cytotoxicity in colorectal cancer cells. *FEBS J.* **2018**. [CrossRef]
35. Pettersen, K.; Monsen, V.T.; Hakvag Pettersen, C.H.; Overland, H.B.; Pettersen, G.; Samdal, H.; Tesfahun, A.N.; Lundemo, A.G.; Bjorkoy, G.; Schonberg, S.A. DHA-induced stress response in human colon cancer cells—Focus on oxidative stress and autophagy. *Free. Radic. Biol. Med.* **2016**, *90*, 158–172. [CrossRef]
36. Eltweri, A.M.; Thomas, A.L.; Metcalfe, M.; Calder, P.C.; Dennison, A.R.; Bowrey, D.J. Potential applications of fish oils rich in omega-3 polyunsaturated fatty acids in the management of gastrointestinal cancer. *Clin. Nutr.* **2017**, *36*, 65–78. [CrossRef]
37. Bathen, T.F.; Holmgren, K.; Lundemo, A.G.; Hjelstuen, M.H.; Krokan, H.E.; Gribbestad, I.S.; Schonberg, S.A. Omega-3 fatty acids suppress growth of SW620 human colon cancer xenografts in nude mice. *Anticancer Res.* **2008**, *28*, 3717–3723. [PubMed]
38. Zou, S.; Meng, X.; Meng, Y.; Liu, J.; Liu, B.; Zhang, S.; Ding, W.; Wu, J.; Zhou, J. Microarray analysis of anti-cancer effects of docosahexaenoic acid on human colon cancer model in nude mice. *Int. J. Clin. Exp. Med.* **2015**, *8*, 5075–5084. [PubMed]

39. Busquets, S.; Marmonti, E.; Oliva, F.; Simoes, E.; Luna, D.; Mathisen, J.S.; López-Soriano, F.J.; Öhlander, M.; Argilés, J.M. Omega-3 and omega-3/curcumin-enriched fruit juices decrease tumour growth and reduce muscle wasting in tumour-bearing mice. *JCSM Rapid Commun.* **2018**, *1*, 1–10. [CrossRef]
40. Larsson, S.C.; Kumlin, M.; Ingelman-Sundberg, M.; Wolk, A. Dietary long-chain n-3 fatty acids for the prevention of cancer: A review of potential mechanisms. *Am. J. Clin. Nutr.* **2004**, *79*, 935–945. [CrossRef] [PubMed]
41. Watson, H.; Mitra, S.; Croden, F.C.; Taylor, M.; Wood, H.M.; Perry, S.L.; Spencer, J.A.; Quirke, P.; Toogood, G.J.; Lawton, C.L.; et al. A randomised trial of the effect of omega-3 polyunsaturated fatty acid supplements on the human intestinal microbiota. *Gut* **2018**, *67*, 1974–1983. [CrossRef]
42. Norwegian Food Safety Authority. Rapeseed Oil, The Norwegian Food Composition Table. Available online: www.matvaretabellen.no (accessed on 5 January 2020).
43. Patterson, E.; Wall, R.; Fitzgerald, G.F.; Ross, R.P.; Stanton, C. Health implications of high dietary omega-6 polyunsaturated Fatty acids. *J. Nutr. Metab.* **2012**, *2012*, 539426. [CrossRef]
44. Rise, P.; Eligini, S.; Ghezzi, S.; Colli, S.; Galli, C. Fatty acid composition of plasma, blood cells and whole blood: Relevance for the assessment of the fatty acid status in humans. *Prostaglandins Leukot. Essent. Fat. Acids* **2007**, *76*, 363–369. [CrossRef]
45. Liu, G.; Muhlhausler, B.S.; Gibson, R.A. A method for long term stabilisation of long chain polyunsaturated fatty acids in dried blood spots and its clinical application. *Prostaglandins Leukot. Essent. Fat. Acids* **2014**, *91*, 251–260. [CrossRef] [PubMed]
46. Harris, W.L.; Polreis, J. Measurement of the Omega-3 Index in Dried Blood Spots. *Ann. Clin. Lab. Res.* **2016**, *4*, 1–7. [CrossRef]

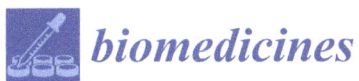

Article

TCox: Correlation-Based Regularization Applied to Colorectal Cancer Survival Data

Carolina Peixoto [1], Marta B. Lopes [2,3], Marta Martins [4], Luís Costa [4,5] and Susana Vinga [1,*]

1. INESC-ID, Instituto Superior Técnico, Universidade de Lisboa, Rua Alves Redol 9, 1000-029 Lisboa, Portugal; anacpeixoto@tecnico.ulisboa.pt
2. NOVA Laboratory for Computer Science and Informatics (NOVA LINCS), FCT, UNL, 2829-516 Caparica, Portugal; marta.lopes@fct.unl.pt
3. Centro de Matemática e Aplicações (CMA), FCT, UNL, 2829-516 Caparica, Portugal
4. Instituto de Medicina Molecular-João Lobo Antunes, Faculdade de Medicina, Universidade de Lisboa, Avenida Professor Egas Moniz, 1649-028 Lisboa, Portugal; marta.martins@medicina.ulisboa.pt (M.M.); lmcosta@medicina.ulisboa.pt (L.C.)
5. Oncology Division, Hospital de Santa Maria, Centro Hospitalar Lisboa Norte, 1649-028 Lisboa, Portugal
* Correspondence: susanavinga@tecnico.ulisboa.pt

Received: 17 September 2020; Accepted: 6 November 2020; Published: 10 November 2020

Abstract: Colorectal cancer (CRC) is one of the leading causes of mortality and morbidity in the world. Being a heterogeneous disease, cancer therapy and prognosis represent a significant challenge to medical care. The molecular information improves the accuracy with which patients are classified and treated since similar pathologies may show different clinical outcomes and other responses to treatment. However, the high dimensionality of gene expression data makes the selection of novel genes a problematic task. We propose TCox, a novel penalization function for Cox models, which promotes the selection of genes that have distinct correlation patterns in normal vs. tumor tissues. We compare TCox to other regularized survival models, Elastic Net, HubCox, and OrphanCox. Gene expression and clinical data of CRC and normal (TCGA) patients are used for model evaluation. Each model is tested 100 times. Within a specific run, eighteen of the features selected by TCox are also selected by the other survival regression models tested, therefore undoubtedly being crucial players in the survival of colorectal cancer patients. Moreover, the TCox model exclusively selects genes able to categorize patients into significant risk groups. Our work demonstrates the ability of the proposed weighted regularizer TCox to disclose novel molecular drivers in CRC survival by accounting for correlation-based network information from both tumor and normal tissue. The results presented support the relevance of network information for biomarker identification in high-dimensional gene expression data and foster new directions for the development of network-based feature selection methods in precision oncology.

Keywords: regularized optimization; Cox regression; survival analysis; TCGA data; RNA-seq data

1. Introduction

Colorectal cancer (CRC) is one of the leading causes of mortality and morbidity in the world. It is the third most commonly occurring cancer in men and the second in women, accounting for approximately 1.8 million new cases in 2018 and 880,792 deaths worldwide [1].

The pathogenesis of CRC results from the accumulation of genetic and epigenetic alterations that lead to the transformation of normal glandular epithelial cells into invasive adenocarcinomas. The majorities of CRCs (75%) are sporadic in origin and occur in people without genetic predisposition or family history of CRC. The other cases are familial or related to inflammatory bowel diseases [2].

Several types of genomic instability have been described in CRCs and may facilitate the acquisition of multiple tumor-associated mutations such as chromosomal instability, which generates gene deletions and duplications and occurs in 70–85% of CRCs, and microsatellite instability, characterized by mutations at nucleotide repeat sequences and accounting for 15% of sporadic CRCs [3,4]. This genomic instability may lead to a higher inter-patient and intra-tumor heterogeneity, being a great challenge for both diagnosis and cancer therapy [5,6]. Thus, it is essential to understand the molecular basis of individual susceptibility to colorectal cancer and to determine factors that initiate tumor development, drive its progression, and determine its responsiveness or resistance to antitumor agents.

During the past few years, high-throughput functional genomics has made notable progress. The development of novel high-throughput sequencing techniques such as RNA sequencing (RNA-seq) provided new methods for mapping and quantifying transcriptomes [7]. Furthermore, RNA-seq allows the study of the gene expression profile of thousands of genes simultaneously, providing a better view of the genetic pathways, showing genes that may be highly correlated or redundant [8]. Moreover, this rising of genome sequencing technologies contributes to more precise medicine, where the molecular information improves the accuracy with which patients are classified and treated [9]. Indeed, molecular data are particularly important in cancer studies, where patients with similar pathologies may show different clinical outcomes and different responses to treatment [10].

However, the high dimensionality of gene expression data makes the selection of novel biomarkers a difficult task, since the number of individuals (N) is typically much smaller than the number of genes (p covariates). In fact, $N \ll p$ leads to a high-dimensional problem that may cause instability in the selected genes [11]. Thus, to lower the dimensionality of the data, feature selection via model regularization has been applied in classification and also Cox survival models in the context of precision oncology [10,12,13]. For instance, in Cox regression, this corresponds to adding a penalty term to the partial log-likelihood of the Cox model, which sets some variables' coefficients to zero. The Elastic Net (EN) penalty [14] and its particular case of the Least absolute shrinkage and selection operator (Lasso) [15] are state-of-the-art strategies for regularization-based feature selection.

Extensions to the above penalties to account for network-based information have been proposed in the context of cancer genomics. Penalty terms based on centrality measures of the nodes (genes) in the network have been suggested, such as the degree, therefore penalizing the variables based on their role in the overall network [12,16], and also by promoting the smoothness of the parameters across adjacent nodes in the network [17]. Network-based regularizers built on the correlation between the variables in different groups have also been proposed [13,18]. The central premise is that biomolecular networks in different cancer or cell types exhibit distinct network-based correlation patterns that might be regarded as biomarkers for disease/cell typing, but also similarities whose relevance might be investigated in the definition of common therapies for distinct disease conditions. Correlation has long been used for feature selection in classification and regression problems [19], in high-dimensional benchmark datasets [20], for early diagnosis and cancer progression based on cancer and normal biomolecular networks [21], for multivariate differential coexpression analysis between two conditions based on the complete correlation structure between genes [22], and for weighted gene co-expression network analysis for the discovery of the relationship between networks/genes and phenotypes in cancer, e.g., disease stage and overall survival [23,24].

In this work, we propose TCox, a correlation-based regularizer for feature selection in Cox regression models applied to transcriptomic data. This regularizer considers the differences in correlation between genes' networks in healthy and in cancer tissues, promoting the selection of genes with different correlation patterns in the two conditions. The key underlying hypothesis of TCox is that a gene with distinct interactions in the normal and tumor groups, given by its correlation with the other genes in the network, might have a potential association with patient survival. This regularizer was applied to colorectal cancer RNA-seq data to identify key genes in the survival outcomes and putative therapy targets of cancer patients.

2. Materials and Methods

To disclose transcriptomic signatures in CRC, the model performances of survival models based on regularized Cox regression were evaluated over a range of different model parameters and data partitions. The analysis pipeline of this study is described in Figure 1.

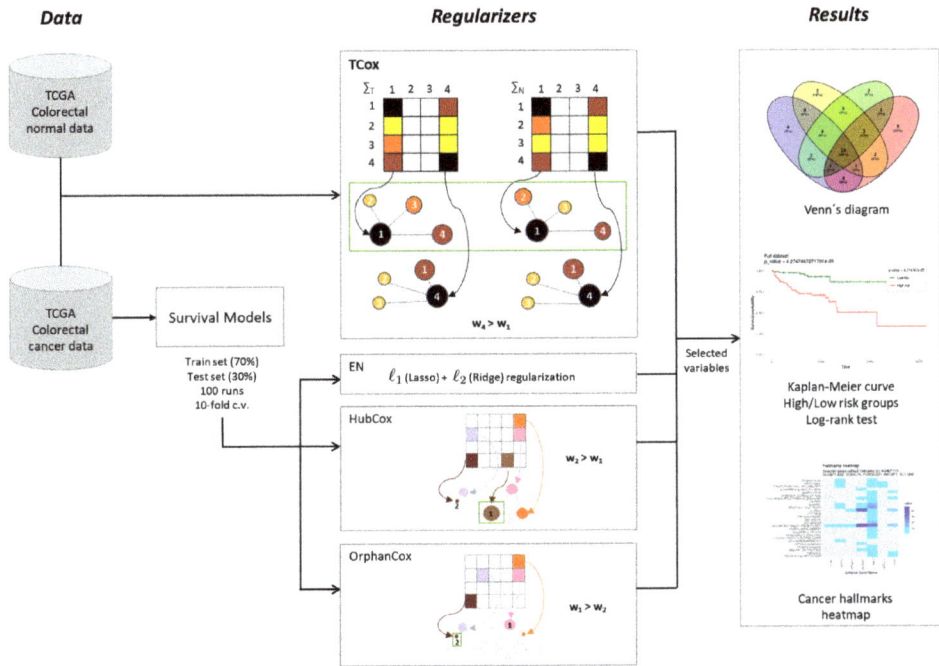

Figure 1. Methodological procedure for the identification of gene signatures in colorectal cancer data.

2.1. Datasets

Transcriptomic and clinical data of colorectal cancer patients were obtained from The Cancer Genome Atlas (TCGA) through the Genomic Data Commons (GDC) data portal [25]. Colon Adenocarcinoma (COAD) and Rectum Adenocarcinoma (READ) RNA-seq Fragments Per Kilobase per Million (FPKM) data were imported using the RTCGAtoolbox R package [26]. The COAD transcriptomic dataset is comprised of 20,501 variables (genes) for a total of 328 samples (patients), 282 corresponding to primary solid tumor and 46 to normal tissue samples; the READ dataset has 20,501 variables for a total of 105 samples, 91 corresponding to primary solid tumor and 14 to normal tissue samples. Both datasets were merged and used for further analysis. Regarding clinical data, the colorectal cancer patient *status* (dead or alive) and *days to death* variables were selected for 595 samples. A total of 357 samples with both clinical and RNA-seq data were used for further analysis.

2.2. Survival Analysis

The analysis of the course of a disease in time is a crucial feature for cancer characterization, including prognosis and optimal therapies' definition [27]. Survival analysis studies the time until an event of interest occurs (such as death) [28]. An inherent feature of survival times is that sometimes, the event of interest is not observed, either because the patient dropped out of the study or the study finished and the event did not occur during that time-frame, thus leading to censored survival times [27]. The Kaplan–Meier method allows the estimation of the population's proportion that would survive given a particular length of time, under the same circumstances, using both complete and censored survival times [28]. The comparison of the survival curves of two groups is often performed using a formal non-parametric statistical test called the log-rank test [29]. To adjust for multiple variables or factors, the proportional hazards regression model was proposed [30] and is briefly described below.

2.2.1. Cox Regression

The Cox regression model is a multiple regression model for the analysis of censored survival data. It is used to study the association between the features and the hazard function through [27]. The hazard function gives the instantaneous potential (per unit time) for the event of interest to occur, given that the individual has survived up to that time [31].

$$h_i(t) = h_0(t) \exp(\mathbf{x}_i^T \boldsymbol{\beta}), \tag{1}$$

where $h_i(t)$ represents the hazard function of individual $i = 1, \ldots, n$, $h_0(t)$ represents the baseline hazard, $\mathbf{x}_i = (x_{i1}, x_{i2}, \ldots, x_{ip})^T$ are the measured covariates, and $\boldsymbol{\beta} = (\beta_1, \beta_2, \ldots, \beta_p)$ are the regression coefficients.

The inference is made by maximizing the partial log-likelihood, given by:

$$l(\boldsymbol{\beta}) = \sum_{i=1}^{n} \delta_i \left(\mathbf{x}_i^T \boldsymbol{\beta} - \log \sum_{j \in R_i} \exp(\mathbf{x}_j^T \boldsymbol{\beta}) \right), \tag{2}$$

where $R_i = R(t_i) = \{j : t_j \geq t_i\}$ denotes the set of all individuals that are at risk at t_i, i.e., with a follow-up time greater than or equal to t_i, and δ_i indicates if the event was observed ($\delta_i = 1$) or not ($\delta_i = 0$) for patient i.

Model regularizers have been proposed to cope with the high-dimensional nature of modern datasets, such as gene expression data, comprising thousands of highly-correlated features. In Cox regression, a penalty term $F(\boldsymbol{\beta})$ is added to the partial log-likelihood $l(\boldsymbol{\beta})$ of the Cox model. In particular, the Elastic Net (EN) penalty, given by:

$$F(\boldsymbol{\beta}) = \lambda \left\{ \alpha \|\boldsymbol{\beta}\|_1 + (1 - \alpha) \|\boldsymbol{\beta}\|_2^2 \right\}, \tag{3}$$

combines two different regularizers, the ridge penalty (ℓ_2-norm regularization), which shrinks the coefficients and helps to reduce the model complexity, and the Lasso (ℓ_1-norm regularization), which can lead the coefficients to zero, therefore performing feature selection [14]. The penalty is controlled by α and bridges the gap between Lasso ($\alpha = 1$) and ridge ($\alpha = 0$).

Network-based regularizers have also been proposed in the context of cancer genomics. The `glmSparseNet` package generalizes sparse regression models including a network-based regularizer when genes show a graph structure [12]. The models are built based on the `glmnet` [32] family of models, by including centrality measures of the network as penalty weights in the regularization term. The resulting network-based penalty is related to the weights attributed to each gene or node, either promoting highly connected genes (hub genes) or isolated genes (orphan genes) [12].

2.2.2. TCox

To identify features (genes) that have distinct roles in cancer and normal tissue, we propose TCox. This new weighted regularizer promotes the selection of genes with distinct correlation patterns across tumor and normal tissue through Cox regression. TCox departs from a recently proposed method that also uses a correlation-based regularizer and exhibits promising results in identifying biomarkers [13]. The `twiner` is based on sparse logistic regression and enables the selection of gene signatures shared by two diseases in breast and prostate cancer. The correlation structure was also relevant to identify heterogeneity factors in glioblastoma [18]. Instead of trying to retrieve similar correlation patterns, TCox promotes genes that exhibit distinct relationships between two groups, thus highlighting potential differences in the corresponding sub-networks.

Given the tumor and normal datasets, TCox builds the correlation matrices, $\Sigma_T = [\sigma_1^T, \sigma_2^T, ..., \sigma_p^T]$, and $\Sigma_N = [\sigma_1^N, \sigma_2^N, ..., \sigma_p^N]$, respectively. Each column σ_j corresponds to the correlation of gene j with the remaining ones. The dissimilarity measure of gene j between the two datasets can be defined as:

$$d_j(T, N) = \arccos \frac{<\sigma_j^T, \sigma_j^N>}{\|\sigma_j^T\| \cdot \|\sigma_j^N\|}, j = 1, \ldots, p. \quad (4)$$

Two patterns are considered identical if the angle between the corresponding vectors is zero. In the context of this work, since we were looking for dissimilarities (tumor vs. normal), angles equal to zero were discarded. The goal is not to select genes that exhibit the same correlation pattern between tumor and normal tissues, but rather identify those that behave very differently in the two tissue types, i.e., being correlated in distinct ways.

The dissimilarity term is then normalized by their maximum value, as follows:

$$w_j = \frac{d_j(T, N)}{\max_k d_k(T, N)}, \quad j, k = 1, \ldots, p. \quad (5)$$

The resulting **w** vector is then used as a weight factor in the EN regularizer, controlling how much the parameter λ affects each coefficient, as follows:

$$F(\boldsymbol{\beta}) = \lambda \left\{ \alpha \|\mathbf{w} \circ \boldsymbol{\beta}\|_1 + (1 - \alpha) \|\mathbf{w} \circ \boldsymbol{\beta}\|_2^2 \right\}. \quad (6)$$

where $\circ$ represents the Hadamard or entry-wise vector product, i.e., $\mathbf{w} \circ \boldsymbol{\beta} = w_1 \beta_1 + \ldots + w_p \beta_p$.

Genes with a larger dissimilarity between the two correlation matrices are less penalized in TCox, which does not hold in the present form of w. With the goal of favoring the selection of the most dissimilar genes across tumor and normal correlation data matrices, several transformations of w were considered and tested, namely $1 - w$, $1 - w^3$, $(1 - w)^3$, $\frac{1}{w}$, $\exp(-w^3)$, and $\exp((1 - w)^3)$.

Among the transformations tested using colorectal RNA-seq data, the $\frac{1}{w}$ transformation was chosen, since it yielded the lowest p-values in the separation of high- and low-risk survival curves, over the values of α evaluated (Figure 2). In the resulting penalty factor, for a certain gene in the network, the more different the correlation pattern across datasets is, the less penalized it will be in the regularization term of the Cox regression.

To evaluate the accuracy of TCox, we compared this approach with the above-mentioned survival methods, namely Cox regression based on the EN penalty, herein called EN, and HubCoxand OrphanCox models. TCox and Cox regression based on EN were built using the glmnet R package and the HubCox and OrphanCox models using the glmSparseNet package.

2.3. Model Evaluation and Comparison

Samples were randomly divided into a training set for model construction and a test set for model evaluation, comprising 70% and 30% of the data, respectively. Both subsets had the same proportion of censored samples.

The survival analysis was performed using four models: EN, HubCox, OrphanCox, and TCox. All models were estimated from 100 randomly generated runs with $\alpha = 0.1$ for both the training and the test sets. Among the 100 runs tested, only a few were statistically significant (Table 1), and none yielded significant results for the four methods simultaneously in the test set. The results presented hereafter were obtained using the run that showed statistically significant results for the test set in three models: TCox, HubCox, and EN. Afterwards, to analyze the level of sparsity of the models using the same partition obtained earlier, the α parameter was set between $\alpha = 0.3$ and $\alpha = 0.05$, which provides a feasible number of features to be further analyzed. To evaluate the performance of the models, the observations were split into two groups defined by the median of the fitted relative risks. This procedure allows performing the log-rank test via the Kaplan–Meier estimator and assessing if the two groups' mortality is the same by evaluating the corresponding p-values. The selected variables using $\alpha = 0.1$ were compared between models and queried in the CHAT (Cancer Hallmarks Analytics Tool [33]) to assess the association between the selected genes and cancer hallmarks based on previous studies.

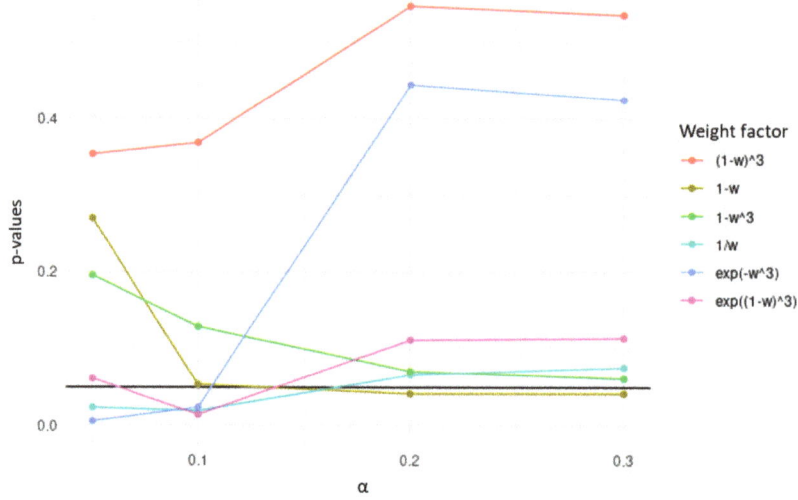

Figure 2. p-values obtained in the separation of high- and low-risk survival curves based on the genes selected by TCox models generated with transformations of w using colorectal RNA-seq data, tested over different α values.

Table 1. Results from 100 runs of training and test sets in all survival models analyzed using $\alpha = 0.1$. S—statistically significant runs (p-value < 0.05); NS—non-statistically significant runs; #—number of runs.

Models	TCox			EN			HubCox			OrphanCox		
Runs Test set	NA	S	NS	NA	S	NS	NA	S	NS	NA	S	NS
#	33	7	60	31	4	65	43	3	54	32	2	66
Mean p-value	–	0.0164	0.4985	–	0.0251	0.5354	–	0.0137	0.5168	–	0.0160	0.4997

2.4. Availability of Data

All the implementations and R code described are freely available at https://github.com/sysbiomed/TCox, thus ensuring full reproducibility of the presented results. To perform all the analysis, we used the following R packages: to download TCGA data, we used RTCGAToolbox; regarding general preprocessing and visualization, we used dplyr [34], ggplot2 [35], and survminer [36]; for differential gene expression analysis, we used edgeR [37]; and for survival analysis and regularization, we used survival [38], glmnet [32], glmSparseNet [12], and biospear [39].

3. Results and Discussion

TCox regression models were built based on the TCGA colorectal RNA-seq data from tumor and normal tissue samples to find a molecular signature comprising genes with a distinct correlation pattern in tumor and normal tissue networks. For biomarker and model evaluation, three different α were considered (0.3, 0.2, and 0.1) for the run chosen, thus selecting a different number of variables (Table 2). Most α values enabled the selection of a set of variables yielding significance (given by a p-value lower than 0.05) in the separation of the survival curves of high- and low-risk patients for the test set. Figure 3 illustrates a representative survival curve based on the variables selected by the TCox model in the training and test datasets, highlighting the significance of the selected gene set in the separation of the two risk groups.

Table 2. Summary of TCox, EN, HubCox, and OrphanCox model results showing the number of selected variables and the p-values obtained for the training and test sets.

Survival Models	α	Selected Variables	p-Value Train	p-Value Test
TCox ($\frac{1}{w}$)	0.3	10	0.002401583	0.0757
	0.2	11	0.000588251	0.0665
	0.1	53	2.66444×10^{-9}	0.0194
EN	0.3	18	8.38703×10^{-7}	0.0088
	0.2	47	2.47428×10^{-8}	0.0717
	0.1	88	5.28787×10^{-9}	0.0492
HubCox	0.3	26	1.78804×10^{-8}	0.0138
	0.2	47	1.18224×10^{-8}	0.0129
	0.1	90	2.74104×10^{-9}	0.0418
OrphanCox	0.3	8	2.48965×10^{-5}	0.1519
	0.2	44	1.20494×10^{-7}	0.0327
	0.1	67	6.80248×10^{-9}	0.0632

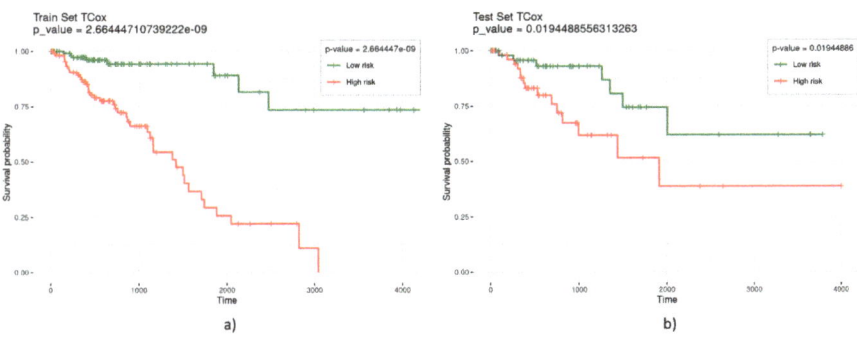

Figure 3. Kaplan–Meier curves obtained from the (**a**) training and (**b**) test sets, based on the variables selected by the TCox model with $\alpha = 0.1$.

The accuracy of the TCox survival model was compared against a Cox model with the EN penalty, HubCox, and OrphanCox survival models. Overall, in most runs, models were not able to significantly separate high- vs. low-risk groups (Table 1). Within the 100 runs tested using $\alpha = 0.1$, only a few runs were statistically significant in terms of the log-rank test using the estimated Cox parameters and median risks. The percentage of data partitions for which the models could not be estimated was 33% (TCox), 31% (EN), 43% (HubCox), and 32% (OrphanCox). Concerning the significant runs (p-value < 0.05), the 4%, 3%, and 2% significant runs were obtained with EN, HubCox, and OrphanCox models, respectively, whereas TCox yielded 7% significant runs. These results may be an indication that the model performance is highly dependent on the data partition and might foster further research directions to cope with this limitation [40]. Besides these techniques, we also tested adaptive Lasso to evaluate other methods that are also based on sparsity and weighted regularization. However, the results were not statistically significant and, therefore, were not included.

Regarding the variables selected by the models, genes that were selected for at least 50% or 75% of the runs are listed in Table 3. One of the genes, *ELFN1*, was selected in at least 50% of the runs by the EN, HubCox, and TCox models. Interestingly, it was demonstrated that this gene enhanced both cell proliferation and migration in CRC [41].

Table 3. List of genes selected for at least 50% or 75% of the runs by all methods tested.

Runs		TCox	EN	HubCox	OrphanCox
75%	#	3	2	2	1
	genes	GABRD, NKAIN4, ZIC3	ELFN1, LOC646498	ELFN1, LOC646498	LOC646498
50%	#	16	16	16	1
	genes	ASB10, ASPHD1, CST2, CT45A3, CYP19A1, DAD1L, ELFN1, FOXS1, GABRD, GH2, HIST1H2BG, HIST1H4H, NKAIN4, RHOXF2B, ZIC3, ZNF676	CLEC18C, EEPD1, ELFN1, HIST2H2BA, HIST2H2BE, KCNMB3, LOC100270710, LOC220930, LOC646498, NELF, ONECUT1, PRRX2, PRSSL1, RFPL4B, SIX2, TAS2R20	EEPD1, ELFN1, HIST1H2AE, HIST2H2BA, HIST2H2BE, KCNMB3, LOC100270710, LOC220930, LOC338758, LOC646498, NELF, ONECUT1, PRRX2, PRSSL1, TAS2R20, ZNF676	LOC646498

Considering the results obtained for the representative run selected, TCox showed the lowest p-value for $\alpha = 0.1$ in the test set (Figure 4). When comparing the genes selected by the models tested using $\alpha = 0.1$ (an α-value that selected a reasonable number of genes to be further evaluated), some of the genes found, i.e., 18 genes, were selected by all four models (Figure 5).

Differential gene expression analysis using the edgeR package was performed to assess which genes were found to be up- or down-regulated in tumor tissue (Table 4).

Table 4. Genes selected by all models evaluated and selected exclusively by EN, HubCox, OrphanCox, and TCox. Arrows indicate if genes were found to be up- (↑) or down-regulated (↓) in tumoral tissue (differential gene expression analysis was performed using the edgeR R package).

All models	CYP7A1 (↓), FAM159A (↓), ZNF883, CLDN9 (↑), LBX2 (↑), MEIG1, PAX5 (↓), NKAIN4 (↓), ZDHHC19 (↓), GRAPL, PCDHB12 (↓), EEPD1 (↑), HPCAL1, PGAM2 (↓), LOC732275, FAM138B (↓), LOC646498, PRCD (↓)
EN	HOTAIR (↑), GJA3 (↑), LOC283663 (↓), DNAI2 (↓), NELF (↑), GUCA1B
HubCox	CYGB (↓), UNC13B, LIPT2 (↑), RFT1 (↑), BEND4 (↓), FAM24B (↑), SLFN11, RASGRP2 (↓)
TCox	ANKRD26P1 (↑), CARKD, IGLON5, OSTN (↓), RAB20, TXNL4B (↑), AOX2P, DCLK3 (↑), FCRL2 (↓), SEPT7P2 (↑), ASPHD1 (↑), COL19A1 (↓), DCP1A, FLJ16779 (↑), LOC100303728 (↓), PCDHA7, SNTG1, COX4I2, NXF2B (↑), TAC3 (↓), C20orf106, LOC285780 (↓), OR2T5, TERF2IP, CAPN7, OSBPL3 (↑), TRIM67 (↓)

Among those, eight genes were found to be associated with the hallmarks of cancer (Figure 6). Specifically, the models identified genes involved in metabolism (*CYP7A1* and *PGAM2*), tight junction formation (*CLDN9*), photoreceptor stability and transduction (*PRCD* and *HPCAL1*, respectively), genomic integrity (*MEIG*), and transcription regulation (*LBX2* and *PAX5*). Furthermore, besides some genes previously uncharacterized (such as *FAM159A*, *ZNF883*, and *LOC646498*), the models also selected non-coding RNA sequences (*LOC732275* and *FAM138B*) and protein-coding genes involved in cellular adhesion (*PCDHB12*) and DNA double-strand break repair (*EEPD1*), processes highly relevant in the context of cancer.

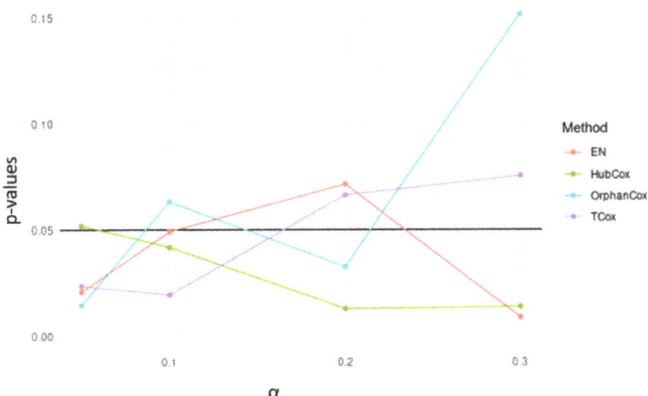

Figure 4. *p*-values obtained for survival models applied to the test sets, using different α-values.

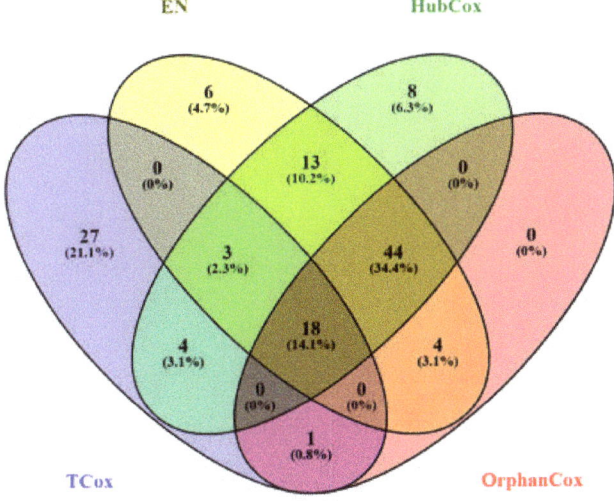

Figure 5. Venn diagram representing the number of genes selected by EN (yellow), HubCox (green), OrphanCox (red), and TCox (blue) using $\alpha = 0.1$.

Nevertheless, specific genes were selected only by HubCox (8 genes), EN (6 genes), and TCox (27 genes), most of them with associations with the cancer hallmarks (Figures 7 and 8). TCox was the model that identified the highest number of genes (Table 4); among them, eleven genes were associated with the hallmarks of cancer. In particular, the *RAB20*, *FCRL2*, *COL12A1*, *DCP1A*, and *OSBPL3* genes were previously shown to have prognostic value in cancer. In addition, pseudogenes (such as *ANKRD26P1*, *AOX2P*, and *SEPTIN7P2*) and genes involved in the integrity of the extracellular matrix (*COL19A1*), cellular adhesion (*IGLON5*, *PCDHA7*), the mitochondrial respiratory chain (*COX4I2*), telomere function (*TERF2IP*), E3 ubiquitination (*TRIM67*), and the export of nuclear RNA (*NXF2B*) suggested important roles in CRC development that should be further investigated. After analyzing each gene independently, we observed that most of the genes were not significantly associated with survival (Figure 9).

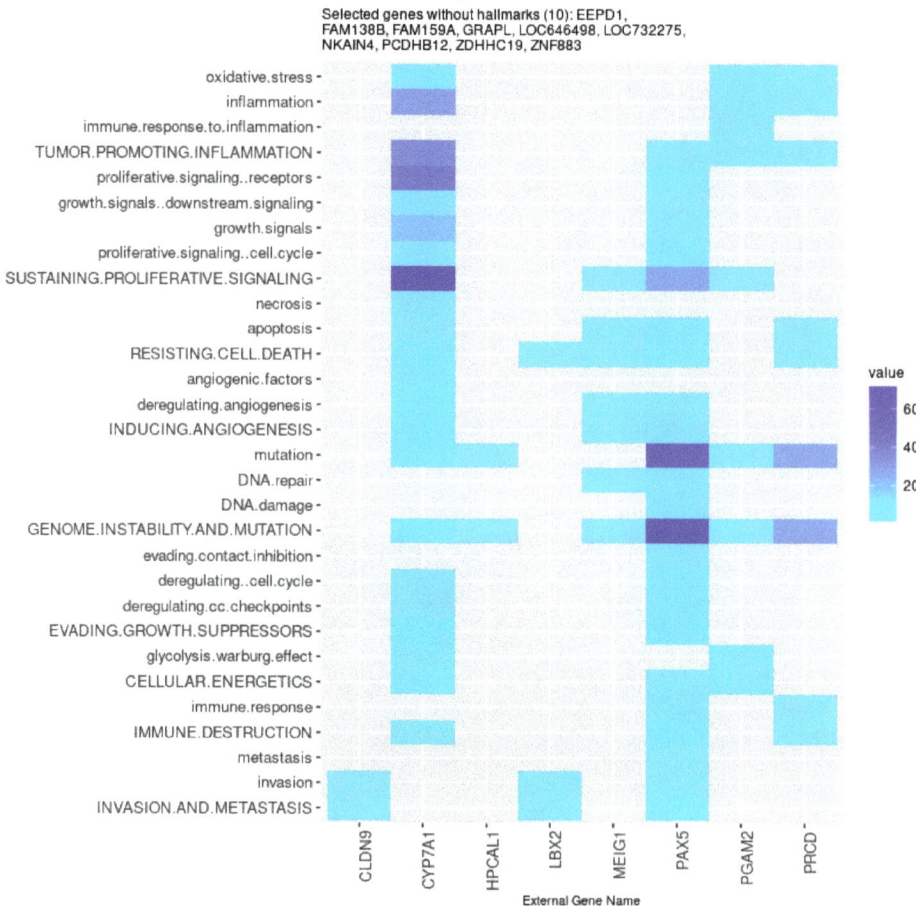

Figure 6. Genes selected by all models tested associated with the hallmarks of cancer, given by the CHAT. Value corresponds to the number of hits found in the literature, where light and dark blue correspond to a low and high number of hits, respectively.

Finally, it is noteworthy that all the novel regularizers—either those favoring or penalizing the selection of hubs (HubCox and OrphanCox) or promoting the genes with distinct correlation patterns in tumor and normal tissue samples (TCox)—added valuable information to the results obtained by the Elastic Net only. Indeed, by significantly expanding the resulting gene sets, TCox generated hypotheses regarding putative targets that may be further tested and experimentally analyzed.

In the present study, we exclusively used RNA-seq data from TCGA. The inclusion of other clinical parameters is expected to improve the performance of the models. For example, the recent classification of CRC tumor subtypes (Consensus Molecular Subtypes (CMS1-4)) [42] may in the future contribute to a better set of biomarkers with higher prognostic value.

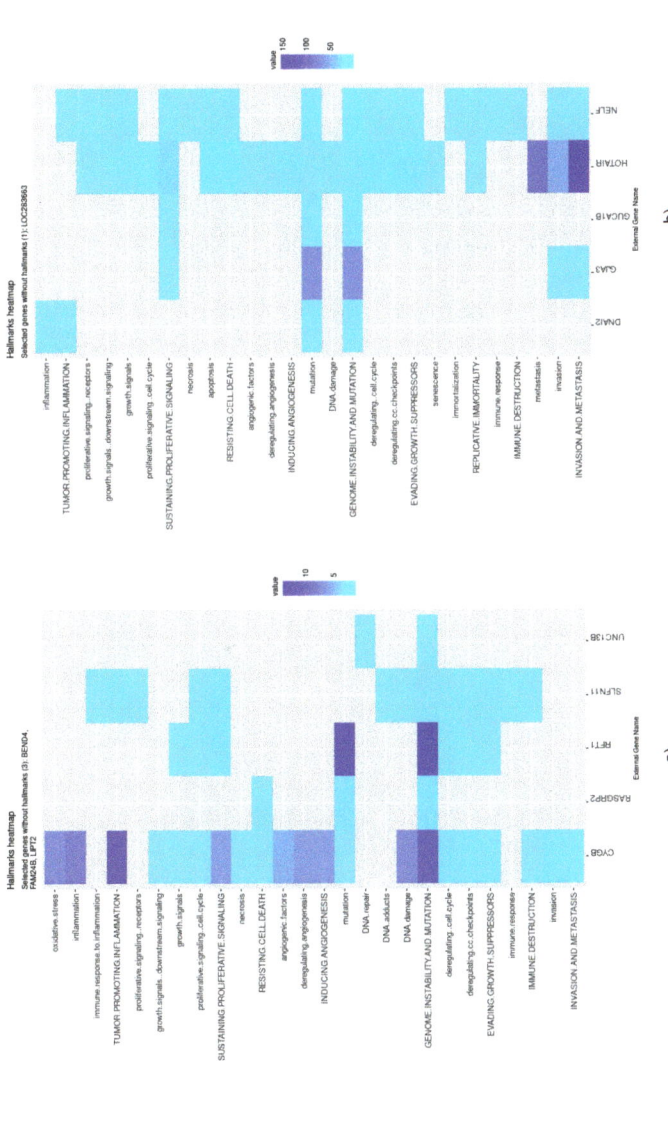

Figure 7. Genes selected by the HubCox and EN models associated with the hallmarks of cancer, given by the CHAT. (**a**) HubCox; (**b**) EN. The value corresponds to the number of hits found in the literature, where light and dark blue correspond to a low and high number of hits, respectively.

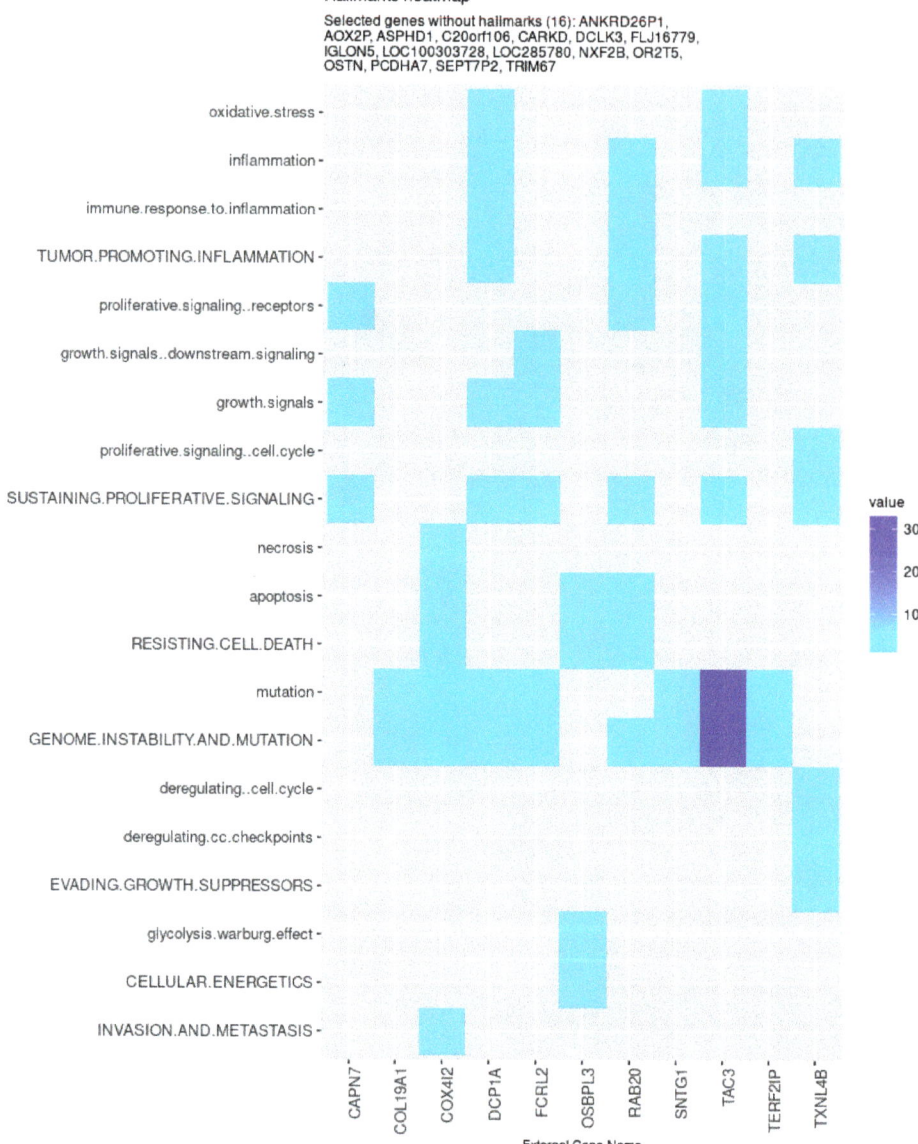

Figure 8. Genes selected by the TCox method associated with the hallmarks of cancer, given by the CHAT. The value corresponds to the number of hits found in the literature, where light and dark blue correspond to a low and high number of hits, respectively.

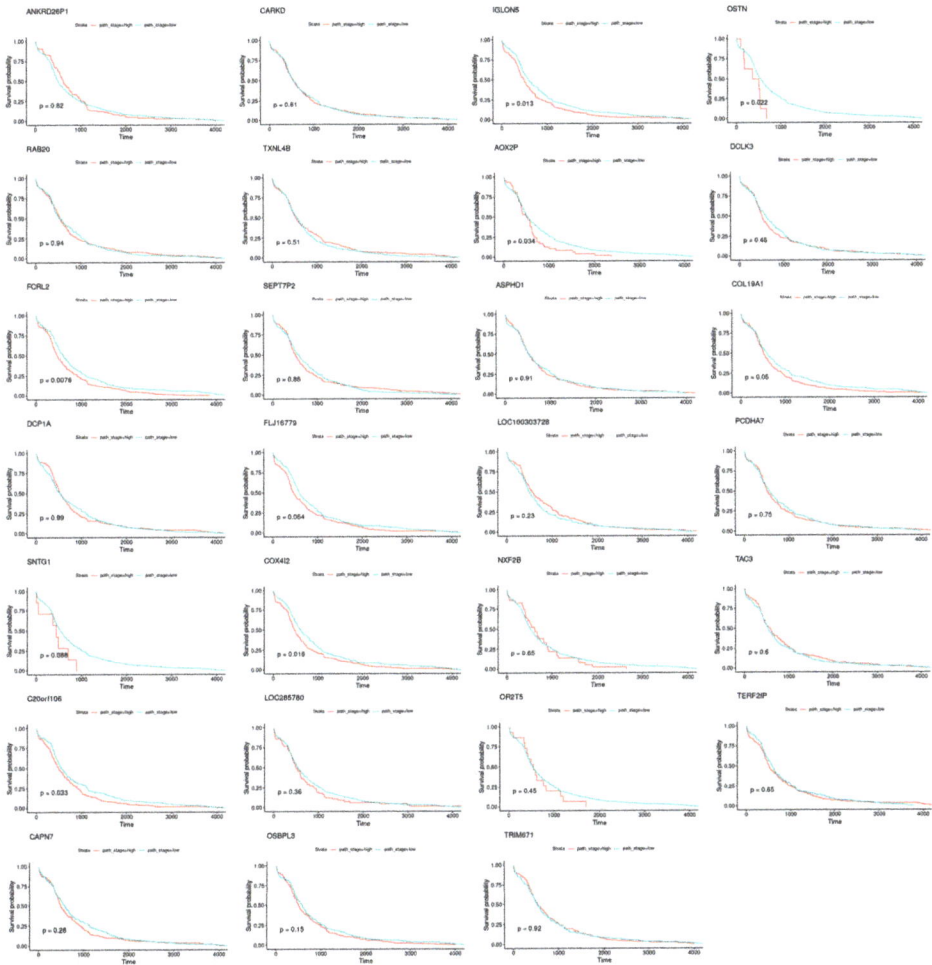

Figure 9. Survival curves obtained for the genes exclusively selected by the TCox method, when analyzed individually.

4. Conclusions

We propose TCox, a new weighted regularizer for Cox regression that penalizes the similarity of gene correlations across tumor and normal tissue samples in the selection of gene signatures associated with the survival outcome of colorectal cancer patients. Comparable model performance was obtained for TCox with respect to previously described methods in the literature, namely Elastic Net (EN), HubCox, and OrphanCox. Besides a consensus list of genes selected by all the regression models tested, with many of them already described to be involved in cancer formation and progression, TCox exclusively selected genes with an established role in colorectal cancer (CRC) and carcinogenesis, being able to categorize patients into significant risk groups. Regularized regression and, in particular, correlation-based Cox models are promising strategies to cope with high-dimensional data derived from multi-omics patient studies and can be useful to identify novel biomarkers in cancer.

Author Contributions: C.P., M.B.L., and S.V. designed the study; C.P. implemented and performed the testing; M.M. and L.C. provided clinical interpretation; C.P., M.B.L., M.M., L.C., and S.V. analyzed the results and wrote the manuscript. All authors read and agreed to the published version of the manuscript.

Funding: This work was partially supported by national funds through Fundação para a Ciência e a Tecnologia (FCT) with references PD/BD/139146/2018, IF/00409/2014, UIDB/50021/2020 (INESC-ID), UIDB/50022/2020 (IDMEC), UIDB/04516/2020 (NOVA LINCS), and UIDB/00297/2020 (CMA) and projects PREDICT (PTDC/CCI-CIF/29877/2017) and MATISSE (DSAIPA/DS/0026/2019).

Acknowledgments: The authors thank André Veríssimo and Massimo Amicone for providing insights on the glmSparseNet package and GTEx data, respectively. This article is based on work from COST action CA17118, supported by COST (European Cooperation in Science and Technology, www.cost.eu).

Conflicts of Interest: The authors declare no conflict of interest.

Abbreviations

The following abbreviations are used in this manuscript:

CHAT	Cancer Hallmarks Analytics Tool
COAD	Colon Adenocarcinoma
CRC	Colorectal Cancer
EN	Elastic Net
FPKM	Fragments Per Kilobase per Million
GDC	Genomic Data Commons
READ	Rectum Adenocarcinoma
RNA-seq	RNA sequencing
TCGA	The Cancer Genome Atlas

Reference

1. Global Cancer Observatory. Available online: http://gco.iarc.fr/ (accessed on 1 July 2020).
2. Grady, W.M.; Markowitz, S.D. The molecular pathogenesis of colorectal cancer and its potential application to colorectal cancer screening. *Dig. Dis. Sci.* **2015**, *60*, 762–772. [CrossRef] [PubMed]
3. Markowitz, S.D.; Bertagnolli, M.M. Molecular basis of colorectal cancer. *N. Engl. J. Med.* **2009**, *361*, 2449–2460. [CrossRef] [PubMed]
4. Yamagishi, H.; Kuroda, H.; Imai, Y.; Hiraishi, H. Molecular pathogenesis of sporadic colorectal cancers. *Chin. J. Cancer* **2016**, *35*, 4. [CrossRef]
5. Molinari, C.; Marisi, G.; Passardi, A.; Matteucci, L.; De Maio, G.; Ulivi, P. Heterogeneity in Colorectal Cancer: A Challenge for Personalized Medicine? *Int. J. Mol. Sci.* **2018**, *19*, 3733. [CrossRef] [PubMed]
6. Sagaert, X.; Vanstapel, A.; Verbeek, S. Tumor Heterogeneity in Colorectal Cancer: What Do We Know So Far? *Pathobiology* **2018**, *85*, 72–84. [CrossRef]
7. Wang, Z.; Gerstein, M.; Snyder, M. RNA-Seq: A revolutionary tool for transcriptomics. *Nat. Rev. Genet.* **2009**, *10*, 57. [CrossRef]
8. Yegnasubramanian, S.; Isaacs, W.B. *Modern Molecular Biology: Approaches for Unbiased Discovery in Cancer Research*; Springer Science & Business Media: New York, NY, USA, 2010.
9. AZIM, F.S.; Houri, H.; Ghalavand, Z.; Nikmanesh, B. Next Generation Sequencing in Clinical Oncology: Applications, Challenges and Promises: A Review Article. *Iran. J. Public Health* **2018**, *47*, 1453.
10. Lopes, M.B.; Veríssimo, A.; Carrasquinha, E.; Casimiro, S.; Beerenwinkel, N.; Vinga, S. Ensemble outlier detection and gene selection in triple-negative breast cancer data. *BMC Bioinform.* **2018**, *19*, 168. [CrossRef]
11. Marx, V. The big challenges of big data. *Nature.* **2013**, *498*, 255–260. [CrossRef]
12. Veríssimo, A.; Carrasquinha, E.; Lopes, M.B.; Oliveira, A.L.; Sagot, M.F.; Vinga, S. Sparse network-based regularization for the analysis of patientomics high-dimensional survival data. *bioRxiv* **2018**, 403402. [CrossRef]
13. Lopes, M.B.; Casimiro, S.; Vinga, S. Twiner: Correlation-based regularization for identifying common cancer gene signatures. *BMC Bioinform.* **2019**, *20*, 356. [CrossRef] [PubMed]
14. Friedman, J.; Hastie, T.; Tibshirani, R. Regularization paths for generalized linear models via coordinate descent. *J. Stat. Softw.* **2010**, *33*, 1. [CrossRef] [PubMed]
15. Tibshirani, R. Regression shrinkage and selection via the Lasso. *J. R. Stat. Soc. Ser. B (Methodological)* **1996**, *58*, 267–288. [CrossRef]

16. Veríssimo, A.; Oliveira, A.L.; Sagot, M.F.; Vinga, S. DegreeCox–a network-based regularization method for survival analysis. *BMC Bioinform.* **2016**, *17*, 449. [CrossRef] [PubMed]
17. Zhang, W.; Ota, T.; Shridhar, V.; Chien, J.; Wu, B.; Kuang, R. Network-based survival analysis reveals subnetwork signatures for predicting outcomes of ovarian cancer treatment. *PLoS Comput. Biol.* **2013**, *9*, e1002975. [CrossRef]
18. Lopes, M.B.; Vinga, S. Tracking intratumoral heterogeneity in glioblastoma via regularized classification of single-cell RNA-Seq data. *BMC Bioinform.* **2020**, *21*, 59. [CrossRef]
19. Hall, M.A. Correlation-based Feature Selection for Discrete and Numeric Class Machine Learning. In Proceedings of the 17th International Conference on Machine Learning (ICML-2000), Stanford, CA, USA, 29 June–2 July 2000; pp. 359–366.
20. Yu, L.; Liu, H. Feature selection for high-dimensional data: A fast correlation-based filter solution. In Proceedings of the 20th International Conference on Machine Learning (ICML-03), Washington, DC, USA, 21–24 August 2003; pp. 856–863.
21. Ling, B.; Chen, L.; Liu, Q.; Yang, J. Gene expression correlation for cancer diagnosis: A pilot study. *Biomed Res. Int.* **2014**, *2014*, 253804. [CrossRef]
22. Rahmatallah, Y.; Emmert-Streib, F.; Glazko, G. Gene Sets Net Correlations Analysis (GSNCA): A multivariate differential coexpression test for gene sets. *Bioinformatics* **2014**, *30*, 360–368. [CrossRef]
23. Li, S.; Liu, X.; Liu, T.; Meng, X.; Yin, X.; Fang, C.; Huang, D.; Cao, Y.; Weng, H.; Zeng, X.; et al. Identification of biomarkers correlated with the TNM staging and overall survival of patients with bladder cancer. *Front. Physiol.* **2017**, *8*, 947. [CrossRef]
24. Liu, R.; Zhang, W.; Liu, Z.Q.; Zhou, H.H. Associating transcriptional modules with colon cancer survival through weighted gene co-expression network analysis. *BMC Genom.* **2017**, *18*, 361. [CrossRef]
25. Grossman, R.L.; Heath, A.P.; Ferretti, V.; Varmus, H.E.; Lowy, D.R.; Kibbe, W.A.; Staudt, L.M. Toward a shared vision for cancer genomic data. *N. Engl. J. Med.* **2016**, *375*, 1109–1112. [CrossRef] [PubMed]
26. Samur, M.K. RTCGAToolbox: A new tool for exporting TCGA Firehose data. *PLoS ONE* **2014**, *9*, e106397. [CrossRef] [PubMed]
27. Christensen, E. Multivariate survival analysis using Cox's regression model. *Hepatology* **1987**, *7*, 1346–1358. [CrossRef] [PubMed]
28. Walters, S.J. *What is a Cox Model?*; Citeseer: Princeton, NJ, USA, 1999.
29. Jager, K.J.; Van Dijk, P.C.; Zoccali, C.; Dekker, F.W. The analysis of survival data: The Kaplan–Meier method. *Kidney Int.* **2008**, *74*, 560–565. [CrossRef] [PubMed]
30. Cox, D.R. Regression models and life-tables. *J. R. Stat. Soc. Ser. B (Methodological)* **1972**, *34*, 187–202. [CrossRef]
31. Kleinbaum, D.G.; Klein, M. *Survival Analysis : A Self-Learning Text*, 3rd ed.; Statistics for Biology and Health; Springer: New York, NY, USA, 2012; 700p.
32. Simon, N.; Friedman, J.; Hastie, T.; Tibshirani, R. Regularization Paths for Cox's Proportional Hazards Model via Coordinate Descent. *J. Stat. Softw.* **2011**, *39*, 1–13. [CrossRef]
33. Baker, S.; Ali, I.; Silins, I.; Pyysalo, S.; Guo, Y.; Högberg, J.; Stenius, U.; Korhonen, A. Cancer Hallmarks Analytics Tool (CHAT): A text mining approach to organize and evaluate scientific literature on cancer. *Bioinformatics* **2017**, *33*, 3973–3981. [CrossRef]
34. Wickham, H.; Francois, R.; Henry, L.; Müller, K. Dplyr: A Grammar of Data Manipulation. R Package Version 0.4.3. 2015. Available online: https://CRAN.Rproject.org/package=dplyr (accessed on 1 July 2020).
35. Yin, T.; Cook, D.; Lawrence, M. ggbio: An R package for extending the grammar of graphics for genomic data. *Genome Biol.* **2012**, *13*, R77. [CrossRef]
36. Kassambara, A.; Kosinski, M.; Biecek, P.; Fabian, S. Survminer: Drawing Survival Curves Using 'Ggplot2'; R Package Version 0.4.8. 2020. Available online: https://CRAN.R-project.org/package=survminer (accessed on 1 July 2020).
37. Robinson, M.D.; McCarthy, D.J.; Smyth, G.K. edgeR: A Bioconductor package for differential expression analysis of digital gene expression data. *Bioinformatics* **2010**, *26*, 139–140. [CrossRef]
38. Therneau, T.M. A Package for Survival Analysis in R; R Package Version 3.2-7. 2020. Available online: https://CRAN.R-project.org/package=survival (accessed on 1 July 2020).
39. Ternès, N.; Rotolo, F.; Michiels, S. biospear: An R package for biomarker selection in penalized Cox regression. *Bioinformatics* **2018**, *34*, 112–113. [CrossRef]

40. Simon, R.M.; Subramanian, J.; Li, M.C.; Menezes, S. Using cross-validation to evaluate predictive accuracy of survival risk classifiers based on high-dimensional data. *Briefings Bioinform.* **2011**, *12*, 203–214. [CrossRef] [PubMed]
41. Lei, R.; Feng, L.; Hong, D. ELFN1-AS1 accelerates the proliferation and migration of colorectal cancer via regulation of miR-4644/TRIM44 axis. *Cancer Biomark.* **2020**, *27*, 433–443. [CrossRef] [PubMed]
42. Guinney, J.; Dienstmann, R.; Wang, X.; De Reyniès, A.; Schlicker, A.; Soneson, C.; Marisa, L.; Roepman, P.; Nyamundanda, G.; Angelino, P.; et al. The consensus molecular subtypes of colorectal cancer. *Nat. Med.* **2015**, *21*, 1350–1356. [CrossRef] [PubMed]

Publisher's Note: MDPI stays neutral with regard to jurisdictional claims in published maps and institutional affiliations.

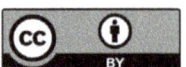

© 2020 by the authors. Licensee MDPI, Basel, Switzerland. This article is an open access article distributed under the terms and conditions of the Creative Commons Attribution (CC BY) license (http://creativecommons.org/licenses/by/4.0/).

MDPI
St. Alban-Anlage 66
4052 Basel
Switzerland
Tel. +41 61 683 77 34
Fax +41 61 302 89 18
www.mdpi.com

Biomedicines Editorial Office
E-mail: biomedicines@mdpi.com
www.mdpi.com/journal/biomedicines

www.ingramcontent.com/pod-product-compliance
Lightning Source LLC
LaVergne TN
LVHW070140100526
838202LV00015B/1863